Contact Dermatitis

Contact Dermatitis

ALEXANDER A. FISHER, M.D.

Clinical Professor, Department of Dermatology
New York University Post-Graduate Medical School
Associate Attending in Dermatology
University Hospital
New York University Medical Center
New York, New York

SECOND EDITION

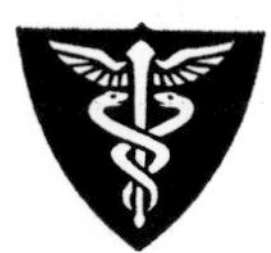

Lea & Febiger • *1973* • *Philadelphia*

Library of Congress Cataloging in Publication Data

Fisher, Alexander A.
Contact dermatitis.

Includes bibliographical references.
1. Contact dermatitis. [DNLM: 1. Dermatitis, Contact. WR175 F533c 1973]
RC592.F5 1973 616.9'73 73–5553
ISBN 0–8121–0411–0

ISBN 0–8121–0411–0

Library of Congress Catalog Card Number 73–5553

Published in Great Britain by Henry Kimpton Publishers, London

Printed in the United States of America

To Lillian

Preface

Since the first edition of this book was published, a North American Contact Dermatitis Research Group has been formed, and membership includes William E. Clendenning, Ernst Epstein, Alexander A. Fisher, Otis Field Jillson, William P. Jordan, Jr., Norman Kanof, Walter G. Larsen, Howard Maibach, John C. Mitchell, Silas E. O'Quinn, Earl J. Rudner, William F. Schorr and Marion B. Sulzberger. As a member of this group, I wish to express my appreciation to my colleagues for their expert help in writing this second edition.

This North American Group is patterned after, and cooperates with, the International Contact Dermatitis Research Group, which publishes the *Contact Dermatitis Newsletter* under the editorship of Prof. C. D. Calnan of London. It is a great asset to be alerted, through the Newsletter, to contact allergens long before such material appears in the formal literature. It is a veritable treasure chest for those with a special interest in contact dermatitis.

The material in the Newsletter may be reprinted only with the author's permission. I am indebted to many European colleagues for allowing me to quote from their contributions to the Newsletter, which is indicated in this edition by the notation "personal communication." Consequently, I wish to express my appreciation to the following members of the International Group and contributors to the Newsletter: Prof. C. D. Calnan (England), Dr. P. Bonnevie (Denmark), Dr. E. Cronin (England), Dr. K. D. Crow (England), Dr. S. Fregert (Sweden), Dr. E. Hegyi (Czechoslovakia), Dr. N. Hjorth (Denmark), Dr. B. Magnusson (Sweden), Dr. C. L. Meneghini (Italy), Dr. G. Verspyck Mijnssen (Holland), Dr. J. P. Nater (Holland), Dr. J. S. Pegum (England), Dr. V. Pirila (Finland), Dr. E. Rudzki (Poland), Dr. B. F. Russell (England), Dr. W. G. Van Ketel (Holland), Dr. J. L. Verbov (England), Dr. C. F. H. Vickers (England), Dr. K. Wereide (Norway), Dr. D. S. Wilkinson (England), Dr. H. Wilson (England) and Dr. G. Zina (Italy).

This new edition contains a wealth of new material; all the chapters have been extensively rewritten to incorporate new developments in the field, and several chapters have been added. For example, Chapter 1, "Allergic Contact Dermatitis," now includes the terminology and definitions of the sensitization processes recommended by the International Group, and Chapter 2, "Irritant Reactions to Chemicals, Excretions, Secretions and Tear Gas," includes a discussion of dermatitis due to tear gases (lacrimators).

In Chapter 3, "The Role of Patch Testing in Allergic Contact Dermatitis," patch test materials are discussed, and the designations of patch test readings recommended by the International Group are given. Chapter 4, "The Use of Patch Test Series," is new and includes standard test series recommended by the North American Group as well as a vehicle test series. Also discussed are the patch test allergens studied by the International Group. The recently introduced aluminum patch test is described, and sources of patch testing material at home and abroad are given. Chapter 5, "Hand Dermatitis Due to Contactants," includes recent investigations of perfumes, enzymes and phenolic compounds in soaps and detergents as causes of hand dermatitis. The hazard of acrylic bone cement to the orthopedic surgeon's hands is discussed, and herpetic paronychia is noted.

In Chapter 6, "Dermatitis and Discolorations from Metals," stainless steel and its safety for metal-sensitive individuals is stressed. The usefulness of the dimethylglyoxime spot test in the management of nickel sensitivity is emphasized, and allergic contact reactions to gold in jewelry are described. In Chapter 7, "Contact Dermatitis in Childhood," new aspects of management of diaper (napkin) dermatitis, with and without psoriasiform complications, are discussed. Bubble bath and detergent dermatitis in children also is presented.

Drs. William Schorr and William Jordan were kind enough to review Chapter 8, "Dermatitis from Clothing," and inform me of the results of their extensive studies of the role of formaldehyde and formaldehyde resins in clothing dermatitis. Lichenoid and purpuric eruptions from rubberized clothing are also discussed. Dr. Silas O'Quinn reviewed Chapter 9, "Shoe Dermatitis," and recommended a shoe company that will make, to order, shoes that are free of sensitizers proved by patch tests.

In Chapter 10, "Dermatitis from Rubber, Adhesives and Gums," many new rubber accelerators and antioxidants, including isopropyl paraphenylenediamine, are discussed. An analysis is made of the significance of the penetration of rubber gloves by acrylic monomer in bone cement used by orthopedic surgeons. Dr. Gerald Gellin made many valuable contributions to Chapter 11, "Industrial Dermatitis." Several recently introduced industrial contactants are discussed, and the role of protective clothing is brought up to date. I was again fortunate in having Dr. Leonard Harber collaborate with me in the writing of Chapter 12, "Contact Photodermatitis." The role of many new sunscreening agents in the *prevention* and *production* of photosensitivity is presented.

Dr. Earl Brauer reviewed Chapter 13, "Cutaneous Reactions to Cosmetics." His expert knowledge of cosmetics was of great value in describing new products. A discussion of feminine hygiene sprays, cosmetic dermatitis in males, and sensitizers in perfumes has been added. Dr. Otis Jillson reviewed Chapter 14, "Dermatitis Due to Plants and Spices," and helped clarify the subject of plant photosensitizers. The role of lactones as specific plant sensitizers is considered, and a section on dermatitis from spices has been added.

In Chapter 15, "Contact Dermatitis in Atopic Individuals," a study by the International Group is reviewed. The Scholtz regimen in the management of atopic dermatitis is presented, and contact urticaria due to lichens and canine saliva is described. Chapter 16, "Noneczematous Contact Dermatitis," includes many recently documented causes of contact urticaria, contact granulomas and contact purpuric and petechial eruptions. In Chapter 17, "Systemic Eczematous Contact-Type Dermatitis," the increasingly important role of topical sensitization to ethylenediamine in systemically produced drug eruptions is stressed.

Chapter 18, originally entitled "Contact Stomatitis and Cheilitis," has been expanded to include contact conjunctivitis, vulvitis, proctitis and balanitis. The sensitizing ingredients of popular dentifrices and mouthwashes are detailed, and irritants and sensitizers in douches, feminine hygiene sprays and contraceptives are discussed. Ophthalmic preparations containing the ubiquitous preservative benzalkonium chloride (BAK) are listed, and BAK-free preparations are given. Chapter 19, "Aquatic Contact Dermatitis," is new and was written in collaboration with Dr. William L. Orris, Medical Director of The Chester W. Nimitz Marine Faculty, Scripps Institute of Oceanography, University of California, San Diego.

The more than 600 contact allergens listed in the Appendix of the first edition have been increased to more than 800. Combinations of allergens are enumerated, and sources of them, both at home and abroad, are given. Dr. Ernst Epstein, in reviewing the Appendix, made many valuable suggestions concerning patch test concentrations.

We wish to thank the following organizations whose financial aid made possible the inclusion of a great many color plates. We are indebted to them for their generosity. Dermik Laboratories, Inc.; Doak Pharmacal Company, Inc.; H & A Enterprises; Johnson & Johnson; Schering Corporation; Science and Medicine Publishing Company; Stiefel Labs, Inc.; Syntex Laboratories, Inc.; Westwood Pharmaceuticals.

In addition, appreciation is expressed to the following individuals: Dr. Rudolf Baer, for creating an ambience at the New York Skin and Cancer Unit that is most conducive to the study of contact dermatitis; Dr. Norman Kanof, a colleague whom I consulted on many aspects of this edition; and Dr. Jerome Z. Litt, for his indefatigable eagle-eyed proofreading, for his constructive literary criticisms, for his numerous valuable facts and figures, and for his unflagging enthusiasm—all of which add up to a labor of love.

ALEXANDER A. FISHER

New York, New York

Contents

Contact Dermatitis

1

Allergic Contact Dermatitis

In the preface, some results of the cooperation between the International and North American Contact Dermatitis Research Groups were noted. In this chapter will be presented the recommendations of a committee appointed by the International Group to define and standardize the terminology of contact dermatitis.[1]

The International and North American Contact Dermatitis Research Groups are cooperating to standardize the terminology of contact dermatitis and the technique of patch-testing procedures

TERMINOLOGY RECOMMENDED BY THE INTERNATIONAL GROUP

Sensitization. This is the process of being sensitized.

Sensitivity. This is an indication that the process has occurred, and the individual is fully sensitized.

Latent Sensitivity. This is a confusing term that has been used to describe a state in which a patient is sensitized (clinically or by patch test) but has not had sufficient contact with the allergen to develop clinical signs of sensitivity. The term *unrevealed sensitivity* would be more accurate.

Allergen and *Sensitizer.* These terms are synonymous. The Committee has expressed no preference; the choice depends on context, style and euphony. The term *Allergenic* is self-evident.

Primary Allergen. This term refers to the prime substance inducing sensitization.

Secondary Allergen. This is a substance immunologically related to the primary allergen.

Hapten. This word indicates an incomplete allergen and should be used only to convey this exact meaning.

Sensitizing Index (*or Potential*). This refers to the relative capacity of a given agent to induce sensitization in a group of human beings and animals. It has been my clinical experience that the five most common causes of allergic eczematous contact dermatitis[2] in order of frequency are as follows:

1. Rhus (poison ivy, oak or sumac)
2. Paraphenylenediamine
3. Nickel compounds
4. Rubber compounds
5. Ethylenediamine

It should be noted that ethylenediamine has replaced the dichromates, which were listed as fifth in the previous edition.

Ethylenediamine has joined poison ivy, paraphenylenediamine and nickel and rubber compounds as a most common cause of allergic eczematous contact dermatitis

Index of Sensitivity. This is an index of incidence of sensitivity to a substance in a given population at a given time. It is of particular value as far as externally applied therapeutic agents are concerned. The following medications have a high index of sensitivity and should either be avoided or used with great caution: benzocaine, nitrofurazone (Furacin), antihistamines, ammoniated mercury, neomycin (particularly on eczematous skin), penicillin and the sulfonamides.

Latent Period. This is the interval between first contact with a sensitizer and observed onset of sensitization.

Refractory Period. This refers to a period of patch test unresponsiveness following a severe allergic reaction.

Reaction Time. This is the time between exposure of a previously sensitized subject to the specific sensitizing allergen and the development of the clinical reaction. This may vary from 8 to 120 hours, but I have found that the reaction usually takes place in 12 to 48 hours, occasionally from 4 to 72 hours, and rarely as early as an hour following exposure. I have seen the most rapid allergic reaction occur when solvents such as alcohol or acrylic monomer were sensitizers.

Multiple Nonspecific Reactions. These are multiple reactions that occur especially in patients with active eczema, damaged skin or abnormally enhanced reactivity.

Multiple Primary Specific Sensitivities (also referred to as *concomitant sensitivity*). These are multiple sensitivities to substances that are unrelated chemically, e.g., lanolin and neomycin. One sensitivity may predispose the patient to another, e.g., by treatment, or he may have a genetic or constitutional predisposition to sensitivities.

Multiple Secondary Specific Sensitivities. Allergic sensitization engendered by one compound, the primary allergen, extends to one or more compounds, the secondary allergens. The allergens are related chemically or are converted to substances that are identical or closely related, and the sensitized cells are unable to distinguish between them.

Multiple reactions to compounds containing an identical allergen include the following types:

1. (*False cross-sensitivity*). This involves positive reactions to substances that are apparently unrelated but that contain an identical or closely related substance, which is the sensitizer. For example, cobalt may contain traces of nickel, and balsams and other natural substances may contain related or identical substances; i.e., the same impurity may exist in widely differing products.

2. *Single sensitization.* Substance A induces sensitization. Substances A_1 and A_2 are the same as A but occurring in different products and under different guises, e.g., chrome in cement, matches and anticorrosive agents.

3. *Multiple sensitization.* Substances A and B occur in different products and usually induce sensitization at different times. Although A_1 and B_1 are the same substances as A and B, they occur in different products, and they may elicit sensitization simultaneously or at different times, e.g., nickel and rubber additives.

4. *Concomitant sensitization.* Here, A and B are present in the same product and both induce sensitization. Substances A_1 and B_1 are the same as A and B but are present in different products and may elicit contact dermatitis simultaneously or at different times, e.g., chrome and cobalt in cement or mercaptobenzothiazole and tetramethyl thiuram in rubber gloves.

5. *Simultaneous sensitization.* Substances A and B are present in different products but may induce sensitization simultaneously. Substances A_1 and B_1 are the same as A and B and are present in different products and elicit contact dermatitis separately, e.g., chrome in cement and additives in rubber gloves.

6. *Cross-sensitization.* In this instance, A is the primary allergen, inducing sensitivity; A_a is the secondary allergen, chemically related to A and also capable of eliciting contact dermatitis, e.g., neomycin and kanamycin.

7. *Combination of cross-sensitization and concomitant sensitization.* Both A and B are present in the same substance and induce sensitization. Substances A_1 and B_1 are the same as A and B, but they are present in different substances and may also elicit contact dermatitis. Likewise, A_a and B_b are cross-reacting substances, i.e., secondary allergens, present in different substances, but capable of eliciting contact dermatitis. For example, balsams may contain many unknown allergens. The distinction between cross-sensitization and concomitant sensitization is often difficult to make.

Other terms used to describe allergic contact dermatitis include:

Incubation Period. After an initial sensitizing exposure to a contactant there is an incubation period of 5 to 21 days during which changes develop in the skin, which lead to clinical dermatitis on reexposure to the specific allergen. It is presumed that antibodies are being formed during this period.

"Spontaneous" Flare-up. A "spontaneous" flare-up of dermatitis, without apparent reexposure to the specific allergen, may occur at the site of the sensitizing exposure if sufficient allergen remains *in situ* to react with the now sensitized skin after the incubation period has elapsed. Another type of "spontaneous" flare-up may occur after a lapse of weeks to years in healed areas of allergic eczematous contact dermatitis, even though these sites are not directly exposed to the specific allergen. For example, a positive patch reaction to poison ivy on the back may flare into a neat square of dermatitis if the sensitized individual acquires poison ivy dermatitis of the hands years after the patch test was performed.[3]

Persistence of Sensitivity. Once allergic hypersensitivity to common contactants, such as poison ivy, paraphenylenediamine and nickel, has been established, sensitization usually persists for many years.[4] With some allergens, however, it may be lost after a few years. When individuals are sensitized deliberately under experimental conditions with 2,4-dinitrochlorobenzene, there usually is loss of contact sensitivity after a few weeks.[5]

Contact Sensitizers. Almost any contactant, particularly a simple chemical such as a dye, a plant, a medication or a natural or synthetic resin, may be a cutaneous sensitizer. Protein substances rarely cause allergic eczematous contact dermatitis. Contactants vary greatly in their ability to initiate sensitization.

ALLERGIC ECZEMATOUS CONTACT DERMATITIS

Allergic eczematous contact dermatitis, sometimes called dermatitis venenata, results from exposure of sensitized individuals to contact allergens or sensitizers. It is a delayed hypersensitivity reaction in contrast to dermatoses that are of the immediate urticarial variety.[2]

Clinical Appearance

In its acute phase, allergic eczematous contact dermatitis is characterized by redness, edema, papules, vesiculation, weeping and crusting and is accompanied by pruritus. If it becomes chronic, the involved skin may become thickened, lichenified, fissured and pigmented. Occasionally, dermatoses such as Duhring's disease or erythema multiforme may be confused with it.

"Dermal" Contact Dermatitis. Certain contactants, particularly neomycin, nickel and ragweed, have been reported to produce an allergic "dermal" contact dermatitis in which the eczematous element is minimal or absent. The eruption remains edematous and erythematous throughout its course. Histologically, there is a normal epidermis with edema and dense perivascular small round cell infiltrate in the dermis. Occasionally, "dermal" contact dermatitis is combined with the usual papulovesicular eczematous variety, in which case one can usually demonstrate both a positive patch and an intracutaneous reaction with the specific allergen.[6]

Allergic contact dermatitis can occur at any age and is usually eczematous. Edema and erythema <u>without</u> vesiculation may also occur with certain contactants

Osmundsen[7] has described an atypical contact dermatitis consisting of a pigmented petechial eruption from Tinopal, a detergent whitening agent used in Denmark for nylon textiles.

Differential Diagnosis. The clinical picture may be closely simulated by other eczematous dermatoses, such as primary irritant dermatitis, nummular eczema, atopic dermatitis, seborrheic eczema, and eczematous eruptions due to fungi and bacteria. Furthermore, many dermatoses that are usually noneczematous may become so, and many dermatoses may be complicated by a superimposed allergic eczematous contact dermatitis. The location, clinical course and appearance of the eruption together with the history of exposure to contactants and the proper evaluation of patch tests usually help differentiate these conditions.

FACTORS INFLUENCING ALLERGIC ECZEMATOUS CONTACT DERMATITIS

The extent of dermatitis that develops on exposure to a contactant in a sensitized individual depends on many factors including:

1. *The intensity, duration and frequency of exposure to the allergen.*[8]

2. *The degree of allergic sensitivity.* For example, some individuals exposed repeatedly and intensively to poison ivy develop only a slight dermatitis.

3. *The presence of infected, inflamed, burned or eczematized skin.* The area around a varicose ulcer or the site of varicose eczema is notoriously easy to irritate and sensitize. Furthermore, irritation of an eczematous dermatitis on the lower extremities is often complicated by an autosensitization phenomenon with the production of a symmetrical eruption on the upper extremities and sometimes the face.[9]

Rowe and Warnzensk[10] found that the number of significant positive patch tests in patients with stasis dermatitis is twice that of those with psoriasis or atopic dermatitis.

4. *The area exposed to the contactant. The eyelids* are one of the most sensitive areas. Any substance used on the scalp, face or hands may produce allergic eczematous contact dermatitis of the eyelids, while those primary sites remain unaltered. Airborne pollen and dust and all types of volatile agents may affect the eyelids first and exclusively. Eyelash curlers may produce eyelid dermatitis because of sensitivity to the rubber edge of the nickel-plated portion of the appliance. Marked edema of the eyelids is often a feature of poison ivy and hair dye dermatitis.

The face may also react to substances applied to the scalp and hands. In fact, the face and the eyelids are the most common sites of photocontact and other photosensitizing reactions.

The scalp is particularly resistant to contactants. Allergens applied to this area often produce dermatitis of the eyelids, ears, neck and hands, while the scalp remains unaffected.

The ears, particularly their helix, may be the site of the disease due to hair sprays, shampoos and dyes. Ear lobe dermatitis is a cardinal sign of nickel-sensitivity in women wearing costume jewelry earrings. Otitis externa may be caused by sensitizing medications applied to the ear canals, particularly neomycin.[11] Habitual insertion of metallic objects (hairpins, pens and pencils) into the canals may produce the dermatitis in nickel-sensitive individuals. The piercing of ear lobes is often a precipitating factor in nickel and gold sensitivity.

The neck, like the eyelids and genitalia, is a very reactive site. Cosmetics applied to the face, scalp or hair, and topical acne medications often initially affect the neck. Berloque and nail polish dermatitis also commonly involve this area.

The trunk, periaxillary region and antecubital spaces may be the sites of perfume dermatitis or of a symmetrical type of dermatitis due to the finishes and dyes in clothing.

The forearms also may be the site of dermatitis due to sensitizers that splash above protective gloves. It must not be forgotten that loose bracelets may have considerable excursion on the forearm and thereby produce dermatitis from the wrist to the antecubital spaces.

Allergic eczematous contact dermatitis may appear in areas distant from the site of application of contact allergens. This is particularly likely on the eyelids and neck

The penis and scrotum may react to sensitizers conveyed to these areas by the hands. Marked dermatitis from poison ivy oleoresin is not uncommon, and airborne substances may be funneled up to the genitals via the trousers. Rubber condom dermatitis may result in depigmentation.

The vulvar and perivulvar areas may be the sites of reaction to sensitizers in bubble baths and similar preparations. Rubber-sensitive patients may acquire vaginitis and vulvar dermatitis from the use of rubber pessaries. Sensitizers carried by the hands eventually contact these areas.

Perianal dermatitis from benzocaine and other medicaments in suppositories is not uncommon. Oral hyposensitization with plant oleoresins may also cause it.

The palms and soles are resistant to this type of dermatitis. Lynfield et al.,[12] however, readily sensitized the palms to dinitrochlorobenzene (DNCB).

5. *Mechanical factors.* Pressure and friction increase the intimacy of contact of the sensitizer with the skin and thus may initiate and prolong the disease.

6. *Perspiration.* Sweat can dissolve certain sensitizing chemicals from contactants, thereby releasing them for the production of allergic dermatitis. Some sensitized individuals develop nickel, dye or dichromate dermatitis only when they perspire excessively.

7. *Alkalinity of the skin.* A shift of normal acid skin pH toward alkalinity seems to enhance allergic eczematous contact dermatitis.

8. *Cachexia, lymphomas and sarcoidosis.* These conditions appear to decrease reactivity to allergic eczematous contact dermatitis.[13,14] Johnson et al.[15] concluded that failure of advanced cancer patients to be sensitized to DNCB may be due to a defective inflammatory response and not to a defect in delayed hypersensitivity response.

9. *Genetic factors.* Children whose parents have been sensitized to dinitrochlorobenzene become sensitized at a higher rate than do children whose parents have not been sensitized. This tends to support the hypothesis that genetic factors play a role in susceptibility to human allergic contact dermatitis, at least when experimentarily produced.[16] In another study,[17] relatives of patients suffering from allergic eczematous contact dermatitis were patch tested with common contact allergens. Preliminary results indicated an increased incidence of atopic diseases and of positive patch tests among the siblings and children of these patients. Such findings, in my opinion, should not be taken to suggest that atopic diseases are connected to the same genetic constitutions as the allergic eczematous dermatoses, if indeed there are genetic factors in human allergic contact dermatitis.

AGE AS A FACTOR IN ALLERGIC CONTACT DERMATITIS

Although allergic dermatitis may develop from early infancy to old age, the patient's age does modify the appearance and course of the eruption. The special features of contact dermatitis in early life are considered in Chapter 7 (Contact Dermatitis in Childhood). As far as the older age group is concerned, it has been my experience that the common potent sensitizers such as paraphenylenediamine, nickel, the dichromates, poison ivy and rubber compounds produce as many instances of A.E.C.D. with strongly positive patch test reactions in patients over 65 as in younger age groups.

Dryness of the skin of elderly individuals may be aggravated through normal use of toilet soaps and detergents, predisposing them to allergic contact sensitization. To relieve the dryness the patient may use lubricants and bath oils containing lanolin products or surfactants, which may be sensitizers.[18]

In tracking down the cause of contact dermatitis in the older age group, not only must the patient be questioned concerning new contactants, but a thorough investigation also must be made of substances to which there has been exposure for decades. It is surprising how frequently the older patient becomes sensitized to a contactant to which there has been intermittent exposure throughout life without any previous reaction. Properly performed patch tests are reliable in finding the causative agents in allergic contact dermatitis in persons of this age group.[19]

Features in the Aged. In older people, the disease, even during the acute stage, may show relatively little vesiculation or inflammation. Scaling is regularly a prominent features in all phases of dermatitis in the elderly. Thickening, hyperpigmentation and lichenification take place readily, and itching is usually pronounced. Both allergic and irritant eruptions tend to persist and be more resistant to therapy in the aged than in younger persons.

If the older patient is improperly managed or reexposed to irritants or sensitizers, the eruption readily becomes widespread and intractable, particularly if intercurrent disease is present.

In industry, older workers who may have handled certain substances in their occupation for decades without difficulty can suddenly develop a severe allergic contact dermatitis. Such occurrences are likely for cement workers, painters, tile setters and bakers. Even the prompt retirement of such older workers and the avoidance of irritants or specific allergens do not necessarily prevent the dermatitis from persisting or becoming generalized. Such widespread involvement may be due to an increased nonspecific irritability of the entire skin surface, which becomes hyperreactive to many irritants and even to bland substances.

In the elderly, autosensitization may also play a role in the development of widespread eruptions, particularly those resulting from injudicious treatment of varicose ulcers and eczema on the lower extremities. A combination of sensitization to bacteria, the absorption of modified protein from inflamed or ulcerated skin and topical medications appears to take part in the production of such autosensitization.

Plant, Dye and Wearing Apparel Dermatitis in the Older Age Groups

Ragweed Dermatitis. This airborne allergic eruption seems to be more common in elderly than in younger individuals. It may masquerade as neurodermatitis or even lymphoblastoma. Men seem to acquire sensitization to ragweed much more readily than do women. This dermatitis occurs most commonly in farmers between the ages of 40 and 75, but people in other occupations and in suburban areas not infrequently acquire sensitization to ragweed oil. Even in the older age group, hyposensitization procedures with ragweed oil should be attempted, because spontaneous cure usually does not occur and exposure to the oil-laden pollen is unavoidable in certain areas.

Rhus Dermatitis. Although there is experimental evidence that the capacity to become sensitized to the oleoresin of poison ivy, oak and sumac appears to be diminished after the age of 50, I have found that, with adequate exposure, Rhus dermatitis occurs readily even in octogenarians. Not infrequently elderly persons acquire ivy poisoning during visits to cemeteries. Hyposensitization procedures for protection against Rhus dermatitis are not indicated for the elderly because they can usually learn to avoid contact with the offending plants.

Hair Dye Dermatitis. Allergic eczematous contact dermatitis due to paraphenylenediamine (PPDA) hair dyes is not uncommon in elderly women. In my series of 30 individuals sensitive to it, 10 were over 60 years of age. Furriers sensitized to it show positive patch test reactions long after they have retired.

Wearing Apparel Dermatitis. Dermatitis due to the finishes and dark dyes of clothes is not uncommon in women at the menopause and those going into mourning ("widow's dermatitis"). Obesity and hyperhidrosis in older age groups are important factors in the production of wearing apparel dermatitis.

Travel abroad exposes the individual to unusual contactants

Dermatitis from Hobbies. Older people may acquire contact dermatitis from materials used in various hobbies, including gardening, carpentry, bookbinding, painting, ceramics and enameling. Turpentine is a frequent irritant and sensitizer. Gardening may expose the elderly individual to plants, insecticides and fertilizers. Pyrethrum and Malathion can readily sensitize individuals of all ages. Many of the most severe cases of contact dermatitis due to insecticides that I have observed have been in elderly persons. The epoxy resins, glues and adhesives used in carpentry, sculpture and collages may cause the disease at all ages. In England, primroses are a common cause of this disease in the elderly.

PRACTICAL AIDS IN THE DETECTION OF CONTACTANTS IN ANY AGE GROUP

1. Since allergic eczematous contact dermatitis may resemble other types of eczematous dermatitis, one should suspect contactants as either causing or aggravating any eczematous eruption.

Plate 1. Five Common Contact Allergens

1. Rhus

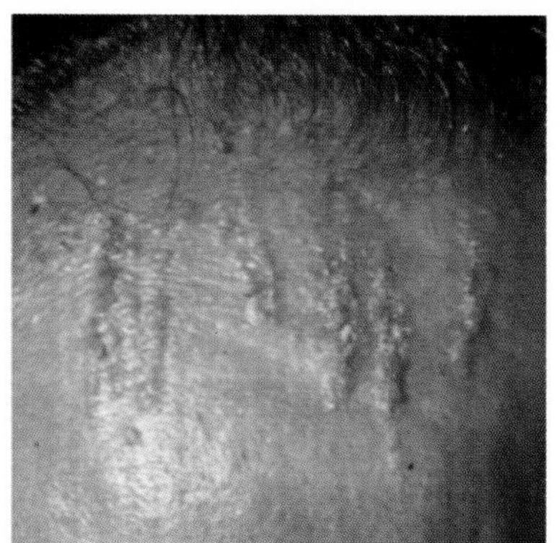

Poison Ivy Dermatitis of Forehead

2. Paraphenelenediamine

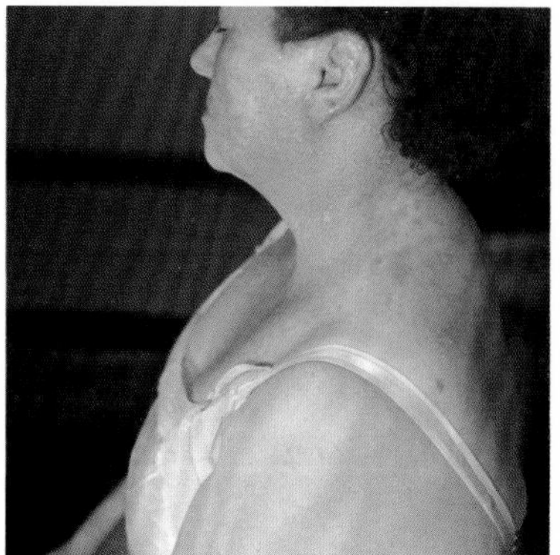

Hair Dye Dermatitis

3. Nickel

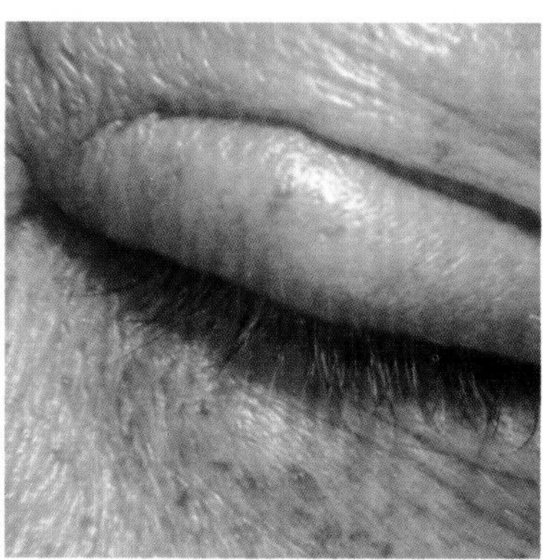

Eyelid Dermatitis Caused by Nickel-plated Eye Lash Curler

4. Rubber

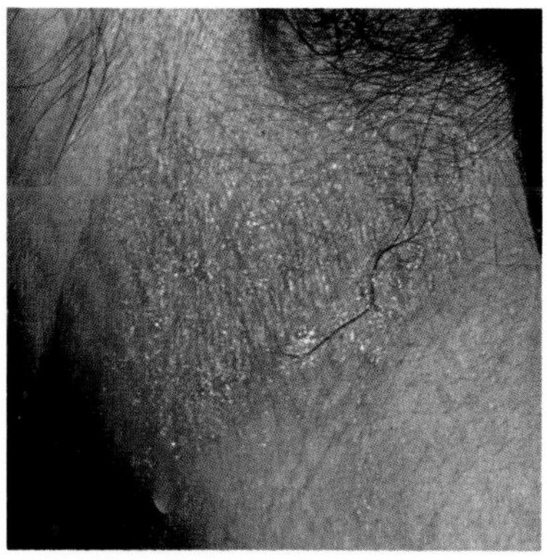

Dermatitis of Neck From Beauty Parlor Rubber Head Rest (New York Skin and Cancer Unit)

5. Ethylenediamine

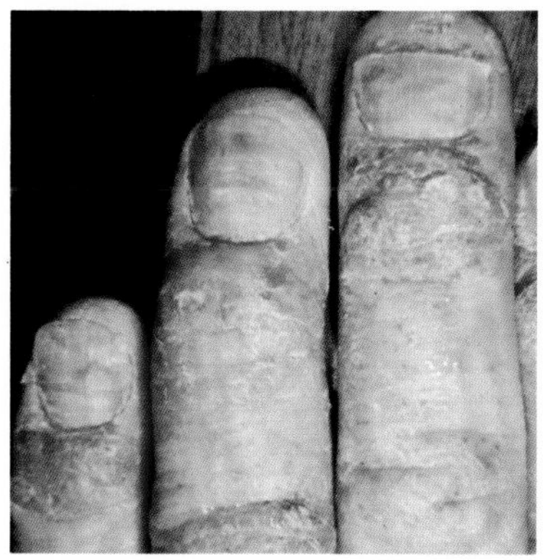

Allergic Contact Dermatitis of the Hands due to Ethylenediamine in Mycolog Cream Applied for Tinea of the Nails

2. Although exhaustive questioning may be necessary to detect the culprits, the most productive leads often follow from answers to the following questions: What kind of work do you do? What are your hobbies? Are you allergic to any drugs? What medications do you use externally or internally? What purchases have you made recently? What gifts have you received? Are you wearing new clothing or using new cosmetics? Has your house been sprayed recently with an insecticide? Have you been abroad recently?

3. Since atopic eczema may resemble or be complicated by contact dermatitis, it is important to inquire about associated conditions such as hay fever or asthma.

4. Always examine the feet of patients having hand dermatitis. Certain hand eczemas may be the result of id reactions from active fungal or bacterial foci on the feet. Even shoe dermatitis may produce chemical ids of the hands. When an eruption of the feet accompanies a hand eczema, it is unlikely that the hand involvement is due solely to external contactants.

5. Keep in mind that the five most common causes of contact dermatitis are plants, nickel, dyes, rubber and topical medicaments.

6. If the history and observation do not reveal the cause of the disease, patch tests with a standard group of allergens may be helpful. Remember that a positive patch test reaction is not absolute proof that the presenting dermatitis is produced by the test substance causing the positive reaction. The positive patch test reaction must fit the clinical picture.

7. When there is a positive reaction to a patch test or a history of allergic hypersensitivity to a particular compound, consider the possible role of immunochemically related compounds in the production of the dermatitis.

8. Wilkinson[20] has reviewed certain techniques to identify the allergens in allergic contact dermatitis.

The *spot test for nickel* is a 1 per cent alcoholic solution of dimethylglyoxime, which gives a raspberry color in ammoniacal solution in the presence of available nickel (see chapter on metals). This reaction is inhibited when the nickel is chelated by ethylenediaminetetraacetic acid (EDTA). Experiments are being performed to determine whether this acid can be incorporated into barrier creams to prevent nickel dermatitis in sensitized individuals.

Another chemical test for nickel, which is based upon the violet color of nickel diphenylcarbazine, can also be used to detect hydrazines.

Textile allergens may be detected with chromotropic acid, which indicates *formalin* in fabrics. If stockings are steam heated before pieces are applied for patch testing, a negative or doubtful reaction may be converted into a positive one. Nylon dyes can be extracted for patch tests by soaking the fabric in hot alcohol for an hour (see also chapter on clothing).

Fluorescent contact sensitizers can be detected by Wood's light.

GUIDES TO PROPHYLACTIC MANAGEMENT AND PREVENTION OF CHRONICITY

1. Avoid the use of topical medications with a high index of sensitivity. Before such agents are used, it may be advisable to perform a preliminary patch test to ascertain whether the patient had already acquired allergic hypersensitivity to them.

Irritating and sensitizing medicaments are becoming a more prevalent cause of chronicity of contact dermatitis. Not only the active ingredients but also the inert preservatives and stabilizers of creams and lotions are potent allergens.

2. Do not give poison ivy oleoresin injections in the presence of poison ivy dermatitis. Desensitization procedures involving an injection of protein substances for asthma or hay fever should be avoided during the acute phases of the disease.[21]

3. Whenever possible, instruct the patient how to obtain suitable nonsensitizing substitutes for topical medications or other contactants that previously produced the dermatitis.

4. At times, even when the contact allergen has been identified, the dermatitis persists because the patient is exposed to occult forms of the allergen. For example, the dichromate-sensitive individual is exposed to the

allergen in diverse substances such as cement, matches and leather.

5. The patient may be exposed systemically by ingesting the sensitizer in the form of medication. For example, if he was originally sensitized to a thiuram in rubber, subsequent administration of Antabuse (tetramethylthiuram disulfide) may perpetuate the dermatitis.[22]

6. Cross-sensitivity reactions may produce chronicity. A patient who has become sensitized to benzocaine may react to hair and fur dyes, such as paraphenylenediamine.

7. Have the patient avoid exposure to sunlight in the acute phase of the dermatitis.

8. Treat acute dermatitis of the lower extremities with utmost gentleness. Rough removal of crusts may cause a widespread autosensitization eczema, particularly in individuals with varicose veins or impaired circulation.

9. Thus far, protective or barrier creams have failed to prevent allergic eczematous contact dermatitis, although Decaspray or Kenalog or Valisone spray may prevent nickel dermatitis for short periods.

10. Do not rely on spontaneous hyposensitization or specific hardening to occur, since, once sensitization to a chemical occurs, it usually persists for many years.

11. Aside from moderately successful prophylactic treatment of poison ivy and ragweed oil sensitivity, do not expect specific desensitization therapy to be of much aid in this type of dermatitis.

Chronicity in allergic eczematous contact dermatitis may be due to sensitizing or irritating topical medication, to occult exposures to the allergen or chemically related chemicals and to secondary infection

Lowney[23] has shown that there is a low incidence of sensitization and low intensity in those who are sensitized following buccal application of dinitrochlorobenzene. If unresponsiveness to contact sensitizers can be confirmed for other compounds, buccal application may become of practical importance.

12. Secondary infection often leads to chronicity, particularly when strong or sensitizing antiseptics or antibiotics are applied.

13. Itching and scratching of a contact dermatitis not infrequently lead to lichenification of the site with subsequent localized neurodermatitis or even hypertrophic scarring, particularly following nickel dermatitis.

TOPICAL TREATMENT

In all stages, topical therapy is used to alleviate itching and inflammation and to prevent scratching. Some patients obtain relief by gently rubbing the inflamed skin with an ice cube held in a piece of cloth, thereby avoiding the trauma caused by scratching. Spraying localized areas of eczema with Valisone aerosol may give relief from itching.

Acute Stage

Cold, wet dressings are usually soothing in acute eczematous eruptions and help to stop the oozing. The colder the dressing, usually the more efficacious it becomes. The addition of finely cracked ice to the water often enhances the antipruritic effect. Wet dressings consisting of water with ice, made to the consistency of a sherbet and applied with a cotton cloth for 5 to 15 minutes and reapplied as necessary, are often well-tolerated and beneficial. They must not be used over a wide area in elderly or debilitated patients, however, because such persons may get a chill. One extremity or one quarter of the body may be treated at a time with wet dressings fairly safely. The dressings may be supplemented at night by zinc oxide paste applied on closely woven cotton cloth. On the scalp, the zinc oxide paste may be replaced by a mixture of equal parts of olive oil and lime water.

Medicated Wet Dressings. Burow's solution (liquor aluminum acetatis) may be used routinely as a wet dressing in the acute stages by diluting it 1:20 with cold tap water or by dissolving 1 Domeboro tablet (Dome) or 1 Domeboro packet (Dome) in a pint of water. For use about the *eyelids*, 2 per cent boric acid solution is preferable to Burow's solution.

For *infected* dermatitis, potassium permanganate solution, prepared by thoroughly dissolving a 2-grain potassium permanganate tablet in a quart of water, may be used as a wet dressing. When there is *persistent oozing*, a 0.05 per cent solution of silver nitrate, made by adding 1 teaspoonful of 10 per cent silver nitrate solution to a quart of water, may be employed as an astringent.

Baths. Soothing baths are useful both as anti-inflammatory agents and as a means to soak off ointments and other medications. Sitz baths may be used as substitutes for wet dressings in intertriginous areas and the genitalia. Colloidal oatmeal (Aveeno [Cooper]), 2 cupfuls to a tub of water, is acceptable to most patients, but it should be used cautiously, because it makes the tub slippery.

Rest. When the disease is widespread, confinement to bed for a few days may be necessary. Immobilization of an extremity that is acutely inflamed and edematous may be indicated.

Subacute Stage

Topical corticosteroid medications, which are not particularly effective in the acute stage, in which there is weeping and vesiculation, are helpful in the subacute stage. Every physician has his favorite preparation. As Sulzberger and his colleagues state, "In a great many instances, it makes little difference which preparation is selected. The therapeutic response is excellent with almost any of them."[24]

There is no doubt, however, that the bases and vehicles of topical corticosteroids play a role in therapeutic efficacy. Certainly, one preparation that feels good to one patient may be uncomfortable for the next. Furthermore, the preservatives, particularly the parabens and ethylenediamine, may be sensitizers. Paraben-sensitive individual should use Hytone, Aristocort, Valisone or Lidex cream, all of which are paraben-free. Great caution should be used in prescribing Mycolog cream, because ethylenediamine, the stabilizer in this preparation, is a potent sensitizer.

In additon, topical application of strong corticosteroids, such as betamethasone or the fluorinated corticosteroids, appears to cause a nonallergic perioral or rosacea type of dermatitis.[25] In such instances, hydrocortisone (i.e., Hytone cream) may be well-tolerated.[26]

Chronic Stage

The skin is usually dry and thickened in the chronic stage. Corticosteroid creams or ointments with or without 3 per cent iodochlorhydroxyquin (Vioform) may be helpful. If there is secondary infection in any phase of the dermatitis, broad-spectrum antibiotic ointments, such as erythromycin (Ilotycin), chlortetracycline hydrochloride (Aureomycin), tetracycline hydrochloride (Achromycin), oxytetracycline hydrochloride (Terramycin), or chloramphenicol (Chloromycetin Cream), are indicated. In my experience, neomycin is much more sensitizing and less effective than these antibiotics.

Persistent lichenified areas may be painted with a solution of coal tar or Arning's tincture. Intralesional injections of steroid suspensions are sometimes successful in localized areas. Spraying the lesions with aerosols containing steroids may be cooling and healing.

Castellani's carbolfuchsin paint, diluted with 3 parts water, is often effective in chronic intertriginous dermatitis accompanied by maceration and excessive sweating. After the paint has dried, a corticosteroid cream may be applied.

Table 1–1 is the formula for a modified carbolfuchsin solution that is free of phenol, has less alcohol than commercial preparations, does not sting, and is usually well-tolerated.

Table 1-1.
Modified Carbolfuchsin Solution

Combine:	(cc.)
Fuchsin	2.6
Alcohol	20.0
Water	190.0
Filter and add:	
Boric Acid	2.0
Let stand 2 hours and add:	
Acetone	10.0
Resorcin	20.0
Filter solution	

SYSTEMIC TREATMENT

Corticosteroids. The ability of corticosteroids to allay inflammation has radically changed the outlook in severe, widespread and disabling cases of allergic eczematous contact dermatitis and has made the need for hospitalization of such patients largely unnecessary. Provided there are no contraindications, especially an active peptic ulcer, systemic corticosteroid therapy is indicated in acute disease, because it usually need only be given for 3 weeks. In adults, an initial intramuscular injection of 40 mg. of Aristocort suspension or its equivalent may be given. Twenty-four hours later, oral corticosteroid therapy is begun with the administration of 60 mg. of prednisone or its equivalent for 2 days. This dose is gradually decreased so that by the end of the first week of therapy 30 mg. of prednisone are being given daily. Twenty mg. are administered daily during the second week, and 10 mg. given daily during the third and final week of treatment.

Corticosteroid therapy is tapered off gradually over a 3-week period in order to avoid a rebound of the dermatitis, which may take place if the corticosteroid therapy is stopped before the patient's own immune mechanism can take over.

Antipruritic and Sedative Therapy. In the initial phase, while the corticosteroids are beginning to exert their anti-inflammatory effect or when systemic corticosteroids are not given, sedation with phenobarbital ($\frac{1}{2}$ grain and aspirin 5 grains, 3 or 4 times daily) may be helpful. Upon retiring, hydroxyzine hydrochloride (Atarax, 25 mg.), cyproheptadine hydrochloride (Periactin, 4 mg.) or diphenhydramine hydrochloride (Benadryl, 50 mg.) may be given for their sedative and antipruritic effects.

REFERENCES

1. Wilkinson, D. S., et al.: Terminology of Contact Dermatitis. Acta Dermatovener., *50,* 287, 1970.
2. Baer, R. L.: Allergic Eczematous Sensitization in Man. J. Invest. Derm., *43,* 223, 1964.
3. White, W. A., Jr., and Baer, R. L.: Failure to Prevent Experimental Eczematous Sensation: Observations on the "Spontaneous" Flare-Up Phenomenon. J. Allergy, *21,* 334, 1950.
4. Fisher, A. A., Pelzig, A., and Kanof, N.: The Persistence of Allergic Eczematous Sensitivity and the Cross-Sensitivity Pattern to Paraphenylenediamine. J. Invest. Derm., *30,* 9, 1958.
5. Harber, L. C., Rosenthal, S. A., and Baer, R. L.: Actively Acquired Tolerance to Dinitrochlorobenzene. J. Immun., *88,* 66, 1962.
6. Epstein, S.: Contact Dermatitis Due to Nickel and Chromate, Observations on Dermal Delayed (Tuberculin-Type) Sensitivity. Arch. Derm., *73,* 236, 1956.
7. Osmundsen, P. E.: Pigmented Contact Dermatitis. Brit. J. Derm., *83,* 296, 1970.
8. Calnan, C. D.: The Climate of Contact Dermatitis. Acta Dermatovener., *44,* 34, 1964.
9. Baer, R. L.: Multiple Eczematous Sensitizations. J.A.M.A., *170,* 1041, 1959.
10. Rowe, R. J., and Warnzensk, C. M.: Comparative Studies of Patch Testing. Ann. Allergy, *27,* 117, 1969.
11. Jensen, C. O., Allen, H. J., and Mordecai, L. R.: Neomycin Contact Dermatitis Superimposed on Otitis Externa. J.A.M.A., *195,* 175, 1966.
12. Lynfield, Y. L., Wininger, M., and Frank, L.: Allergic Contact Dermatitis of the Palms. J. Invest. Derm., *51,* 494, 1968.
13. Schier, W. W., et al.: Hodgkin's Disease and Immunity. Amer. J. Med., *20,* 94, 1956.
14. Rostenberg, A., Jr.: Etiologic and Immunologic Concepts Regarding Sarcoidosis. Arch. Derm., *64,* 385, 1951.
15. Johnson, M. W., Maibach, H. I., and Salmon, S. E.: Skin Reactivity in Patients with Cancer. New Eng. J. Med., *284,* 1255, 1971.
16. Walker, F. B., Smith, P. D., and Maibach, H. I.: Genetic Factors in Human Allergic Contact Dermatitis. Int. Arch. Allergy, *32,* 453, 1967.
17. Forsbeck, M., Skog, E., and Ytteborn, K.: The Frequency of Allergic Diseases Among Relatives to Patients with Allergic Eczematous Contact Dermatitis. Acta Dermatovener., *46,* 149, 1966.
18. Tindall, J. P., and Smith, J. G.: Skin Lesions of the Aged and Their Association With Internal Changes. J.A.M.A., *186,* 1039, 1963.
19. Smith, J. G., Jr., and Kiem, I. M.: Allergic Contact Sensitivity in the Aged. J. Geront., *16,* 118, 1961.
20. Wilkinson, D. S.: Contact Dermatitis. XVIII—Ancillary Aids in Elucidation of Causes of Contact Dermatitis. Brit. J. Derm., *86,* 445, 1972.

21. Derbes, V. J., and Caro, M. R.: Localized Eczema Induced by House Dust Extract Injections. Arch. Derm., *75*, 804, 1957.
22. Calnan, C. D.: Studies in Contact Dermatitis. XXII—Chronicity. Trans. St. John Hosp. Derm. Soc., *54*, 170, 1968.
23. Lowney, E. D.: Dermatologic Implication of Immunologic Unresponsiveness. J. Invest. Derm., *54*, 355, 1970.
24. Sulzberger, M. B., et al.: *Dermatology Diagnosis and Treatment* (Ed. 2). Chicago, Year Book Medical Publishers, 1961, p. 174.
25. Weber, G.: Rosacea-Like Dermatitis: Contraindications or Intolerance Reaction to Strong Corticosteroids. Brit. J. Derm., *86*, 253, 1972.
26. Fisher, A. A.: Facial Papular Dermatitis Due to Topical Fluorinated Steroids. Cutis, *10*, 459, 1972.

2

Irritant Reactions from Chemicals, Excretions, Secretions and Tear Gas

The International Contact Dermatitis Research Group is of the opinion that the term *Primary Irritant Dermatitis* is redundant and that the word *Primary* should be omitted. According to this group, " '*Irritant* (*contact*) *dermatitis*' describes the effect caused by a strong irritant on the skin, *e.g.* that caused by a strong alkali. The term 'acute irritant dermatitis' may be used in contrast to 'cumulative insult dermatitis,' which, though cumbersome, is exact in the description of a dermatitis developing 'after repeated insults by weak primary irritants over a long period.' It is to be preferred to 'traumiterative dermatitis.' 'Wear and tear dermatitis' is an acceptable alternative."

> **The word primary may be dropped from the term primary irritant dermatitis. The word irritant is preferred to toxic**

Irritants are substances that "damage the skin by direct toxic action."[1] In their study of irritants, Kligman and Wooding[2] stressed the difficulties of assessing irritant results because the reactions may be influenced by age, sex, race and season of the year. They emphasized that the findings are relative and that the usefulness of the test is contingent upon the selection of an appropriate reference for comparison. For strong irritants, they deduced statistically the concentration that would produce a reaction in 50 per cent of patients tested. For weak irritants, they estimated the number of days for 50 per cent of those tested to develop a threshold irritant response.

Bandman and Dohn[3] have demonstrated that the histopathology of irritant reactions differs markedly from substance to substance. Bjornberg[4] has shown that irritant patch test reactions do not necessarily subside rapidly. They may be petechial or follicular and leave scarring and hyperpigmentation.

> **The rapidity of disappearance of a patch test reaction cannot be the basis for differentiating an irritant from an allergic reaction. Severe irritant reactions tend to increase over the first 72 hours**

In general, the intensity of reaction to irritants is proportional to the concentration and exposure time. It is impossible to differentiate statistically between a patient with normal skin and one with eczema or to establish criteria by which predisposition to eczema may be defined. Bjornberg did, however, find that patients with active hand eczema have an increased susceptibility to irritants on the thighs. Once the hand eczema has healed, the patient shows normal reactivity to most irritants.

No test is available to predict hypersusceptibility to irritants. Patients with active hand eczema have a hyperirritable skin, which makes it difficult to assess such testing

Hyperirritable skin in the presence of eczema may cause false positive allergic reactions and explain so-called hardening of the skin and allergic patch test reactions that become negative when the dermatitis has healed. There is no general agreement, however, on this interpretation.

TESTS FOR IRRITANCY

Tests for primary cutaneous irritancy in laboratory animals are unreliable indicators of irritancy in man because the anatomical and physiological differences between the skin of man and of laboratory animals are great.

Open contact and closed patch tests in a limited number of subjects usually are sufficient preliminary screening procedures. If such tests do not produce undesirable reactions, one should do usage tests in several hundred persons, applying the preparation under study to all areas of the body where it might reasonably be used and under foreseeable conditions. It is particularly important that the preparation be used under various climatic conditions because of the possibility of differences in primary irritancy and because extremes of climate might emphasize otherwise undetected reactions.

SKIN REACTIONS FROM IRRITANT CHEMICALS

Strong or Absolute Irritants. These chemicals produce severe inflammatory skin changes on first exposure by immediate and direct destruction. Strong acids and alkalies in sufficient concentrations and for long enough periods always produce changes in the skin varying from redness to vesiculation or necrosis by coagulating skin protein or by dehydrating tissue.

The irritants may vary from strong, absolute or obvious to mild, relative or insidious

Mild or Relative Irritants. These chemicals produce inflammatory skin changes in most individuals provided there is repeated exposure or overexposure. Occasionally, bland substances are irritating when the skin is hyperirritable.

Soaps, detergents and solvents are mild irritants, which produce dryness, fissuring and dermatitis in most individuals who are sufficiently exposed. After an eczematous eruption, the skin becomes alkaline with resulting impairment of alkali neutralization, which in turn enhances the damaging effect of irritants. Some detergents produce an acanthosis, which increases skin susceptibility to primary irritants.[5]

Certain conditions heighten the susceptibility of the skin to primary irritants.[6] For example, skin that has healed from an eczematous eruption or a burn may remain hyperirritable for several months. Excessive humidity, friction, pressure, hyperhidrosis and maceration may allow many usually nonirritating substances to produce inflammation. Sweat is capable of dissolving chemical dusts, which may dissociate to produce skin irritation. Disturbances in sweating (dyshidrosis) and infection may also make the skin hyperirritable.

Bland substances may become primary irritants when the skin is eczematous or has been subjected to maceration, friction, pressure, infection ann excessive perspiration

Patch tests performed on such irritable skin may result in nonspecific reactions to normally nonirritating substances.

Mild irritation may be cumulative, resulting in "skin fatigue." In this state, the skin may be irritated by even the blandest of substances. Occasionally, however, after daily exposure to irritants, localized adaptive changes such as hyperplasia and pigmentation permit the individual to handle harsh agents without further reaction. This type of "skin hardening" occurs fairly frequently when mild irritants are factors but only rarely in the case of allergens. As far as primary irritants are concerned, hardening is strictly local. The hardened skin may withstand primary irritants while adjacent unhardened skin remains susceptible to irritation. When hardening occurs with allergic sensitizers, the hyposensitization takes place over the entire skin surface.

Repeated exposures to irritants may be cumulative, leading to "skin fatigue," characterized by hyperirritability, or to thickening and "hardening"

There is a great variation in the damaging effects of irritants from one individual to another and from one area of skin to another. Individuals who are thin-skinned are more susceptible to primary irritants than those whose skin is thicker. Indeed, acquired thickening of the skin may be a form of hardening. Individuals with inactive sweat glands and dry skin are more susceptible to dehydrating chemicals than those with active sweat glands and moist skin. People with excessively oily skins may be more susceptible to chemical compounds that have a high affinity for fats.

Urine and feces may produce irritant dermatitis in the presence of bacteria that form ammonia. This type of irritant dermatitis is not unusual in infants and in incontinent individuals. In addition, the skin around stomas or fistulas may become inflamed from contact with enzymes and bacteria in intestinal fluids or body secretions.

The presence of hair follicles and sebaceous and sweat glands may determine the type of irritant reaction that a particular chemical produces on the skin. Thus, tetryl and TNT (trinitrotoluene) dusts may collect in hair follicles and produce a typical follicular irritation.

The sebaceous glands of the hair follicles are particularly vulnerable to fat solvents, and certain chlorinated compounds, such as the chlornaphthalenes, chlordiphenyls, chlordiphenyloxide, chlorbenzols and chlorphenols, may cause straw-colored noninflammatory cysts, pustules, inflamed follicles and comedones.

Such occupational chloracne may be produced not only by exposure to chlorinated compounds but also by prolonged contact with vapors or with clothing saturated with insoluble cutting oils, crude petrolatum, paraffin, coal tar and coal tar pitch. Acneiform eruptions from tars may be complicated by melanosis and photosensitivity reactions.

The control of occupational acneiform eruptions may be difficult. Precipitated sulfur, 10 per cent in calamine lotion, may be used therapeutically and prophylactically for industrial acne.

Relation of Primary Irritant and Allergic Contact Dermatitis. Clinically and microscopically, primary irritant and allergic dermatitis may be difficult to differentiate.[7] Occasionally, contact with a chemical produces a primary irritant reaction that simultaneously sensitizes the individual to the compound. For example, the first exposure to phenol may not only burn but also sensitize the skin so that subsequent exposures to low concentrations of phenol, such as carbolated petrolatum, may produce an allergic eczematous reaction.

Whenever there is difficulty in distinguishing between a primary irritant and an allergic reaction, patch testing with a proper nonirritating concentration of the chemical indicates whether the individual has become allergenically sensitized to the chemical.

Primary irritant and allergic dermatitis may be difficult to differentiate, and certain chemicals may be both irritants and sensitizers

Although this chapter is concerned particularly with the irritating effect of chemicals, it must be remembered that skin irritation and dermatitis can result from mechanical action (friction or repeated pressure), physical agents (heat, cold or electricity), sunlight, ultraviolet radiation between 2800 and 3200 Å, x-rays, radiation from radioactive materials and biological agents (bacteria, fungi and parasites).

Chemical burns differ from thermal burns in that the chemical may continue to act for an indefinite period if not removed by copious washing with water. The blisters from a second degree thermal burn, if left undisturbed, allow more physiologic healing.

With certain chemical burns, however, the prompt removal of the blister fluid and the overlying skin may result in more rapid healing. For example, blister fluid caused by skin burns due to alkyl mercury compounds contains mercury and should be removed to prevent further damage.[8]

Immediate cooling of burns, usually by immersion in ice water, decreases pain and edema and may actually decrease the extent of the burn.[9]

Chemical burns differ from thermal burns in that the chemical continues to act if not removed or neutralized

DERMATITIS AND BURNS FROM STRONG IRRITANTS

Strong acids, alkalies, fluorine, phosphorus, phenol, resins, mercury compounds, titanium tetrachloride and dimethyl sulfate can produce severe inflammation and burns of the skin requiring special treatment.[10]*

REACTIONS DUE TO ACIDS

Strong Acids. Such acids can combine with water in the skin causing marked dehydration. They may also form albuminates in combination with the skin protein. Acid burns are usually not as extensive as those caused by strong alkalies. Even weak acids or their fumes entering abrasions or wounds, however, can cause ulcerations, and certain acids can produce burns as severe as those produced by alkalies.[10]

Mineral Acids. Hydrochloric acid, nitric acid and particularly sulfuric acid are corrosive. Concentrated nitric acid and concentrated hydrochloric acid give off fumes that are extremely irritating to the respiratory tract and the skin. Nitric acid colors tissues a deep yellow. People coming in contact with concentrated solutions of the mineral acids may be severely burned and scarred.

Any body surface that has had contact with mineral acids should be treated with prolonged washing with water or weak alkalies

The local treatment of mineral acid burns consists of removing the acid as quickly as possible from the skin by prolonged washing with water or with one of the following:

Magnesia magma (milk of magnesia)
Sodium bicarbonate (dilute solution)
Calcium hydroxide solution (lime water)
Aluminum hydroxide gel
Precipitated calcium carbonate (chalk)
Soap solution

Time should not be lost searching for these alkalies if they are not readily available, since plain water used abundantly and thoroughly is almost as efficacious. Special care should be given to the eyes, which should be kept open under running water for 20 minutes. After all traces of acid are removed, systemic therapy may be necessary for alleviation of pain and prevention of shock and infection.

The burns resulting from oxalic acid and hydrofluoric acid require special treatment.[10]

Oxalic Acid. Prolonged contact of the hands with solutions of oxalic acid may result in paresthesias, cyanosis of the fingers and pale yellow discoloration of the fingernails. Gangrene of the fingertips may even occur.

The usual alkalies cannot be used as antidotes for oxalic acid because the salts formed from the union of alkalies and oxalic acid are strong and soluble irritants. Magnesium and calcium salts, however, can be used in the treatment of oxalic acid exposure, because these salts form precipitates of magnesium oxalate and calcium oxalate, which are insoluble and nonirritating.

* This reference is especially valuable for plant physicians and others engaged in industrial medicine.

Burns due to oxalic or hydrofluoric acid require special treatment

Hydrofluoric Acid. Contact of hydrofluoric acid with the skin may initially produce a slight reaction that progresses to severe injury. Low concentrations produce erythema. Higher concentrations produce blanching and edema, which may be followed by vesication and extensive necrosis. Such damaged tissue heals extremely slowly. Involvement about the nail causes the nail bed to become inflamed. The nail may be destroyed and the destruction may extend to the bone.

Hydrofluoric acid burns of the skin are treated with wet dressings of a mixture of magnesium oxide and magnesium sulfate. Severely inflamed areas should be infiltrated with 3 per cent calcium gluconate solution to prevent gangrene.

Reinhardt[11] suggests an alternative treatment for hydrofluoric acid burns, which consists of thorough and immediate flushing with water, followed by iced alcohol or aqueous soaks with a high molecular weight quaternary ammonium compound (Hyamine), at intervals varying from 1 to 4 hours. The solution consist of 2 grams of the ammonium compound in 1 liter of Formula 46 alcohol or a liter of distilled water. If blisters form, complete debridement is necessary; an ointment composed of fibrinolysin and desoxyribonuclease (Elase) keeps the areas free of debris. A compression dressing with an ointment containing vitamins A and D should then be applied for several days.

DERMATITIS AND BURNS FROM ALKALIES

Compounds of potassium, sodium, ammonium and calcium are the most common causes of alkali burns. Sodium hydroxide, potassium hydroxide, sodium carbonate and potassium carbonate may produce deep caustic burns on contact with the tissues.

Sodium Hydroxide. This alkali is a powerful keratin solvent and in concentrated solution causes severe burns and ulcerations. In lower concentrations, various grades of dermatitis are produced. Sodium hydroxide is present in cleaning and sanitizing agents such as Drano Disinfectant, Easy-Off Oven Cleaner, Holly Pine Cleaner, Lycons Cleaner, N.S.C. Detergent, Plumite Drain Opener, Prouton Detergent, Quick-'N-Brite and SuperAlkali Detergent.

Skin exposed to strong alkalies should be thoroughly cleaned with running water until it is free of alkali as indicated by disappearance of soapiness. After this treatment, the following weak acids may be applied to neutralize the alkali in deeper tissue:

1. Vinegar diluted with 4 parts water; or 2% acetic acid
2. Lemon juice
3. Orange juice
4. Dilute (0.5%) hydrochloric acid.

All alkali burns may be treated by this method with the exception of calcium oxide.

Alkalies should be removed from the skin by copious washing with water or weak acids, except calcium oxide (quicklime), which should be removed by an oil or grease or by a strong stream of water under pressure

Calcium Oxide. Quicklime absorbs water to form slaked lime with the creation of a great deal of heat. Unslaked lime is strongly alkaline, a powerful keratin solvent and a dehydrating agent. Since the heat generated by the solution of 1 gm. of calcium oxide is 18,330 calories, the particles should be removed if possible with oil or grease *before* the lime is wetted. A *rapid copious* stream of water under pressure, which will immediately mechanically remove the calcium oxide particles, may also be used. This agent can also produce burns, fissuring of the skin and brittleness of the nails.

SPECIAL TREATMENT OF SKIN BURNS DUE TO CHEMICALS

Other chemicals that cause severe damage to the skin and that need special handling include fluorine, phosphorus, hot and activated resins, phenol, titanium tetrachloride and dimethyl sulfate.

Fluorine. This chemical, used in organic

synthesis, together with the related hydrogen fluoride which is used in etching glass and in the petroleum industry, can produce corrosive ulcers on contact with the skin. Exposed skin should be thoroughly washed under a stream of water for 15 minutes. A paste of 20 per cent magnesium oxide in glycerine should be applied to the burnt area for at least an hour.

Fluorine burns, particularly around the fingernails, are extremely painful and require special care to relieve pain as well as to prevent infiltration into the deeper structures, which may result in destruction of deep tissue and bone and necessitate amputation. The nails should be split from the distal end to the nail bed to allow free drainage. A 10 per cent calcium gluconate solution should be injected around and beneath the nail. The affected part should then be soaked in iced alcohol or iced magnesium sulfate for 2 hours.

Phosphorus. White phosphorus burns should be treated by placing the part immediately under water for 15 minutes. The area then should be covered with a 3 per cent copper sulfate solution to coat the phosphorus with a layer of copper phosphide. The copper salt particles can then be removed with tweezers. Complete removal is essential because the phosphorus will ignite again as soon as it dries.

Resins, Asphalts and Thermoplastics. Burns from these chemicals in the heated state should be treated by cooling the affected part rapidly with ice cold water. Tannic acid jelly is then applied and covered with a loose dressing. No attempt is made to remove the resin or asphalt at once. It may be removed later, when the surrounding skin is less inflamed, by applying a solvent such as methyl ethyl ketone. Soap and water is then employed to remove the solvent.

Phenol (Carbolic Acid). Phenol is a general protoplasmic poison entering into a loose combination with protein. It can penetrate tissue deeply and is readily absorbed from all surfaces of the body. Local gangrene occurs from prolonged contact of phenol with tissue. Irritation is soon replaced by anesthesia due to the death of nerve endings. The skin becomes white and necrotic.

Skin and mucosal areas exposed to phenol should be washed with large amounts of water for 15 minutes followed by the application of castor oil or 10 per cent ethyl alcohol.

Titanium Tetrachloride. This compound is an important intermediate in the production of titanium metal and certain pigments. It is a colorless liquid that fumes strongly in moist air and reacts violently with water to liberate heat and produce hypochloric acid. Serious injuries have resulted when workers have been sprayed with water after being splashed with the chemical. It should be removed from the body by *dry* wiping before any water is applied. Burns resulting from its action are deep and slow to heal.

Dimethyl Sulfate. This agent hydrolyzes in the presence of water to methyl alcohol and sulfuric acid and is used for methylation in the chemical industry. Skin corrosions should be treated with weak alkaline wet dressings. In contaminated areas, dimethyl sulfate should be deactivated by spraying with water or a 5 per cent sodium hydroxide solution.

Alkyl Mercury Compounds. Ethyl mercury phosphate and methyl mercuric acetate may cause burns attended with no initial discomfort; pain, redness, fissuring and blistering, however, may occur in 6 to 10 hours. The fluid in the bulla should be evacuated promptly and the overlying skin removed to prevent the mercury in the fluid from producing a third degree burn.

Other Chemicals. Many other chemicals may produce severe inflammation and burns of the skin. Aside from quicklime, all these compounds should be removed from the skin with copious washings of water. If the clothing has been contaminated, it should be removed while the patient is under a cool shower.

MILD IRRITANTS

The type of dermatitis encountered in handling detergents, solvents and household cleansers is discussed in the chapter on hand dermatitis.

Soaps, detergents, solvents and household cleansers are insidious irritants, which act by defatting and drying the skin

Plate 2. Some Unusual Irritants

1. Occluded Tincture Iodine

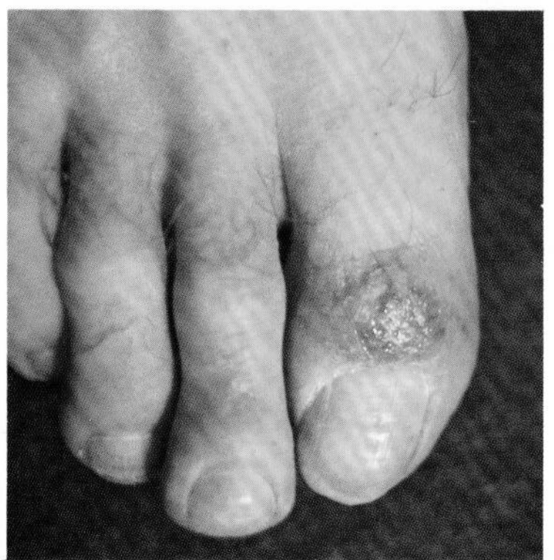

Applied to Abrasion and Covered

2. Mace

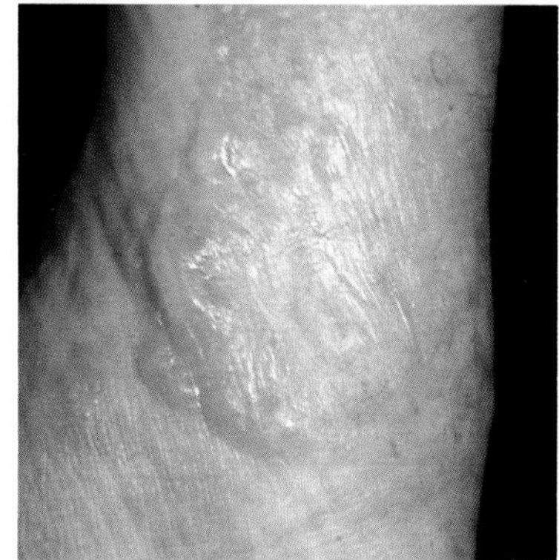

Tear Gas Bulla

3. Cantharadin

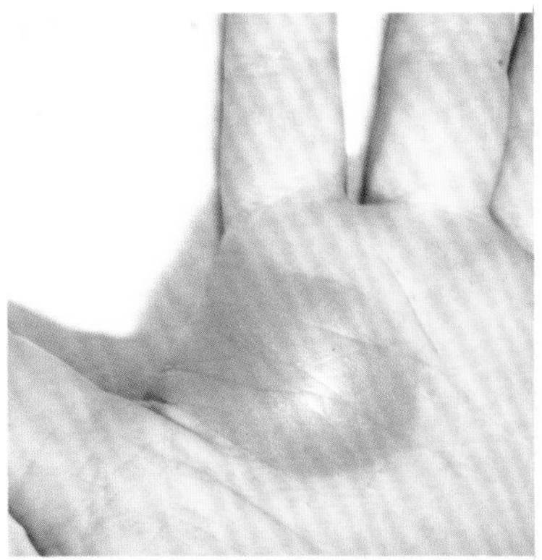

Blister Beetle Bulla

4. Fluorinated Corticosteroid

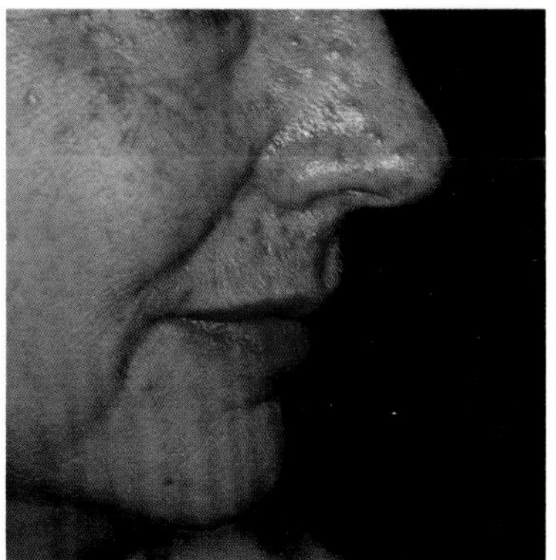

"Facial Papular Eruption"

5. Ethylene Oxide

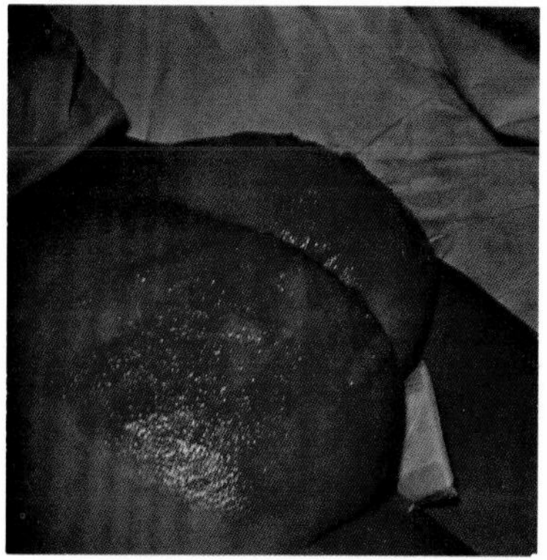

Severe Bullous Dermatitis of the Buttocks due to Improperly Aerated Drape Sheets (Courtesy Dr. L. Biro)

DERMATITIS DUE TO URINARY AND FECAL INCONTINENCE

In adult incontinent patients the changes of the skin closely resemble those seen in infants with diaper dermatitis.[12] The eruption in adults, however, usually covers a much wider area and also has more of a tendency to unilateral involvement, being apt to localize on the side on which the patient habitually lies. In hemiplegics the eruptions usually are on the paralyzed side because this is the side upon which the subject generally lies. Incontinent patients who rest mainly on the back usually exhibit a more symmetrical eruption. The skin involvement may become widespread, extending along the thighs and over the back up to the scapular area with points of pressure showing the most marked changes.

The patients who suffer from urinary incontinence alone may present a follicular eruption resembling miliaria rubra or may show areas of the skin that are smooth and shiny with scaly borders.

Contamination of the skin with urine and feces may produce follicular and erosive lesions

Patients with both urinary and fecal incontinence often have small round erosions in the involved areas resembling the erosive eruption sometimes seen in infantile diaper dermatitis.

The miliaria-like or smooth eruption of urinary incontinence and the erosive dermatitis from fecal incontinence are usually superimposed on skin that is purplish red from chronic pressure.

The dermatitis of incontinent patients is managed by changing the soiled bedsheets as often as possible. At least three changes daily are ideal. The skin may be washed with a nonalkaline soap, such as Dove (Lever Bros.), and powdered. Not infrequently there is a superimposed moniliasis which may be treated by painting the lesions, twice daily with a dilute solution of Castellani's carbolfuchsin paint (1 part paint to 6 parts water).

The ammonia formed by the excretions of the incontinent patient may not only give off a strong odor, but may also be sufficiently concentrated to irritate the skin. Sodium acid phosphate (20 grains, given 3 times daily) will help to acidify the urine and prevent the formation of such ammonia.

CIRCUM-ILEOSTOMY AND COLOSTOMY DERMATITIS

Skin irritation around a stoma may be due to leakage under an appliance, an improper appliance or irritation or sensitivity to the appliance adhesive or to the solvent used to remove it.[13] The cause may be determined by removing the appliance and inspecting the site. A patch test should be done on every adhesive or karaya product before it is used with an ileostomy appliance.

Occasionally contact dermatitis results from allergic hypersensitivity to the cement, which usually contains rubber compounds. In this case, karaya gum is used either as a substitute or as a protective layer between the skin and the cement.

Karaya gum powder is made from the resin of the tree *Sterculia urens* found in India and becomes gummy when water is added. Calamine lotion may be added instead of water, because it is soothing and binds the powder more securely.

Neo-Karaya is a combination of karaya and aluminum hydroxide gel, which is more efficient than karaya with water in allaying inflammation and in forming a protective coating to insulate skin that is allergic to cement. For patients who are allergic to karaya, Orabase (Squibb), which contains pectin, may be used.

Temporary, disposable ileostomy pouches are satisfactory postoperatively and when one has a problem with his stoma. Permanent appliances, however, are more economical, can be worn for longer periods between changes and usually fit the stoma better.

Skin excoriation around the ileostomy is usually corrected initially by putting a large karaya ring or, preferably, a Collyseel ring around the stoma and then sticking a temporary appliance over it. Adhesive extending beyond the karaya ring is cut away. The appliance can be held in place with a belt or with a porous, hypoallergenic adhesive tape if the patch test shows it to be safe.[14]

A permanent appliance should be used as soon as all skin excoriation has healed. It can be used with a karaya ring and an adhesive (latex, spray or double-faced) known not to cause irritation.[15]

Once irritation becomes established beneath the appliance disc, it is difficult to cement it to the abdominal skin without increasing the dermatitis. Even when the appliance fits properly, great care must be exercised in the proper use of the various cements. In addition, any solvents employed to remove the cement should be used as sparingly as possible.

The following instructions may help prevent dermatitis about a stoma:

1. If possible, the faceplate of the appliance should be removed *without* use of solvent by gently and persistently peeling it away from the skin.
2. Accumulated cement on the faceplate need not be removed. As long as the appliance is cleaned and thoroughly dried, accumulated cement will not interfere with adherence of fresh cement.
3. A thin roll of absorbent cotton or lamb's wool may be placed around the base of the stoma after the cement has been applied. This "washer" fills in the area between the stoma and the disc opening and helps protect the skin.

When a solvent has to be used, it should be applied between the skin and the bag with a medicine dropper, one drop at a time, so that no puddles accumulate on the skin. The solvent must be completely evaporated from the cement film on the skin and on the disc before the appliance is reapplied.

Patients with colostomies and ileostomies may benefit from ileostomy clubs, which offer valuable information concerning proper use of various appliances. Information about these clubs may be obtained from the Ileostomy Association of New York, Inc., Suite 536, 152 West 42nd Street, New York, N. Y. 10036.

A physician may receive help with stoma problems from his local chapter of the United Ostomy Association and by consulting an enterostomal therapist. United Ostomy Association offices and all enterostomal therapists in the United States are listed in *Ileostomy Care*.[16]

The treatment of acute dermatitis about a stoma is essentially the same as for acute dermatitis in other areas. Some patients obtain quick relief by applying aluminum hydroxide in the form of Amphojel from which the supernatant liquid has been removed. Hydrocortisone, 1 per cent in plain Lassar's paste, is usually healing. This paste may be covered with plastic food wrap and the appliance reapplied.

DERMATITIS FROM OILS, TARS AND CUTTING FLUIDS

Oils and tars may produce acneiform eruptions at the sites of contact, and the lesion may be identical to that seen in acne vulgaris, with the formation of comedones, papules, pustules and even cysts. The distinguishing characteristics are age of the patient, sites of eruption and history of exposure to oils or tars.[17]

Topical medications commonly contain oils and tars, but an acneiform eruption from use of these preparations is infrequent. Ointments have a greater tendency to cause such a reaction than do creams and oily lotions, and hairy areas of the skin are considerably more susceptible. The reaction sometimes occurs in small children from the protracted use of baby oils, but is more commonly seen in adults, especially in the hirsute, from the use of tar-containing ointments for dermatologic disorders. Oily cosmetics also occasionally cause it.

Occupational exposure to oils and tars is of much greater significance, and this possibility must always be considered when an individual with the possibility for such exposure develops an acneiform eruption. Contact with heavy oils, waxes, cutting oils and chlorinated hydrocarbons occurs universally among machinery operators. The eruptions appear most frequently on the forearms and thighs, especially if the clothing becomes impregnated with the substance. If the industrial process leads to dispersion of the oil in the air, however, the worker may develop a facial eruption that closely resembles spontaneous acne vulgaris. Electrical insulating materials that contain chloronaphthalenes and related compounds are capable of producing the same phenomenon.

Acneiform eruptions may occur from oils and tars in topical medications and from industrial exposure. Such chloracne is often difficult to eradicate

Chloracne and acneiform dermatitides caused by oils, tar and greases are extremely recalcitrant. Systemic antibiotics, such as tetracycline, and topical acne preparations may offer periodic improvement, but they are poor substitutes for avoidance of contact and better hygiene. Workmen with occupational acne must wash with soap and water—not naphtha or mineral spirits—several times a day, and they must discontinue using oil-saturated waste for removal of oil from the skin. Their clothes must be changed, if necessary, each day to avoid body contact with oils and should not be laundered with the family wash.

Even when the patient is no longer in contact with the tars and oils, the chloracne may remain recalcitrant to treatment, causing pigmentary and acneiform disfigurement and even serious hepatotoxicity. As long as exposure to the chloracnegen continues, the disease will remain and generally progress. Comedone extraction, meticulous cleansing of the skin, acne preparations, acne surgery, antibiotics and sometimes intralesional steroids are useful, but if exposure continues, a job change is the only alternative. Even then months may be required for recovery.

Cutting fluids are widely used in manufacturing processes involving metals and are categorized as insoluble oils, emulsion oils and synthetic coolants.[18]

Contact with insoluble oils causes occlusion of pilosebaceous follicles, which is presumably mechanical but may possibly be caused by oil-induced alterations in follicular keratinization. The clinical counterparts are comedones (oil acne), perifollicular inflammation and, at times, secondary pyogenic folliculitis and furunculosis (oil boils). These lesions are found most often on the dorsum of the hands, face, forearms and thighs.

The most common problem resulting from exposure to emulsion oils and synthetics is primary irritant contact dermatitis. Repeated immersion in these alkaline, soaplike fluids leads to dryness, erythema, scaling and fissuring. Some additives, such as excess bacteriostatic agents, sulfur, chlorine, rancid fatty acids and acroleates from overheated oils, may also act as irritants. The common mechanism is presumably damage to the stratum corneum, with all other effects following this initial injury. Allergic contact dermatitis is rare and has been related to corrosion inhibitors, bacteriostatic agents and breakdown products, nickel salts from machined metals or chromates.

DERMATITIS DUE TO TEAR GASES (LACRIMATORS)

The term *tear gases* includes not only gases but also liquids and solids that at ordinary temperatures give off vapors which produce so much irritation of the conjunctivae with lacrimation and photophobia that the affected individual is temporarily blinded and can more readily be subdued.[19]

Most of the tear gas used by military and law enforcement officers are synthetic organic compounds. Recently citizens in the United States have been arming themselves with tear gas containing the oleoresin of capsicum.

THE CHEMICAL NATURE OF TEAR GASES

1. *Chloracetophenone.* This lacrimator, known in America as CN, was first used in World War I and has become a tear gas weapon used worldwide by the military and the police. Chloracetophenone ($C_6H_5COCH_2Cl$) is made by chlorinating acetic acid to form monochloracetic acid, which is further chlorinated with sulphur monochloride and chlorine gas to form chloracetyl chloride. This compound is treated with benzene in the presence of aluminum chloride. It consists of colorless crystals that melt at 59° C and smells like apple blossoms.[20,21]

2. *Mace.* Chloracetophenone is available in a compound called Mace, which is an acronym derived from the chemicals *m*ethyl-chloroform and chlor*ace*tophenone. Methylchloroform, a solvent, is 1,1,1-trichloroethane.[22] Mace also contains kerosene. The chemical mixture is dissolved in an ether-alcohol combination and emitted under pressure from a grenade cartridge by one of the Freons.

A billy club that sprays Mace out of its end is also available.

3. *C.S.* This term refers to the lacrimator ortho-chlorbenzolmalonitrile,[23] a white powder that is often combined with ethyl bromacetate, a dispersing agent. The letters are rumored to represent *C*arson and *S*toughton, the chemists who invented the chemical. It has been used in thermal grenades by the United States military in Vietnam, by American police in domestic disturbances and by British forces in Northern Ireland.

Recently C.S. has become available in the United States in aerosol form.

4. *Miscellaneous Synthetic Tear Gases.* Much less widely used lacrimators include the following:[21]

A. *Brombenzyl cyanide* ($C_6H_5CHBrCN$) is known as C.A. in America and as Chamite in France.
B. *Ethyliodoacetate* ($CH_3ICOOC_2H_5$) is the British SK.
C. *Bromacetone* (CH_3COCH_2Br) is the American BA, the French Martinite, and the German B-Stoff.
D. *Xylyl bromide* ($C_6H_4CH_3CH_2Br$) is the German T-Stoff.
E. *Benzyl iodide* ($C_6H_5CH_2I$) is the French Fraissite.
F. *Ethyl bromoethanoate* ($CH_2Br \cdot COOC_2H_5$).
G. *Phenyl carbylamine chloride* ($C_6H_5CNCl_2$).
H. *Benzyl bromide* ($C_6H_5CH_2Br$) is the French Cyclite.
I. *Acrolein* (CH_2CHCHO) is the French Papite.
J. *Bromo methyl ethyl ketone* ($BrCH_2COC_2H_5$).
K. *Chloracetone* (CH_3COCH_2Cl) is the French Tonite.
L. *Iodoacetone* (CH_3COCH_3I) is the French Bretonite.

5. *The Oleoresin of Capsicum.* For some time, the United States Government has issued aerosol sprays containing this oleoresin to postal carriers for repelling animals, particularly dogs. Recently, individuals have been similarly arming themselves with capsicum aerosols in containers varying in size from that of a lipstick to a fountain pen.

The oleoresin is a dark red, extremely acrid and pungent liquid that is extracted from cayenne pepper pods with alcohol or ethyl ether. It irritates the conjunctivae and the nasal and oral mucosa and can be classified as a tear gas or lacrimator.[24] Although organic synthetic lacrimators do not affect dogs and horses as much as they do humans, the oleoresin of capsicum is an efficient repellent for both man and beast.

Cayenne pepper (*Capsicum frutescens*), from which the oleoresin of capsicum is extracted, is distributed worldwide and has the following names in different countries: *pimenton* (Spain); *poivre rouge* (France); *cayennepferrer* (Germany); *kajennepeppar* (Sweden); *cayennepeper* (Holland); *pepe di caienna* (Italy); *pimentao-de-caiena* (Portugal); *kayenski pyerets* (Russia); *la-chiao* (China); and *filfil ahmar* (Arabic). In Japan, cayenne pepper is not known, but the closely related chili pepper (*togarashi*) is available. Cayenne pepper may colloquially be called Guinea pepper, Spanish pepper, African pepper, chilies or bird pepper.

PRIMARY IRRITANT REACTIONS TO TEAR GASES

All lacrimators in high concentrations are powerful skin irritants and can produce first and second degree burns. Third degree burns with ulceration may result, particularly with C.S., in the presence of moisture and occlusion. Stinging and erythema are produced when C.S. is wetted.

People who are blond or have light pigmentation acquire irritant dermatitis most readily. Under proper conditions, however, people of all colors and races are affected. Mace dermatitis particularly can cause disfiguring depigmentation of black skin, which may persist for many months.

Technicians and others handling lacrimators, particularly C.S., acquire an irritant dermatitis, especially where there is constriction from wearing apparel, such as at the neck and waist. In addition, moist areas, such as the axilla and vulva, may be subject to irritant dermatitis from C.S.

The irritation from CN and oth er chlorinated lacrimators may be d ue to the release of hydrochloric ac id from such compounds

ALLERGIC CONTACT DERMATITIS FROM TEAR GASES

For the past three decades allergic contact dermatitis from chloracetophenone has been reported.[23–28] It has recently been reemphasized that the CN in Mace is a potent sensitizer, which cross-reacts with dichloracetophenone but not with para-chloracetophenone or bromoacetophenone.[29] Although C.S. is also a sensitizer, it is not as potent as CN.

Many sensitized individuals acquired an allergic eczematous contact dermatitis not only during deliberate exposure by the military or police, but also in the manufacture or in other handling of tear gas.

Allergic contact dermatitis from synthetic tear gas is typical eczematous dermatitis, often accompanied by marked edema. Contact sensitization to the oleoresin of capsicum is not common, but it suggests the possibility that ingestion of foods containing capsicum (pickles, liqueurs and ginger ale) may produce an eczematous contact-type dermatitis. Diffuse erythema has been reported from the ingestion of capsicum.[30]

PATCH TEST WITH TEAR GASES

Great care must be taken in performing patch tests with tear gases, because the minimum irritating concentration is as low as 1 part in 100,000.[21]

Patch tests with tear gases should be started with a 1 to 100,000 dilution

In Mace, CN is present in an 0.9 per cent concentration. Patch tests may be performed with chemical Mace diluted 1 part with 100 parts acetone, which gives a 0.009 per cent concentration of chloracetophenone. This concentration is not an irritant under a closed patch test and is sufficient to produce a positive allergic eczematous patch test reaction in sensitized individuals.[29]

Patch tests with C.S. should be commenced with a 1 to 100,000 dilution in acetone. (It should be noted that C.S. dissolves with difficulty.) The other tear gases should be tested in a 1 to 100,000 dilution in alcohol in order to determine a concentration that is not irritating under a closed patch.

Capsicum may be tested in a 1 per cent alcoholic solution.[31]

MANAGEMENT OF TEAR GAS DERMATITIS

In sensitized individuals, Mace must be removed from the skin with soap and water within 1 minute or dermatitis is inevitable.[29] The lacrimator C.S. should also be removed with water as soon as possible. Although dry skin initially is unharmed by it, prolonged exposure produces first and second degree burns and even ulceration. As soon as the individual begins to wash the powder off, a burning sensation and erythema occur but usually subside in an hour or so.

Barrier creams and petrolatum do not offer much protection from tear gas. Plastic clothing, including plastic helmets and visors, are the best protective devices available.

The treatment of primary irritation, burns or allergic dermatitis from the tear gases is similar to the treatment of these conditions from other causes.

The United States Surgeon General's report concerning chemical Mace states: "It is generally agreed that flushing of the agent from the contact point is the most effective treatment and that the application of salves, creams or ointments should be discouraged since these substances aid in localizing the active material at the site of injury."

REFERENCES

1. Hjorth, N., and Fregert, S.: Contact Dermatitis. In A. J. Rook et al. (eds.): *Textbook of Dermatology.* London, Blackwell, 1968.
2. Kligman, A. M., and Wooding, W. M.: A Method for the Measurement and Evaluation of Irritants on Human Skin. J. Invest. Derm., *49*, 78, 1967.
3. Bandman, H. S., and Dohn, W.: Die Epicutantestung. Munich, Bergman, 1967, p. 36.
4. Bjornberg, A.: Skin Reactions to Primary Irritants in Patients with Hand Eczema. Goteberg, Oscar Isaacson, 1968.

5. Cooke, M. A.: The Problem of Skin Cleansing. Trans. St. John Hosp. Derm. Soc., *51*, 137, 1965.
6. Baer, R. L.: Multiple Eczematous Sensitivities. J.A.M.A., *170*, 1041, 1959.
7. Rostenberg, A., Jr.: Primary Irritant and Allergic Eczematous Reactions: Their Interrelations are Discussed. Arch. Derm., *75*, 547, 1957.
8. Berkhout, P. G., et al.: Treatment of Skin Burns Due to Alkyl Mercury Compounds. Arch. Environ. Health, *3*, 592, 1960.
9. King, T. C., Zimmerman, J. M., and Price, P. B.: Effect of Immediate Short-Term Cooling on Extensive Burns. Surg. Forum, *13*, 487, 1962.
10. Fleming, A. J., D'Alonzo, C. A., and Zapp, J. A.: Modern Occupational Medicine (Ed. 2). Philadelphia, Lea & Febiger, 1960, pp. 365–411.
11. Reinhardt, C. F.: Hydrofluoric Acid Burn. Amer. Industr. Hyg. Ass. J., *27*, 166, 1971.
12. Kogsard, E.: Skin Complications of Urinary and Fecal Incontinence. Cutis, *1*, 178, 1965.
13. Lenneberg, E., and Rowbotham, J. L.: *The Ileostomy Patient, A Descriptive Study of 1,425 Persons*. Springfield, Ill., Charles C Thomas, 1970.
14. Rowbotham, J. L.: Current Concepts: Stomal Care. New Eng. J. Med., *279*, 90, 1968.
15. Rowbotham, J. L.: Skin Excoriation around Ileostomy. Questions and Answers. J.A.M.A., *22*, 514, 1972.
16. Sparberg, M.: *Ileostomy Care*. Springfield, Ill., Charles C Thomas, 1971.
17. Hitch, J. M.: Acneiform Eruptions Induced by Drug and Chemicals. J.A.M.A., *200*, 878, 1967.
18. Arndt, K. A.: Cutting Fluids and the Skin. Cutis, *5*, 143, 1969.
19. Fisher, A. A.: Dermatitis Due to Tear Gases (Lacrimators). Int. J. Derm., *9*, 91, 1970.
20. Stein, A. A., and Kerwin, W. E.: Chloracetophenone (Tear Gas) Poisoning: A Clinico-Pathological Report. J. Forensic Sci., *9*, 379, 1964.
21. Schwartz, I., Tulipan, L., and Birmingham, D. J.: *Occupational Diseases of the Skin* (Ed. 2). Philadelphia, Lea & Febiger, 1957, p. 466.
22. Fisher, A. A.: Mace, A Modern Acronym and An Ancient Nomenclature. J.A.M.A., *212*, 320, 1970.
23. Gleason, M. N. et al.: *Clinical Toxicology of Commercial Products* (Ed. 3). Baltimore, Williams and Wilkins, 1969, p. 301.
24. Rosengarten, F.: *The Book of Spices*. Wynnewood, Pa., Livingston Publishing Co., 1969, p. 129.
25. Queen, F. B., and Stander, T.: Allergic Dermatitis Following Exposure to Tear Gas (Chloracetophenone) (CN). J.A.M.A., *117*, 1879, 1941.
26. Kissin, M., and Mazar, M.: Cutaneous Hypersensitivity to Tear Gas (Chloracetophenone), Bulletin 81. U.S. Army Medical Department, 1944, pp. 120–121.
27. Madden, J. F.: Cutaneous Hypersensitivity to Tear Gas (Chloracetophenone). Arch. Derm., *63*, 133, 1951.
28. Ingram, J. T.: Dermatitis from Exposure to Tear Gas. Brit. J. Derm., *54*, 319, 1942.
29. Penneys, N. S., Israel, R. M., and Indgin, S. M.: Contact Dermatitis Due to 1-Chloracetophenone and Chemical Mace. New Eng. J. Med., *281*, 413, 1969.
30. Ormsby, O. S., and Montgomery, H.: *Diseases of the Skin* (Ed. 8). Philadelphia, Lea & Febiger, 1954, p. 239.
31. Fisher, A. A.: *Contact Dermatitis*. Philadelphia, Lea & Febiger, 1967, p. 266.

3

The Role of Patch Testing in Allergic Contact Dermatitis

The patch test is indispensable in proving the cause of allergic contact dermatitis.

It is an exact scientific method of investigation with rules, regulations and established fundamentals. The patch test, which seems so simple to apply and read, may in reality be tricky and should not be attempted until one has practiced the method under the supervision of experienced personnel. Furthermore, modification of the standard procedure should not be undertaken lightly, because it may lead to confusion and misinterpretation.

There is no substitute for the patch test in management of allergic contact dermatitis

The patch test admittedly is artificial and does not necessarily duplicate clinical exposure in which sweating, maceration and pressure may play roles in producing the dermatitis. In most instances in which a contactant is the cause of allergic eczematous dermatitis, however, the patch test does reveal the culprit. Patch testing is safer and quicker than clinical trial and error, which may produce a widespread dermatitis.

The patch test exposes only a small portion of skin and may be performed on covered parts of the body, so that even strongly positive reactions need not be disabling or disfiguring. Finally, if positive reactions are properly interpreted, they are scientific proof of the causation of a dermatitis and may be of medicolegal importance.

When a contact dermatitis is acute, spreading or widespread, it is wise to postpone patch testing until the eruption is under control, since under such circumstances the entire skin may be irritable and false positive reactions may be obtained. Furthermore, a strongly positive patch test reaction may cause a flare-up of the dermatitis.

Topical application of corticosteroids suppresses patch test reactions more than systemic administration

Effects of Corticosteroids on Patch Test Results. The *systemic* administration of corticosteroids is not a contraindication to patch testing. Patients with allergic eczematous contact dermatitis can be studied by patch testing with suspected allergens while they are receiving corticosteroid therapy without great risk of masking or altering significant reactions to allergens applied in standard concentration. This is true even when hormones are given in doses sufficient to completely suppress the clinically visible eruption. Corticosteroids might mask weak patch test responses, which are probably not of clinical significance.[1] Similarly, antihistaminics do not significantly influence the patch test reaction. The presence of a corticosteroid in a *topical* medicament, however, is much more likely to suppress a response.[2]

SITE OF APPLICATION OF PATCH TESTS

Patches should be placed on grossly normal, nonhairy skin. It is preferable to utilize areas that are usually covered by clothing so that strongly positive reactions, which may persist for a week or so, will not embarrass the patient. In rare instances, hyperpigmentation, depigmentation and even slight scarring may occur.

Some investigators feel that the back is the most reliable site for patch tests, since the pressure to which this area is subjected when the patient is sitting and lying down enhances reactions.[3] When more than four tests are made, the back is usually the site selected. When only a few tests are done, the upper inner aspect of the arm may be employed, because it enables the patient to readily remove any patch that itches or burns excessively. In general, if it is suspected that a test substance may cause a severe reaction, it should be tested at a separate site so that the patient can remove the reacting test without disturbing the other patches.

For patients who are in hot, humid climates or who perspire so profusely that the adhesive does not adhere to the skin, the arms may be used as the site and the patch tests are held in place with a bandage.

Patients should be given the following instructions after the patch tests have been applied.

1. You may remove any patch that causes severe itching or burning, but try not to disturb the other patches. Keep the remaining patch test areas dry.
2. Avoid rubbing or scratching any test site. If you have to remove a patch, cold water compresses will help allay itching or burning and will not affect the reading of the reaction provided you keep the other patches dry. You may take aspirin or a sedative if necessary.

In regions that are so hot and humid and for patients who perspire so excessively that the patch test loosens or falls off, the tests should be applied to the arm and held in place with a bandage

APPLICATION OF PATCH TESTS

The International Contact Dermatitis Research Group has adopted the aluminum patch test as the standard. It consists of a cellulose disc fastened to polyethylene-coated aluminum. The North American group is comparing the aluminum test with other patch tests. Magnusson and Hersle[4] compared six types of patch tests and could not determine which one was best.

The 2-inch square Band-Aid (Johnson & Johnson) is readily available, inexpensive and generally useful for routine patch testing. Patients who are allergic to or irritated by the rubber-adhesive mass in Band-Aids will tolerate patches made of Dermicel (Johnson & Johnson) or Blenderm (Minnesota Mining), both of which contain an acrylic mass adhesive.

There seems to be a general agreement that petrolatum (U.S.P.), also known as Vaseline or yellow soft paraffin, is the best vehicle for test substances in patch tests.[5] Petrolatum is nonsensitizing, nonirritating and so occlusive that it permits fixation of the patches with nonocclusive, nonirritant adhesive tape and thus may prevent adhesive reactions from interfering with test readings.

Petrolatum (Vaseline) should be used whenever possible as a patch test vehicle since it is nonallergenic, nonirritating and occlusive. Test substances in petrolatum remain allergenic for at least a year

Dr. K. E. Malten (personal communication, 1969) studied a patient with positive reactions to yellow petrolatum but not to the white variety.

Hjorth[6] has devised a time-saving patch test antigen dispenser. Epstein[7] uses mixtures ("chem-mixes") to permit screening of many compounds with a limited number of tests. Paschoud[8] objects to mixtures: "Since the mixed tests give only a general orientation, it is necessary to use individual substances in a second series, although this is not always feasible. Moreover, the chemical reactions which interfere in these substances once they are mixed in a single excipient are unknown." He dissolves test substances in alcohol and acetone and then incorporates them into laceranum anhydricum, an excipient of lanolin. MacLeod and Frain-Bell[9] use a glycogelatin patch test.

PATCH TEST SUBSTANCES

The gauze cotton or disc is covered with the test material. The International Group obtains its material from K. Trolle-Lassen, Laboratory for Dermatologic Patch Tests, Hoyrups Alle 1, 2900 Hellerup, Copenhagen, Denmark. The North American Group also uses the material from Denmark and is comparing these substances with ones obtained from other sources.

Many contactants mentioned in this text may also be obtained from Hollistier Laboratories with headquarters in Spokane, Washington, and branches in California, Illinois, Georgia, Texas, Pennsylvania and Canada.

Unstandardized Substances

Solids. These substances are made into fine shavings, scrapings or powder and applied to the water-moistened gauze or disc.

Solid objects may cause false positive reactions, particularly at their margins, because of the pressure of a cutting edge. If sufficient pressure is exerted, the reaction can cover the entire site. Such effects may be minimized by beveling the edges and using objects that are round. The uneven surfaces of a solid object, particularly spurs and depressions, may produce nonspecific papules under a patch. Pressure can also potentiate a patch test reaction,[10] particularly with higher dilutions of allergens and in persons with a low degree of sensitivity. When pressure is deliberately applied to a patch test, it is no longer considered standard and requires special interpretation. Blisters and even bullae may occur under solid objects, and such reactions may be entirely nonspecific.[11] Traumatic blisters and bullae tend to dry quickly and usually become inconspicuous within 24 hours, whereas a vesicular or bullous allergic reaction persists for several days.

Patch test results from testing with solid objects should be evaluated with care since such objects often produce false positive reactions

Even an elastic substance such as sponge rubber, if thick enough and sufficiently compressed, can produce a nonspecific traumatic effect. Patch tests with dentures, coins, buttons, wooden objects, chips, scrapings, and fine sawdust may produce erythema, papules, vesicles and bullae, which are nonspecific reactions.

Vesicles and bullae produced by large patch tests with hard objects, such as dentures, have been found in the subepidermal zone, with little reaction in the cutis or epidermis, whereas vesicles produced by chips, scrapings or coarse powders have been found in the epidermis and contain many polymorphonuclear cells. Occasionally, a foreign body giant cell has been seen in the cutis.

Liquids. Certain liquids tend to become concentrated at the edge of the gauze; in such instances, an augmented reaction may be seen at the periphery of the patch. A true allergic response occurs throughout the patch test site.

Gases. Fumes emanating from liquids are tested by pouring a small amount of the liquid into cotton placed in the bottom of a small glass cup or a thimble. The container is then inverted and strapped onto the skin,

Table 3-1. Artificial Sweat

Sodium chloride	3.0 Gm.
Sodium sulfate	1.0 Gm.
Urea	2.0 Gm.
Lactic acid	2.0 cc.
Olein	2.0 Gm.
Stearin	2.0 Gm.
Aq. dist. q.s. ad	1000.0 cc.

Note: To make the solution acid, add a drop of acetic acid; to make it alkaline, add a drop of ammonia. It is used to moisten fabrics and other contactants prior to patch testing in order to simulate clinical exposure when hyperhidrosis may be a factor.

but the liquid-soaked cotton should not touch the skin.[12]

Fabrics. Textiles may be cut into ½-inch squares, moistened with water and covered with patches. Occasionally a positive reaction is obtained only if the fabric is soaked in artificial sweat (Table 3–1), which leaches out sensitizing dyes or other chemicals from the material.

> **Soaking fabric, metals and other contactants with artificial sweat prior to patch testing may help leach out sensitizers, producing positive reaction that otherwise might not be obtained**

SAFE AND STANDARD TEST SUBSTANCES

It is relatively safe to perform patch tests with materials such as topical medications, cosmetics and clothing, which were intended by the manufacturer to come in contact with skin. Great caution must be taken, however, when testing with chemicals or other substances that were not intended for use on or near the skin. The concentration of any test substance must be such that it does not cause a reaction on nonsensitized skin. Lists of correct concentrations and proper vehicles for patch testing are available for many contact allergens (see Appendix). Hjorth[13] points out that the optimal strength of patch test reagents is a matter of accumulated experience.

A substance may be allergenic because of impurities, the importance of which retailers and even manufacturers are often unaware. When natural products are used in patch testing, the difficulties are increased, because oxidation, degradation, storage, ultraviolet light and heat may radically alter the nature or proportion of sensitizers in a substance.

> **Clinical patch testing should be a standardized procedure**

THE TIME OF READING OF PATCH TESTS

This is usually given as 48-hour (1st) reading and 72-96 hour (2nd) reading after application. The joint European study showed that the first reading is often performed at 72-hour and that this might be regarded as a "first reading" (equivalent to a 48-hour reading) and the "second reading" after 96 hours. It was, therefore, decided to recommend the day of reading instead of the hours, to avoid giving a misleading impression of an exact time of reading which, in fact, was not always the case. Thus:

D1: 24 hours (particularly for phototests)
D2: 48 hours
D4: 96 hours
D7: 1 week

RECORDING AND EVALUATION OF POSITIVE PATCH TEST REACTIONS

The patch test reaction depends on the sensitivity of the patient, the concentration of the substance and the length of time it remains on the skin. Usually, the patch test is kept in place for 48 hours, then removed and a reading made.

The patient is instructed to keep the site dry and to remove any patch that causes great discomfort, such as burning or itching. When the patch is removed, it is wise to mark the location on the skin with a skin-marking pencil or pen, especially if the results are slight or doubtful and may have to be read later.

Readings should be made 20 to 60 minutes after removal of the patch so that the skin may recover from the effects of *pressure* of patch test substances, which may produce a mild erythema or even dermographia, which is usually *transient.* The true erythema of the specific reaction to the test agent *persists* for hours or days. Instead of erythema, the pressure may produce a *blanching* effect at the test site and cause a temporary negative reaction, which becomes positive only when the effect of the pressure wears off and allows edema and the eczematous response to come through the cutis into the epidermis.

Read patch test results 20 to 60 minutes after removal of the patch to allow effects of pressure to wear off. Doubtful reactions should be read again in 24 hours

Significant reactions to patch tests present the changes in the skin characteristic of eczema. As a rule, the site of a positive reaction itches. A typically significant positive reaction consists of vesicles on an edematous, red area. When a single bulla occurs, it is usually due to a primary irritant, but there are exceptions. When there is a questionable reaction, such as a mild erythema, it is wise to reexamine the site the following day. Redness, which persists or increases, is probably significant for an allergic reaction. Erythema at the test site, which fades in 24 hours, is probably not associated with an allergic reaction of *clinical significance.*

Signs for recording degrees of patch test reactions:

1. No reaction	0
2. Erythema	+
3. Erythema and papules	++
4. Erythema, papules and vesicles	+++
5. Marked edema and vesicles	++++

Unless one is dealing with weak sensitizers, such as fabrics and cosmetics, a 1+ reaction (simple erythema) is usually not of clinical significance. Corticosteroids in proprietary ointments, however, may mask a reaction, so that in testing with such medications, a 1+ reaction can be of clinical significance.

The International Contact Dermatitis Research Group points out that the notations used in recording patch test results vary throughout the world and even within one nation. It is usual to describe results in terms of − and +, but there is no universal agreement on the exact meaning of the symbols used, particularly the signs ± and +++. In the United States, these algebraic symbols are replaced by the Arabic 0 to 4+; these save space but are difficult to translate into visual terms and may invite confusion with numbers used to denote the subject involved. The International Group recommends the following symbols for patch test results:

NT	not tested
?+	doubtful reaction
+	weak (nonvesicular) reaction
++	strong (edematous or vesicular) reaction
+++	extreme reaction, e.g., markedly bullous or ulcerative
IR	irritant reaction

The minus sign should be used for negative reactions in preference to 0, which may be construed as meaning "not tested."

SIGNIFICANCE OF WEAK PATCH TEST REACTIONS

In my experience, weak patch test reactions in many cases are of *no clinical significance.* A follow-up of many patients with weakly positive patch test reactions to sensitizers such as paraphenylenediamine and the dichromates for as long as 20 years revealed that the patch test reactions continue to remain weak and the patients remained free of clinical dermatitis attributable to the allergens in question. Further studies are in progress to evaluate more fully weak patch test reactions.

A long follow-up of patients with weak patch test reactions reveals that such reactions are not usually clinically significant

It is conceivable that such weak reactions are an expression of a fixed level of sensitivity, which actually prevents stronger sensitization. For example, many patients with a weak patch test reaction to paraphenylenediamine continue to dye their hair for many years with no or minimal dermatitis.

REACTIONS DUE TO PERSPIRATION

Excessive perspiration under a patch may produce maceration, sweat retention, miliaria or folliculitis, any of which may complicate a true reaction or produce a false positive one. In such instances, reexamination of the site the day after patch removal is indicated because effects due to hyperhidrosis are much less marked while true allergic reactions are more prominent.

As mentioned previously, sweating may be so profuse that the patch test is loosened and adequate contact is prevented. Such patches can be held in place with a bandage.

REACTIONS DUE TO THE ADHESIVE PORTION OF THE PATCH

Prior to the application of a patch, the patient should be asked if he is allergic to or irritated by ordinary adhesive tape. If he is, the aluminum patch or one made with Dermicel or Blenderm should be employed and held in place with the Dermicel or Blenderm. Allergic reactions to the acrylic mass adhesive (Dermicel or Blenderm) are extremely rare, and irritation is usually minimal.

Removal of the patch may cause an erythema of the site, which usually fades in an hour or so. Irritant and allergic reactions from the adhesive in the patch are usually most marked at the periphery, while the portion covered by the gauze shows little or no reaction. Irritant adhesive reactions usually fade within 24 hours, but allergic reactions to adhesive persist for several days and may mask a positive patch test reaction. In such instances, the test should be repeated, using gauze held in place with Dermicel or Blenderm tape.

STAINS AND DISCOLORATIONS

Stains and discolorations due to dyes or colored substances (lipstick, nail polish, silver nitrate and potassium permanganate may cause confusion. Paraphenylenediamine is colorless when applied, but oxidation on the skin results in a colored compound, which is of no clinical significance. Often it darkens in the test bottle or syringe, because of partial oxidation, but this does not interfere with the dye's ability to produce an allergic response. The completely oxidized compound is not a sensitizer.

ISOMORPHIC AND COINCIDENTAL PATCH TEST REACTIONS

Patients who have or have had psoriasis or lichen planus may develop patches of the lesion at patch test sites a week or so following a positive eczematous patch test reaction.

Rarely, a lesion of a dermatosis, such as pityriasis rosea, or a drug eruption may coincidentally appear on the patch test site. In such instances, the patch test may have to be repeated when the eruption has disappeared.

The application of a drug to the site of a healed fixed drug eruption often leads to a false positive reaction, because the site may remain irritable for several weeks. If this method of proving the cause of a fixed drug eruption is employed, unrelated drugs should first be applied as controls.

False positive patch test reactions may be produced by solids, pressure, perspiration, stains and isomorphic eruptions

PUSTULAR PATCH TEST REACTIONS

Not infrequently the salts of *heavy metals*, particularly nickel, mercury and arsenic, and the halogens produce a pustular reaction without any erythema.

Pustular reactions to nickel salts are common but not exclusive in individuals with atopic dermatitis. These pustules are usually small, measuring from 1 to 2 mm. in diameter. Occasionally ammonium fluoride produces large, milky pustules, which heal with slight, depressed scars. Pustular reactions seem to be distinct from ordinary irritant reactions.[14]

Stone and Johnson[15] regularly produced pustular patch test reactions with 5 per cent nickel sulfate patches in areas of inflammation induced by injections of *Corynebacterium acnes*. Eberhartinger et al.[16] obtained papulopustular reactions mostly with arsenic and nickel, but occasionally with formalin. They concluded that these reactions depend on the condition of the skin and the concentration of the test substances and classified them as "sensitivity reactions distinct from the toxic or allergic variety."

Pustular patch test reactions seem to be distinct, clinically and histopathologically, from allergic and irritant patch test reactions. Such pustular reactions have no clinical significance as far as allergic sensitization is concerned but represent an irritable or nonspecific hypersensitivity

All the positive patch test reactions I have obtained have been in apparently normal (noninflamed) skin of the back.

Symptoms. Pustular patch test reactions are usually without symptoms, but allergic eczematous patch test sites often itch. Primary irritant patch test reactions may cause a burning sensation.

Reproducibility. Pustular patch test reactions cannot be regularly reproduced and occur in few patients. Allergic eczematous patch test reactions usually can be regularly reproduced once the patient has become sensitized. The ordinary primary irritant patch test reactions occur in the majority of persons and usually can be regularly reproduced.

Patch test results may not be reproduced if the original test was performed when the skin was inflamed or hyperirritable.

Persistence. Pustular patch test reactions and mild primary irritant reactions fade quickly. Allergic eczematous reactions may be evident for several days to weeks and often increase in intensity after removal of the patch. Reactions due to primary irritants may occasionally be so severe that they persist for several days or longer and cause scarring. Mild scarring is occasionally a sequela of the large pustules produced by ammonium fluoride.

Microscopic Appearance. Intercellular edema (spongiosis) is usually slight or absent in pustular patch test reactions, but it is usually prominent in allergic eczematous and primary irritant eczematous patch test reactions.

Etchings or erosions can be caused by ordinary primary irritants, but in such instances spongiosis usually is present. Etchings or erosions of the epidermis without spongiosis appear to be a feature of pustular patch test reactions. In addition, large pustules produced by ammonium fluoride show marked acantholysis and changes resembling "ballooning degeneration" of the epidermal cells.

The pustules contain many polymorphonuclear and mononuclear cells in equal quantities. The vesicle fluid of allergic eczematous patch test reactions characteristically contains a greater proportion of mononuclear cells, whereas that of a primary irritant patch test reaction usually shows a predominance of polymorphonuclear cells.

Eberhartinger[16] found considerable leukocytic infiltration of the "sebopilar" apparatus only.

FALSE POSITIVE (PSEUDO-POSITIVE) PATCH TEST REACTIONS

These are patch test reactions not due to allergic sensitivity but usually to irritants.

The established techniques of patch testing, including use of standard concentrations and vehicles, cannot be varied without careful planning and thorough investigation, because such modifications may result in reactions not significant for an allergic reaction. Investigators who scarify or strip the skin before applying a patch or who apply unusual pressure to the site introduce variables that may result in pseudo-positive reactions or in readings that cannot be compared with standard reactions. The clinical significance of altered tests is still obscure.

Stripped, scarified, scratched or inflamed skin or contactants to which penetrants are added may yield false positive reactions

IRRITANT PATCH TEST REACTIONS

False positive readings may be due to irritant effects of substances applied in too high a concentration. Volatile substances that are not irritants when applied to the skin uncovered may be irritants under a covered patch. Many medications can be applied to the thick skin of the palms, soles, corns, calluses, warts or scalp without causing dermatitis but may be irritants when occluded by a patch.

In general, irritants burn rather than itch and produce skin reactions sooner than do sensitizers. A strong irritant may cause a reaction in a few minutes to several hours, whereas a sensitizer usually requires 24 to 48 hours to produce its effect. Epoxy resins and solvents such as acrylic monomer and alcohol may produce a true allergic patch test reaction within a few hours. Mild or insidious irritants such as soaps, detergents and solvents, which act by defatting the skin over a period of several days or weeks, may not produce an irritant reaction.

A primary irritant reaction tends to remain confined to the site of application and fades rapidly after the site has been uncovered, unless the irritant is so strong that it causes a burn or ulcer. Many allergic reactions tend to spread beyond the site and to persist and even become more marked for several days after the patch is removed.

Except for reactions produced by too strong a substance, irritant patch reactions tend to fade rapidly after the patch is removed, whereas allergic reactions may increase in size and severity

HISTOPATHOLOGICAL FEATURES OF IRRITANT AND ALLERGIC REACTIONS

Certain histopathological features theoretically establish a difference between an allergic eczematous and a primary irritant reaction,[17] but there is no general agreement that one can rely on them.

Features Favoring Diagnosis of an Allergic Eczematous Reaction

Epidermis: Intercellular edema (spongiosis) and vesicle formation usually starting in the lower part of the prickle cell layer.

Dermis: Edema and perivascular cellular infiltration, predominantly with mononuclear cells.

Vesicle fluid: A considerable number of mononuclear cells.

Features Favoring Diagnosis of a Primary Irritant Reaction

Epidermis: Intercellular edema (spongiosis) and vesicle formation usually starting near the surface. Erosion of the surface may take place.

Dermis: Progression of necrosis. Perivascular reaction is variable.

Vesicle fluid: Predominance of polymorphonuclear cells.

SIGNIFICANCE OF POSITIVE PATCH TEST REACTIONS

A positive patch test reaction does not necessarily mean that the presenting dermatitis is caused by the substance that produced a positive patch test reaction. Investigation must show that the patient actually came in contact with the particular substance and that the presenting dermatitis could indeed be produced in the involved areas by the incriminated contactant. Positive patch test reactions must always fit the clinical picture in order to be significant for the dermatitis under investigation.

A positive patch test reaction is considered *relevant* if the allergen is traced. If it reflects a past episode of contact dermatitis, it may be referred to as *sensitivity with past relevance.* If the source of a positive test is not traced, the term *unexplained positive* may be used.

A positive patch test reaction may have relevance to the present or past or may be unexplained

SIGNIFICANCE OF NEGATIVE PATCH TEST REACTIONS

True Negative Reactions. In this case a properly applied patch test in the proper concentration nearly always means an *absence* of allergic hypersensitivity to the contactant.

False Negative Reactions. An individual with an allergic hypersensitivity to a contactant may give a negative reaction because the eliciting threshold concentration was not used; i.e., the concentration was too low or the substance was a photosensitizer requiring an open test with exposure to sun or ultraviolet light.

Lost Reactions. This is a negative reaction that was previously positive under identical environmental and experimental conditions. Such reactions have been rare in my experience.

Other Theoretical Causes of Negative Reactions

1. *The skin is sensitized in a localized area only.* It is sometimes advised that the patch test be repeated closer to the original eruption. A positive patch test reaction obtained by such repetition may be false positive, since the grossly normal skin adjacent to an area of dermatitis may be physiologically abnormal and irritable. The standard sites, such as the extremities or the back, usually are reliable for testing no matter where the original dermatitis is located.

Negative patch test reactions may be true, false or lost. False results may be due to too low a concentration, to the need for exposure to light or to spoiled test materials

2. *A refractory period is present.* Following an allergic reaction in the immediate type of hypersensitivity, a refractory period may occur. In the delayed eczematous type of hypersensitivity, however, it is infrequent. Indeed, the skin more often is hyperirritable following an acute dermatitis and reacts nonspecifically to many substances.

3. *The test substance has spoiled.* To avoid oxidation, test substances should be kept in dark containers and be renewed at least once a year.

4. *The pathology is mainly in the dermis.* Epstein[18] and others[19] have called attention to a type of allergic dermal contact sensitivity in which the clinical picture is a chronic papular dermatitis, patch tests produce a papular dermatitis or give negative results and intradermal tests produce a delayed and often persistent reaction.

Neomycin, nickel and the dichromates may produce a papular dermal type of contact dermatitis. The concentrations recommended for intradermal testing are as follows: neomycin sulfate, 1:100; nickel sulfate, 1:10,000; and potassium dichromate, 1:10,000.

Epstein[18] has stated that one cannot assume that negative patch test reactions to neomycin, nickel and the dichromates indicate lack of hypersensitivity to the tested material. Occasionally, contact allergy to these chemicals may be present in spite of negative reactions, and that it often can be demonstrated by intradermal tests.

In my own material, patch testing has proved reliable in detecting allergic contact sensitivity to neomycin, nickel and the dichromates.

SIGNIFICANCE OF DELAYED REACTIONS

1. *Low order of sensitivity.* Occasionally a patch test reading is negative at the end of 48 hours but becomes positive the following day, probably indicating a low order of sensitivity. In most instances, when an allergen causes clinical dermatitis, a positive patch test reaction occurs within 48 hours.

2. *Active sensitization induced by patch testing.* A reaction that occurs 7 days or later with no preceding reaction is a late reaction caused by the interaction of residues of the allergen with the newly sensitized tissues. This type of reaction is sometimes called a "spontaneous flare."

Agrup[20] states that sensitization is commonly produced by p-aminoazobenzene, p-phenylenediamine, diaminodidiphenylmethane, cobalt and chromium, necessitating reevaluation of the procedure.

In our material these substances do not sensitize as frequently as reported by Agrup.

The following test substances, however, do sensitize frequently:

Dinitrochlorobenzene
Poison ivy extract, primrose and other plant resins
Methyl salicylate (synthetic oil of wintergreen)
Nitroso-dimethyl aniline
Phthalic anhydride
Picryl chloride
Trinitrobenzene

A delayed patch test reaction may occur when there is a low order of sensitivity (a delay of less than 5 days), active sensitization by the patch test procedure (delay of more than 7 days) or the test substance is a photosensitizer

There is general agreement that patch testing should not be performed unnecessarily because of the hazard of sensitizing the patient. The knowledge gained, however, usually outweighs such risks. Moreover, the sensitization may be no great disadvantage, since clinical exposure would also cause a sensitization dermatitis, which would probably be more widespread than the dermatitis localized to a patch test site.

3. *The tested substance may be a photosensitizer.* Another type of delayed reaction is due to photosensitization. In this, the patch test reaction is negative at the end of 48 hours, but on exposure to sunlight or ultraviolet radiation the site becomes reactive. Such a reaction may be due to a photoallergic or a phototoxic dermatitis and is called a pseudo-delayed reaction because light is necessary to form the whole antigen with the contactant.

Properly performed patch test procedures are so helpful in the management of allergic contact dermatitis that the advantages outweigh the inherent risk of active sensitization

INDICATIONS FOR OPEN PATCH TESTING

1. *Potential photosensitizers.*

2. *Volatile substances.* Vapors, mists, fumes or gases may be tested by exposing the forearms to an open vessel containing the suspected contactant for 10 minutes and observing the test site over a period of 48 hours. Volatile hair tonics, hair lacquers and perfumes may be tested in this fashion. Controls are necessary.

3. *Antiperspirants, shaving creams and dentifrices.* The substance may be gently massaged into the forearm 3 times daily for 3 days. If there is a positive reaction, 3 normal individuals must be tested by the same method.

4. *Strong topical medicaments.* The following substances may act as primary irritants under closed patch tests and, therefore, are best tested by the open method: tincture of iodine, Whitfield's ointment, ammoniated mercury and salicylic acid combinations and anthralin ointment. (A 0.03 per cent anthralin ointment may be used by the closed patch test technique.)

Use the open patch test method with photosensitizers, volatile substances, strong medications and possible primary irritants as well as when in doubt

PATCH TESTING WITH NEW UNTESTED SUBSTANCES

When a contactant that is not listed in any table or list of standard patch test materials is used, the following precautions should be followed whenever possible:

1. Ascertain the toxicity and irritation potential of the substance and the results of animal experiments from the manufacturer. As a rule, he will furnish such information whenever available.

2. If the substance to be tested is not intended for contact with the skin, it should be diluted at least 100 times in a proper vehicle and tested by the open method. The patient should be observed in the office for at least 1 hour, and if no reaction has occurred, the patch test site may be covered. If a positive reaction occurs with the 1:100 dilution, the substance should be similarly tested on 3 normal controls to ascertain whether it is a primary irritant in this concentration.

3. If no reaction occurs with the 1:100 dilution, prepare and test with progressively greater concentrations. A positive patch test reaction is significant only when the patient has an eczematous reaction but the controls do not.

4. If the suspected contactant is a solid and cannot be dissolved readily, a few granules or shavings may be placed on the skin and the patient observed in the office for 1 hour. If a reaction occurs within this time, the sub-

Plate 3. Patch Test Reactions

1. Strong Allergic

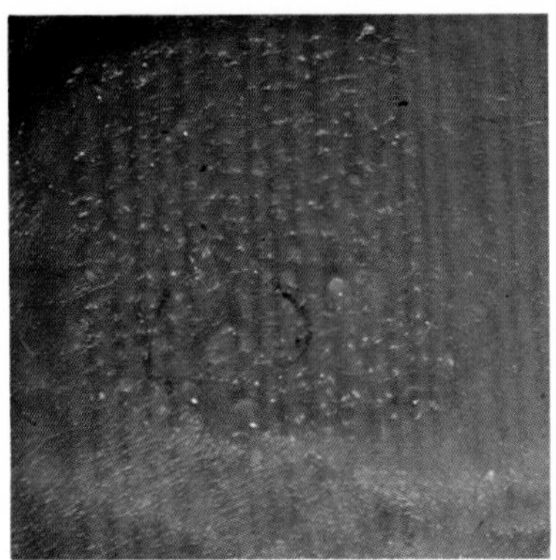

Edema and Vesiculation

2. Weak Allergic

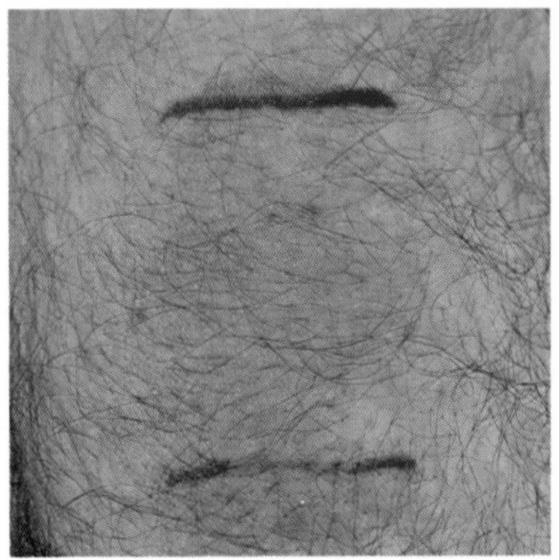

Erythema

3. Non-specific Pressure Bulla

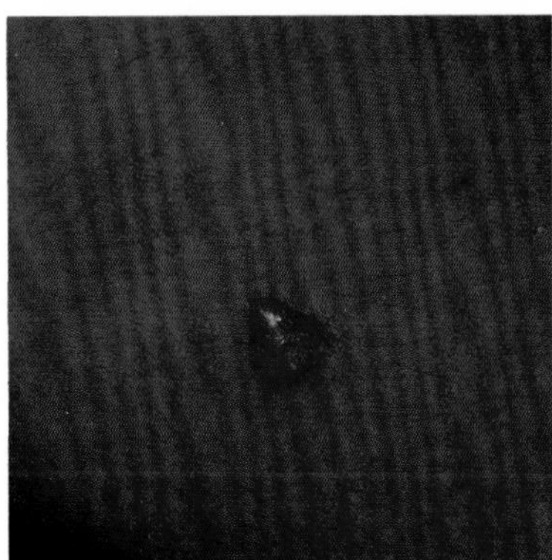

From Strapping Denture to Forearm

4. Non-specific Irritant Bulla

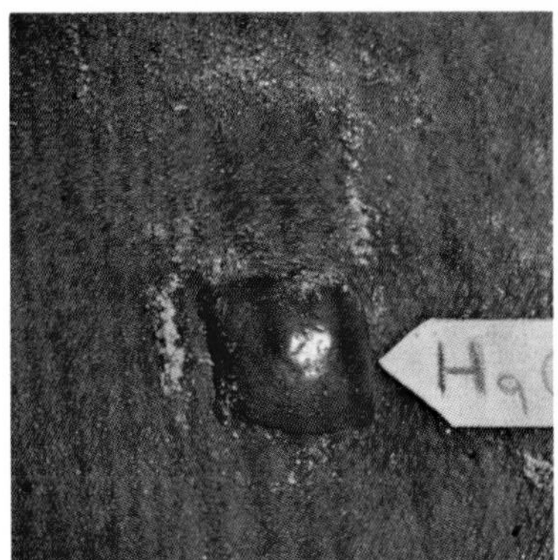

Non-irritant Concentration of Bichloride to Inflamed Skin

5. Non-allergic Pustular Reaction

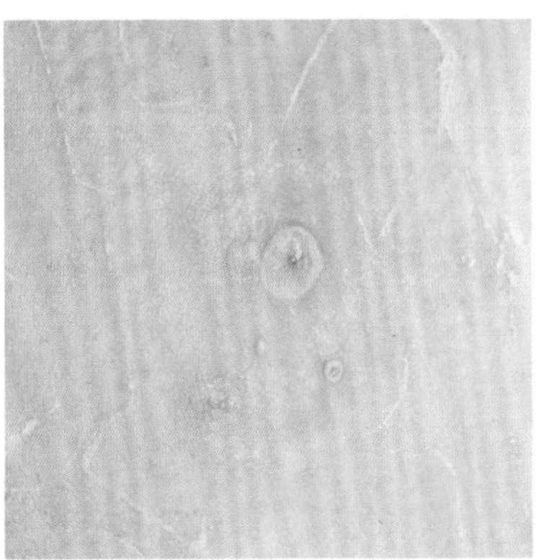

5% Nickel Sulfate Solution

6. Non-allergic Erosive Reaction

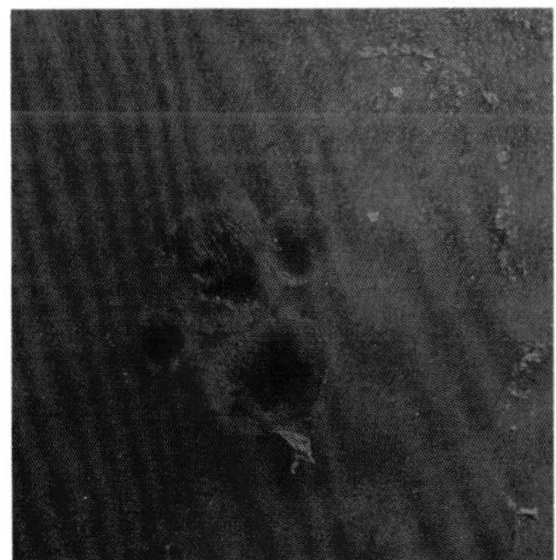

1% Ammonium Fluoride Solution

stance is a primary irritant and, although it may also be a sensitizer, further testing may not be done unless proper dilutions can be made. If no reaction occurs at the end of an hour, the test site may be covered; if a reaction occurs at the end of 48 hours, 3 controls must be similarly tested to rule out a primary irritant reaction.

5. If the test substance is intended to be used in contact with the skin, it may be tested as is by the closed patch test method provided it is not primarily intended for use on thick skin, such as the palms, soles or hairy scalp. Preparations such as corn cures, callus removers, wart medications and volatile hair tonics should be tested by the open method.

Testing with substances that are not listed in any standard table and that are not intended for contact with the skin is an investigative procedure and must be performed with great caution

PROPHETIC OR PREDICTIVE PATCH TESTS

These tests are designed to assess the sensitization potential of a new substance or to compare it with the known potential of similar substances. The techniques used should be exactly specified.

Brunner[21] points out that all test procedures in current use involve repeated application of the agent and evaluation of any inflammatory reaction. Preliminary screening of new agents may be carried out in experimental animals but, because of species differences in reactivity, human subjects must be used for final evaluation. Ordinary patch testing, however, is not adequate. Irritancy of the new product must be compared with that of a control preparation that has shown a satisfactory level of mildness in usage. To develop enough reactions so that the comparison is statistically meaningful, it is often necessary to intensify the reactivity by repetitive application, generally with occlusion. Similar considerations apply to sensitization tests. A preliminary screening test first may be run in animals.

Definitive tests for humans include the Schwartz-Peck, Brunner, Draize, Shelanski, Traub and Kligman procedures. Repetitive applications are required because maximal sensitization occurs only after a number of contacts. Occlusion of the test site, pretreatment of the skin with surface-active agents, damage to the skin with CO_2 snow, or repeated application of the product to the same site without rest periods may increase the number of sensitizations. These intensifying procedures become necessary only when simple repeated contact fails to provide a sufficient number of reactions with the control of statistical comparison with the new formulation.

Results of laboratory investigation of irritancy and sensitization must be supported by usage studies. A logical program includes, successively, preliminary animal screening tests, irritancy and sensitization tests in humans, use of the product by small panels of subjects under controlled conditions and, finally, limited trial sale of the product with follow-up. The trial period must be long enough for a sufficient number of contacts to cause possible sensitization reactions.

With composite preparations, it is necessary to determine the irritating and sensitizing potentials not only of each component but also of the whole product because they may not be the same.

Kligman[22–26] reviewed the methods of detecting allergies by predictive testing and found all except his own to be seriously wanting. The predictive patch test is merely a coarse screening procedure and indicates only in a limited manner the sensitizing potential of the tested material. Even one sensitization reaction in several thousand persons may be a serious hazard if millions of people will use the product on or near the skin. It is, therefore, of great importance to be certain that the predictive procedure is properly interpreted. Great confusion results if the tests are done haphazardly.

Predictive patch tests for sensitizing potential of new products are useful but not infallible and should be checked by adequate usage tests. Serious errors occur if the tests are not performed with the total formulation that will actually be used

Furthermore, a patch test procedure should be followed by an adequate usage test. The tested material should be put on trial in a small community for several months to ascertain whether actual usage with exposure to light, sweat, friction and pressure confirms the favorable results of the patch test procedure.

REPEATED INSULT (PROVOCATIVE) PATCH TESTS

The repeated insult patch test is a modification of the predictive patch test.[27–31] In this technique, the tested material is applied every other day or 3 times weekly for a total of 10 to 15 applications, and it is allowed to remain on the skin for 24 hours. Some investigators use the same site for each application; others prefer to use random sites.

Because of a greater number of applications, the repeated insult method is more capable of detecting sensitizing substances that have a lower threshold of sensitivity than those that can be detected by the original prophetic patch test technique. For this reason, fewer subjects (50 to 100) are usually employed in this method.

The repeated insult patch test has also been adapted to measure a type of primary irritant reaction called a fatigue or exhaustion reaction. In this technique, the reaction is elicited by consecutive applications of the test material at the same site rather than at random sites. Theoretically, the fatigue type of irritant reaction is not elicited if the testing material is not placed on the same site as previous tests. It is claimed that a reaction on a site adjacent to the original reaction would tend to show that it was an allergic rather than an irritant response.

Repeated insult patch tests may not be clinically significant because the threshold of skin irritability has marked individual differences

PATCH TEST TERMINOLOGY ADVOCATED BY THE INTERNATIONAL GROUP

This group suggests that the term *patch test* be written without a hyphen.[3] If qualification is needed, the word *standard* or *conventional* can be used without confusion, but the term *open* must be used when this exceptional method of testing is used.

Photo-patch and *phototest*, though coined adjectives, are the shortest terms in English to describe a patch test irradiated by natural or artificial light. The terms do not imply a particular method.

The terms *patch test reading* and *patch test results* are self-evident.

Patch refers to the single piece of material or unit on which the allergen is applied to the skin. It should be fully described; e.g., "Al-test IMECO, Stockholm, in strips of five patches was used."

The vehicle and concentration of allergen must be specified. Vaseline and yellow soft paraffin are best abbreviated as *pet.* (yellow petrolatum).

Test substance is the preferred term for the agent used in testing and does not prejudice the issue of sensitization.

COMPARISON OF PATCH TEST RESULTS IN VARIOUS COUNTRIES

Comparative patch test results indicate that nickel, paraphenylenediamine, formaldehyde, dichromates, benzocaine and rubber compounds are common sensitizers at home and abroad.[32] The incidence of significant patch test results for other sensitizers varies from country to country. The Contact Dermatitis Newsletter gives valuable information concerning patch test results in various countries and makes possible the following comparison of contact allergens at home and abroad.

Metals

Nickel is one of the most common contact allergens in most countries, except Poland.[33] The *dichromates*, present in high concentration in European cements, are more common sensitizers abroad than in the United States. In Israel, they are a common cause of housewives eczema. *Cobalt*, a common sensitizer in Europe, rarely gives positive patch test reactions in the United States. (See also chapter on Dermatitis and Discolorations from Metals.)

Plant Substances

Balsam of Peru, *colophony* (rosin) and *turpentine* are more common sensitizers in Scandinavian countries than elsewhere.[34] In the Orient, *Tiger Balm*, a popular proprietary medication containing balsams that cross-react with balsam of Peru, is a common allergen. *Primula*, a common sensitizer in England, may show cross-reactions with members of our daisy family (*compositae*). The *Rhus poison plants* in the United States cause many cases of dermatitis and cross-react with the mango and cashew of the Philippines and tropical America and with the ink of the marking nut tree of India (*Bella gutti*), which produces dhobi itch when used as a laundry mark. (See also chapter on Dermatitis Due to Plants and Spices.)

Lanolin

First emphasized as a common sensitizer in England and Scandinavia, lanolin is now included in the North American Contact Research Group's standard patch test series (see next chapter).

Topical Medications

Dr. E. Cronin (personal communication, 1971) points out that wherever *Mycolog cream* is used, its stabilizer, ethylenediamine, has become a common contact allergen. In England, it is called Triacortyl cream.

In France, Mycolog cream is not used but the ointment, which is free of ethylenediamine, is prescribed. *Phenergan cream* (not used in the United States) produces many instances of allergic reactions in France. It is significant that Phenergan (promethazine) cross-reacts with ethylenediamine. Patients sensitized to Phenergan cream in France, therefore, simultaneously become sensitized to the ethylenediamine in Mycolog cream.

Balsam of Peru, used for the treatment of burns in Scandinavia, is a common sensitizer abroad.

Sodium perborate is high on the list of sensitizers in Spain.

Benzocaine is a worldwide sensitizer and its use should be avoided. Dr. E. Hegyi (personal communication, 1969) states that its use is prohibited in Czechoslovakia.

Neomycin is also a common worldwide sensitizer, and in Finland it is the most common contact allergen. (For details and references see next chapter.)

REFERENCES

1. O'Quinn, S. E., and Isbell, K. H.: Influence of Oral Prednisone on Eczematous Patch Test Reactions. Arch. Derm., *99*, 380, 1969.
2. Fisher, A. A. et al.: Allergic Contact Dermatitis Due to Ingredients of Vehicles. Arch. Derm., *104*, 288, 1971.
3. Magnusson, B., and Hersle, K.: Patch Test Methods. Regional Variations of Patch Test Response. Acta Dermatovener., *45*, 260, 1965.
4. Magnusson, B., and Hersle, K.: Patch Test Methods. I. A Comparative Study of Six Different Types of Patch Tests. Acta Dermatovener., *45*, 123, 1965.
5. Magnusson, B., and Hersle, K.: Patch Test Methods. III. Influence of Adhesive Tape on Test Response. Acta Dermatovener., *46*, 275, 1966.
6. Hjorth, N., Trolle-Lassen, C., and Wilkinson, D. S.: Time-Saving Patch Test Antigen Dispenser. Arch. Derm., *102*, 300, 1970.
7. Epstein, E.: Simplified Patch Test Screening with Mixtures. Arch. Derm., *95*, 269, 1967.
8. Paschoud, J. M.: Routine Patch Tests, Composed Tests and Specialized Tests. Dermatologica, *136*, 193, 1968.
9. MacLeod, T. M., and Frain-Bell, W.: The Advantages of the Glycogelatin Patch Test Over Traditional Testing Methods. Brit. J. Derm., *81*, 536, 1969.
10. Anderson, W. A., Shatin, H., and Canizares, O.: Influence of Varying Physical Factors on Patch Tests Responses. J. Invest. Derm., *30*, 77, 1958.
11. Fisher, A. A.: Allergic Sensitization of the Skin and Oral Mucosa to Acrylic Denture Materials. J.A.M.A., *156*, 238, 1954.
12. Fernstrom, A. B.: A New Technique for Epicutaneous Testing with Vapor Emitted by Liquids or Solid Substances. Acta Dermatovener., *44*, 97, 1964.
13. Hjorth, N.: The Critical Strength of Patch Test Reagents. Brit. J. Derm., *80*, 22, 1968.
14. Fisher, A. A., et al.: Pustular Patch Test Reactions. Arch. Derm., *80*, 742, 1959.
15. Stone, O. J., and Johnson, D. A.: Pustular Patch Test Experimentally Induced. Arch. Derm., *95*, 618, 1967.
16. Eberhartinger, C., Ebner, H., and Klotz, L.: Knowledge and Interpretation of Follicular Papulo-Pustular Reactions in Patch Tests. Berufsdermatosen, *17*, 241, 1969.

17. Baer, R. L., and Yanowitz, M.: Differential Cell Counts in the Blister Fluid of Allergic Eczematous and Irritant Bullous Lesions. J. Allergy, *23*, 95, 1952.
18. Epstein, S.: Detection of Chromate Sensitivity: Intradermal Teating. Ann. Alergy, *24*, 68, 1966.
19. Marcussen, P. V.: Comparison of Intradermal Test and Patch Test Using Nickel Sulfate and Formaldehyde. J. Invest. Derm., *40*, 263, 1963.
20. Agrup, G.: Sensitization Induced by Patch Testing. Brit. J. Derm., *80*, 631, 1968.
21. Brunner, M. J.: Pitfalls and Problems in Predictive Patch Testing. J. Soc. Cosmetic Chem., *18*, 323, 1967.
22. Kligman, A. M.: The SLS Provocative Patch Test in Allergic Contact Sensitization. J. Invest. Derm., *46*, 573, 1966.
23. Kligman, A. M.: The Identification of Contact Allergens by Human Assay. I. A Critique of Standard Methods. J. Invest. Derm., *47*, 369, 1966.
24. Kligman, A. M.: The Identification of Contact Allergens by Human Assay. II. Factors Influencing the Induction and Measurement of Allergic Contact Dermatitis. J. Invest. Derm., *47*, 375, 1966.
25. Kligman, A. M.: The Identification of Contact Allergens by Human Assay. III. The Maximization Test. A Procedure for Screening and Rating Contact Sensitizers. J. Invest. Derm., *47*, 393, 1966.
26. Kligman, A. M., and Wooding, W. M.: A Method for the Measurement and Evaluation of Irritant on Human Skin. J. Invest. Derm., *49*, 78, 1967.
27. Klauder, J. V.: Patch Test Study to Determine Cutaneous Reaction to New Compounds. Arch. Environ. Health, *1*, 407, 1960.
28. Smeenk, G., and Polano, M. K.: Methods for Comparative Estimation of the Irritancy of Various Detergents on Human Skin. Trans. St. John Hosp. Derm. Soc., *51*, 220, 1965.
29. Maibach, H. I., and Epstein, W. L.: Predictive Patch Testing for Allergic Sensitization in Man. Toxic. Appl. Pharmacol., 7, 39, 1965.
30. Justice, J. D., Travers, J. J., and Winson, L. J.: The Correlation Between Animal Tests and Human Tests in Assessing Product Mildness. Proc. Sci. Sect. Toilet Goods Assoc., *35*, 12, 1961.
31. Finkelstein, P., Laden, K., and Miechowsky, W.: New Methods for Evaluating Cosmetic Irritancy. J. Invest. Derm., *40*, 11, 1963.
32. Fregert, S., et al.: Epidemiology of Contact Dermatitis. Trans. St. John Hosp. Derm. Soc., *55*, 17, 1969.
33. Rudzki, E., and Kleniewska, D.: The Epidemiology of Contact Dermatitis in Poland. Brit. J. Derm., *83*, 543, 1970.
34. Magnusson B., et al.: Routine Patch Testing. V. Acta Dermatovener., *49*, 556, 1969.

4

The Use of Patch Test Series

Allergens grouped together for patch testing are referred to as a test series or battery. The series may be *general*, i.e., a standard group, or *specific*, such as a therapeutic, metal or rubber series. Such groupings often overlap, because the standard series may contain metals, rubber chemicals and topical therapeutic agents that are common sensitizers.

STANDARD PATCH TEST SERIES

A group of chemicals that have proved to be frequent causes of allergic contact dermatitis may be included in a standard patch test series variously labeled as diagnostic, scout, basic, screening, etiologic, key routine or battery. Testing with a standard group of substances is of great value when allergic contact dermatitis is suspected and the offending agents cannot be pinpointed by a careful history or by trial and error.

Epstein et al.[1] emphasized that patch test screening only supplements, but never supplants, patch testing with suspected environmental agents. No screening series could ever encompass the many allergens encountered in cosmetics, industry and gardening, for example.

Screening with a standard patch test series often reveals a contactant that otherwise would remain undetected

Screening by a series of standard patch tests revealed that as many as half of all cases of contact dermatitis may be caused or complicated by an allergic contact sensitivity.[2] Hence, patch testing may be useful in any case of dermatitis. The examination is also useful as a guide to substances that should be avoided in order to reduce the risk of a relapse. Admittedly, there is risk of sensitization, but the patch test is so valuable in tracing the causes of contact dermatitis that the screening series is an indispensable diagnostic tool.

New sensitizing chemicals and products are continuously being introduced. Hence, the selection of substances for a standard test series cannot be rigidly defined. Constant revision and additions are needed to adapt the standard series to the sensitivities currently prevalent in the population served by a clinic. For this reason, ethylenediamine has recently been added to most standard screening series.

Agrup et al.,[3] testing with a routine series of 20 compounds in 140 patients with suspected allergic contact dermatitis, found 97 positive patch test reactions in 49 patients. The number of expected and unexpected test reactions was about the same. The allergens could be traced in one half of the unexpected reactions, demonstrating the diagnostic value of testing. These authors state that there is a risk of sensitization in the patch test procedure.

A positive patch test reaction to one or more substances included in the standard series gives the physician and patient a lead and may help to determine in retrospect how contact could have been made with the substance. It also enables the physician to investigate the possibility that the dermatitis was produced by a chemical that cross-reacts with the substance. For example, a positive patch test reaction to paraphenylenediamine not only may incriminate the dye, but also may alert the physician to the possibility that a group of immunochemically related substances, such as local anesthetics and other chemicals with an amino group in the para position, may have to be investigated.

When a clinically significant patch test reaction is obtained, the patient must be given the following written information about the substance to which he has shown a sensitivity:

1. Synonyms and various names and guises under which the substance could possibly masquerade.
2. Immunochemically related substances that might cross-react with the sensitizer.
3. Methods of avoiding clinical exposure to the contactant.
4. When available, the names of suitable nonsensitizing substitutes. Unless such information is obtained, the patient may be doomed to repeated attacks of allergic contact dermatitis.

Once the offending contactant is detected, the patient must be told under what guises it may masquerade and cross-react. Suitable substitutes should be given

TEST SUBSTANCES IN THE STANDARD SERIES

The list of substances in Table 4-1 is slightly modified from the one recommended by the North American Contact Dermatitis Group, and in my experience has yielded the greatest number of clinically significant patch test reactions. All test substances are dispersed in *petrolatum* unless otherwise designated.

The contactants in the standard screening tray yield many positive patch test reactions of clinical significance

Table 4-1. Standard Test Tray

1. Nickel sulfate 2.5% aqueous
2. Ethylenediamine 1%
3. Paraphenylenediamine 1%
4. Benzocaine 5%
5. Paraben mixture 15%
   (5% each of methyl, ethyl and propyl)
6. Thimerosal (Merthiolate) 0.1%
7. Ammoniated mercury 1%
8. Lanolin (natural)
9. Formaldehyde 2% aqueous
10. Mercaptobenzothiazole 2%
11. Tetramethylthiuram disulfide 2%
12. Potassium dichromate 0.025% aqueous
13. Turpentine 10% in olive oil
14. Neomycin sulfate 20%

NICKEL SULFATE

Nickel is ubiquitous, but its presence in stainless steel does not present a hazard to the nickel-sensitive individual. The dimethylglyoxime spot test is extremely useful in detecting it in objects believed to be nickel-free. The details and significance of a positive test to nickel are discussed in the chapter on metals.

Both at home and abroad, nickel is a common sensitizer

ETHYLENEDIAMINE HYDROCHLORIDE

This substance is a stabilizer because it is dibasic.

Ethylenediamine, a stabilizer in Mycolog cream, constituent of aminophylline and the parent substance of certain antihistamines, now rivals nickel as a sensitizer

In a study[4] of 100 patients suspected of having allergic eczematous contact dermatitis due to topically administered medications, it was the most potent sensitizer, accounting for 18 of 40 reactions. Twelve of the 18 patients had used Mycolog cream prior to testing and presumably were sensitized to ethylenediamine hydrochloride as a result.

Sensitization to ethylenediamine has also followed exposure to aminophylline, a combination of theophylline and ethylenediamine,[5,6] and topical use of ethylenediamine-related antihistaminics, namely, antazoline hydrochloride (Antasan) ophthalmic solution, promethazine (Phenergan) cream and tripelennamine (Pyribenzamine) cream.[7,8] Incidentally, tripelennamine cream is no longer available in the United States but is still used abroad.

Ethylenediamine tetraacetate (EDTA), a preservative frequently found in ophthalmic solutions, may be another source of exposure and sensitization.[9] Systemic administration of aminophylline, tripelennamine or promethazine to ethylenediamine-sensitive individuals may result in widespread eczematous eruptions.

Provost and Jillson[10] administered aminophylline to two ethylenediamine-sensitive individuals with resulting exacerbation of their generalized eczematous eruptions, which cleared following the use of hydrocortisone cream and avoidance of Mycolog cream.

Epstein and Maibach[11] reported 10 patients with ethylenediamine sensitivity and confirmed that patients allergic to ethylenediamine frequently have false negative patch test reactions to the ethylenediamine-containing medicament. Adequate patch testing requires a 1 per cent concentration of ethylenediamine, approximately five times that in the commercial product. Nearly all cases were discovered as a result of routine patch testing, reemphasizing the value of a screening patch test series in the diagnosis of occult eczematous disorders.

Patients with allergic dermatitis from ethylenediamine in Mycolog cream may give false negative patch test reactions to the cream on normal skin. Tests should be done with 1 per cent ethylenediamine in petrolatum

Ethylenediamine joins neomycin and the paraben preservatives as medicaments that may cause dermatitis and yet elicit false negative patch test responses when the commercially available topical preparation is used. This paradox is probably a consequence of differing skin barrier functions, because it is suspected that the skin barrier is severely impaired in inflamed skin. The presence of a topical corticosteroid also may produce a false reaction.

It is not certain whether the presence of ethylenediamine as a chelating agent in Tincture of Merthiolate (Lilly) presents any hazards to the ethylenediamine-sensitive individual.

Industrial Exposure. Ethylenediamine exposure also occurs in industry. This chemical is widely used in the preparation of dyes, inhibitors, rubber accelerators, fungicides, synthetic waxes, resins, insecticides and asphalt wetting agents. Because of its dibasic nature, ethylenediamine is valuable for neutralizing oils, preparing casein and shellac solutions, stabilizing rubber latex, inhibiting corrosion and controlling alkalinity.

Although ethylenediamine is a potent sensitizer, industrial exposure rarely leads to sensitization and dermatitis because exposure is not prolonged or intimate and normal skin usually is involved. In clinical practice, the ethylenediamine in Mycolog Cream is rubbed into damaged skin, which is more readily sensitized than the relatively normal skin of most industrial workers.

PARAPHENYLENEDIAMINE (PPDA)

In England and the Western Hemisphere, this stubstance is widely used as a hair dye, but in Scandinavian countries it is forbidden and *paratoluenediamine* substituted. A related dye, *para-aminodiphenylamine*, is sometimes used in Europe and the United States, but its use is forbidden in Denmark. Schonning[12] states that the sensitizing properties of para-aminodiphenylamine seem to be greater than those of paraphenylenediamine.

Blohm and Rajka[13] concluded from their experiment that benzoquinone and its derivatives play a decisive role in paraphenylenediamine-sensitization, and Mackie and Mackie[14] warn that antihistamines, which are potential quinone-imine formers, may show cross-reactions with it. In addition, paraphenylenediamine may show cross-reactions with azo and aniline dyes.

Paraphenylenediamine, widely used as a hair dye in the United States and England, is forbidden in continental Europe and in Scandinavian countries

Cross-Reacting Therapeutic Agents. These substances include the esters of para-aminobenzoic acid, local anesthetics such as benzocaine and procaine, the sulfonamides, carbutamide, para-aminosalicylic acid and HydroDIURIL. (For details of the significance of such cross-reactions, see the chapter on Systemic Eczematous "Contact-type" Dermatitis.)

In countries where the use of topical sulfonamides is outlawed and lidocaine (Xylocaine) or mepivacaine (Carbocaine) is substituted for procaine, the incidence of paraphenylenediamine-sensitivity appears to be less.

Industrial Exposure. Such exposure occurs in hair dressers, furriers, leather processors, rubber vulcanizers, printers, lithographers and x-ray technicians. (For details of patch testing and significance of paraphenylenediamine in hair dyeing, see chapter on Cutaneous Reactions to Cosmetics.)

BENZOCAINE

This topical anesthetic (Anesthesin, Anesthone, Parathesin, ethyl aminobenzoate) is still widely used even though it is a common and potent sensitizer, which can produce allergic dermatitis from infancy to old age. In my opinion, its use should be prohibited, as it is in Czechoslovakia (E. Hegyi, personal communication, 1969).

Any topical liquid, spray, cream or ointment that has the term *anesthetic* or *caine* on its label should be suspected of containing benzocaine.

Table 4–2 is a list of topical medicaments that contain benzocaine and must be avoided by people who are allergic to it and chemicals with which it cross-reacts.

Table 4-2. Topical Agents Containing Benzocaine*

Antitussives

Duad (Hoechst)
Romilar Chewable Cough Tablets for Children (Sauter)
Vick's Cough Silencers (Vick)
Vick's Formula 44 Cough Discs (Vick)

Liquid topical oral antibacterial preparations

Dalidyne (Dalin)

Solid topical oral antibacterial preparations (troches or lozenges)

Axon Throat Lozenges (McKesson)
Bio-Tytra (Approved Pharmaceutical)
Cēpacol Troches (Merrell)
Colrex Troches (Rowell)
Isodettes (International Playtex)
Iso-Thricin (Approved Pharmaceutical)
Junior Isodettes (International Playtex)
Medicated Isodettes (International Playtex)
Nymore (Durst)
Semets (SeMed)
Spec-T (Squibb)
Super Isodettes (International Playtex)
Tripac (Person and Covey)
Trokettes (Bryant-Vitarine)

Table 4-2. *(Continued)*

Astringents

Benadex (Fuller)
Dalidyne (Dalin)
Osmopak (Neisler)

External analgesics (liquid)

Ger-O-Foam Aerosol (Geriatric)

Burn remedies

Americaine (Arnar-Stone)
Burn-a-lay (Kendall)
Burntone (McKesson)
Foille (Carbisulphoil)
Kip First Aid Spray and Sunburn/Windburn Lotion (Kip)
Kip Sunburn Soap (Kip)
Kip Sunburn Spray (Kip)
McKesson Burn Lotion and Spray (McKesson)
Morusan (Semed)
Solarcaine (Plough)
Unburn (Leeming)
Unburn Spray (Leeming)
Unguentine Spray (Norwich)

Athlete's foot remedies

McKesson Spray for Athlete's Foot (McKesson)

Corn, callus and wart remedies

Blue Jay Corn Pad Treatment (Kendall)
Noxacorn (Fougera)

Hemorrhoidal products

Americaine Suppositories and Ointment (Arnar-Stone)
Anoroid Hemorrhoidal Suppositories (Bryant-Vitarine)
Benadex (Fuller)
Eucupin (Rare-Galen)
Eudacaine Compound Rectal Suppositories (Rexall)
Kip Hemorrhoid Relief Ointment (Kip)
Kip Hemorrhoid Relief Suppositories (Kip)
Lanacane Cream (Combe)
Mentholatum Suppositories (Mentholatum)
Pazo Ointment and Suppositories (Bristol-Myers)
Rectalgan Liquid (Ayerst)
Rectal Medicone Suppositories and Unguent (Medicone)
Rectodyne Rectal Suppositories (SeMed)
Wyanoid Ointment (Wyeth)

Poison ivy products

Calamatum (Blair)
Calamatum Spray (Blair)
Caligesic (Quinton)
Hista-Calma (Rexall)
Ivarest (Carbisulphoil)
Ivy Super Dry (Ivy)
Poison Ivy Cream (McKesson)
Poison Ivy Spray (McKesson)
Rhulicream (Lederle)
Rhulihist (Lederle)
Rhulispray (Lederle)

Table 4-2. *(Continued)*

[illegible]r sore, cold sore and denture irritation preparations

[illegible] (Vick)
Campho-Blis (Rabin-Winters)
CKA-Can Aid (Pannett Products)
Dalidyne (Dalin)
Dalidyne Jel (Dalin)
Jiffy (Hamilton Drug)
Mumzident (PurePac)
Ora-Jel (Commerce Drug)
Baby Ora-Jel (Commerce Drug)
Tanac (Commerce Drug)

Miscellaneous compounds containing benzocaine

A–C Troches (Abbott)
Auralgan Otic Solution (Ayerst)
Bradosol Lozenges (CIBA)
Dentalgia Drops (SeMed)
Derma Medicone Ointment (Medicone)
Dermoplast Aerosol (Ayerst)
Epinephricaine Ointment (Upjohn)
Synthaloids Lozenges (Tilden-Yates)
Teeds Lozenges (Warren-Teed)
Thriocaine Lozenges (Lemmon)
Tyoben Throat Lozenges (Elder)
Tanurol (Durst)
Topocide (Lilly)
Achromycin Powder for Ear Solution (Lederle)
Chloromycetin Otic Ointment (Parke, Davis)
Myringacaine Ear Drops (Upjohn)
Tympagesic Ear Drops (Warren-Teed)
Tigan Rectal Suppositories (Roche)
Banausea (Amfre-Grant)
Hurricaine (Beutlich)
Tyzomint (Blue Line)

* This table was prepared with the aid of Dr. J. Litt.

THE PARABENS

The name parabens is applied to the alkyl esters, butyl, ethyl, methyl and propyl, of p-hydroxybenzoic acid, which are widely used as preservatives in the pharmaceutical and cosmetic industries, as well as in foods. The parabens are the most commonly used preservatives in topical dermatologic medicaments, drugs, dentifrices and suppositories.

In our study[4] of paraben sensitivity, patients were tested with a mixture of paraben esters (equal parts of methyl, ethyl and propyl p-hydroxybenzoic acid). In view of the high incidence of cross-reactions among the esters and the frequent use of two or more esters in the same preparation, we felt that a mixture (paraben mix) is desirable for the detection of hypersensitivity to any or all of them.

The relatively high incidence of positive reactions in our series, 3 per cent compared to 0.8 and 1.15 per cent previously reported, may reflect the fewer number of individuals tested by us or indicate an increase in prevalence of hypersensitivity because of more opportunities for exposure. Contrary to the assumption of Hjorth and Trolle-Lassen,[15] our study and those of Schorr[16] indicate that repeated topical applications of relatively low concentrations of parabens in medicaments, cosmetics and dentifrices appear to be sufficient for sensitization. Once paraben sensitivity has been established, the patient may have great difficulty avoiding exposure to this ubiquitous preservative.

The Food and Drug Administration requires that the labels on food and topical prescription drugs indicate the presence of parabens. This does not apply, however, to numerous oral preparations, nonprescription drugs, cosmetics and dentifrices.

Allergic hypersensitivity to the parabens is reported in the United States with increasing frequency because of use in antimicrobial and corticosteroid lotions, creams and ointments, anesthetics, emollients, acne preparations, eye, ear and nose drops, vaginal jellies and suppositories, rectal suspensions and impregnated paste bandages for stasis ulcers.[17–19]

Epstein[20] noted that the parabens are used in a concentration of 0.01 to 0.1 per cent as preservatives in skin creams, hair lotions, suntan preparations, face powder, soaps, lipsticks and toothpastes as well as in syrups, milk preparations, soft drinks, candies, jellies and Sucaryl (an artificial sweetener). Sensitivity reactions to orally ingested parabens, however, have not been reported.

Schamberg[21] has listed American products and Evans[22] British products that contain the parabens.

At present, the following facts concerning topical medications should be taken into consideration when treating a paraben-sensitive individual:[23]

1. All corticosteroid *creams* except Hytone (Dermik), Valisone (Schering), Aristocort (Lederle) and Lidex (Syntex) contain parabens.

The following corticosteroid creams are paraben-free: Hytone, Aristocort, Valisone and Lidex

2. Most corticosteroid *ointments* are *paraben-free* except Cortril and Medrol.

3. Paraben-free antibacterial ointments include Ilotycin, Neosporin, Polysporin and Terra-Cortril.

4. Many cosmetics, hair lotions, suntan preparations, soaps and toothpastes contain parabens.

5. Certain adhesives, glues, and shoe dressings include the parabens.

It has not been established whether the following parenteral medicaments, which contain paraben, are safe for paraben-sensitive individuals: lidocaine hydrochloride, prednisone, Solu-Medrol and penicillin, Syrup of Aristocort, Achromycin Pediatric Drops, Maalox and Terfonyl Suspensions.

I am unaware of any instances of systemic contact-type dermatitis in paraben-sensitive individuals from the injection or ingestion of medications containing this preservative.

The possibility that para-aminobenzoic acid (PABA) may cross-react with the parabens, because of the similarity of structure, has been considered, but at present such reactions have not been proved.

THIMEROSAL (MERTHIOLATE)

Thimerosal, sodium ethylmercurithiosalicylate, is a preservative and antiseptic in topical and parenteral medications. Hypersensitivity reactions may be due to either the mercurial or the thiosalicylate portion of the compound.[24 25]

Thimerosal is present as a preservative in the diluting fluid used for preparation of antigens for scratch or intradermal testing and may give false positive reactions in mercury-sensitive individuals in the form of a delayed papule or occasionally a sterile abscess.

Epstein[26] reported that Merthiolate-sensitive individuals may give positive delayed tuberculin-type reactions to intradermal testing with diluting fluid in which it is a preservative. Reisman[27] showed the need for using control subjects whenever tests are performed with antigens that have been diluted with fluids containing preservatives. Hansson and Moeller[28] stated that Merthiolate should not be added to intracutaneous test solutions because it may interfere with the evaluation of positive reactions.

Tincture of Merthiolate (Lilly) contains ethylenediamine as a stabilizing agent and is colored with a combination of D and C Yellow No. 7 (fluorescein) and D and C Red No. 22 (eosin YS).

Hansson and Moeller[29] reported a high

incidence of positive patch test reactions to Merthiolate in a group of young adult males without previous or current skin disease. In persons tested with a battery, positive reactions occurred, mainly in the younger age groups, while a much older group did not react even to a strong Merthiolate patch test. Although the clinical and histologic features of the reaction are mainly of an allergic type, there is evidence that it should be considered a false positive reaction peculiar to that substance and to young skin.

In our material we have not noted such false positive reactions,[4] or observed cross-reactions between thimerosal and phenylmercuric acetate. The explanation may be either that closely related chemical compounds need not be cross-sensitizing, as with dichlorophene and hexachlorophene, or that our Merthiolate-sensitive patients were allergic to the thiosalicylate and not to the mercury in the compound.

Tincture of Merthiolate (Lilly) contains a mercury component, a thiosalicylate, ethylenediamine, fluorescein and eosin dyes

AMMONIATED MERCURY

Exposure to this compound is principally through its use in psoriasis remedies (Table 4–3) and depigmenting or bleaching agents (Table 4–4).

Inorganic ammoniated mercury may or may not cross-react with organic mercurials, such as Merthiolate or Mercurochrome.

Dr. C. F. H. Vickers (personal communication, 1970) studied a patient who had a widespread allergic eruption because of application of ammoniated mercury ointment to a small area of her body. She had positive patch test reactions to ammoniated mercury and mercury bichloride. Each time she had a tooth filled, she acquired a widespread eczematous eruption. Contact with mercury from a broken thermometer also produced an allergic eczematous flare.

Table 4-3. Psoriasis Remedies Containing Ammoniated Mercury

Unguentum Bossi (Doak)
Sorsis Cream (Ar-Ex)
Riasol (Shield)
Psoriasis Treatment Lotion (Rexall)

Table 4-4. Depigmenting Agents Containing Ammoniated Mercury

Esoterica
Stillman's Freckle Cream
Nadinola Bleach Cream
Peacock's Imperial Cream
Golden Peacock Bleach Cream
Mercolized Cream
Blue Ointment

Iodine and sulfur form a strong primary irritant when coupled with ammoniated mercury.

Topical agents that contain mercurials, but not necessarily ammoniated mercury, are Lanacane, Mycolog cream, Preparation H, Unguentine, Mazon and Bag Balm.

LANOLIN

Lanolin (wool fat, wool grease, wool wax, wool alcohol and adeps lanae anhydrous) and its various esters, fatty acids and aliphatic alcohols are used in many topical medicaments and cosmetics.

Lanolin is a natural product obtained from the fleece of sheep, and its constituents vary from time to time and place to place. It is among the more important causes of cutaneous sensitization, but the exact allergenic fraction awaits clarification. It is still unknown whether or not lanolin-sensitive patients can tolerate modified or purified lanolin and its derivatives.

Lanolin is a natural product that is an important sensitizer. The exact sensitizing component has not been isolated. Lanolin-sensitive patients can sometimes tolerate one lanolin preparation but not another

Composition. *Lanolin* contains sterols, fatty alcohols and fatty acids. The lanolin sterols (lanolin alcohols or wool alcohols) include principally cholesterol, lanosterol and agnesterol, and are built from one or more benzene rings.

Commercially these wool alcohols are called Cerolan, Type HO, Hartolan, Golden Dawn and Nimco. Cholesterol is the major ingredient of lanolin alcohol, and commercial lanolin products list the cholesterol content. Further studies are required to establish whether these lanolin alcohols are the sole or main sensitizers in lanolin.[30]

The fatty alcohols are long chained, and include the closely related stearyl and cetyl alcohols. The fatty acids, the other ingredients of lanolin, have not been found to be sensitizers.

Modifications. *Acetylated lanolin* (Modulan), according to Cronin,[30] is less of a sensitizer than plain lanolin. *Dewaxed lanolin* (*Lantrol*), formed by a solvent crystallization process, is also claimed to cause less sensitization than lanolin.

Another modification is *hydrogenated lanolin.* Vollum[31] has reported that it is being used more frequently in the pharmaceutical and cosmetic industry because it is colorless, odorless, free from tackiness and more hydrophilic than lanolin.

Hydrogenation is carried out by heating lanolin with a catalyst to 330° C at a pressure of 180 atmospheres. The absorption of hydrogen is complete within half an hour and the hydrogenated lanolin contains dihydrocholesterol, other hydrogenated steroids and some saturated alcohol. It was originally hoped that hydrogenated lanolin, or a modification, could be used in cases of lanolin sensitivity, but some patients show a marked sensitivity to hydrogenated lanolin and not to the plain lanolin. Dermatitis due to hydrogenated lanolin may be missed if patients are patch tested with wool alcohols or plain lanolin and not the hydrogenated variety.

Patch Tests for Lanolin Sensitivity. Many investigators routinely test with 30 per cent wool alcohol in petrolatum, but because it may not be the sensitizing substance in lanolin, patch testing should be performed with lanolin. Thune's investigation[32] indicates that the addition of salicylic acid to *lanolin* or Eucerin may cause false positive reactions. Patch tests for wool fat sensitivity should be performed with lanolin without the addition of salicylic acid.

Newcomb[33] emphasizes that lanolin is a complex natural material, which is never completely identified because of the wide variations in purity. The development of new derivatives and further purification may contribute to lowering the incidence of skin reactions to this emollient.[34]

Patch test results with lanolin alcohols should be verified by testing natural lanolin from several sources

FORMALDEHYDE AND FORMALIN

Formalin, a 37 per cent aqueous solution of formaldehyde gas, causes puzzling patch test reactions and clinical evaluation is often difficult. Many individuals have 1+ and 2+ reactions to formaldehyde that are apparently of no clinical significance. Even strongly positive patch test reactions often cannot be correlated with a clinical dermatitis. Marcussen states that "75 per cent of positive formaldehyde tests cannot be explained and that only 20 per cent of such positive reactions can be related with actual instances of formaldehyde dermatitis."[35]

Epstein and Maibach[36] suggest that tests with 4 to 5 per cent formalin give many false positive reactions. Their recommendation that patch tests be done with 2 per cent formalin has been widely adopted.

Allergic contact dermatitis from formalin may occur in sensitized individuals from the following exposures:

1. *Wash and wear apparel* (wrinkle or crease resistant fabrics) treated with formaldehyde resins and in which free formaldehyde remains. When clothing dermatitis is suspected in a formaldehyde-sensitive patient, a positive patch test reaction to a piece of the fabric soaked in artificial sweat confirms the diagnosis.

Table 4–5 indicates fabrics that are free of formaldehyde and formaldehyde resins and that may be worn by formaldehyde-sensitive individuals.

Table 4-5. Formaldehyde-Free Fabrics*

Acetate
Triacetate
Nylon
Polyester
(Dacron, Fortrel, Avlin, Trevera, Quintesse)
Acrylic (Orlon, Creslan, Zephran)

About 80 per cent of all fabrics containing *cotton* or *rayon* have been treated with formaldehyde, a cross-linking reactant that stabilizes the fabric and thereby makes it resist shrinkage and wrinkling. (For details of testing and management of wearing apparel dermatitis due to formaldehyde, see the chapter on clothing.)

2. *Paper.* Formaldehyde and its reactive derivatives are used in the paper industry to improve the wet-strength, water-resistance, shrink-resistance, grease-resistance and other characteristics of paper and paper products. In addition, formaldehyde serves as a disinfectant and preservative in paper manufacture and in the preparation of finishes, sizing agents and parchment paper.

Formaldehyde sensitivity is not necessarily associated with formaldehyde-resin allergy

3. *Cosmetics.* Many shampoos contain formaldehyde as a preservative. At present, the following shampoos are free of preservatives: Neutrogena, Therel (Spence-McCord), Polytar (Stiefel) and Ionil (Owen). Subrosa Cream *Deodorant*, Marvel Finger *Nail Hardener*,[37] Thermodent *Toothpaste* and various permanent wave lotions also contain formaldehyde.

4. *Medical exposure.* Wart remedies, fungicides, insecticides, tissue fixatives, embalming fluid and sterilizing fluid are possible sources of contact.

5. *Industrial exposure.* In industry, there are widespread opportunities for exposure to formaldehyde, such as in the manufacture of synthetic resins, leather, rubber, metals and woods. Exposure may also occur in photography, agriculture, oil-refining, dye synthesis, disinfection and fumigation.

Gaul[38] has shown that there is an absence of formaldehyde sensitivity in individuals sensitized to phenol-formaldehyde.

MERCAPTOBENZOTHIAZOLE AND TETRAMETHYLTHIURAM DISULFIDE

The rubber accelerators mercaptobenzothiazole (MBT) and tetramethylthiuram disulfide (TMTD) account for many instances of allergic rubber dermatitis. Wilson,[39] in a study of 106 rubber-sensitive patients, attributed sensitivity to these substances in all but 2 cases.

Tetramethylthiuram disulfide (TMTD) and mercaptobenzothiazole, both rubber accelerators, are the most common causes of rubber dermatitis

In the rubber industry, TMTD has many commercial designations, such as Vulcacurae TMD, Thiurad Thiuram M, Tuex, Methyl Thiuram, TMT (Henley) Cyruam DS, Aceto TMTD, Pernasaw, Puralin and Pomarsol. In insecticides it has the following commercial designations: Arsan, Naquets, Panoram and Tersan.

In the form of Antabuse tablets, TMTD may produce erythema, urticaria and itching upon the ingestion of alcohol or paraldehyde. Patients with hand eczema from rubber glove allergy due to TMTD may notice a flare after drinking alcohol.

In tablet form (Antabuse), TMTD sensitizes patients to alcohol and paraldehyde. Patients whose dermatitis flares after drinking alcohol should be patch tested with TMTD

POTASSIUM DICHROMATE

The significance of patch test reactions to chromium compounds is discussed in the chapter on metals.

Pirila et al.[40] found that a considerable proportion of dichromate in a patch test of cellulose or linen material is reduced to trivalent chromium during the first few hours, and they investigated the suitability of non-reducing glass fiber paper for patch testing. Mali et al.[41] claimed that chromate ions penetrate a covered patch test as quickly as water does and are quickly absorbed into the body. Pedersen et al.[42] found, however, that chromium may persist for a month or more at patch test sites. They noted that less chromium reached the dermis in allergic subjects than in the controls possibly because more of the epithelium and, therefore, chromium is shed because of the inflammatory reaction. On the other hand, the same quantity of chromium was found at the test site of controls and allergic subjects one month after *intracutaneous* testing.

Dr. J. Fregert (personal communication, 1970) found that chromium-sensitive individuals who have been tested intracutaneously with chromium compounds sometimes show repeated flare-up reactions on the test sites, particularly when trivalent chromium compounds are injected.

Patch Reactions Reported from Abroad. In two large series of routine patch tests reported from Scandinavia by Fregert et al.[43] and Magnusson et al.[44] chromates were the commonest sensitizers in men. The incidence was approximately 12 per cent of all the males tested in the Scandinavian group and nearly 11 per cent of those in the study involving many European countries. The level of sensitivity varied from city to city and reflected the presence of dichromates in the environment. Of all the patients tested in Bari, in southern Italy, 21 per cent reacted positively to chromate, while in both London and Wycombe the incidence was 6 per cent, and it dropped to 3 per cent in Copenhagen. The incidence in Bari was high because many patients were from building and construction trades. Marcussen[45] showed that in Copenhagen during the war years the level of chromate sensitivity decreased because of cessation of chromium imports and increased again in the postwar period when imports were resumed.

In men, chromate is the most frequent industrial sensitizer. The commonest source of exposure is cement, which is used principally in building, construction and plastering, but chromates are also handled in the engineering and printing trades. Its presence in industry is widespread and may not be easy to trace.

Patch test reactions to dichromates are not nearly as frequent in the United States as abroad.

Positive patch reactions to dichromates may be related to clinical dermatitis with difficulty because of subtle, widspread exposure to this metal salt

TURPENTINE

Oil of turpentine is a variable mixture of numerous terpenoid compounds and is derived from various sources, such as balsam of pine trees and is a byproduct in the manufacture of sulfate cellulose. The main components are alpha-pinene, beta-pinene, delta-3-carene and dipentene (limonene). These are monoterpenes with a common chemical formula of $C_{10}H_{16}$.

According to Pirila et al.,[46] practically all oils of turpentine contain large amounts of 2-pinene. On the other hand, the 3-carene content varies in different types, being high (30–40 per cent) in most sulfate oils and low or negligible in many balsam oils, e.g., French oil of turpentine. The eczematogenic effect of 3-carene depends on its hydroperoxide content.

Hjorth and Wilkinson[47] confirmed that with turpentine the patch test reactions provoked by the same dilution are related to the source, the method of manufacture (sulfate process or gum distillation), the amount of delta-3-carene present and the concentration of peroxides formed during storage. These factors vary as do the relative quantities of alpha-pinene and beta-pinene present. Because some patients may be sensitized by alpha-pinene and others by delta-3-carene, turpentine for testing should contain both of these ingredients and a suitable concentration of their peroxides.

The sensitizers in turpentine vary with the sources and both delta-3-carene and alpha-pinene, with their peroxides, should be included in patch testing

Pirila uses a mixture of 3-carene, 2-pinene and limonenes containing 1 per cent peroxides in olive oil for testing turpentine sensitivity.[46]

Turpentine is both a primary irritant and a sensitizer. As an irritant, it usually acts by defatting the skin and causing dryness and fissuring. It is universally used as a cleanser for removing paints and waxes and is one of the most common causes of hand eczema.

Turpentine is an oleoresin obtained from various species of pine. The oleoresin contains a volatile oil (oil of turpentine), which is responsible for its properties and is the form generally used. The irritating and sensitizing property of turpentine varies greatly with the country of origin.

Opportunity for contact with turpentine is widespread, both in industry and elsewhere. It may be applied externally in the form of liniments, ointments and "rubbing" compounds, and in some countries it is prescribed internally as an anthelmintic and laxative. Other compounds containing turpentine include varnishes, lacquers, floor waxes, cleansers, shoe and floor polishes, paint thinners, printer's ink, dry cleaning preparations and various adhesives, including adhesive tape. The skin of citrus fruits contains oleoresins related to turpentine. Topical agents containing turpentine include Mentholatum, Penetro Analgesic Rub, Cloverine Salve, Minard Liniment, Sloan's Liniment, Johnson's Anodyne and Vicks Vaporub.

Old, oxidized turpentine is more irritating and sensitizing than is the freshly made product. When turpentine is allowed to stand, especially with exposure to light, oxidation results in the formation of formic acid and aldehydes, which may be irritating to the skin. Pinenes and limonene, which are also formed in the oxidation process, may cause allergic sensitization and cross-react with the oils in orange peels and other essential oils.

The terpenes in turpentine have also been incriminated as active sensitization agents. Similar terpenes are present in citrus fruits and celery, and the possibility of cross-reaction must be kept in mind. Cross-sensitivity reactions may also occur between turpentine and ragweed oleoresin, chrysanthemum, pyrethrum and various balsams, such as those of pine, spruce and Peru.

The residue remaining after distillation of crude oil of turpentine is rosin, or colophony, which consists mainly of abietic acid and 1-pinearic acid. Rosin obtained from turpentine is present in many adhesives and may cause dermatitis in sensitized individuals. (See chapter on plants for further discussion of turpentine.)

Old, oxidized turpentine is more irritating and sensitizing than the fresh variety

NEOMYCIN SULFATE

Neomycin compounds have become the most widely used topical antibiotics in the United States. Several controversial aspects of the drug are the proper concentration for patch testing, the role of intradermal testing, the incidence of neomycin sensitivity, and cross-reactions with other antibiotics.

Concentration Used for Patch Tests. The North American Contact Dermatitis Group has adopted neomycin sulfate 20 per cent in petrolatum as the standard concentration for testing. Some authorities use 30 to 50 per cent for testing, but such high concentrations may result in primary irritant reactions and sensitize patients to the patch testing procedure.

Intradermal Testing. In this test, 0.05 ml. of a 1 per cent sterile neomycin solution is injected, using the diluent and preservative as a control. A positive reaction is a delayed, tuberculin-type papule, which appears in 24 to 48 hours and persists for 1 or more weeks.

Raab[48] stated that neomycin solutions in concentration exceeding 0.1 per cent are not suitable for intradermal tests, because a nonspecific toxic reaction may occur that mimics a positive delayed type of intradermal reaction.

Patch tests are performed with 20 per cent neomycin in petrolatum

Relationship Between Patch and Intradermal Tests. Epstein[49] stated that neomycin sulfate sensitivity can be detected in more than 90 per cent of all cases with a 48-hour occlusive patch test using a 20 per cent neomycin sulfate concentration, and that an occasional patient has a negative patch test reaction with the 20 per cent concentration but a positive reaction to intradermal testing. Hjorth also stated that the false negative reactions with low concentrations can be largely obviated by increasing the concentration of neomycin sulfate to 20 per cent. Epstein found that intradermal tests with a 1:1000 dilution of neomycin sulfate are usually positive and that those with a 1:100 dilution are apparently always positive in his sensitive patients.

The lack of perfect correlation between patch and intradermal testing may be due to false negative patch test reactions even at the 20 per cent concentration or to different criteria of what constituted a positive patch test reaction.

Neomycin and the Atopic State. Epstein stated that "contact dermatitis from neomycin appears to occur predominantly in atopic persons."[49] Patrick et al.[50] concurred with this view. Wereide,[51] however, concluded that the atopic state does *not* predispose to neomycin sensitivity, but that patients with stasis dermatitis have a higher incidence of neomycin sensitivity than do patients with other types of eczematous dermatitis.

Neosamine sugars are probably the common sensitizers in neomycin, paromomycin and ambutyrosin

Cross-sensitivity with Other Antibiotics. Pirila et al.[52] previously reported simultaneous hypersensitivities to bacitracin, framycetin, kanamycin and paromomycin, the latter three being considered true cross-sensitivities. More recently they found that 40 of 100 patients who were sensitive to neomycin were also sensitive to gentamicin (Garamycin [Schering]).

Schorr (personal communication, 1971) found strong cross-sensitization between neomycin, paromomycin, and ambutyrosin because of the presence of neosamine sugars in all three.

Role of the Vehicle in Neomycin Sensitivity. Hjorth and Thomsen[53] found that neomycin *ointments* are the major cause of sensitization to this antibiotic and recommended that neomycin not be prescribed in this form. The risk of inducing sensitization with neomycin in creams, lotions or powders appears to be significantly less. Occasionally the preservatives in topical neomycin medication may also be sensitizers.

The presence of a corticosteroid in a neomycin preparation may mask neomycin-induced dermatitis.

Neomycin is a common sensitizer, particularly in eczematous and stasis dermatoses and in ointment preparations

Panzer et al.[54] found no sensitization in experimental subjects whose bodies were completely covered with neomycin sulfate ointment for six hours, and there was no percutaneous absorption through intact normal skin.

A VEHICLE PATCH TEST SERIES

From the standpoint of allergenicity of topical preparations, attention has been directed almost exclusively to the sensitizing potential of active agents, without consideration for the possible role of the vehicle. This may have been justified when bases and vehicles consisted primarily of petrolatum or lanolin pastes (zinc oxide, starch and petrolatum), "shake" lotions (zinc oxide, talc, glycerin and water) and tinctures (alcoholic solutions). Many of the current vehicles, particularly washable creams and lotions, are complex formulations, frequently composed of 10 or more chemicals, including solubilizers, antioxidants, emulsifiers, excipients, preservatives, stabilizers and surfactants. There is growing awareness that some of these may induce cutaneous sensitization and clinical episodes of allergic contact dermatitis, but in general, their role is not fully appreciated.

Four substances that were included in a recent study of the incidence of sensitization to vehicles (ethylenediamine, paraben mix, lanolin and Merthiolate) have been recognized as such common sensitizers that they are now included in the standard test series by the North American Research Contact Group.

Ethylenediamine, lanolin, the parabens and Merthiolate, present in many vehicles, are common enough sensitizers to be included in the standard series

In a recent study,[55] 100 patients who had eczematous eruptions following topical application of preparations for other conditions were patch tested with the vehicle tray shown in Table 4–6. These materials are known to be currently present in the vehicles of many topical preparations, including cosmetics. The patients were tested with these substances after it had been determined that they had not become sensitized to the active agents in the preparations they had used. Standardized concentrations and vehicles were employed for testing with already known sensitizers. In some instances, such as for propylene glycol, we determined an appropriate nonirritant concentration after preliminary testing of controls.

As a result of this study and further testing of preservatives, stabilizers and emulsifying agents of vehicles in modern topical medicaments, I now employ the modified vehicle test tray shown in Table 4–1.

Hexachlorophene, sorbic acid and chlorocresol are very rare sensitizers

Table 4-6. The Vehicle Tray: Concentrations and Results of Patch Tests in 100 Cases of Allergic Eczematous Contact Dermatitis

Vehicle Ingredient	*Concentration*	*Number of Positive Reactions*
Ethylenediamine hydrochloride	1% in petrolatum	18
Lanolin	As is	6
Paraben mix	5% in petrolatum	3
Dichlorophene (G-4)	1% in petrolatum	2
Phenylmercuric acetate	0.1% in petrolatum	2
Thimerosal	As is	2
Propylene glycol	10% aqueous	2
*Polyethylene glycol monostearate	As is	2
*Triethanolamine	5% in petrolatum	2
Sorbic acid	5% in petrolatum	1
Hexachlorophene (G-11)	1% in petrolatum	0
Sodium lauryl sulfate	1% aqueous	0
Polysorbate (Tween 20)	5% aqueous	0
Cetyl alcohol	30% in petrolatum	0
Chlorobutanol	As is	0
total		40

* Further study has convinced me that the reactions to polyethylene glycol monostearate and triethanolamine were not clinically significant because the reactions could not be repeated with fresh material.

Table 4-7. A Modified Vehicle Patch Test Tray

Ethylenediamine	1% in petrolatum
Ethylenediamine tetraacetate	1% in petrolatum
Paraben mix	5% in petrolatum
Lanolin	As is
Merthiolate	0.1% in petrolatum
Dichlorophene	1% in petrolatum
Hexachlorophene	1% in petrolatum
Phenylmercuric acetate	0.1% in petrolatum
Propylene glycol	10% aqueous
Sorbic Acid	5% in petrolatum
Chlorocresol	2% in petrolatum
Benzalkonium chloride	1:1000 aqueous solution

THE NECESSITY FOR TESTING WITH THE INDIVIDUAL INGREDIENTS OF A VEHICLE

A topical medication may sometimes give a false negative patch test reaction in a sensitized individual even though it contains chemicals that are sensitizers and have produced a severe allergic contact dermatitis in the patient. Such false reactions may be due to the following:

1. A patch test is performed on normal skin. The dermatitis-producing vehicle is used on inflamed, eczematous or ulcerated skin.

2. The vehicle may contain a corticosteroid, which can suppress a mild allergic reaction on a patch test site but not on abnormal skin.

3. The concentration of the vehicle ingredient that is producing the allergic reaction is too low to produce a positive patch test reaction. For example, the parabens are used in a concentration of less than 0.5 per cent as preservatives in vehicles, but a concentration of at least 3 per cent is necessary to produce a positive patch test reaction on normal skin in the sensitized individual.

In our study there were 6 patients whose clinical picture indicated that nystatin-neomycin - gramicidin - triamcinolone cream exacerbated the dermatosis for which it was prescribed. Patch tests with the cream (Mycolog) were negative, but strongly positive patch test reactions were obtained to ethylenediamine, a stabilizer in the cream.

4. Positive reaction to a patch test with a topically applied agent may be the product of multiple sensitivities. Unless the components of a formulation are tested separately, the dermatitis-inducing ingredients would not be detected.

The concentration of an ingredient may be sufficient to result in contact dermatitis when used repeatedly for treatment, but too low to elicit a positive reaction under ordinary conditions of testing, particularly if a corticosteroid is present in the medication

The significance of positive reactions to ethylenediamine, the parabens, lanolin and Merthiolate were discussed as part of the standard series.

ETHYLENEDIAMINE TETRAACETATE

Raymond and Cross[56] have shown cross-reactions between ethylenediamine tetraacetate (EDTA) and ethylenediamine. It is a widely used preservative present in diverse products such as ear and nose drops, Monocaine and other injectable solutions, salad oils, wines and most ophthalmic solutions.

EDTA, a widely used preservative, particularly in ophthalmic solutions, may cross-react with ethylenediamine, the number one sensitizer of the standard and vehicle trays

Marketed as the calcium disodium salt of ethylenediamine tetraacetic acid and as Edathamil calcium, Versene, Sequestrene and Nullapon, EDTA is well known as a chelating agent with a strong affinity for metals such as calcium, lead and magnesium. It is classed as a sequestering agent and can bind metallic ions.

It prevents discoloration due to traces of metals in antibiotics, antihistaminics and local anesthetics. It prevents oxidation by trace metals in cosmetic creams and lotions. It is used as a stabilizer in solutions of ascorbic acid, hydrogen peroxide, formaldehyde, folic acid and hyaluronidase. It is also used systemically for the treatment of urinary calculi, calciferous corneal deposits, hypercalcemia and lead poisoning. In ophthalmic solutions it enhances the antibacterial activity of benzalkonium chloride, chlorobutanol and thimerosal by disrupting the lipid-protein complexes of cell walls.

DICHLOROPHENE (G-4, CUNIPHEN)

Dichlorophene is a fungicide and bactericide used in dentifrices, shampoos, antiperspirant and deodorant creams, powders, toilet waters and preparations for dermatophytosis of the foot. Compound G-4, dihydroxydichlordiphenylmethane, is extensively employed as a mildewcide to treat and preserve cotton fibers, various fabrics, paper, synthetic leather lattices and some adhesive tape backings.

Allergic stomatitis and cheilitis due to G-4 in dentifrices have been reported,[57,58] and it is now rarely used in such products. Gaul and Underwood[59] reported allergic dermatitis from G-4 used as a fungicide. This compound is still present in numerous over-the-counter preparations for athlete's foot, including Foot Rest (Quality Chemists), Fungi Aerosol (Rexall), K-7 Foot Spray (Gard), Green Frost Foot Lotion (Excello), Hex-Phen (Russell), Antiseptic Food Powder (Raleigh) and Foot Note Astringent (Raleigh).

Schorr[60] reported instances of allergic contact dermatitis from the presence of G-4 in Duke Gelocast Bandage for treatment of stasis ulcers. (Note: The Primer Medicated Bandage [Glenwood] contains glycerin, acacia, zinc oxide, white petrolatum and amylum in a vegetable oil base and is free of preservatives.) Schorr also found instances of allergic dermatitis from the presence of G-4 in Jergens Lotion. (Jergens Extra Dry Skin Formula Lotion contains hexachlorophene instead of dichlorophene.)

Epstein[61] found cross-reactions between dichlorophene and hexachlorophene (G-11). In our material and in that of Schorr, no cross-reactions occurred between these closely related phenolic compounds.

Dichlorophene is a more potent sensitizer than hexachlorophene. Though closely related chemically, they rarely cross-react. The Food and Drug Administration has greatly restricted the use of hexachlorophene for its possible toxic, but not allergic, effect

HEXACHLOROPHENE (G-11, At-7, K-34)

This phenolic compound, closely related to dichlorophene, was formerly used in cosmetics, soaps and pharmaceutical vehicles as an antiseptic. At present, hexachlorophene is present in pHisohex, Surgi-Cen, Gamophen and Surofene. Fact and Ipana toothpastes and Pepsodent mouthwash contained hexachlorophene.

The results of testing with our vehicle tray[55] show that hexachlorophene is a rare sensitizer. Irritant reactions of the scrotum from the British preparation Ster-zac[62] and of the face from pHisohex,[63] both of which contain a soluble form of hexachlorophene, have been reported, but in none was hexachlorophene implicated as a sensitizer.

The Food and Drug Administration's recent restriction of the use of hexachlorophene is related to toxic brain damage and not to marked skin toxicity or sensitivity.

PROPYLENE GLYCOL

Because of its superior solubilizing and humectant properties, propylene glycol has largely replaced glycerin in pharmaceutical preparations and cosmetics. We question whether or not the positive reactions obtained with propylene glycol 10 per cent in 2 of 100 cases in our series are indicative of allergic sensitization. Warshaw and Herrmann[64] studied cutaneous reactivity to diluted and undiluted propylene glycol and found it difficult to decide whether they were dealing with primary irritation or allergic sensitization with concentrations as low as 2.5 per cent.

From our experience with graded dilutions in control subjects, we are of the opinion that an eczematous response to propylene glycol 10 per cent may be interpreted as evidence of allergic sensitization. In support of our view, Braun[65] judged approximately 3 of 78 patients (or 4 per cent) to be sensitive to propylene glycol on the basis of positive reactions to this dilution. Cross-reactions between propylene glycol and polyethylene glycol were not observed in this group.

The *United States Pharmacopeia* has no pH 4 specifications for propylene glycol. Manufacturers of the pharmaceutical grade have acknowledged that this variance from pH 4 to pH 8 is uncontrolled and unavoidable. Accordingly, neither physicians nor pharmacists have any influence over the acidity or alkalinity of the propylene glycol utilized in prescriptions.

Recently the Food and Drug Administration approved the use of topical preparations containing 5-fluorouracil in propylene glycol with sodium hydroxide added to a pH of 9. These preparations, which are advocated particularly for the treatment of actinic keratoses, produce a marked inflammatory reaction. There is a possibility that propylene glycol sensitization may be induced under such circumstances.

Hydrophilic ointment U.S.P. contains propylene glycol, whereas Hydrophilic ointment modified contained glycerin in the place of propylene glycol. The term *ointment* as applied to this product is a misnomer because the preparation is essentially a cream base.

Patch test reactions to propylene glycol are difficult to interpret since the pH varies from 4 to 8

POLYETHYLENE GLYCOL MONOSTEARATE

The monostearate is a nonionic surfactant readily soluble or dispersible in water and is present in Synalar Cream (Syntex) and Fungizone Cream (Squibb).

The polyethylene glycols are condensation or polymerization products of ethylene glycol of relatively high molecular weights. The heavier and more solid of these have been called carbowaxes and are found in many cosmetics and topical medications.

Plastibase is a solution of polyethylene in mineral oil. Plastibase hydrophilic also contains glyceryl mono-oleate, an antioxidant, and preservatives. The following Squibb products are formulated in Plastibases:

Florinef-S Ophthalmic	Mycolog Ointment
Fungizone Ointment	Myconef Ointment
Kenalog Ointment	Mycostatin Ointment
Kenalog in Orabase	Orabase Emollient
Kenalog-S Ointment	Spectrocin Ointment
Kenalog-S Ophthalmic	Spectrocin Ophthalmic

Furacin Ointment (Eaton), Aristocort Ointment (Lederle) and Quinolor Ointment (Squibb) contain the polyethylene glycols. Whitfield's ointment (U.S.P. XVI) utilized polyethylene ointment as its base.

The largest number of cases of allergic hypersensitivity to the polyethylene glycols has been reported by Braun[65] who states that, "Routine tests in 92 dermatological patients with contact allergies gave approximately 4% positive reactions with polyethylene glycol." He found no cross-reaction between the polyethylene glycols and the propylene glycols. Strauss[66] also reported allergic sensitization to the polyethylene glycols in the form of carbowax.

Whether or not the monostearate derivative of polyethylene glycol cross-reacts with polyethylene glycols, particularly those of low molecular weight (300 to 400), needs to be ascertained.

PHENYLMERCURIC ACETATE

This mercury salt is used as a preservative in cosmetics and many topical medicaments, except in Germany where its use is prohibited. Phenylmercuric acetate, nitrate and borate are present as spermicidal agents in many contraceptive preparations (see chapter on metals).

Although Hjorth and Trolle-Lassen[67] indicate that patch tests with a 0.1 per cent concentration of phenylmercuric acetate may give false positive irritant reactions, such reactions did not occur in our series. In sensitized individuals, however, patch test reactions may be obtained in concentrations from 0.01 to 0.16 per cent in petrolatum.

Not infrequently there are cross-reactions between organic mercury compounds, such as phenylmercuric acetate, and the inorganic salts, such as ammoniated mercury and bichloride of mercury. Moreover, an allergic eczematous dermatitis due to external sensitization by a mercurial compound may undergo exacerbation or be reproduced by *systemic* administration of medication containing mercury, such as Mercuhydrin, in sensitized individuals.

In order to avoid irritant reactions, phenylmercuric salts should be tested 0.05 per cent in petrolatum, not in aqueous solutions

TRIETHANOLAMINE

Triethanolamine, a mixture of three alkanolamines, is frequently employed as an excipient in hand and body lotions, shaving creams, soaps, shampoos, bath powders and occasionally in pharmaceutical preparations. An excipient is presumably an "inert" substance that gives a topical agent proper consistency through its action as a dispersant or detergent.

Castelain[68] has reported allergic contact dermatitis due to sensitization to triethanolamine. Suurmond[69] showed cross-reaction between triethanolamine and other tertiary amines, such as Phenergan and promethazine. Schwartz cautioned:

> To place on the skin a patch of triethanolamine and a patch of stearic acid as the ingredients of a vanishing cream would give misleading results, because the triethanolamine would irritate the skin whereas in a vanishing cream these chemicals are combined in the form of an innocuous substance, triethanolamine stearate. On the other hand, in some instances the combined irritant action of chemicals in a cosmetic may be greater than the irritant action of the individual substances.[70]

SORBIC ACID

Sorbic acid is known chemically as 2,4-hexadienoic acid. It is a naturally occurring plant substance obtained from the berries of the mountain ash, *Sorbus aucuparia L.*, *Rosaceae* in which it is present as the lactone (parasorbic acid). It is present in cranberries, strawberries and currants and is used as a preservative in many foods. Hytone Cream (Dermik) and Aristocort Cream (Lederle) contain sorbic acid as a preservative.

Sorbic acid is a white, practically odorless, crystalline powder with a faintly acid taste. Potassium sorbate (popularly used salt form) is also a white, almost odorless powder.

Sorbic acid 0.2 per cent is considered the antimicrobial agent of choice for topically applied vehicles and cosmetics containing fatty acids and polyoxyethylene esters. The sensitizing index of this preservative appears to be low—estimated at 0.3 per cent by Hjorth and Trolle-Lassen[67] and 0.6 per cent by Klaschka and Biersdorff.[71] Sorbic acid appears to compare favorably with the parabens and the organic mercurials from the standpoint of allergenicity.

In one patient that I observed who had a 4+ patch test reaction to sorbic acid there was no flare-up after ingestion of berries.

Hytone Cream (Dermik) and Aristocort Cream (Lederle) contain sorbic acid as a preservative and are paraben-free

Dr. J. R. Simpson (personal communication, 1971) described a patient who acquired a disseminated eruption from the use of a paste bandage that contained sorbic acid as a preservative. A positive patch test reaction was obtained to sorbic acid 5 per cent in petrolatum.

CHLOROCRESOL

Chlorocresol (p-chloro-m-cresol) and chloroxylenol (p-chlor-m-xylenol) are chlorinated phenols that are used as preservatives. In 1969, betamethasone 17-valerate (Valisone) with 4-chloro-m-cresol as a preservative became available.

Hjorth and Trolle-Lassen[67] demonstrated cross-sensitization between chlorocresol and chloroxylenol in three patients. Hjorth stated, "We have had no trouble from the 4-chloro-m-cresol. We tested the compound (2% in petrolatum) in 1962 on 612 consecutive patients. Three patients had positive reactions. This indicates that trouble may occur." No instances of allergic reactions to this preservative, however, have been observed in our series.

Dr. R. G. Park (personal communication, 1970) reported that in New Zealand, a country where chlorocresol is widely used in topical medicaments, after 84 negative routine tests he obtained a strongly positive patch test reaction to this preservative. He also noted that Fregert reported sensitization to chlorocresol in a pesticide.

BENZALKONIUM CHLORIDE

Benzalkonium chloride (BAK), alkylbenzyldimethyl ammonium chloride, is a quaternary ammonium cationic detergent. It is widely used as a preoperative skin disinfectant, for disinfection of surgical instruments and in the treatment of burns, ulcers, wounds and infected dermatoses. It is also present in many cosmetics, deodorants, mouthwashes, dentifrices, lozenges and ophthalmic preparations. It is used industrially in the fabrication of textiles and dyes, and in metallurgy and agriculture.

Benzalkonium chloride has produced allergic contact dermatitis in medical personnel from exposure to instruments soaked in it[72,73] and from its use in the treatment of ulcers, burns and cutaneous infections.[74–77] Recently a bizarre ichthyosis type of dermatitis was reported in Japan[78] to be caused by an ointment containing alkyl benzyl trimethyl ammonium chloride, which differs from BAK only by an additional methyl group. Pandos et al.[79] reported an instance of combined cutaneous and mucous membrane allergic contact reaction from BAK that complicated a tracheostomy procedure.

Benzalkonium chloride (Zephiran), a widely used antiseptic and preservative, is a rare sensitizer

Theodore and Schlossman[80] stated that BAK in ophthalmic preparations may produce allergic reactions, but they did not cite specific cases with confirming patch test proof. Fisher and Stillman[81] reported that one of the authors (M.A.S.) developed a conjunctivitis from acquired hypersensitivity to BAK in an ophthalmic medicament, which was then made worse when an unsuspecting ophthalmologist prescribed another preparation containing BAK.

Dabiez et al.[82] pointed out that the primary preservative of most contact lens soaking solutions is BAK, and in a personal communication Dabiez suggested the ophthalmic preparations shown in Table 4–8 for BAK-sensitive individuals.

An indication for testing with individual ingredients of an ophthalmic preparation containing BAK is inclusion of disodium edetate (EDTA) to enhance the antibacterial effect of the BAK. Not only can EDTA in ophthalmic solutions cause allergic contact sensitivity,[9] but it also may cross-react with ethylenediamine.

Huriez et al.[83,84] reported that allergic contact sensitivity to topically applied quaternary ammonium compounds is common in France, and that generalized reactions may result from systemic administration of chemically related drugs. Such medications include the cholinergic medicaments, hypotensive drugs (e.g., tetraethylammonium chloride), neuromuscular blocking agents (e.g., decamethonium bromide) or heparin antagonists (hexadimethrine bromide).

Table 4-8. Ophthalmic Preparations Free of Benzalkonium Chloride

Soaclens (Burton, Parsons)
Vasocon (Smith, Miller and Patch)

Many topical ophthalmic preparations contain benzalkonium chloride, making it difficult for the sensitized individual to avoid using preparations free of this antiseptic

The following antiseptic solutions contain BAK:

Benkosal (Flar)
Bensept (Blue Line)
Benzalkonium Chloride Solution (Professional Products)
Benz-All (Xttrium Laboratories)
Germicidal (Progress)
Germicin (Consolidated Midland)
Graham Germicidal Concentrate (Graham Chemical)
Hya-Cide Concentrated Germicidal Solution (E. R. Powells)
Hyamine 3500 (Rohm & Haas)
Lorvic Germicidal Concentrate (Lorvic)
Mann Germicidal Solution (Mann Chemical)
Pheneen (Ulmer)
Roccal (Winthrop)
Zalkonium Chloride (Vitarine)
Zephiran Chloride Solution (Winthrop)
Zonium Chloride (Lannett)

(See chapter on mucous membranes for a list of ophthalmic products containing benzalkonium chloride.)

CETYL AND STEARYL ALCOHOL

Cetyl and stearyl alcohol are the prinicpal aliphatic alcohols used as solvents in liquid and semisolid emulsions. Hjorth and Trolle-Lassen[67] tested 1664 consecutive patients with equivalent concentrations of cetyl and stearyl alcohol and found 2 positive reactions to the cetyl and 4 to the stearyl type.

Cetyl alcohol, also known as hexadecyl or palmityl alcohol, is a long chain, solid, fatty alcohol. It is a white crystalline substance used as an emollient, emulsifier and coupling agent in pharmaceutical vehicles of the oil-in-water type, and is present in lanolin. It imparts a velvety feel to the skin. It is also used in the manufacture of sulfate alcohol for textile soap.

Gaul[85] reported an urticarial type of contact dermatitis presumably from the presence of cetyl and stearyl alcohols in clothing materials and canvas. Sulzberger et al.[86] reported two lanolin-sensitive patients who reacted to cetyl alcohol, but in our series there were no reactions to it.

Stearyl alcohol appears as unctuous white flakes used in cosmetic creams, emulsions, textile oil and finishes and as an antifoam agent and lubricant.

Ceramol (Dehydgag Wax SX), a blend of cetyl and stearyl alcohols with sodium lauryl sulfate, is used as an emulsifying agent.

Cera Lanetta (Lanette Wax SX) is chiefly cetyl alcohol plus higher fatty alcohol. Cera Emulsivicans B. P. closely resembles Cera Lanetta.

TWEEN

Tween 20 (sorbitan mono-laurate polyoxyethylene derivative) and Tween 80 (sorbitan mono-oleate polyoxyethylene derivative) are surfactants and act as nonionic synthetic detergents. Tween 20 is slightly less hydrophilic than Tween 80 and usually is the preferred emulsifying agent of the two. Although it is classified as a histamine-releasing agent, in the 50 per cent aqueous solution used in our test series, no immediate erythema and no allergic patch test reactions were recorded.

ISOPROPYL MYRISTATE

Isopropyl myristate is a synthetic fatty alcohol widely used in pharmacy and cosmetology and is regarded as innocuous. Professor C. D. Calnan (personal communication, 1970) observed several cases of allergic contact dermatitis due to this alcohol in an antibiotic-steroid spray.

SODIUM LAURYL SULFATE

Sodium lauryl sulfate (Duponol C, Drene, Dreft, Teel and Gardinol) is an emulsifying agent in many pharmaceutical vehicles, cosmetics and foaming dentifrices. Even a concentration of 1 per cent is a mild primary irritant and may, like most soap solutions, produce erythema under a closed patch test. We regard the numerous positive reactions in our study to be nonallergic irritant reactions.

Sams and Smith[87] cited an instance in which sodium lauryl sulfate may possibly have produced an allergic contact dermatitis, but the general consensus is that it is not a sensitizer, but simply drying and irritating to the skin.[88,89]

Sodium lauryl sulfate does not appear to be a sensitizer, producing mild irritant reactions under a closed patch

CHLOROBUTANOL

This chloral derivate with a pungent odor is used as a preservative in topical pharmaceutical vehicles and for parenteral solutions and has a local anesthetic action. Cross-reaction may occur with chloral hydrate. No positive patch test reaction occurred with this preservative in our series.

TINCTURE OF BENZOIN

The tincture is used as an antioxidant to prevent rancidity in cosmetic creams and pharmaceutical vehicles and as a fixative agent in perfumes.

Benzoin is present in tincture of benzoin in a combination of 10 per cent alcohol. Compound benzoin tincture contains benzoin with styrax, balsam of Tolu, aloe and ethyl alcohol. Arning's tincture contains tincture of benzoin, ammonium tumenol, anthrarobin and ether. Benzonated lard, water-repellent barrier creams, lozenges and some cosmetics also contain benzoin.

Benzoin may cross-react with balsam of Peru, benzyl cinnamate, benzyl alcohol, eugenol, vanilla and alpha-pinene. For patch test purposes a 10 per cent solution in alcohol may be painted on the skin and left uncovered. Benzoin is a very rare sensitizer.

PATCH TESTS WITH CORTICOSTEROIDS

In the past few years several investigators have reported allergic sensitivity to topical hydrocortisone,[90–96] hydrocortisone acetate,[97] hydrocortisone alcohol,[98] methylprednisolone,[99] and triamcinolone.[100,101] Alani and Alani[102] reported 21 patients with allergic patch test reactions to hydrocortisone, 3 to triamcinolone, 2 to betamethasone and 10 to pure hydrocortisone. They recommended a 25 per cent concentration of hydrocortisone in petrolatum for patch testing.

Often proprietary preparations of just triamcinolone or betamethasone induce positive patch test reactions in sensitized individuals.

Allergic contact sensitivity to topical corticosteroids is being reported with increasing frequency

Alani and Alani[102] reported a 0.3 per cent incidence of corticosteroid sensitivity. In the future, the incidence will probably increase because of the tendency to use higher concentrations of steroids in stubborn dermatoses. Such potent corticosteroids applied to stasis ulcers appear to be particularly sensitizing.

Topical corticosteroids are popular in the treatment of dermatitis, because usually there is prompt symptomatic relief and improvement. Persistence or exacerbation of the eczematous dermatitis, however, should cause one to suspect the presence of secondary contactants. Sensitization by a component of the treatment vehicle, such as parabens, lanolin, an antibacterial (neomycin) or other additives, such as humectants and surfactants, should be strongly considered, and if these can be excluded, diagnostic testing may then reveal the parent steroid to be the offending agent. This is especially likely when the dermatitis fails to recede in spite of intensive therapy with topical corticosteroids. In cases of contact sensitivity to one of the constituents of corticosteroid cream, the steroid may modify the patch test reactions or may cause negative results.

Because of the anti-inflammatory activity of corticosteroids, the clinical manifestations of infections or fungal invasion may be masked, and when contact sensitivity to steroids coexists, the usual local response to inflammation and sensitivity may be modified.

Topical corticosteroids may produce a superimposed allergic reaction or an irritant rosacea type of dermatitis

Ingredients of topical vehicles may be sensitizers, which in turn enhance sensitization by corticosteroids that may be present.

Comaish[90] obtained a negative *patch* test reaction using 5 per cent hydrocortisone, but *intradermal* testing with hydrocortisone, prednisone and prednisolone acetate gave positive results.

IRRITANT REACTIONS FROM TOPICAL CORTICOSTEROIDS

Perioral or a rosacea type of dermatitis may be produced by the topical use of *strong* corticosteroids, such as betamethasone valerate and fluocinolone acetonide.[103] Hydrocortisone does not seem to produce this reaction. Systemic treatment with tetracycline and topical application of a simple lotion or hydrocortisone (Hytone) is often effective.

PATCH TESTS WITH OTHER THERAPEUTIC AGENTS

Penicillin. Hjorth[104] described 6 patients who were sensitive to penethamate; 3 had positive patch test reactions only to benzyl penicillin, indicating that patch testing should be performed with penethamate. Sensitivity to penethamate may be the reason some patients with a history of reaction after treatment with penicillin have tolerated later treatment.

Ampicillin sensitivity is an occupational hazard among nurses. A 5 per cent aqueous solution may be used for patch tests.

Gentamicin (Garamycin). Pirila et al.[105] patch tested 100 neomycin-sensitive patients with gentamicin and kanamycin. Forty gave positive reactions to gentamicin despite lack of previous exposure to it. Of these, all but 2 also reacted to kanamycin. These investigators used 30 to 50 per cent neomycin sulfate, 30 to 50 per cent bacitracin, 30 per cent gentamicin, and 30 to 50 per cent kanamycin in petrolatum for their studies. Such concentrations may produce irritant reactions.

Lynfield[106] described a patient who was so sensitive to gentamicin that he gave a positive patch test reaction to a 0.1 per cent concentration. Other cases of gentamicin allergy may be missed, however, because a higher concentration is required for a positive reaction on patch testing. This resembles the many false negative results obtained by testing with neomycin-containing topical preparations, which led to the recommendation of 20 per cent neomycin as the optimal concentration for patch tests.

Bacitracin. Topical application of an ointment containing bacitracin has been reported as producing anaphylactic shock.[107]

Nystatin (Mycostatin, Nilstat, Nysta-Dome). Wasilewski[108] studied a patient who was allergic to nystatin following exposure to two different combination-ingredient topical medications containing this antibiotic. On patch testing, the patient reacted to Mycolog Cream, Nystaform-HC Ointment and ethylenediamine. Although Mycolog Cream contains ethylenediamine, Nystaform-HC Ointment does not. Nystatin is the only ingredient common to both preparations, and a subsequent patch test with nystatin (Mycostatin sterile powder for laboratory use) was strongly positive. (The manufacturer states that this is nystatin powder, free of additives.) The patch test material was prepared in a concentration of 100,000 units/ml (1 mg = approximately 3000 units), and 70 per cent ethanol was used as the vehicle. None of 10 volunteers patch tested with this material showed any reaction.

Aureomycin. Professor C. D. Calnan (personal communication, 1969) reported a contact dermatitis due to Aureomycin Ointment (Lederle). A patch test was positive to this antibiotic but negative to parabens and wool alcohols. This patient was also positive to chlortetracycline and dimethylchlortetracycline, but negative to oxytetracycline, tetracycline and cymecycline.

Benzoyl Peroxide. Contact sensitization has been observed occasionally among acne patients treated with topical preparations of benzoyl peroxide.[109] Poole et al.[110] found benzoyl peroxide to be a potent sensitizer in repeated insult patch tests. Similar results were obtained in tests with guinea pigs. (Note: Acneiform skin in no way resembles the skin that was insulted in these experiments.)

Tolnaftate. Drs. G. H. Gellin and H. Maibach (personal communication, 1970) reported contact allergy to tolnaftate (Tinactin [Schering]). This preparation contains a 1 per cent solution of tolnaftate in a vehicle of polyethylene glycol 400 and a preservative, butylated hydroxytoluene. Tolnaftate is n-N-dimethylthiocarbanilic acid, 0-2-naphthyl ester.

Ichthyol (ichthammol, ammonium ichthosulphonate). Professor C. D. Calnan (personal communication, 1970) had one case and Bandmann (personal communication, 1971) had two cases of allergic contact dermatitis due to Ichthyol.

This product is obtained by the sulfation and ammoniation of a distillate from mineral deposits (bituminous schists) originally found near Seefeld (Tyrol). It contains about 10 per cent sulfur, saturated and unsaturated hydrocarbons, nitrogenous bases, acids and thiophene derivatives. Its composition, however, is variable (Martindale).

Tar. Both wood and coal tars can produce allergic reactions. Some tar fractions are photosensitizers. The emulsifying agent *Quillaja bark* in a solution of coal tar (liquor carbonis detergents) was a sensitizer in one case I studied.

Probably no active topically applied medicament is entirely free of sensitizing potential

Erythromycin. Allergic reactions to this antibiotic appear to be extremely rare, and I have not personally encountered any.

BURN REMEDIES

Such remedies often contain *Benzocaine* or *Furacin*, both of which are potent sensitizers.[111]

Mafenide Acetate. Topical application of mafenide acetate (Sulfamylon Cream) has reduced the mortality rate due to burn wound sepsis. Recent studies have shown that it is probably more effective than silver nitrate solution in suppressing the growth of *Pseudomonas aeruginosa.* Allergic reaction to this burn remedy, however, has been reported.[112] Velasco and Afrikus[113] described cutaneous reactions to mafenide acetate in three adults. All had a strongly positive patch test reaction to the 8.5 per cent mafenide acetate and 5 per cent mafenide hydrochloride solution but not to sulfonamides. They believe the critical antigenic site of the mafenide molecule is the methyl group in the para position.

Thermal Contact Burns. Berens[114] pointed out that accident victims sustain cutaneous burns upon contact with highway pavement in the summer. Such persons should, therefore, either be moved or provided with insulation, such as a blanket, paper or car seat.

THERAPEUTIC DYES

Triphenylmethane (TPM) Dyes. In all instances of sensitization to these dyes, therapy was employed for eczema or ulcer of the leg. In these conditions, allergic sensitization occurs so frequently with apparently innocuous medications that not only dye therapy but also medicaments containing neomycins, the parabens, ethylenediamine and lanolin are contraindicated.

In instances in which the erythematous patch test reaction is obscured by the color of the tested dye and papules or vesicles are not evident, an intradermal test with 0.05 ml. of a 1:500 dilution of the dyes may be performed. A delayed tuberculin-type reaction indicates sensitivity.

Triphenylmethane dyes have produced anaphylactic reactions when used during lymphography.

Bielicky and Novak[115] observed 11 patients with eczema mainly on the legs and due to allergic sensitization to brilliant green. A simultaneous sensitivity to gentian violet and crystal violet was found in 8 and to malachite green in 6 patients. Patch tests with various triphenylmethane dyes have shown the possibility of cross-sensitization between crystal violet (contained in gentian violet), brilliant green and malachite green. The probable determinant groups of sensitization are $N(CH_3)_2$ or $-N(C_2H_5)_2$ in the para position of the benzene ring structure. Cross-reactions are limited only to substances with

Table 4-9. Patch Test Concentration for Dyes

Triphenylmethane (1% in petrolatum)
Pararosaniline (saturated solution)
Rosaniline or basic fuchsin (2% in water)
Crystal violet (2% in water)
Malachite green (2% in water)
Brilliant green (2% in water)
Gentian violet (2% in water)

amino groups substituted with at least two alkyl groups. The test reactions to pararosaniline were all negative.

The concentrations of dyes for patch testing are given in Table 4–9.

Bjornberg and Mobacken[116] described 3 patients in whom a necrotic, painful and slowly healing skin reaction developed after topical treatment with 1 per cent gentian violet in aqueous solution. The reaction could be reproduced in stripped but not in nonstripped skin in normal humans and in guinea pigs with both gentian violet and brilliant green. These adverse reactions to triphenylmethane dyes may be erroneously diagnosed as exacerbations of the underlying skin disease for which treatment was given. Treatment with 1 per cent aqueous solutions of these dyes is not as harmless as supposed.

Epstein[117] studied a patient who was treated for a resistant stasis dermatitis of the lower part of her right leg. After a period of time, gentian violet seemed to irritate the skin. Patch tests with this drug were negative, but an intradermal test with 0.5 ml. of a 1:5000 dilution produced a positive delayed tuberculin type of reaction.

Glutaraldehyde. This is a tanning agent with strong bactericidal and fungicidal properties. Topical application of a 10 per cent solution has been used with good effect against hyperhidrosis of the feet. In one study, no cross-reaction was found between glutaraldehyde and formaldehyde.[118]

Gordon and Maibach[119] pointed out that glutaraldehyde is a sensitizer. Several instances of allergic contact dermatitis from this agent in nurses have been described.[120] Jordan et al.[121] have shown that allergic contact dermatitis can result from occasional or incidental contact with glutaraldehyde used for sterilization of medical and dental equipment, as well as from topical application of the compound in dermatologic treatment. Glutaraldehyde can be patch tested as a 1 per cent solution in water. Some sensitized patients had positive reactions to a 0.25 per cent aqueous solution. A slight wrinkling and yellow discoloration of the skin were seen in some nonallergic persons patch tested with a 1 per cent aqueous solution, but these do not interfere with proper interpretation of the reaction.

Fluorouracil. Sams[122] obtained allergic reactions to 5-fluorouracil or the vehicle. Acquired sensitivity occurred in a little more than 1 per cent of all patients treated. Sunlight increased discomfort at the reactive stage but did not appear to increase sensitization.

Precautions are necessary in testing 5-fluorouracil. The marketed ampule is highly alkaline because an unknown quantity of sodium hydroxide is used in solubilizing and buffering the compound. In addition, 5-flu-

Table 4-10. The North American Contact Dermatitis Research Group Standard Series as of July 1, 1972

Medicaments and preservatives
Neomycin
Caine (mixture)
Ammoniated mercury
Thimerosal (Merthiolate)
Ethylenediamine
Parabens (mixture)
Lanolin
Metals
Potassium dichromate
Nickel sulfate
Rubber chemicals
Mercaptobenzothiazole (mixture)
Thiuram (mixture)
Naphthyl (mixture)
p-Phenylenediamine (mixture)
Carba (mixture)
Others
Turpentine
Formaldehyde
Paraphenylenediamine
Epoxy resin
Balsam of Peru

Table 4-11. The International Contact Dermatitis Research Group Patch Test Allergens

Materials available from Trolab Karen Trolle-Lassen, M. Pharm., 1 Hoyrups Alle-2900 Hellrup, Denmark	
Primula	
Special patch tests containing 1 mcg. primin each (on Al-test)*	
European Standard	
Potassium dichromate	0.5%
Cobalt chloride	1%
Nickel sulfate	2.5%
Formaldehyde (in water)	2%
Paraphenylenediamine (PPDA)	2%
Balsam of Peru	25%
Turpentine peroxides (in olive oil)	0.3%
Neomycin sulfate	20%
Benzocaine	5%
Parabens (methyl, ethyl, propyl, butyl and benzyl) 3% each	15%
Chinoform	5%
Colophony	20%
Coal tar	5%
Wood tars (pine, beech, juniper, birch) 3% each	12%
Wood alcohols	30%
Epoxy resin	1%
Mercapto mix	1%
Thiuram mix	1%
Paraphenylenediamine mix	0.60%
Naphthyl mix	1%
Antimicrobial agents	
Bithionol (photo allergen)	1%
Hexachlorophene (photo allergen)	1%
Tetrachlorosalicylanilide (photo allergen)	0.1%
Tribromsalicylanilide (photo allergen)	1%
Chlorquinaldol	5%
Baking	
Cinnamon oil	0.5%
Benzoyl peroxide	1%
Hairdressing	
p-Aminodiphenylamine	0.25%
o-Nitro-p-phenylenediamine	2%
Resorcinol	2%
p-Toluenediamine sulfate	1%
Local Anesthetics	
Procaine chloride	1%
Cinchocaine chloride (dibucaine, Percaine)	1%
Amethocaine chloride (tetracaine, Pantocaine)	1%
Cyclomethycaine chloride (Surfacaine)	1%
Caine mix	8%

* Al-test is a neutral patch test unit used by the International Contact Dermatitis Research Group. Available from IMECO Astra Agency Co. AB, Box 42 070, S-126 12, Stockholm 42, Sweden.

Table 4-11. *(Continued)*

Organic dyes	
Benzidine (out of stock)	
p-Aminoazobenzene	0.25%
Disperse orange 3 (C.I. 11005, nylon dye)	1%
Disperse yellow 3 (C.I. 11855, nylon dye)	1%
Organic mercury chemicals	
Thimerosal (thiomersalate, Merthiolate)	0.1%
Phenylmercuric nitrate	0.05%
Ammoniated mercury	1%
Mercury	0.5%
Pesticides	
Zineb ((ethylene bis(dithiocarbamato))zinc)	1%
Malathion	0.5%
Lindane (hexachlorocyclohexane, gammexane)	1%
DDT (dichlorodiphenyltrichloroethane)	1%
Photographic chemicals	
Hydroquinone	1%
p-Methylaminophenol sulfate (Metol)	1%
Hydrazine sulfate	1%
C.D. 2. (color developer)	1%
C.D. 3. (color developer)	1%
Plastics and Glues	
Phenol formaldehyde resin	5%
p-Tertiary butylphenol formaldehyde resin	1%
Dibutyl phthalate	5%
Tricresyl phosphate (tritotyl phosphate)	5%
Triethylenetetramine (epoxy curing agent)	0.5%
Diaminodiphenylmethane (epoxy curing agent)	0.5%
Ethylenediamine	1%
Rubber chemicals	
n-Cyclohexylbenzothiazylsulphenamide (CBS)	1%
Hydroquinone monobenzylether	1%
1,3-Diphenylguanidine (DPG)	1%
Phenyl-beta-naphthylamine (PBN)	1%
Isopropylaminodiphenylamine identical with phenylisopropyl-p-phenylenediamine (IPPD)	0.1%
4,4′-Dihydroxydiphenyl (DOD)	0.2%
2-Mercaptobenzimidazole (2-benzimidazolethiol)	1%
Hexamethylenetetramine (methenamine)	1%
Tetramethylthiurammonosulfide (TMTM)	1%
Bis(diethyldithiocarbamato)zinc (ZDC)	1%
Mercaptobenzothiazole (MBT)	1%
Tetramethylthioramidisulfide (TMTD)	1%
Phenylcyclohexyl-p-phenylenediamine (CPPD)	1%
Diphenyl-p-phenylenediamine (DPPD)	1%
Dibenzothiazyldisulfide (MBTS)	1%
Morpholinylmercaptobenzothiazole (MOR)	1%
Tetraethylthioramdisulfide (TETD)	1%
Dipentamethylenethiuramdisulfide (PTD)	1%
Di-beta-naphthyl-p-phenylenediamine (DBNPD)	1%
Bis(dibutyldithiocarbamato)zinc (ZBC)	1%
Sun screen agents	
2-Ethoxyethyl-p-methoxycinnamate (photo allergen)	5%
Isobutyl-p-aminobenzoate (photo allergen)	5%

Table 4-11. *(Continued)*

Miscellaneous agents	
Emulsifying wax	20%
Isopropyl myristate	20%
Chlorpromazine chloride (photo allergen)	1%

The substances are dispersed in petrolatum Ph. Nord. 63 if no other medium is mentioned.

The concentrations stated are subject to corrections in accordance with experience from the research group.

Test allergens used infrequently should be stored away from light in a cool place.

It is recommended that the European Standard series be renewed every 6 months.

Patch test materials available from Hollister-Steir	
Coal tar	5%
Cobalt sulfate	2.3%
Formalin	5%
Mercuric chloride, ammoniated	5%
Merthiolate, sodium	0.1%
Neomycin	20%
Nickel sulfate	3%
Paraphenylenediamine	2%
Potassium dichromate	0.25%
Turpentine	10%
Benzocaine (Mix C)	5%
Bithionol (Mix A)	0.5%
Dichlorophene (Mix A)	0.5%
Diphenylguanidine (Mix R)	0.1%
Furacin (Mix H)	0.2%
Hexachlorophene (Mix A)	0.5%
Histadyl (Mix H)	1%
Mercaptobenzothiazole (Mix R)	1%
Nupercaine (Mix C)	1%
Paraben, ethyl (Mix P)	5%
Paraben, methyl (Mix P)	5%
Paraben, propyl (Mix P)	5%
Polybrominated salicyanilide	1%
Pyribenzamine (Mix Hl)	2%
Surfacaine (Mix C)	1%
Tetrachlorosalicylanilide (Mix A)	0.25%
Tetramethylthiuram disulfide (Mix R)	1%
Tribrominated salicylanilide	1%
Vioform (Mix H)	3%
Lanolin	

Mixtures of allergens

- Antiseptic mix (bithionol, dichlorophene, hexachlorophene and tetrachlorosalicylanilide)
- Caine mix (Benzocaine, Nupercaine and Surfacaine)
- Hista mix (Furacin, Histadyl, Pyribenzamine and Vioform)
- Paraben mix (ethyl, methyl and propyl parabens)
- Rubber mix (diphenylguanidine, mercaptobenzothiazole and tetramethylthioramdisulfide)

orouracil alone under a covered patch test in proper concentration could give a false positive reaction, possibly because of inhibition of normal cellular growth and ensuing inflammatory reaction.

In testing the 5 per cent aqueous solution of 5-fluorouracil in 1:20, 1:200 and 1:2000 dilutions, Sams used the lower part of the back to avoid exposure to light. In a patient who was sensitive to the drug, he obtained only a slight response with a more dilute solution but a good response with the 1:20 solution.

Patch test 5-fluorouracil in a 1:20 aqueous solution preferably on the lower part of the back where there is no exposure to light

THE ALUMINUM (Al) PATCH TEST

Al-test (*available from* IMECO Astra Agency Co. AB, S-151 85 Sodertalje, Sweden) is a new design of patch test units, which is claimed to facilitate effective, simple and convenient patch testing in suspected allergic contact dermatitis. It was developed in the Section of Occupational Dermatology at the University of Lund in Sweden and consists of aluminum foil covered with polythene onto which a disc of paper is welded without using glue. The paper disc to which the allergen is applied is surrounded by an area of polythene-coated aluminum, which separates the test site from the area to which the adhesive plaster is applied to the skin. The Al-test units are fixed by a reliable adhesive plaster, e.g., Blenderm or Dermicel.

The International Contact Dermatitis Research Group has used the Al-test in a joint study of about 5000 patients and, therefore, has used more than 100,000 test units. I have found it to be satisfactory, except that the discs sometimes slip off the aluminum paper.

The North American Contact Dermatitis Research Group is evaluating an Al-test patch mounted on Dermicel Tape as well as patch materials in special plastic bottles developed by Dr. William Jordan and supplied through Johnson & Johnson.

REFERENCES

Ethylenediamine

1. Epstein, E., Rees, W. J., and Maibach, H. I.: Recent Experience with Routine Patch Test Screening. Arch. Derm., *98*, 18, 1968.
2. Fregert, S., et al.: Epidemiology of Contact Dermatitis. Trans. St. John Derm. Soc., *55*, 17, 1967.
3. Agrup, G., et al.: Value of History and Testing in Suspected Contact Dermatitis. Arch. Derm., *101*, 212, 1970.
4. Fisher, A. A., Pascher, F., and Kanof, N. B.: Allergic Contact Dermatitis Due to Ingredients of Vehicles. Arch. Derm., *104*, 286, 1971.
5. Tas, I., and Weissberg, H.: Allergy to Aminophylline. Acta Allerg., *12*, 39, 1958.
6. Baer, R. L., Cohen, H. J., and Neideroff, A. H.: Allergic Eczematous Sensitivity to Aminophylline. Arch. Derm., *79*, 647, 1959.
7. Rajka, G., and Pallini, O.: Sensitization to Locally Applied Antistine. Acta Dermatovener, *44*, 255, 1964.
8. Suurmond, D.: Patch Test Reactions to Phenergan Cream, Promethazine and Triethanolamine. Dermatologica, *133*, 505, 1966.
9. Raymond, J. Z., and Cross, P. R.: EDTA: Preservative Dermatitis. Arch. Derm., *100*, 436, 1969.
10. Provost, T. T., and Jillson, O. F.: Ethylenediamine Contact Dermatitis. Arch. Derm., *96*, 231, 1967.
11. Epstein, E., and Maibach, H. I.: Ethylenediamine—Allergic Contact Dermatitis. Arch. Derm., *98*, 476, 1968.

Paraphenylenediamine

12. Schonning, I.: Sensitizing Properties of p-Amino-Diphenylamine. Acta Dermatovener., *49*, 501, 1969.
13. Blohm, S. G., and Rajka, G.: The Allergenicity of Paraphenylenediamine. Acta Dermatovener., *50*, 49, 1970.
14. Mackie, B., and Mackie, L. E.: Cross Sensitization in Dermatitis Due to Hair Dyes. Aust. J. Derm., *7*, 189, 1964.

Parabens

15. Hjorth, N., and Trolle-Lassen, C.: Skin Reactions to Ointment Bases. Trans. St. John Hosp. Derm. Soc., *49*, 127, 1963.
16. Schorr, W. F.: Paraben Allergy—A Cause of Intractable Dermatitis. J.A.M.A., *204*, 859, 1968.

17. Schorr, W. F., and Mohajerin, A. H.: Paraben Sensitivity. Arch. Derm., *93*, 721, 1966.
18. Hjorth, N.: p-Hydroxybenzoic Acid Esters (Paraben Esters, Nipagin Esters). Acta Dermatovener., *41*, 97, 1961.
19. Sarkany, I.: Contact Dermatitis from Paraben. Brit. J. Derm., *72*, 345, 1960.
20. Epstein, S.: Paraben Sensitivity: Subtle Trouble. Ann. Allergy, *25*, 185, 1969.
21. Schamberg, I. L.: Allergic Contact Dermatitis to Methyl and Propyl Paraben. Arch. Derm., *95*, 626, 1967.
22. Evans, S.: Epidermal Sensitivity to Lanolin and Parabens: Occurrence in Pharmaceutical and Cosmetic Products. Brit. J. Derm., *82*, 625, 1970.
23. Fisher, A. A.: Management of Selected Types of Allergic Contact Dermatitis Through the Use of Proper Substitutes. Cutis, *3*, 498, 1967.

Thimerosal

24. Ellis, F. A.: The Sensitizing Factor in Merthiolate. J. Allergy, *18*, 212, 1947.
25. Gaul, L. E.: Sensitizing Component in Thiosalicylic Acid. J. Invest. Derm., *31*, 91, 1958.
26. Epstein, S.: Sensitivity to Merthiolate: A Cause of False Delayed Intradermal Reactions. J. Allergy, *34*, 225, 1963.
27. Reisman, R. E.: Delayed Hypersensitivity to Merthiolate Preservative. J. Allergy, *43*, 245, 1969.
28. Hansson, H., and Moeller, H.: Intracutaneous Test Reactions to Tuberculin Containing Merthiolate as a Preservative. Scand. J. Infect. Dis., *3*, 169, 1971.
29. Hansson, H., and Moeller, H.: Patch Test Reactions to Merthiolate in Healthy Young Subjects. Brit. J. Derm., *83*, 349, 1970.

Lanolin

30. Cronin, E.: Lanolin Dermatitis. Brit. J. Derm., *78*, 617, 1966.
31. Vollum, D. I.: Sensitivity to Hydrogenated Lanolin. Letters to the Editor. Arch. Derm., *100*, 774, 1969.
32. Thune, P.: Allergy to Wool Fat. The Addition of Salicylic Acid for Patch Test Purposes. Acta Dermatovener., *49*, 282, 1969.
33. Newcomb, E. A.: Lanolin Allergy. J. Soc. Cosmetic Chemists, *17*, 149, 1966.
34. Peter, C., Schropl, F., and Franzwa, H.: Experimental Investigation Regarding Allergenic Effects of Wool Wax Alcohols. Hautarzt, *20*, 450, 1969.

Formaldehyde

35. Marcussen, P. V.: Contact Dermatitis Due to Formaldehyde in Textiles. 1934–1958. Preliminary Report. Acta Dermatovener., *39*, 349, 1959.
36. Epstein, E., and Maibach, H. I.: Formaldehyde Allergy. Incidence and Patch Test Problems. Arch. Derm., *94*, 186, 1966.
37. Danto, J. L.: Finger Nail Hardeners. Canad. Med. Ass. J., *98*, 652, 1968.
38. Gaul, L. E.: Absence of Formaldehyde Sensitivity in Phenol-Formaldehyde. J. Invest. Derm., *48*, 485, 1967.

Rubber

39. Wilson, T. H.: Rubber Dermatitis. An Investigation of 106 Cases of Contact Dermatitis Caused by Rubber. Brit. J. Derm., *81*, 175, 1969.

Chromium

40. Pirila, J., Forstrom, L., and Virtamo, M.: Reduction to Trivalent Chromate in Connection with Patch Testing. Dermatologica, *135*, 451, 1967.
41. Mali, J. W. et al.: Quantitative Aspects of Chromium Sensitization. Acta Dermatovener., *44*, 44, 1964.
42. Pedersen, N. B., et al.: Patch Testing and Absorption of Chromium. Acta Dermatovener., *50*, 431, 1970.
43. Fregert, S., et al.: Epidemiology of Contact Dermatitis. Trans. St. John Hosp. Derm. Soc., *55*, 17, 1969.
44. Magnusson, B., et al.: Routine Patch Testing IV. Acta Dermatovener., *48*, 110, 1968.
45. Marcussen, P. V.: Variations in the Incidence of Contact Hypersensitivities. Trans. St. John Hosp. Derm. Soc., *48*, 40, 1962.

Turpentine

46. Pirila, V., et al.: Chemical Nature of Eczematogens in Oil of Turpentine. Dermatologica, *139*, 183, 1969.
47. Hjorth, N., and Wilkinson, D. S.: Turpentine Sensitivity. Brit. J. Derm., *80*, 22, 1968.

Neomycin

48. Raab, W. P.: Allergic and Anaphylactic Inflammation. Letters to the Editor. J.A.M.A., *201*, 143, 1967.
49. Epstein, S.: Neomycin Sensitivity and Atopy. Dermatologica, *130*, 280, 1965.

50. Patrick, J., Panzer, J. O., and Derbes, V. J.: Neomycin Sensitivity in the Normal (Non-atopic) Individual. Arch. Derm., *102*, 532, 1970.
51. Wereide, K.: Neomycin Sensitivity in Atopic Dermatitis and Other Eczematous Conditions. Acta Dermatovener., *50*, 114, 1970.
52. Pirila, V., Forstrom, L., and Rouhunkoski, S.: Twelve Years of Sensitization to Neomycin in Finland: Report of 1,760 Cases of Sensitivity to Neomycin and/or Bacitracin. Acta Dermatovener., *47*, 419, 1967.
53. Hjorth, N., and Thomsen, K.: Patch Test with Neomycin. Acta Allergy, *21*, 487, 1966.
54. Panzer, J. D., and Epstein, W. L.: Percutaneous Absorption Following Topical Application of Neomycin. Arch. Derm., *102*, 536, 1970.

Vehicles

55. Fisher, A. A., Pascher, F., and Kanof, N. B.: Allergic Contact Dermatitis Due to Ingredients of Vehicles. Arch. Derm., *104*, 286, 1971.
56. Raymond, J. Z., and Cross, P. R.: EDTA: Preservative Dermatitis. Arch. Derm., *100*, 436, 1969.

Dichlorophene

57. Fisher, A. A., and Lipton, M.: Allergic Stomatitis Due to "BAXIN" in a Dentifrice. Arch. Derm., *64*, 640, 1951.
58. Fisher, A. A., and Tobin, L.: Sensitivity to Compound G-4 ("Dichlorophene") in Dentifrices. J.A.M.A., *151*, 998, 1953.
59. Gaul, L. E., and Underwood, G. B.: The Cutaneous Toxicity of Dihydroxydichlordiphenylmethane: A New Fungicide for Athlete's Foot. J. Indiana Med. Ass., *42*, 22, 1949.
60. Schorr, W. F.: Dichlorophene (G-4) Allergy. Arch. Derm., *102*, 515, 1970.
61. Epstein, E.: Dichlorophene Allergy. Ann. Allergy, *24*, 437, 1966.

Hexachlorophene

62. Baker, H., et al.: Primary Irritant Dermatitis of the Scrotum Due to Hexachlorophene. Arch. Derm., *99*, 693, 1969.
63. Watt, T. L., and Baumann, R. R.: Primary Irritant Dermatitis Caused by pHisohex. Cutis, *10*, 363, 1972.

Glycols

64. Warshaw, T. G., and Herrmann, F.: Studies of Skin Reaction of Propylene Glycol. J. Invest. Derm., *19*, 423, 1952.
65. Braun, W.: Contact Allergies Against Polyethylene Glycols. Z. Haut Geschlechtskr., *44*, 385, 1969.
66. Strauss, M. S.: Sensitization to Polyethylene Glycols (Carbowax). Arch. Derm., *61*, 420, 1950.

Phenylmercuric Salts

67. Hjorth, N., and Trolle-Lassen, C.: Skin Reactions to Preservatives in Cream with Special Regard to Paraben Esters and Sorbic Acid. Amer. Perf., *77*, 43, 1962.

Triethanolamine

68. Castelain, P.: Generalized Diffuse Eczema Due to Sensitization to Triethanolamine. Bull. Soc. Franc. Derm. Syph., *74*, 562, 1967.
69. Suurmond, D.: Patch Test Reactions to Phenergan Cream, Promethazine and Triethanolamine. Dermatologica, *133*, 503, 1966.
70. Schwartz, L.: Sensitivity Testing in Cosmetics. *Science and Technology*. New York, Interscience Publishers, 1967, p. 1247.

Sorbic Acid

71. Klaschka, F., and Biersdorff, H.: Allergic Eczematous Reaction from Sorbic Acid Used as a Preservative in External Medicaments. Munchen. Med. Wschr., *107*, 185, 1965.

Benzalkonium Chloride

72. Von Herff, D.: So-Called Drug Idiosyncrasies. Deutsch. Med. Wschr., *63*, 1044, 1937.
73. Appel, B.: A Dermatologist Looks at the U.S.P. and the N.F. Amer. Profess. Pharm., *21*, 913, 1955.
74. Gaul, L. E.: Overtreatment Dermatitis. Ann. Allergy, *13*, 642, 1955.
75. Saunders, W.: Contact Dermatitis Due to Benzalkonium Chloride, New York J. Med., *53*, 2700, 1953.
76. Norrlind, R.: Two Cases of Hypersensitivity to Benzalkonium Chloride. Svensk. Lakartidn., *50*, 2442, 1953.
77. Wahlberg, J. E.: Two Cases of Hypersensitivity to Quaternary Ammonium Compounds. Acta Dermatovener., *42*, 230, 1962.
78. Seiji, M., and Mizuno, F.: Unusual Cornification in Ichthyosis-Like Dermatitis. Acta Derm., *50*, 338, 1970.

79. Pandos, E., Horowitz, I. D., and Wunder, G.: Contact Dermatitis Complicating Tracheostomy. Amer. J. Dis. Child., *109*, 90, 1965.
80. Theodore, F. H., and Schlossman, A.: *Ocular Allergy.* Baltimore, Williams and Wilkins Co., 1958, p. 188.
81. Fisher, A. A., and Stillman, M. A.: Allergic Contact Sensitivity to Benzalkonium Chloride (BAK). Cutaneous, Ophthalmic and General Medical Implications. Arch. Derm., *106*, 169, 1972.
82. Dabiez, O. H., Naugle, B. S., and Reich, L.: Evaluation of a Stronger Concentration of Preservative (Benzalkonium Chloride) in Contact Lens Soaking Solution. Eye Ear Nose Throat Monthly, *45*, 78, 1966.
83. Huriez, C., et al.: Frequences des Sensibilisations aux Ammoniums Quaternaires. Bull. Soc. Franc. Derm. Syph., *72*, 106, 1965.
84. Huriez, C., et al.: L'Allergie Aux Sels D'Ammonium Quaternaire. Sem. Hop. Paris, *41*, 2301, 1965.

Cetyl Alcohol

85. Gaul, L. E.: Dermatitis From Cetyl and Stearyl Alcohols. Arch. Derm., *99*, 598, 1969.
86. Sulzberger, M. B., Warshaw, T., and Herrmann, F.: Studies of Skin Hypersensitivity to Lanolin. J. Invest. Derm., *20*, 33, 1953.

Sodium Lauryl Sulfate

87. Sams, W. M., and Smith, J. G.: Contact Dermatitis to Hydrocortisone Ointment. J.A.M.A., *164*, 1212, 1960.
88. Harrold, J. P.: Denaturation of Epidermal Keratin by Surface Active Agents. J. Invest. Derm., *32*, 581, 1959.
89. Van Scott, E. J., and Lyon, M. D.: A Chemical Measure of the Effects of Soaps and Detergents on the Skin. J. Invest. Derm., *21*, 199, 1953.

Corticosteroids

90. Comaish, S.: A Case of Hypersensitivity of Corticosteroids. Brit. J. Derm., *81*, 919, 1969.
91. Burckhardt, Von W.: Kontaktekzem Durch Hydrocortison. Hautarzt, *10*, 42, 1959.
92. Dorn, Von H.: Kontaktallergie gegenuber Salben-Konservierungsmittein und Hydrocortison. Z. Haut. Geschlechskr., *27*, 305, 1959.
93. Kooij, R.: Hypersensitivity to Hydrocortisone. Brit. J. Derm., *71*, 392, 1959.
94. Bonu, G., and Zima, G.: Sensibilizzazione da Contatto a Cortisonici. Minerva, *42*, 513, 1967.
95. Wilkinson, R. D., McGarry, E. M., and Solomon, S.: Allergic Contact Dermatitis to Hydrocortisone, J. Invest. Derm., *43*, 295, 1967.
96. Sams, W. M., and Smith, J. G., Jr.: Contact Dermatitis Due to Hydrocortisone Ointment. J.A.M.A., *164*, 1212, 1957.
97. Church, R.: Sensitivity to Hydrocortisone Acetate Ointment. Brit. J. Derm., *72*, 341, 1960.
98. Edwards, M., and Rudner, E. J.: Dermatitis Venenata Due to Hydrocortisone Alcohol. Cutis, *6*, 757, 1970.
99. Coskey, R. J.: Contact Dermatitis Due to Methylprednisolone. J.A.M.A., *199*, 136, 1967.
100. Bandmann, H. J., Huber-Riffeser, G., and Woyton, A.: Kontaktallergie gegen Triamcinolonacetonid. Hautarzt, *17*, 183, 1966.
101. Wulf, K.: Beitrag zur Triamcinolon-Kontaktallergic. Z. Haut. Geschlechskr., *42*, 19, 1967.
102. Alani, M. D., and Alani, S. D.: Allergic Contact Dermatitis to Corticosteroids. Ann. Allergy, *34*, 181, 1972.
103. Weber, G.: Rosacea-Like Dermatitis: Contraindication or Intolerance Reaction to Strong Steroids. Brit. J. Derm., *86*, 253, 1972.

Therapeutic Agents

104. Hjorth, N.: Penicillin: Occupational Dermatitis Among Veterinary Surgeons Caused by Penethane. Berufsdermatosen Monogr., *15*, 163, 1967.
105. Pirila, V., Hirvonen, M. L., and Rouhunkoski, S.: The Pattern of Cross-Sensitivity to Neomycin. Secondary Sensitization to Gentamicin. Dermatologica, *136*, 321, 1968.
106. Lynfield, Y. L.: Allergic Contact Sensitization to Gentamicin. New York J. Med., *56*, 2238, 1970.
107. Roupe, G., and Strannegard, O.: Anaphylactic Shock Elicited by Topical Administration of Bacitracin. Arch. Derm., *100*, 450, 1969.
108. Waisilewski, C.: Allergic Contact Dermatitis from Nystatin. Arch. Derm., *102*, 216, 1970.
109. Eaglstein, W. H.: Allergic Contact Dermatitis to Benzoyl Peroxide. Arch. Derm., *97*, 527, 1968.
110. Poole, R. L., Griffith, J. F., and MacMillan, F. S. K.: Experimental Contact Sensitization with Benzoyl Peroxide. Arch. Derm., *102*, 635, 1970.

111. Hall, N. A.: O-T-C Burn and Sunburn Remedies. Cutis, *4*, 889, 1968.
112. Yaffee, H. S., and Dressler, D. P.: Topical Application of Mafenide Acetate: Its Association with Erythema Multiforme and Cutaneous Reactions. Arch. Derm., *100*, 277, 1969.
113. Velasco, J. E., and Afrikus, J. A.: Contact Dermatitis to Mafenide Acetate. Arch. Derm., *103*, 61, 1971.
114. Berens, J. J.: Thermal Contact Burns from Streets and Highways. J.A.M.A., *214*, 2025, 1970.
115. Bielicky, T., and Novak, M.: Contact-Group Sensitization to Triphenylmethane Dyes—Gentian Violet, Brilliant Green, and Malachite Green. Arch. Derm., *100*, 540, 1969.
116. Bjornberg, A., and Mobacken, H.: Necrotic Skin Reactions Caused by 1 Per Cent Gentian Violet and Brilliant Green. Acta Dermatovener., *52*, 55, 1972.
117. Epstein, S.: Dermal Contact Dermatitis. Dermatologica, *117*, 291, 1958.
118. Juhlin, L., and Hansson, H.: Topical Glutaraldehyde for Plantar Hyperhidrosis. Arch. Derm., *97*, 327, 1968.
119. Gordon, B. I., and Maibach, H.: Eccrine Anhidrosis Due to Glutaraldehyde, Formaldehyde and Iontophoresis. J. Invest. Derm., *53*, 436, 1969.
120. Sanderson, K. V., and Cronin, E.: Glutaraldehyde and Contact Dermatitis. Brit. Med. J., *3*, 802, 1968.
121. Jordan, W. P., Dahl, M. V., and Albert, H. L.: Contact Dermatitis from Glutaraldehyde. Arch. Derm., *105*, 94, 1972.
122. Sams, W. M.: Untoward Response with Topical Fluorouracil. Arch. Derm., *67*, 14, 1968.

Hand Dermatitis Due to Contactants

Patch testing with the standard and vehicle series usually reveals most contact allergens that may be significant in hand dermatitis. In addition, particularly in women, patch tests should be performed with balsam of Peru, because European studies[1] have shown a surprisingly high number of positive reactions to the balsams. Hjorth[2] suggested the cause may be greater exposure to perfumes, essential oils and spices.

Patch tests with the standard and vehicle series plus balsam of Peru reveal relevant contactants in about 25 per cent of cases of hand dermatitis

Authorities differ markedly concerning the relevance of patch test reactions in hand dermatitis. Wilkinson et al.[1] considered 66 per cent of patch test reactions to be relevant, but in my experience, the significance is closer to 25 per cent.

ROLE OF IRRITANTS IN HAND DERMATITIS

Bjornberg[3] analyzed the skin reactions to 11 primary irritants in patients with eczema and in normal persons. It has been generally assumed that an irritant reaction observed after a 24-hour patch test rapidly subsides. This assumption, which has been used to differentiate allergic from irritant patch test reactions, was found generally to be incorrect. Severe reactions, especially, tend to increase over the first 72 hours.

The average concentration of an irritant causing a faint erythema can be taken as a measure of the skin irritancy of a compound. Only 0.2 per cent of croton oil in Vaseline was necessary to evoke this erythema, whereas 0.9 per cent of sodium lauryl sulfate and the surprisingly high figure of 17.5 per cent of potassium soap were necessary. There was no marked difference between patients and controls. Many authors have described the irritant reaction as an "all-or-none" response, but phenol was the only substance that conformed to this pattern. With all other substances, the intensity of reaction increased in proportion to concentration and exposure time.

A finding of fundamental importance was the increased skin susceptibility to irritants in remote body regions in patients with hand eczema. This is the first proof of the validity of the commonly used term *status eczematicus* and must be taken into account in establishing the concentration of substances used for patch testing and in assessing the reaction to substances that are at the same time allergens and irritants. This increased reactivity may cause nonspecific patch test reactions, add to the risk of accidental patch test sensitization and cause unexpected side effects from therapeutic agents.

Patients with *healed* (in contrast to *active*) hand eczema showed a normal reactivity to most irritants, but both groups gave stronger reactions to soap, sodium lauryl sulfate and benzalkonium chloride than did the controls.

The entire skin of many patients with active hand eczema exhibits increased susceptibility to irritants

DIAGNOSIS OF HAND DERMATITIS

Contact dermatitis of the hands may be difficult to distinguish from atopic eczema, psoriasis and nummular eczema. In addition, dyshidrosiform eruptions (pompholyx), dermatophytosis and various ids may confuse the diagnostic picture. Distinctive primary lesions and familiar patterns of involvement are more apt to be found in widespread eruptions than in those limited to the hands, where superimposed factors may easily distort the clinical picture. Etiologically different hand eczemas may closely resemble each other. Frequently, a definite etiologic diagnosis cannot be made, and symptomatic treatment is all that can be employed.

The perspiring wrist, in contact with an impervious object, such as a wrist band, may become the site of localized miliaria resembling allergic contact dermatitis. Often only a patch test will reveal the true nature of the dermatitis.

Psoriasis of the palms and fingers may closely resemble the dry type of contact dermatitis. Indeed, trauma and contact dermatitis of the hands often precipitate psoriasis in this area in psoriatics (Kobner phenomenon).

Atopic dermatitis of the hands is often complicated by a superimposed contact dermatitis. In individuals with an eczematous diathesis, contact dermatitis tends to be complicated by marked weeping, crusting and dissemination of the eruption to other parts of the body.

Hand dermatitis often becomes secondarily infected. Sensitization to bacteria may produce an infectious eczematoid dermatitis with dissemination to the forearms and more distant areas.

Patterns of hand dermatitis tend to become modified and obscured by eczematization, infection, and spreading from the original sites of involvement

Procedures. Discovery of the responsible irritant or sensitizer may be facilitated by the following procedures:

1. In the event that the eruption has not remained sharply localized, an attempt should be made to ascertain the original site and the contactants.
2. The feet should be examined for psoriasis, dermatophytosis, dyshidrosis, nummular eczema or pustular bacterid. Discovery of an eruption on the feet in a patient with hand eczema indicates that the hand eruption may not be a simple contact dermatitis.
3. Chronic paronychia, particularly of the monilial variety, is usually evidence that the hands are wet much of the time. Occasionally, paronychia may be due to wax, hair, bristles, threads and scales, which enter the paronychial tissues as foreign bodies.[4]
4. Abnormalities of the nails should be noted, particularly for evidence of fungous infections and psoriasis. The role of such dermatoses in the hand dermatitis must be evaluated. Subungual hemorrhages may be caused by excessive exposure to a combination of water, detergents and trauma, such as in professional dishwashers.[5]
5. A history of atopic dermatitis may also be of importance in differential diagnosis and prognosis. In adults, uncomplicated atopic dermatitis of the hands tends to be dry with sharply defined borders. Work in which the hands are wet, however, causes eczema. Housework often precipitates atopic dermatitis with superimposed contact dermatitis of the hands in women who have been free of atopic dermatitis since childhood.

Examine the feet of every patient having hand dermatitis and search for evidence of psoriasis, tinea or atopic dermatitis on the rest of the body

6. A study of the distribution of the eruption may be helpful. A vesicular eruption on the palms and sides of fingers that is symmetrical and bilateral is not as likely to be a contact dermatitis as is one on the back of the hands and fingers with little palmar involvement. The palms usually have greater resistance to irritants and sensitizers than do the dorsal aspects of the hands.

7. A listing by the patient of all previously used medications, hand creams and lotions is necessary to evaluate the role of these preparations in alleviating or exacerbating the dermatitis.

8. A detailed history of contactants encountered in work, play or hobbies is of prime importance.

9. Patch tests may facilitate the pinpointing of offending contactants and may be of decisive value in concluding whether the dermatitis is due to primary irritants or to specific sensitizers.

10. While the search for the cause of the dermatitis is being made, the inflamed hands are protected as much as possible from trauma, strong cleansers and irritating and sensitizing medications.

HOUSEWIFE'S ECZEMA

This is probably the most common type of contact dermatitis of the hands encountered in clinical practice. It occurs principally on fingers, webs and dorsa of the hands of women who do housework and laundry, which entail regular exposure to soaps, detergents and other household cleansers. Housewife's eczema, however, may also affect others whose professions or activities involve excessive exposure to soaps and detergents, including surgeons, medical personnel, dentists, soda clerks, bartenders, kitchen workers and canners. The eruption usually begins with mild dryness, redness and scaling. With continued exposure to soap and water, fissuring, crusting and eventually chronic eczema are produced.

Hand eczema often begins in cold weather with chapping of the hands. Frequently the young mother's hands remain in fairly good condition until 3 to 6 months after childbirth, at which time increased exposure to soaps and water in care of the infant causes a breakdown of the skin. Such eczemas may be intensified by common household irritants, such as bleaches, waxes, polishes and turpentine. The tense, tired housewife not infrequently excoriates the itchy skin, causing secondary infection and lichenification.

SPECIFIC ALLERGENS IN HOUSEWIFE'S ECZEMA

Calnan et al.[6] reported a series of 4000 patients patch tested in 5 European clinics; 1000 were engaged in domestic work only and included 281 women with contact dermatitis of the hands. Half of the 281 had a positive patch test reaction. The responsible allergens in order of prevalence were balsams, nickel, medicaments, cobalt, rubber, chromate, benzocaine and paraphenylenediamine. An allergic basis (42 per cent) was as frequent as an irritant (45 per cent) among those with contact dermatitis. Our patch results are similar, except that the balsams and cobalt are less significant.

Nickel. As a rule, dermatitis due to nickel-plated objects is not confined to the hands, because other sites also are usually exposed to nickel-containing jewelry, clips and zippers. This type of dermatitis occurs principally from handles, knobs, pencils, scissors and surgical instruments, knitting needles, thimbles and coins. Traces of nickel in detergents probably are not significant in the United States, although in some countries the nickel content may be high enough to cause dermatitis (see chapter on metals).

Considering the objects causing hand eczema in housewives, it might be expected that it would mainly affect the palms and palmar surfaces of the fingers, but clinically it is not so since hand eczema in a housewife is as likely to affect the backs of the hands and the sides of the fingers. The significance of a positive patch test reaction to nickel in a patient with hand eczema is undetermined.

Rubber. Patients with hand dermatitis due to irritants may become sensitized to rubber gloves,[7] and this should be suspected when a hand dermatitis stops abruptly at the wrists. Patch tests may be performed with a ½-inch square cut from the rubber glove and supple-

tape and bandages may also cause allergic rubber dermatitis of the hands and complicate housewife's eczema.

Potassium Dichromate. Aside from industrial exposure, individuals sensitized to potassium dichromate may acquire dermatitis of the hands from leather gloves and other leather objects, matches, bleaches, antirust compounds, varnishes, yellow paints, spackling compounds and glues that contain dichromates. Traces of chromates are present in soaps but are not as important in hand dermatitis in the United States as abroad.

Paraphenylenediamine (*PPDA*). Dermatitis of the hands due to allergic sensitization to this chemical occurs mainly in hairdressers and furriers. Occasionally, however, hairdyeing is done at home by nonprofessionals who may develop allergic contact dermatitis of the hands from the procedure.

If the patient has a positive patch test reaction to paraphenylenediamine and apparently has not handled the dye, patch tests should be performed with other para-amino compounds, such as benzocaine, procaine and para-aminobenzoic acid, with which it may cross-react.

In addition, paraphenylenediamine-sensitive individuals who handle certified azo dyes incorporated into foods, drugs and cosmetics should be tested with such dyes because cross-reactions may occur. Allergic dermatitis of the hands from ballpoint pens containing azo dyes may occur in patients sensitized to paraphenylenediamine.[8]

Topical Medications. Housewife's eczema is sometimes made worse by self-prescribed medication or by sensitization to topical agents. Patch tests with these medications and the vehicle tray are valuable in such instances.

Rubber gloves, instead of affording protection for hand dermatitis, may cause irritation due to maceration or a superimposed allergic rubber dermatitis

Rothenberg and Hjorth[9] point out that housewife's eczema is caused by a multiplicity of factors. Among these, soaps and detergents may be important in providing exposure to and promoting absorption of low grade allergens through the skin.

Perfumes in soap and detergents may produce allergic reactions. Sensitization may be enhanced because these cleansers promote absorption of allergens through the skin

Patients with positive reactions to perfumes often show positive reactions to balsam of Peru, wood tars and benzyl salicylate. Some perfumes contain phenylacetaldehyde, which is a sensitizer.[10]

Allergic Reactions to Antibacterial Agents. Many bacteriostatic agents added to soaps and cleansers are photosensitizers. These substances may produce photosensitization[11] and depigmentation.[12]

Rosin (*Colophony*). Yellow (soft) laundry bars owe their properties to the presence of rosin, which is the solid resin residue remaining after the distillation of spirits of turpentine derived from the crude oleoresin of certain species of pine. Rosin consists of a mixture of complex abietic acids and esters. It makes laundry bars more soluble and hastens sudsing in cool water. Some toilet soaps also contain a small percentage of this agent. Rosin may be a sensitizer. For patch test purposes, rosin N.F. 10 per cent in olive oil may be used.

IRRITATION FROM SOAPS AND DETERGENTS

The role of soaps and detergents in hand eczema is controversial. Wechsler[13] and Blohm and Lodin[14] suggested that the term *detergent hands* is a misnomer because of the limited role of soaps and detergents as irritants. Indeed, Suskind[15] found that immersion of hands in solutions of soaps or synthetic detergents in the concentrations recommended by the suppliers actually *improves* the hand dermatitis.

Kligman and Wooding[16] pointed out that hand eczema in housewives was once attributed to soap, but since World War II, synthetic detergents have been incriminated. Their introduction, however, has not led to any notable increase in housewife's eczema, and widespread use of dishwashers and washing machines over the last 10 years has not led to any conspicuous decline.

All investigating methods distinguish between detergents causing a low and a high degree of irritancy. The results, however, show unexplained discrepancies that suggest detergents are by no means homogeneous and that the damage may be produced by different mechanisms.

Wood and Bettley,[17] who studied the denaturing action of detergents upon keratin and irritancy on human skin, also found considerable differences among detergents.

Glickman and Silvers[18] found that 82 per cent of patients with hand eczema have a history of atopy.

Although it is not certain that soaps and detergents play a major role in hand eczema, contact with them should be minimized, especially in atopic persons

The incidence of housewife's eczema, "dishpan hands" and "detergent hands" is low compared to the number of people exposed. Washerwomen, scrubwomen, dishwashers and others who earn their living by having their hands immersed in solutions of these detergents, however, do frequently develop dermatitis. In many instances the inflamed skin does not tolerate soap and detergents well, and contact with these compounds should be avoided, at least until the acute phase has subsided.

Under appropriate circumstances, excessive exposure to water and soap and detergents leads to changes in the skin. The amount of damage depends on traumatic and environmental influences, such as cold weather, low humidity, impairment in alkali neutralization capacity, emotional stress, hyperhidrosis, exposure to other contactants (such as vegetables, fruits, meat juices and other foods) and contact with cleansing and polishing products containing bleaches, abrasives, alkalies and solvents.

Soaps and detergents probably damage skin by the following mechanisms:

1. Alkali-induced damage of the keratin layer of the epidermis, which increases the permeability of the horny layer.
2. Irritative effects of certain fatty acids.
3. Removal of lipids and the protective mantle of the skin and prevention of reestablishment of the mantle and its normal acidity.
4. Alteration of the buffering capacity of the skin.
5. Removal of amino acids with damage to the water-holding capacity of the horny layer. This is particularly likely with synthetic detergents.

Often irritation by soaps and detergents is heightened by concentration of the detergent solution on the skin, such as when cleansers become trapped under rings or when, during dishwashing, dishes are held tightly for a period of time in the detergent-moistened hand. Soaps for fine fabrics are probably the least irritating of the detergent cleansers.

Builders. Practically all laundry soaps contain additives, such as sodium carbonate, sodium phosphate, ash, borax or sodium silicate, which may irritate but not sensitize.

Abrasive Agents. Many powdered industrial hand cleansers have ingredients to increase the mechanical cleansing action. The inorganic scrubbers include pumice, talc, sand and borax; the organic agents include ground nut shells, cornmeal and wood flours. These agents are effective in removing heavy oil, greases, tar and other stubborn dirt from the hands, but the inorganic variety is particularly rough on the skin.

ENZYMES IN DETERGENTS

Currently 70 to 75 per cent of laundry detergents sold in the United States contain enzymes. Depending on the brand and type, these products contain as much as 0.1 per cent active enzymes, which are prepared by fermentation with the widely distributed nonpathogenic soil organism *Bacillus subtilis*.

The Food and Drug Administration made

public a study in which the average enzyme detergent laundry product in normal use by consumers did not produce more primary irritation of the skin than did similar products containing no enzymes. Ducksbury and Dave,[19] however, reported that 12 women in the home help service in Nottingham developed an irritant dermatitis after using enzyme detergents. A survey based on a questionnaire showed an incidence of dermatitis of 5 per cent among people using these products. Onychia may result from their use.

ALLERGIC REACTIONS TO ENZYME DETERGENTS

Exposure to the concentrated enzyme in industry has caused dermatitis, allergic rhinitis and asthma.[20]

Patch tests can be done with a 0.25 per cent aqueous solution of the commercial product. The "pure subtilisins" can be patch tested with a 0.1 per cent solution in water.

Belin et al.[21] stated that sensitization to enzyme detergents can also occur in consumers of enzyme-containing washing powder and in every situation in which these enzymes are dust particles. These investigators obtained positive scratch tests in sensitized patients.

Enzymes in detergents can occasionally cause irritation and sensitization

PATCH TESTING WITH SOAPS AND DETERGENTS

Patch testing with soaps and detergents is usually performed with a 1 to 2 per cent aqueous solution. The test site occasionally becomes slightly red, desquamates and wrinkles or appears glazed. These reactions are not indicative of allergic sensitization but are merely due to the irritant effect of soap or detergent solutions under the covered patch. Patch test reactions with these agents should always be checked on at least three control subjects.

The irritant reactions under a covered patch may interfere with the interpretation of allergic reactions. Whenever possible, therefore, patch tests should be performed with the suspected ingredient. Occasionally, however, photosensitivity reactions due to antiseptics in soaps are clear even when the testing is done with the soap solutions.

The alkalies and fatty acids of soaps are not sensitizers. Any white, unscented soap that is free of antiseptics, other medication or lanolin is nonallergenic, and patch testing, except for investigative purposes, is usually unrewarding. Similarly, the synthetic detergents without additives are nonsensitizing and do not usually yield patch test results of clinical significance.

Numerous methods have been devised for testing new soaps and detergents before they are introduced for general use. Such testing may be of value in detecting unusual irritant qualities of new products.

ROLE OF FOOD AND FOOD ADDITIVES IN CONTACT DERMATITIS

Preservatives, flavoring agents and dyes used as food additives may produce contact dermatitis in sensitized individuals.

Mitchell[22] pointed out that some of the sensitizing preservatives used in topical agents, such as the parabens and ethylenediamine, are also used as preservatives for foods. Table 5–1 is a list of skin sensitizers which can be added to foods.

Sodium Bisulfite in Salads. Dr. E. Epstein (personal communication, 1970) described hand eczema in a saladmaker due to "Veg-White," an antioxidant used to prevent discoloration of fruit and vegetables used in salads. The specific sensitizer in this preparation was sodium bisulfite. Patch tests can be performed with a 10 per cent aqueous solution of sodium bisulfite.

Mitchell[22] suggested the possibility that exposure to vanilla in various flavorings could account for many unexplained positive patch test reactions to balsam of Peru with which vanilla cross-reacts. Vanilla also cross-reacts with benzoin, rosin, benzoic acid, orange peel, cinnamon and clove.

Hjorth and Weisman (personal communication, 1972) reported that chefs and sand-

Table 5-1. Sensitizers Added to Foods

Sensitizer	*Food*
Parabens	Tomato, meat and fish products, pickles, relishes, sauces
Benzoyl peroxide	Flour
Karaya	Confectionery
Gum arabic (acacia)	Creams and cheeses
Lanolin	Chewing gum
Quillaja	Soft drinks
Vanillin	Artificial flavors
Nickel	Hydrogenated fats
Synthetic organic dyes	Many foods
Sodium bisulfite	Fruit and vegetable salads

wichmakers may acquire hand dermatitis from contact with fish and shellfish. Some individuals had positive patch test reactions; others had positive scratch test reactions to these seafoods.

Brun[23] reported contact dermatitis in a baker from lauryl gallate added to margarine as an *antioxidant*.

Preservatives added to foods like those added to topical creams may produce hand dermatitis in cooks, bakers and housewives

INSTRUCTIONS FOR PATIENTS WITH HOUSEWIFE'S ECZEMA

1. Use long handled brushes for dishwashing and for cleansing and scouring pots, pans and stoves. Use brushes in place of rubber gloves for household chores.
2. Heating and sweating inside a rubber glove may be as bad for the hands as is the irritation from soap and cleansers. White cotton gloves must be worn inside the rubber gloves and talcum powder or cornstarch must be dusted into the cotton gloves. Loose fitting gloves may be more comfortable and less irritating than gloves that fit snugly. Try not to wear rubber gloves for more than a half hour at a time. Do not put your hands into very hot water when wearing rubber gloves, because the heat may penetrate the gloves and irritate the hands. Soak dishes in hot soapy water for 30 minutes and let cool before washing so that the hands will not be overheated by the hot water.
3. Bathe babies with the bare hands, because soaps used for this purpose are mild and not irritating. If the hand dermatitis is acute and rubber gloves are worn, however, put a pair of cotton gloves *over* the rubber gloves so that the baby can be handled without danger of slipping because of the wet rubber gloves.
4. Handling of diapers, which contain much ammonia, may irritate the hands. Pick up such diapers with forceps or tongs, place them into a basin containing 1 teaspoon of boric acid powder to 1 quart of water and allow them to remain in this solution for about 1 hour to neutralize the ammonia.
5. While doing dry, dusty and dirty housework, wear cotton gloves to prevent the hands from getting excessively soiled. This makes the need for excessive cleaning of the hands unnecessary. If the fingertips are free from dermatitis, cut off the tips of the gloves to allow air to circulate about the hands and thereby prevent excessive sweating.
6. Contact of the hands with fruit juices, fruits, vegetables and raw meats may be irritating to the skin. Until the hands are better, use canned or frozen products. Avoid direct contact of the inflamed skin with irritating juices of onions and garlic.
7. Wool causes itching and irritation in many individuals and contact with it should be minimized.
8. Avoid exposure of the hands to hair tonics and lotions. Use a brush or cotton-tipped swab to apply such preparations to the scalp.
9. When pouring or measuring detergents or bleaches be careful that they do not splash onto the hands and forearms. Patients with hand eczema should use bleaches in

tablet form or those that are premeasured and packaged in plastic containers.

[illegible]

A. Do not use household cleansers on the hands. These products are made to remove dirt from dishes, clothes, walls and floors and are too harsh for use on the skin. Also avoid the use of waterless cleansers, which are essential organic solvents and often irritate and inflame the skin.
B. Avoid prolonged or too frequent washing of the skin. Gently pat the skin dry with a soft washcloth or tissues. Avoid vigorous rubbing. Remember that some people seem to tolerate unlimited washings of the hands with soap and water, whereas others get dry and irritated skin even with minimal washing. Do not use soaps that sting and are excessively drying. Use superfatted soaps and soap substitutes when this occurs.
C. Even the mildest soap must be *gently* and *thoroughly* rinsed off the hands.
D. In the acute stage, when the hands are swollen and red, avoid cleansing the skin with soap. Bathe the hands in Burow's solution, 1 part to 20 parts water. If the skin feels dry after this procedure, gently swab it with olive oil and apply the prescribed medication. Remove rings from fingers when washing the hands.

PATCH TESTS IN MEMBERS OF THE MEDICAL AND ALLIED PROFESSIONS

Physicians, surgeons, nurses and dentists develop contact dermatitis confined to the hands. In addition to tests with compounds discussed in connection with hand dermatitis in the general population, patch tests performed with benzalkonium chloride (Zephiran), mercury, formalin, local anesthetics, iodine compounds and alcohol are of value in hand eczema in this professional group.

> **Medical personnel with hand eczema should be tested for sensitivity to mercury, formalin, local anesthetics, alcohol, benzalkonium chloride and glutaraldehyde**

Mercury. Aside from producing [illegible] dermatitis, metallic mercury from a broken thermometer can produce a granulomatous response.

Formalin. Members of the medical and allied professions may be exposed to formaldehyde when it is used for sterilizing purposes, as a disinfectant or as a fixing solution for tissues. Formaldehyde is not only a powerful sensitizer but also a potent primary irritant. A strong solution of it can coagulate the protein of the skin and produce necrosis and scarring. Prolonged contact, even with weak solutions, may cause extreme dryness of the skin with fissuring. Formalin may cause the nails to become discolored, soft or brittle. Paronychia and even suppuration of the matrix may follow exposure to this chemical.

When allergic sensitization to formalin occurs, the dermatitis may become widespread. In extremely sensitive individuals, the mere presence of formaldehyde gas in a room in which a bottle of it was previously opened is sufficient to cause dermatitis. A minute amount of formaldehyde on thermometers, instruments, slides and biopsy containers is also sufficient to produce dermatitis in sensitized individuals.

Local Anesthetics. Allergic contact dermatitis of the hands due to local anesthetics may occur among medical and dental personnel.[24]

Even the slightest contact with solutions containing local anesthetic agents may cause dermatitis in sensitized individuals. A large proportion of dentists who have dermatitis after contact with procaine (Novocain) solutions are also hypersensitive to other local anesthetics that are derived from paraaminobenzoic acid or PABA (Table 5–2).

The anesthetics listed in Table 5–3 are not based on PABA and may be used as substitutes for Novocain-sensitive individuals.

Table 5-2. Local Anesthetics Based on PABA

Procaine (Novocain)
Butethamine (Monocaine)
Tetracaine (Pontocaine)
Butacaine (Butyn)
Benzocaine (Anesthesin)
Propoxycaine (Ravocaine)

Table 5-3. Local Anesthetics Not Based on PABA (Amide Type)

Lidocaine (Xylocaine)
Metabutoxycaine (Primacaine)
Meprylcaine (Oracaine)
Meprivacaine (Carbocaine)

Table 5-5. Topical Anesthetics Chemically Related to Benzocaine

Butacaine
Naepaine (Amylsine)
Orthoform
Neo-Orthoform

Since the potential danger of sensitization to procaine and benzocaine is great, particularly among dentists, it is recommended that medical and dental personnel with hand eczema, regardless of cause, employ Xylocaine as a local anesthetic.

Table 5–4 lists anesthetics derived from benzoic acid that occasionally cross-react with the anesthetics based on PABA.

Table 5–5 lists topical anesthetics chemically related to benzocaine.

These anesthetics should be avoided by individuals sensitized to benzocaine. Topical Xylocaine and diclonin are not related to benzocaine.

Iodine Compounds. Tincture of iodine and Ioprep (1 per cent iodine and 10 per cent nonionic surfactants) are primary irritants when covered and should be tested by the open method. Betadine (iodine in polyvinylpyrrolidine) may be tested by the usual closed method.

Medical personnel sensitized to inorganic iodine compounds may also develop dermatitis from handling or injecting radiopaque iodized contrast media.

Alcohol. Although it is widely recognized that alcohol can dry and irritate the skin, the possibility of it being a cutaneous sensitizer is usually overlooked. Externally applied alcohol is usually ethyl alcohol, which for this purpose is denatured or unfit for drinking because of the addition of chemicals. For industrial use, 5 per cent methyl alcohol or acetone is often added to denature ethyl alcohol; for ordinary or medicinal use about 40 chemicals are available for denaturing it. Most of these substances have a bitter taste or cause emesis. Rubbing alcohol is 70 per cent ethyl alcohol with a denaturing agent. In alcohol used in cosmetics, the added chemicals are odorless and nontoxic. Denatured alcohols used for perfumes and other cosmetics often contain diethyl phthalate.

Table 5-4. Local Anesthetics Based on Benzoic Acid Derivatives

Cocaine
Surfacaine
Piperocaine (Metycaine)
Meprylcaine (Oracaine)
Methabutethamine (Unacaine)

The most popular denaturing agents in rubbing alcohol include tartar emetic, salicylic acid, quinine sulfate, colchicum extract, brucine (an alkaloid resembling strychnine), quassia (the bitter principle of a Jamaica wood), and sucrose octa-acetate (an anhydrous adhesive used in lacquers). Isopropyl alcohol, which has a slight odor resembling that of acetone, may also be used as a denaturing agent. Pure ethyl alcohol is used in some hospitals, but coloring matter, such as methylene blue or amaranth pink (an azo dye used to color elixir phenobarbital), is added to discourage drinking it.

The chemicals added to denature alcohol are neither potent nor frequent sensitizers. Allergic contact dermatitis may, however, occasionally be caused by pure ethyl alcohol, and the allergic sensitivity usually extends to amyl, butyl, methyl and isopropyl alcohols. Some individuals having allergic contact sensitivity to alcohol may react to the ingestion of alcohol with a generalized erythema.

Reports[25–29] indicate that allergic reactions to the alcohols are not as rare as formerly believed.

Richardson[29] reported an allergic eczematous contact dermatitis to a commercially available prepackaged alcohol sponge (Preptic Swab). The dermatitis appeared on the hands of nurses and at the sites of electrocardiogram electrode placement (where the sponges were used as conductors) on cardiac patients. Patch tests indicated that the allergen is probably a volatile substance added to sterilize the swab. The actual sensitizer was not discovered.

Allergic contact dermatitis from various alcohols is not rare

Alcohol may be tested undiluted. The reaction to topical application of ethyl alcohol may occur within 15 minutes in the form of a bright red erythema, which may persist for 2 hours or more and become vesicular after several hours. It is, therefore, advisable to test for contact sensitivity to alcohol by the open patch test method and to keep the patient under observation for an hour or so. Similar prompt patch test reactions have also occurred with acrylic monomer and epoxy resins in highly sensitized individuals and may be related to quick diffusion of these chemicals into the skin.

HAND DERMATITIS IN NURSES

Aside from exposures while in pursuit of their medical duties, nurses may be exposed to detergents, other cleansers and alcohol, which can lead to dryness and eczematization of their hands. Such irritated skin may be more readily sensitized to the medications and chemicals that nurses handle in their work than is nonirritated skin.

When a nurse has an intractable hand dermatitis, patch tests should be performed with the chemicals and medications listed under housewife's eczema and under eczema in the professional group. In addition, it is of value to perform patch tests with streptomycin, penicillin and chlorpromazine.

Streptomycin. This drug is an especially important occupational hazard to nurses and a frequent cause of allergic contact sensitization.[30] The allergic dermatitis may first be noted at the tips of the thumb and the index and middle fingers where there is contact with streptomycin from a leaking syringe or needle. Prolonged contact in the sensitized individual may produce deep fissures and hyperkeratoses with superimposed eczematization. Once dermatitis has developed, several weeks of treatment may be required before the hands return to normal, even if contact with streptomycin is avoided.

For patch test purposes, a 2.5 per cent aqueous solution of streptomycin is used. In most instances, sensitized individuals show a strongly positive patch test reaction. Occasionally the reaction is negative, but a scratch test may produce an urticarial wheal within 15 minutes, which may remain for an hour or so and be replaced by a papule or vesicle after 24 to 48 hours. Although scratch testing with streptomycin is a relatively safe procedure, the intracutaneous test is hazardous and may cause a generalized urticaria and anaphylactoid shock. Desensitization to streptomycin is dangerous and usually fails.

Nurses with hand dermatitis should be tested with streptomycin, penicillin, chlorpromazine and glutaraldehyde in addition to other substances

Glutaraldehyde. This antiseptic may produce hand dermatitis in nursing, dental and medical personnel.[31]

Penicillin. Allergic sensitization to penicillin may be initiated by external contact with various forms of penicillin, and dermatitis may be produced in sensitized individuals by contact with penicillin used for injections or by cleaning syringes contaminated with it. Allergic contact sensitivity to penicillin is usually combined with the immediate anaphylactic variety. Inhalation of penicillin from powder or aerosols or molds may produce asthma and anaphylactoid shock in individuals with contact sensitivity.

Patch tests may be performed with penicillin powder, ointment (500 units per gram) or topical medications. The usual positive reaction occurs in 24 to 48 hours. In extremely sensitive individuals, however, an immediate reaction may occur within half an hour consisting of an erythematous wheal, sometimes with pseudopods.[32] A positive patch test reaction of the delayed type may be significant, because the allergic eczematous contact sensitivity is frequently accompanied by the immediate anaphylactic reaction. If there be a compelling need for penicillin in a patient who has a positive patch test reaction to it, scratch and intracutaneous tests must be performed to determine the presence or absence of the immediate type of sensitivity before systemic administration is attempted. Furthermore, systemic administration to an individual with a positive patch test reaction can produce a severe eczematous contact-type dermatitis medicamentosa, which may be widespread and disabling.

Medical personnel who have allergic contact sensitivity to penicillin often also develop the immediate anaphylactic variety as well

Nurses and others with known sensitivity to penicillin must avoid handling all preparations containing this drug. Desensitization is extremely hazardous and should be attempted with great caution.

Chlorpromazine (Thorazine). This drug is a common cause of contact dermatitis in nurses who inject it.[33] Pharmacists and others who handle chlorpromazine powder or tablets may also become sensitized.[34,35] Three types of sensitivity are seen with the phenothiazine drugs:[36]

1. The usual allergic contact eczematous variety in which the covered patch test reaction is positive.
2. A photoallergic reaction in which the covered patch reaction is negative when the drug is used alone but becomes positive when the patch test site is irradiated.
3. A photoallergic reaction in combination with an allergic eczematous contact-type sensitization in which the patch test reaction is positive with the phenothiazine derivative alone, but a stronger response is elicited if the site is irradiated with a suberythematous dose of ultraviolet rays or exposed to strong sunlight for 20 minutes.

Thorazine and other phenothiazines may produce both allergic eczematous dermatitis and persistent photoallergy

The increased sensitivity of the skin to light sometimes persists for months. The patient sensitized to chlorpromazine, therefore, should avoid exposure to sunlight for at least several weeks after recovering from the dermatitis. If exposure is unavoidable, a sunscreen should be used to protect the involved skin.

Sensitivity to chlorpromazine may cause cross-reactions with other phenothiazine drugs, such as prochloroperazine, chlorpromethazine, promazine and promethazine hydrochloride (Phenergan).

HERPETIC PARONYCHIA

Rosato et al.[37] observed 5 physicians and nurses who acquired herpetic paronychia from extensive contact with patients with herpetic stomatitis. Topical idoxuridine was successfully used in some cases.

Herpetic paronychia is an occupational hazard of medical personnel

HAND DERMATITIS IN DENTISTS

Since dentists usually work without gloves, their unprotected hands are constantly being washed and routinely subjected to contact with many primary irritants and sensitizers.[38] In dentists, it is often difficult to distinguish an allergic contact dermatitis from that caused by primary irritants. Indeed, not infrequently a combination of irritants and allergens produces the dermatitis.

The tips and volar aspects of the fingers and the palms may become dry, fissured and hyperkeratotic from exposure to both irritants and sensitizers. The fingers may become leathery, with loss of fine tactile perception. When the dorsal aspect of the fingers and hands become involved, erythema, edema and vesiculation may occur.

Patch tests are of great value not only in distinguishing between an allergic and an irritant hand dermatitis, but also in quickly pinpointing responsible allergens.

A strongly positive patch test reaction alerts the dentist to the risk of contacting even minute amounts of a material. Frequently they protest that they hardly touch or rarely use a chemical that produced a positive reaction, but it must be emphasized that a single exposure in a sensitized individual may produce a dermatitis that persists for a week or more. Even exposure once weekly may produce a chronic dermatitis. The dentist must not only avoid contact with the sensitizer but also become aware of the guises under which it may appear and the chemicals that cross-react with it.

Some causes of allergic contact dermatitis in dentists are local anesthetics (Novocain, benzocaine), acrylic monomer, antiseptics, essential oils, formaldehyde and balsam of Peru

The dentist with an intractable hand dermatitis should be tested with all the chemicals mentioned in this chapter, with the possible exception of streptomycin and chlorpromazine. Particular attention should be paid to the local anesthetics, which are major causes of allergic dermatitis in dentists. In addition, patch tests should be performed with the acrylic monomer, essential oils and quaternary ammonium compounds discussed in the following paragraphs.

Local Anesthetics. Samitz and Shmunes[39] showed that dentists use local anesthetics in two ways: (1) by injecting a "caine" compound into the buccal areas, in which case the solution may spill on the fingers holding the syringe; (2) by rubbing a solution, spray or ointment containing a "caine" onto the gums with his finger prior to the injection of the local anesthetic or for treating oral diseases.

Acrylic Monomer. In the United States, 95 per cent of dentures are made of acrylic resin by mixing the acrylic liquid monomer methyl methacrylate with polymethyl methacrylate powder. Polymerization and hardening of the resin may take place by heating or by self-curing at room temperatures. For self-curing acrylic resins, polymerization of the mixture of liquid monomer and polymethyl powder is induced with an organic peroxide and an accelerator or promoter. The self-cured resin normally contains much more residual monomer than does the heat-cured resin.

As a rule, dentures are cured by heat, but when the dentist has to repair or build up a portion of the denture, the self-curing acrylic resin is employed. In addition, self-curing acrylic material is extensively used in creating small temporary bridges, crowns and fillings.

Uncured acrylic monomer is a sensitizer; when completely polymerized, acrylic compounds no longer produce dermatitis

Acrylic monomer alone is a powerful sensitizer, but the polymer and the heat-cured resin are not.[40] Enough residual acrylic monomer is present in the self-cured portion of a denture, however, to cause reactions on the skin and the oral mucosa in sensitized individuals.

Excessive exposure of the dentist to acrylic monomer may cause not only an allergic contact eczematous reaction but also dryness and fissuring of the fingertips by a defatting action on the skin. It is, therefore, advisable for dentists with hand dermatitis to avoid direct contact with liquid acrylic monomer and self-cured dentures and acrylic teeth. Dentists with marked allergic sensitivity to the acrylic monomer, proved by strong patch test reactions, may, nevertheless, wear heat-cured acrylic dentures.

Unfortunately, rubber gloves do not afford protection against acrylic monomer. Pegum and Medhurst[41] reported on an orthopedic surgeon who developed dermatitis from acrylic materials that had penetrated surgical rubber gloves. Cases of rubber glove dermatitis with negative patch test reactions may have a similar explanation. Laboratory tests suggest that monomer does not damage rubber sufficiently to allow bacteria to penetrate gloves, but it remains possible that this could happen.

Acrylic monomer can penetrate rubber gloves

Plate 4. Allergic Hand Dermatitis in Medical and Allied Personnel

1. Orthopedic Surgeon

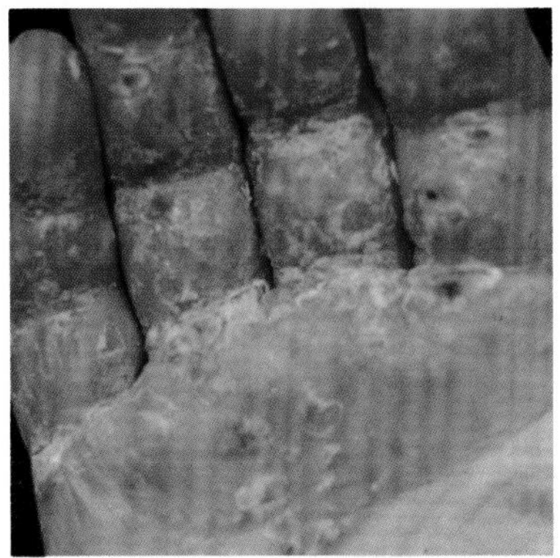

Acrylic Bone Cement

2. Dentist

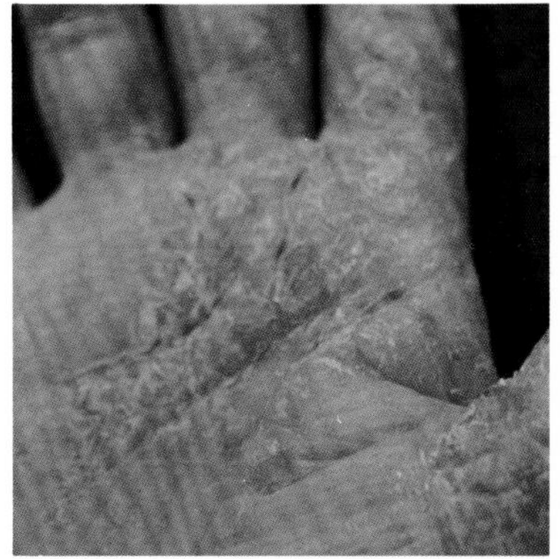

Acrylic Monomer

3. Nurse

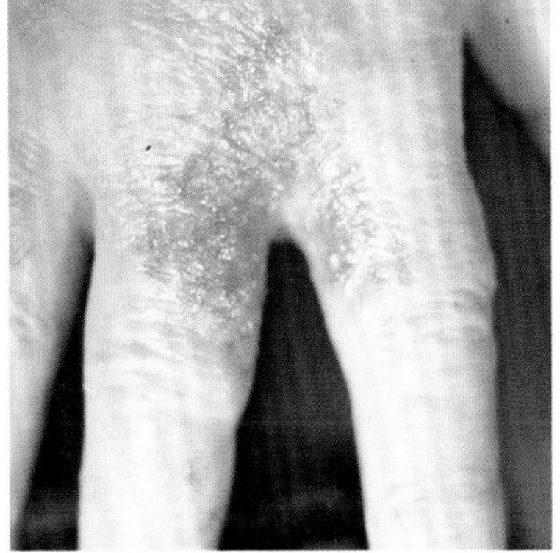

Chlorpromazine

4. Veternarian

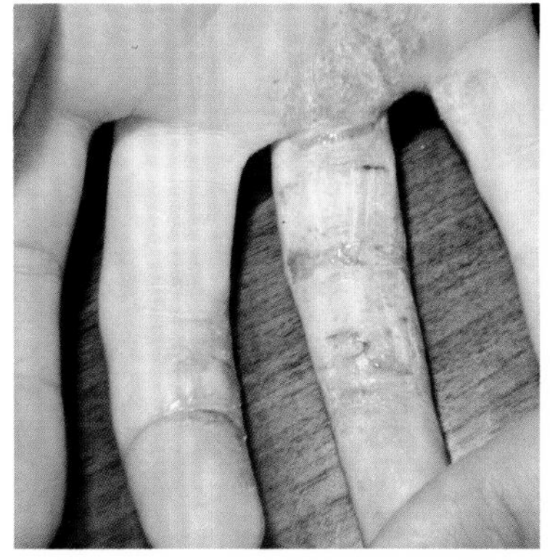

Ethylenediamine Added to Animal Feed

Acrylic resin sealers and adhesives may produce hand dermatitis in sensitized individuals.[42]

Patch Tests with Acrylic Monomer. Patch tests may be performed with 10 per cent acrylic monomer in olive oil. Since some monomers contain benzoyl peroxide (test 10 per cent in petrolatum), hydroquinone (test 2 per cent aqueous solution) or dimethyl-p-toluidine (test 2 per cent in petrolatum), patch tests with these chemicals should also be done to determine whether a positive reaction is due to the monomer or these additives.

Occasionally, pronounced patch test reactions take place in sensitized patients within a few hours. It is, therefore, advisable to test the acrylic monomer separately so that if a marked reaction occurs, the patient can remove the acrylic monomer patch without disturbing the others.

Formaldehyde. Exposure to this disinfectant occurs during sterilization of dental instruments and use for the reduction of ammoniacal silver nitrate.

Essential Oils. In dentistry, essential oils are chiefly used as pharmaceutical aids and as mild antiseptics and anodynes. Those to which the dentist is exposed and that are sensitizers include the following:

1. Eugenol. This pale-yellow liquid with a strong smell of carnation is employed in the widely used zinc oxide–eugenol dental cement. It may also be combined with rosin and zinc oxide. It is the essential chemical constituent of clove oil and is also present in cinnamon oil, perfumes, soaps and bay rum. Individuals sensitized to eugenol should avoid exposure to such products. Eugenol is both a primary irritant and a sensitizer. For patch testing, a 5 per cent solution in olive oil or petrolatum is used.

2. Clove oil. This oil is used mainly in dentistry as an anodyne. For patch tests, a 25 per cent concentration in castor oil is employed.

3. Cinnamon oil (cassia oil). This oil is an antiseptic and a flavoring agent. For testing, a 5 per cent solution in olive oil is used. Bakers may acquire hand dermatitis from cinnamon. Vermouths that are flavored with it are also possible sources.

4. Peppermint and anise oil. These oils are flavoring agents and are tested as a 25 per cent dilution in castor oil.

5. Spearmint oil. This flavoring agent is tested in a concentration of 1 per cent in alcohol.

6. Balsam of Peru. This substance is used in dentistry as a component of cement liquids. It is tested as a 10 per cent solution in petrolatum.

Essential oils, particularly eugenol, cinnamon oil and clove oil, may cross-react with balsam of Peru, benzoin, rosin and vanilla and may be present in or cross-react with perfumes in soap and toilet water.

7. Eucalyptus Oil. This oil is used mainly as a solvent for gutta percha in root canal fillings. It is tested as a 1 per cent solution in alcohol.

QUATERNARY AMMONIUM COMPOUNDS

These foaming antiseptic detergents, which include compounds such as Zephiran (benzalkonium chloride) and Phemerol (benzethonium chloride), are rare sensitizers and may be tested in a 1:1000 aqueous solution.

RINGS IN HAND DERMATITIS

Hand eczema frequently begins under a ring. In many instances when it appears on the left fourth finger, the patient changes the ring to the right hand, thereby producing a dermatitis on both hands. If a dermatitis due to rings is not properly treated, the eruption may spread onto the hand and other fingers. The irritated skin produced by a recurring ring dermatitis is subject to secondary infection and sensitization to other chemicals.

Hand eczemas may be initiated by the accumulation of irritants under rings and by the corrosive action of salt on certain rings. Smog-tarnished rings may irritate the skin

Soaps, detergents, waxes, polishes and even cosmetic creams may accumulate under the ring and cause a primary irritant dermatitis.

Whenever possible, therefore, rings should be removed when washing the hands with soaps or exposing them to detergents. Rings must be cleaned at regular intervals to remove such accumulated material.

Certain rings, especially alloys of copper and silver, can corrode readily and form primary irritants in the presence of an adequate concentration of salt.[43]

Industrial smog contains sulfides (from the burning of low grade, sulfur-laden coal and fuel oil) and other corrosive chemicals, such as phosphates, which can attack gold alloys, even when not being worn. When a tarnished ring is slipped on the finger, or a bracelet is placed on the arm, the thin film of tarnish rubs off in a black smudge and may irritate the skin. Allergic reactions to various metals may occur (see chapter on metals).

Radioactive Rings. Simon and Harly[44] reported that radiodermatitis of the fingers is produced by gold rings contaminated with gold seeds containing decayed radon. Leone[45] found that a radioactive gold ring made from improperly salvaged gold radon seeds caused a long-standing radiodermatitis.

TOBACCO SMOKE AND MATCHES IN HAND DERMATITIS

Tobacco smoke contains tar, nicotine, collidine, picoline, pyridine, ammonia salts, cyanogen, arsenic, lead and carbon monoxide.

Cormia and De Gara[46] found a vesiculobullous eruption of the hands due to sensitivity to an ingredient in tobacco smoke. Weary and Wood[47] observed a patient who had chronic dermatitis of the opposing surfaces of the index and middle fingers. Patch tests showed he reacted to the tobacco smoke residues deposited on the filter and to crude coal.

Phosphorus trisulfide in matches has been implicated as a cause of dermatitis.[48]

PAPER IN HAND DERMATITIS

Allergens in high speed duplicating papers include azo dyes, hydroquinone, aniline dyes and p-tertiary-butyl-catechol.[49] The sensitizer in typewriting paper appears to be the abietic acid in the rosin, which is a component of the size. Perfumed toilet paper was implicated by Keith et al.[50] as a cause of contact dermatitis. Paper towels may contain melamine resin to increase resistance to water. This formaldehyde resin also may produce contact dermatitis.

GENERAL MEASURES IN THE MANAGEMENT OF HAND DERMATITIS

In addition to the special measures and instructions already suggested in this chapter, most patients with contact dermatitis of the hands require anti-eczematous and antibacterial therapy and may benefit from the following:

1. Wet dressings. In the acute phase, when itching, edema and oozing are features, compresses with cold water to which crushed ice has been added are valuable, except in the presence of vascular disease of the hands, particularly Raynaud's syndrome. In the presence of infection, the addition of Burow's solution (1 tablespoonful to a pint of cold water) is indicated. In most instances, it is inadvisable to use wet potassium permanganate dressings on the hands because it produces uncomfortable drying and crusting and discoloration of the nails, which may be embarrassing to the ambulatory patient.

2. Proper cleansing. Avoid all soap in the acute stage. Gentle swabbing of the hands with olive oil is permitted for cleansing purposes. The skin does not have to be completely cleansed before each application of a topical remedy. Only scales, crusts and debris that come away easily with gentle cleansing should be removed.

3. Topical medications. Following the use of the wet dressings, topical corticosteroid medications may be applied. For ambulatory patients, creams may be used in the daytime and ointments overnight. Often ointments are more effective on the palms than are creams.

Practically all fissured, crusted hand eczemas are secondarily infected and benefit from topical treatment with corticosteroid preparations combined with broad-spectrum antibiotics. Terra-Cortril ointment is safe and efficient. I often prescribe a corticosteroid cream for the daytime and Ilotycin (erythromycin) ointment for use at night. Ilotycin ointment is a nonstaining, efficient, nonsensitizing antibiotic topical preparation in a simple petrolatum base that is free of preservatives.

Many hand eczemas are secondarily infected. These conditions and fissured and excoriated eruptions require a combination of a corticosteroid and antibiotic topical medication

4. Systemic treatment. Systemic corticosteroid therapy may be indicated when the dermatitis of the hands is severe and spreading and does not respond quickly to topical remedies. In the absence of contraindications, particularly a history of peptic ulcer, 60 mg. of prednisone or its equivalent may be given in divided doses for 2 days. The dose is gradually decreased so that by the end of the first week 30 mg. are given, 20 mg. daily are given for the second week, and 15 mg. daily during the third week of therapy. Gradual tapering prevents the rebound of the contact dermatitis that occurs when therapy is stopped too abruptly. Meanwhile, the offending contactant is sought and eliminated to prevent recurrences.

5. Treatment of fissures. Fissures of the fingers or hands may be painted with 2 per cent silver nitrate, tincture of benzoin or Arning's tincture.

6. Occlusive dressings. In the chronic phase, corticosteroid ointments covered with an occlusive dressing, such as plastic food wrap, may expedite healing. It should be avoided in individuals with an atopic background and with hyperhidrosis.

7. Protective bandages. The patient should avoid the use of Band-Aids and other adhesives directly on the skin. Light, white cotton gloves are useful to protect the hands and keep topical remedies in place. Even ordinary gauze bandages may irritate the hands. Soft, closely woven cotton or linen dressing is preferable.

8. Sedation. For the tense, pruritic, sleepless patient, 4 mg. of Periactin twice a day, or 10 mg. of Atarax 3 times daily and 25 mg. on retiring, may be prescribed for the antipruritic and sedative effects.

REFERENCES

1. Wilkinson, D. S. et al.: The Role of Contact Allergy in Hand Eczema. Trans. St. John Hosp. Derm. Soc., *56*, 19, 1970.
2. Hjorth, N.: Eczematous Allergy to Balsams. Acta Dermatovener., Suppl. 46, 1961.
3. Bjornberg, A.: *Skin Reactions to Primary Irritants in Patients With Hand Eczema.* Goteborg, Sweden, Oscar Isacson, 1968.
4. Stone, O. J., and Head, S. H.: Chronic Paronychia-Occupational Material. Arch. Environ. Health, *9*, 587, 1964.
5. Long, P. I., Jr.: Subungual Hemorrhage in Pan Washers. J.A.M.A., *168*, 1226, 1958.
6. Calnan, C. D., et al.: Hand Dermatitis in Housewives. Brit. J. Derm., *82*, 543, 1970.
7. Wilson, H. T. H.: Rubber Glove Dermatitis. Brit. Med. J., *2*, 21, 1960.
8. Sidi, E., and Arouete, J.: Sensitization to Azo Dyes and the Para Group. Presse Med., *67*, 2067, 1959.
9. Rothenberg, H. W., and Hjorth, N.: Allergy to Perfumes From Toilet Soaps and Detergents in Patients With Dermatitis. Arch. Derm., *97*, 417, 1968.
10. Fregert, S.: Sensitization to Phenylacetaldehyde. Dermatologica, *141*, 11, 1970.
11. Osmundsen, P. E.: Contact Dermatitis Due to An Optical Whitener in Washing Powders. Brit. J. Derm., *81*, 799, 1969.
12. Kahn, G.: Depigmentation Caused by Phenolic Detergent Germicides. Arch. Derm., *102*, 172, 1970.
13. Wechsler, A. L.: Soaps, Detergents and Hand Eruptions. Cutis, *6*, 525, 1970.
14. Blohm, S. G., and Lodin, A.: Eczema of the Hands in Women—"Housewives' Eczema." Acta Dermatovener., *48*, 7, 1968.
15. Suskind, R. R.: Cutaneous Effects of Soaps and Synthetic Detergents. J.A.M.A., *163*, 943, 1957.
16. Kligman, A. M., and Wooding, W. M.: A Method for the Measurement and Evaluation of Irritants on Human Skin. J. Invest. Derm., *49*, 78, 1967.
17. Wood, D. C., and Bettley, L.: The Effect of Various Detergents on Human Epidermis. Brit. J. Derm., *84*, 320, 1971.
18. Glickman, F. S., and Silvers, S. H.: Hand Eczema and Atopy in Housewives. Arch. Derm., *95*, 487, 1967.
19. Ducksbury, C. F. L., and Dave, V. K.: Contact Dermatitis in Home Help Following the Use of Enzyme Detergents. Brit. Med. J., *1*, 537, 1970.
20. Weill, H., Waddell, L. C., and Ziskind, M.: A Study of Workers Exposed to Detergent Enzymes. J.A.M.A., *217*, 425, 1971.

21. Belin, L., et al.: Enzyme Sensitization in Consumers of Enzyme-Containing Washing Powder. Lancet, *684*, 1153, 1970.
22. Mitchell, J. C.: The Skin and Food Additives. Letter to the Editor. Arch. Derm., *104*, 329, 1971.
23. Brun, R.: Eczema de contact a un antioxydant de la margarine (gallate) et changement de metier. Dermatologica, *140*, 390, 1970.
24. Burdick, K. H.: Dermatitis Involving the Dentist's Hands. J.A.M.A., *60*, 643, 1961.
25. Wasilewski, C.: Allergic Contact Dermatitis from Isopropyl Alcohol. Arch. Derm., *98*, 502, 1968.
26. Fregert, S. et al.: Alcohol Dermatitis. Arch. Derm., *49*, 493, 1969.
27. Fregert, S., et al.: Hypersensitivity to Secondary Alcohols. Acta Dermatovener., *51*, 271, 1971.
28. Hicks, R.: Ethanol, A Possible Allergen. Ann. Allergy, *26*, 64, 1968.
29. Richardson, D., et al.: Allergic Contact Dermatitis to "Alcohol" Swabs. Cutis, *5*, 1115, 1969.
30. Sidi, E., Longueville, R., and Hincky, M.: Occupational Eczema in Therapists. Springfield, Ill., Charles C Thomas, 1958, p. 196.
31. Jordan, W. P., Dahl, M. V., and Albert, H. L.: Contact Dermatitis from Glutaraldehyde. Arch. Derm., *105*, 94, 1972.
32. Blanton, W. B., and Blanton, F. M.: Unusual Penicillin Hypersensitiveness. J. Allergy, *24*, 405, 1953.
33. Calnan, C. D., Frain-Bell, W., and Cuthbert, J. W.: Occupational Dermatitis from Chlorpromazine. Trans. St. John Hosp. Derm. Soc., *48*, 49, 1962.
34. Lewis, G. M., and Sawicky, H. H.: Contact Dermatitis from Chlorpromazine. J.A.M.A., *157*, 909, 1955.
35. Goodman, D., and Cahn, M. M.: Contact Dermatitis to Phenothiazine Drugs. J. Invest. Derm., *33*, 27, 1959.
36. Epstein, S.: Allergic Photo Contact Dermatitis from Promethazine (Phenergan). Arch. Dermat. & Syph., *81*, 175, 1960.
37. Rosato, F. E., Rosato, E. F., and Plotkin, S. A.: Herpetic Paronychia. An Occupational Hazard of Medical Personnel. New Eng. J. Med., *283*, 804, 1970.
38. Paffenbarger, G. C.: Dental Materials 1956–1958: A Review. J. Amer. Dent. Assn., *60*, 601, 1960.
39. Samitz, M. H., and Shmunes, E.: Occupational Dermatoses in Dentists and Allied Personnel. Cutis, *5*, 180, 1969.
40. Fisher, A. A.: Allergic Sensitization of the Skin and Oral Mucosa to Acrylic Denture Materials, J.A.M.A., *156*, 238, 1954.
41. Pegum, J. S., and Medhurst, F. A.: Contact Dermatitis from Penetration of Rubber Gloves by Acrylic Monomer. Brit. Med. J., *2*, 141, 1971.
42. Allardice, J. T.: Dermatitis Due to an Acrylic Resin Sealer. Trans. St. John Hosp. Derm. Soc., *53*, 86, 1967.
43. Gaul, E. G.: Primary Irritation from the Action of Salt on Jewelry Alloys. Arch. Derm., *77*, 526, 1958.
44. Simon, W., and Harly, J.: Skin Reactions from Gold Jewelry Contaminated with Radon Deposit. J.A.M.A., *200*, 254, 1967.
45. Leone, R. A.: Radiodermatitis Caused by a Radioactive Gold Ring. J.A.M.A., *206*, 2113, 1968.
46. Cormia, F. E., and De Gara, P. F.: Vesiculobullous Dermatitis from Tobacco Smoke. J.A.M.A., *193*, 391, 1965.
47. Weary, P. E., and Wood, B. T.: Allergic Contact Dermatitis from Tobacco Smoke Residues. J.A.M.A., *208*, 1905, 1969.
48. D'Angelo, I.: Remarks on 15 Cases of Topical Eczema from Phosphorus Trisulphide (So-called Eczema from Matches). Arch. Ital. Derm., *35*, 277, 1968.
49. Wikstrom, K.: Allergic Contact Dermatitis Caused by Paper. Acta Dermatovener., *49*, 547, 1969.
50. Keith, L., Reich, W., and Bush, I. M.: Toilet Paper Dermatitis. J.A.M.A., *209*, 269, 1969.

6

Dermatitis and Discolorations from Metals

Nearly all commercially available metal salts are contaminated with other metals. Nickel, the chromates and mercury are the most common causes of metal dermatitis in the United States. In Europe,[1,2] cobalt is also a major cause.

Allergic sensitivity to a metal is usually highly specific and cross-sensitivity reaction with other metals is exceptional. Many reports of cross-reactions between metals are more apparent than real, because no person is exposed to a pure metal and testing is usually not done with pure metals. This is particularly the case with cobalt, nickel and chromium.[3,4]

There is a possibility that sensitization to trace metallic elements in detergents, tattoo marks, dental amalgam fillings, metallic foreign bodies and metals of osteosynthesis appliances may produce allergic metal dermatitis.[5]

Most metallic salts are contaminated with other metals. Nickel, mercury and chromium are most common causes of metal dermatitis in the United States. In Europe, cobalt is a common sensitizer. Cross-reactions between these metals are rare

Many individuals tolerate metals in the solid state and acquire allergic metal dermatitis only if the metal salts are in solution, or if they perspire. It is, therefore, not unusual for individuals who show marked allergic contact sensitivity to a chromate solution to be able to handle chrome-plated objects without difficulty. Similarly, contact with stainless steel containing nickel does not produce nickel dermatitis in the most nickel-sensitive individual, because the alloy binds the nickel so firmly that sweat cannot liberate nickel salts.

Metallic chrome or chrome-plated objects are not a hazard to chromate-sensitive individuals. Metallic nickel, nickel-plated and chrome-plated objects containing nickel readily produce dermatitis in nickel-sensitive individuals. Stainless steel is non-allergenic

PLATED METALS

So-called plated metals consist of electrodeposited metallic coatings embracing about 18 metals and alloys with widely varying physical and chemical properties.[6] The metals range in hardness from soft materials, such as lead and tin, to those as hard as nickel and chromium. Chemically, these substances range in reactivity from electronegative (anodic) metals, such as zinc and cadmium, to the relatively inert nodal metals, exemplified by gold and platinum. In color, electrodeposited coatings vary from the white of zinc, cadmium and silver, through the yellows of brass, and the greens and reds of the gold alloys, to the black of platinum black and black nickel.

Small, inexpensive metallic items, such as garter clips, zippers and other cheap fasteners, generally are simply nickel-plated. On the other hand, metallic wrist watch bands and most costume jewelry usually are flashed with bright chromium (or some other electro-deposit, e.g., gold, silver or rhodium) after nickel-plating. In general, the thin deposits of chromium and other metals over the nickel are not continuous but contain many microscopic discontinuities, sometimes referred to as pinholes or pores. The nickel in a *chrome-plated* object, for example, may come through the pinholes of the plated object after being dissolved out by sweat and produce dermatitis in individuals with allergic hypersensitivity to nickel. The extent to which the underlying nickel may be attacked by sweat will, of course, depend upon the degree of porosity of the overlying metal coating. Accordingly, one cannot assume that the underlying nickel will not come through a chrome-plated object, even though it appears not to have been worn off.

It is probable that most instances of allergic contact dermatitis from chrome-plated objects are due to the presence of nickel in such objects coming into contact with nickel-sensitive individuals.

Except for industrial plating in which the chrome coating is used because of its own unique mechanical and chemical properties, chrome-plated objects generally carry a much thicker deposit of nickel than of chromium, the ratio generally being at least 100:1. Nickel-plated objects are pinkish white, whereas chrome-plating imparts a bluish white color.

STAINLESS STEEL

The dermatologist, the allergist and often the orthopedic surgeon are concerned with stainless steel because it may contain sensitizing metals, such as chromium, nickel and occasionally cobalt.

Stainless steel is an iron-based alloy containing at least 12 per cent chromium. Basically, the chromium content imparts the stainless property. The addition of nickel is said to create a hard, smooth surface, which increases resistance to corrosion, wear and abrasion. Some stainless steels contain as much as 26 per cent chromium; others contain as much as 37 per cent nickel.

Various other ingredients may be added, such as molybdenum, magnesium, silicon, carbon, phosphorus, cobalt and sulfur. The molybdenum helps prevent pitting by body chlorides.

The term *solid solution* as applied to stainless steel means that an element is dispersed homogeneously and is not a separate phase, such as a precipitant.

When stainless steel is manufactured, all the metals are contained in a solution at a temperature of 2400° C. As it cools, a crystalline lattice is formed, which *locks in* the various metals.

Stainless steel is basically an iron-chromium solid solution alloy with nickel and other ingredients added to increase resistance to corrosion and pitting

Corroded steel may show pit marks, which are produced by acids and sodium chloride. Even though sodium chloride produces *grains* of stainless steel, the lattice framework is preserved with the metals locked into it.

Rust may be formed when there is high humidity in the presence of salt, and chromic oxide may be formed, but its role in chrome sensitivity has not been established.

ORTHODONTIC STAINLESS STEEL

Stainless steel is better than alloys of precious metals for orthodontic purposes because it has complete resistance to corrosion in the mouth. Stainless steel is now used extensively for bands and almost universally for arch wires.[6]

In Russia and other Iron Curtain countries, stainless steel dentures containing 18 per cent chromium and 8 per cent nickel are still being used. According to the London International Nickel Company Research Department, allergic reactions to such dentures have not been reported.

STAINLESS STEEL SUTURES

Several nickel-sensitive individuals have had stainless steel sutures inserted for surgical procedures without reacting. Ethicon stainless steel sutures contain approximately 10 per cent nickel. Dr. J. P. Jones, Director of Medical Affairs of Ethicon, Inc., has informed me that no allergic reactions relating to stainless steel sutures have been referred to him since 1961.

DERMATITIS FROM METALLIC SURGICAL IMPLANTS (PROSTHETIC METALS)

Many metallic foreign bodies, such as screws, bolts, splints, bullets and shells, which are alloys containing nickel and chromium, have been reported to cause sensitization and dermatitis. The removal of such orthopedic appliances or military missiles has resulted in the clearing of dermatitis in nickel-sensitive individuals.[5] The findings of such reports, however, do not always prove that the dermatitis was due to an allergic reaction.

Table 6–1 lists currently used metallic implant materials.

When employed as implants, these alloys are exposed to tissue fluid, which resembles dilute sea water and can cause corrosion.

Table 6–2 gives the composition of Hank's solution, which is a physiologic salt solution designed to simulate the body fluids to which the metallic implants are exposed.

Investigations are in progress to determine whether prolonged immersion of stainless steel objects in such a solution will leach out nickel or chromium, which can produce dermatitis in chromate- or nickel-sensitive individuals. Thus far there is no evidence that corroded stainless steel is a hazard to patients sensitized to various metals.

Table 6-1. Metallic Implant Materials

Stainless steel. The most commonly employed implant material is made of this product.
Vitallium. This is a cobalt-chromium-molybdenum alloy that is free of nickel.
Titanium
Tantalum
Zirconium
Ticonium. This alloy contains nickel, cobalt, chromium, beryllium and molybdenum.
Elgiloy. This complex cobalt-based alloy has been used in the repair of heart valves.

Table 6-2. Hank's Solution

	(%)
$NaCl$	8.00
$CaCl_2$	0.14
KCl	0.40
$NaHCO_3$	0.35
$MgCl_2 6H_2O$	0.10
Na_2HPO_4	0.06
$MgSO_4 \cdot 7H_2O$	0.06
NaH_2PO_4	0.10
Glucose	1.00

Corrosion of a metallic implant may result in nickel along with chromium leaving the implant and entering the tissues as ions or as corrosion products. The nickel, however, does not seem to be *selectively* leached from stainless steel in any environment and is probably still in combination with the chromium within the lattice framework.

When a metallic foreign body corrodes, the corrosion products may produce inflammation of the surgical site, and an irritancy or sensitization dermatitis may develop.

Removal of a metallic object from the tissues with subsequent clearing of a related dermatitis is no proof that the dermatitis was due to allergy.

The clearing of a dermatitis subsequent to the removal of a metallic foreign body is not proof that the eruption was allergic in nature

The following criteria should be fulfilled in order to prove that a nickel-containing metallic implant produced an allergic nickel dermatitis:

1. The patient has a strongly positive patch test reaction to nickel.
2. The corroded metal implant gives a positive reaction to dimethylglyoxime, proving that nickel was leached from the alloy and has become available to produce an allergic reaction.

3. The corroded stainless steel object causes a positive patch test reaction while the noncorroded steel does not.

Brettle,[7] who has surveyed the literature on surgical implants, has informed me that he is unaware of allergic reactions to stainless steel implants that fulfill these criteria.

Nickel-sensitive individuals tolerate contact with stainless steel objects containing nickel without difficulty, because the nickel is so firmly bound in the alloy that it is not available to produce allergic reactions or give a positive dimethylglyoxime test

Investigations are under way to determine whether corroded stainless steel implants yield enough nickel to give a positive dimethylglyoxime test.

METALS IN COINS

Coins contain other metals beside the metal from which they take their names.

The Coinage Act, passed July 23, 1965, changed the composition of the dime, quarter and half dollar. These denominations formerly contained 90 per cent silver and 10 per cent copper. All silver was eliminated from the dime and quarter and the percentage substantially reduced in the half dollar.

The dime and quarter are manufactured from strips composed of three layers of metal bonded together and rolled to the required thickness. This is called cladding. The face is 75 per cent copper and 25 per cent nickel and the core is pure copper, which is visible on the edges of the coins.

The half dollar is also a composite coin with the silver content reduced from 90 to 40 per cent. The face contains an alloy of 800 parts silver and 200 parts copper, and the core is an alloy of silver and copper in a lesser amount.

Since 1965, "silver" coins, such as dimes and quarters, have contained only nickel and copper. The half dollar still contains a small amount of silver

For students of numismatics and handlers of old coins who may be nickel-sensitive, it is of interest that nickel is present in the following coins:[8]

1. Flying Indian Head cent series from 1856–1864.
2. Three-cent pieces issued from 1865 to 1888.
3. Five-cent nickels issued from 1866 to date, except for those issued during the years of 1942 to 1945.[8]

Coins containing nickel readily give a positive dimethylglyoxime test for nickel and can produce dermatitis in nickel-sensitive individuals

METAL SALTS IN COSMETICS

The following metallic salts are permitted color additives, according to the Federal Drug and Cosmetic Act regulations:

Iron oxide—brownish yellow, ochre
Chlorophyllin color complex—green
Chromium oxides—olive, bluish green
Cobalt blue—blue
Lapis lazuli—reddish blue
Ultramarine blue—reddish blue
Manganese violet—violet
Potassium ferrocyanide—yellow solution

Many metal salts, including trivalent chromium oxide, are safe color additives for cosmetics

I have encountered no instances of allergic contact dermatitis from such metallic salts in cosmetics. Even so-called hypoallergenic cosmetics may contain metallic salts. Chromium dermatitis is usually due to the dichromates, but trivalent chrome salts may also be sensitizers. Chromium oxide, a trivalent chrome salt, however, is a permitted color additive in cosmetics, but no instances of sensitization due to its presence have been reported.

METALS IN FOODS

Nickel is permitted as a catalyst for hydrogenated fats in "an amount sufficient for the purpose" (Encyclopedia of Food Chemicals, in *Food in Canada*, Toronto, McLean Hunter, Ltd., 1971). Aluminum sulfate also is permitted in canned fish, pickles, relishes and starch. Recently, mercury in fish has become a source of concern. It is possible that the recent increase in incidence of mercury sensitization may be related to the presence of mercury in seafood.

METAL SALTS IN HAIR DYES

Hair dyeing with metallic dyes is incompatible with permanent waving and coloring with the oxidation type of dyes. The great popularity of such hair treatments has noticeably curtailed the use of the metallic dyes by women. Large quantities of all types of metallic dyes, however, are still used by men. In America, the most popular metallic dyes are lead, silver and copper. Nickel is rarely used alone but may be combined with silver, iron and copper. Silver dyes in the form of a 5 per cent silver nitrate solution are still widely used at home and in beauty shops for dyeing eyebrows and lashes. Allergic reaction or argyria very rarely occurs from the use of metallic silver hair dyes. Abroad, cobalt and manganese are still fairly commonly used as hair dyes.

Metallic salts in hair dyes are not toxic on intact skin and rarely cause dermatitis

The Federal Drug and Cosmetic Act imposes no restriction on the use of metallic hair dyes, because such products are generally considered harmless to the intact skin. Metallic dyes may be absorbed through abrasions, however, and produce toxic effects. Men who use metallic color restorers on mustaches should be warned about the danger of accidental ingestion.

Allergic reactions to metallic hair dyes are extremely rare. In this sense, they are safer than the oxidation-type dyes.

Nickel, magnesium, copper, cobalt, lead, zinc, cadmium and chromium have been found in trace amounts in hair of certain individuals, most of whom patronized a barber shop. The significance, however, is not apparent.[9]

BLACK DERMOGRAPHISM

Black dermographism, the most common cause of skin discoloration from metal jewelry, literally means "black writing on the skin." The discoloration is a thin deposit of metallic powder produced by the friction of a metallic object on skin contaminated by powders or abrasives.

Black dermographism is explained on the basis of the relative hardness of powders dusted on the skin and of metals rubbing on it. (Hardness is defined as the capacity of a substance to abrade another.) By plotting common powders used in cosmetics and medications with metals used in jewlery, it is noted that zinc oxide and pumice are harder than nickel, iron, platinum, silver, gold, copper and tin. Carbon is the hardest of all and is abundant in urban and industrial dust. Carbon is dirtying in itself and adds to the discoloration of metals by abrading them. In general, any powder listed in Table 6–3 will abrade any metal on the scale below it, and the effect will be streaks of color in the pattern of the friction.[10]

Only stainless steel and chromium are harder than cosmetic powders and other make-up, and black dermographism cannot be produced with jewelry made of these cheaper metals. Often the more expensive the jewelry and the more precious the metal, the more discoloration produced by make-up. Twenty-four karat (pure) gold and platinum readily produce black dermographism.

Calamine lotion, face powders containing zinc oxide, titanium dioxide and ferric oxide, and certain dentifrices (both toothpastes and powders) readily remove a fine metallic powder from jewelry and other metallic objects, staining the skin black. The powder is always black, because the particles are so fine that they do not reflect light.

Putting zinc oxide powder or pancake make-up containing it or titanium dioxide on the skin and rubbing with a gold or silver ring immediately produces black lines on the skin. No such effect is obtained with zinc stearate, which is a soft powder.

Black dermographism is really a misnomer because the phenomenon is not confined to the skin and is not physiological. It is purely a *physical* phenomenon, which can readily be produced on paper or fabrics.

Table 6-3. Comparison of the Hardness of Metals and Powders

Powders	*Scale of Hardness*	*Metals*
Carbon	10	
	9.5	Chromium
	7	Steel
Zinc oxide, pumice	5.5	
	5	Nickel
	4.5	Iron
	4	Platinum
Boric acid	3	Antimony
Magnesium, bismuth	2.5	Silver, gold and copper
Kaolin, aluminum, sulfur	2	Tin
Calcium salts	1.5	Lead
Talcum, zinc stearate	1	

When an individual applies make-up to the face or body, or uses a dentifrice (containing pumice), some of the substance may lodge under rings or other jewelry worn on the neck or wrist. In order to avoid black dermographism, metallic ornaments should be removed and the skin that will be in contact with the jewelry should be cleansed with soap and water to make certain that no make-up or dentifrice remains at these sites.

Black dermographism is a physical phenomenon produced by friction of substances in cosmetics that are harder than nickel, gold or silver, which remove fine metallic particles from jewelry and other metallic objects

REACTIONS TO METAL SALTS IN TATTOOS

Allergic reactions to metal salts used for tattooing are not infrequent. *Mercury, chromium, cobalt* and *cadmium* have been reported as producing various types of reactions in tattooed areas in sensitized individuals.

The salts of tattoo metals that may have an allergic effect and the corresponding colors are as follows:

Red—mercury sulfide
Green—chromium and chromic oxide
Blue—cobalt aluminate
Yellow—cadmium

Mercury. In the form of *red cinnabar* in a tattoo, mercury may produce itching, swelling, eczematous granulomatous and sarcoid reactions in sensitized individuals. Often the red tattooed areas are quiescent for many years, and then suddenly an acute allergic reaction occurs. In one instance, the red portions of a tattoo began to itch and swell following intradermal injections of a vaccine containing thimerosal, a complex organic mercurial compound used as a preservative.[11] In another instance, I observed an itchy swelling of the red areas in an individual who ingested calomel (mercurous chloride) and who showed a positive patch test reaction to ammoniated mercury and Mercurochrome. A generalized eczematous eruption may result from laceration of a tattoo in a mercury-sensitive patient.[12]

Chromium. Chromium oxide powder is one of the principal green dyes used in tattooing. This powder is known as *chrome green* or *Casalic green,* and it is very stable, resistant to acids and insoluble in water, alcohol and acetone. *Guignet's green* is a closely related green pigment that contains a mixture of hydrous chromium oxides. Lowenthal[13] cited a case of persistent eczema of the extremities that did not clear until 5 green areas were excised from a tattoo on the arm.

These chrome salts are probably not the sensitizers, but it is suspected that the cause is hexavalent chrome, which is an impurity.

Apparently these chrome particles may lie latent in tattoos for 20 years or more and then suddenly produce an allergic eczematous dermatitis.

Cobalt. In the form of *cobalt blue* (*azure blue, cobaltous aluminate*), cobalt has been reported as causing a sarcoid type of allergic reaction in areas in which it was used as a light blue tattoo pigment.[14] A patch test with cobalt evoked a positive reaction, and cobalt was also demonstrated in the pathologically altered parts of the tattoo. A tattoo test with cobalt blue elicited an inflammatory tissue reaction.

Cadmium. This substance, in the form of *cadmium sulfide*, is sometimes used as a yellow pigment in tattoos, and these areas may itch and swell on exposure to sunlight. Experimental areas tattooed with cadmium sulfide showed an edematous reaction only when exposed to light of 3800, 4000 and 4500 Å wavelengths.[15] The swelling reaction to cadmium sulfide in yellow tattoos seems to be *phototoxic.* Occasionally commercial red tattoo pigment shows traces of cadmium sulfide, which may induce a photosensitive reaction after exposure to sun.[16]

In tattoos, mercury red, chrome green, cobalt blue or cadmium yellow may produce localized or generalized eczematous eruptions in sensitized individuals. Granulomatous and photosensitive reactions can also occur

Iron. The medicinal use of *ferric chloride* (*copperas*) or *Monsel's solution* (iron subsulfate), a brown and highly styptic substance, may occasionally produce permanent stain in the skin due to a deposit of iron in the cutis. For this reason, some physicians avoid the use of iron salts, particularly on the face. Allergic reaction to such salts has not been reported. In addition, rusty needles used by narcotic addicts may produce bluish tattoos from a deposit of rusty iron in the skin.

Lead Pencil Tattoos. Accidental puncture of the skin with deposition of a piece of pencil can produce a nonmetallic tattoo due to *graphite.*

GRANULOMATOUS REACTIONS TO METALS

Many metals are capable of inducing a granulomatous reaction when introduced into the skin of sensitized individuals. *Mercury, chromates* and *cobalt* in tattoos often produce sarcoid-type granulomas. *Mercury* granulomas of the skin can be caused by a broken thermometer. *Beryllium* may produce not only a localized, but also a systemic, sarcoid-type reaction.[17] Zirconium compounds, used in poison ivy medications, readily induce a granulomatous response. Silicon in powders can form granulomas in injured skin.

Intralesional injection of corticosteroids in the concentration of 5 to 10 mg. per milliliter often causes involution of such metal granulomas.

Mercury, chromium, zirconium, beryllium, cobalt and silicon can produce sarcoid-type granulomas, which may be treated with intralesional corticosteroids

METALS IN SOAP AND DETERGENTS

Several European studies stressed that nickel and chromium present in detergents are factors in the production of dermatitis, particularly hand eczemas, in individuals sensitized to these metals. Nickel was found in amounts as great as 9 mg. per kilogram in Dutch phosphate-containing detergents.[18] In order to eliminate nickel-sensitization from detergents, ethylenediamine tetraacetic acid (EDTA) was added during manufacture, because the nickel-EDTA complex has no sensitizing properties.[19] The Dutch investigators concluded that nickel in detergents plays a minor role in nickel dermatitis. A Spanish report, however, concluded that there are sufficient nickel and chromium in detergents to account for the persistence of contact dermatitis due to these metals after the more obvious contacts have been eliminated.[20]

Feuerman[21] concluded that traces of chromates in detergents and bleaching agents are the most frequent cause of contact dermatitis in housewife's eczema in Israel.

Malten and Spruit[19] estimated that the amount of nickel in detergent suds is too small to elicit a reaction, even in nickel-sensitive women, and concluded that nickel in detergents is less important than other sources of nickel as a cause of sensitivity, particularly if they contain a chelating agent, such as EDTA.

I performed the dimethylglyoxime spot test for nickel on several concentrated solutions of American detergents with negative results.

Chromic acid or chromates may be added to brushless shaving creams to prevent rusting of razor blades.

The source of nickel in American detergent compounds is the raw materials used in manufacture, and the most likely source of chromates in trace quantities (up to 5 parts per million) is principally phosphates.[22]

Reports from abroad differ greatly as to the significance of nickel and chromates in detergents. Thus far, American detergents have not been implicated in nickel or chromate sensitization or dermatitis

METALS IN TOOTH FILLINGS AND DENTURES

Dental amalgams all contain mercury and, in addition, may contain copper, silver and tin. According to the number of metals they contain, amalgams are classified as binary, tertiary, quaternary and so forth.

Metal dentures, containing chromium and nickel (rarely used at present), may produce dermatitis and stomatitis,[23] and copper used as a dental restorative has produced a lichen planus type of stomatitis.[24]

THE ACTION OF SODIUM CHLORIDE AND SWEAT ON METALS

A ring dermatitis due to primary irritation from the action of salt on jewelry alloys may be produced.[25] The sodium chloride acting on the metal may come from sweat or from table salt that has become trapped between the ring and the finger. The salt discolors and corrodes the metal, which may produce a primary irritant type of dermatitis.

In addition, a greenish black smudge due to sulfur in the sweat of some people may be produced with all types of metallic jewelry. These persons should remove rings frequently and powder their fingers with an absorbent powder that is free of zinc oxide to prevent both black dermographism and sulfide discoloration.

Sweat and table salt trapped under a ring may produce an irritant dermatitis and dissolve out nickel and gold to produce an allergic dermatitis in sensitized individuals. A high sulfur content of sweat also may corrode metal and produce a greenish sulfide smudge

A "ruster" is an individual who produces a corrosive effect by fingering a freshly polished metallic surface. It has been shown that abnormally high concentrations of chloride ion in sweat are responsible for these adverse effects.[26] Some "rusters" have been found to have cystic fibrosis of the pancreas, although no instances of dermatitis were seen. Many individuals sensitized to nickel or gold acquire contact dermatitis with such metallic objects only when they perspire freely, showing the importance of the leaching action of sweat.

The sodium chloride content of the sweat of perspiring fingers of certain individuals is high enough to corrode and rust freshly polished metallic surfaces

PATCH TESTS WITH METALS AND THEIR SALTS

Table 6–4 lists the concentrations of aqueous solutions of metal salts recommended for patch test purposes. Such solutions should be kept in dark bottles.

In performing patch tests with metal salts, one must be careful not to interpret the pustular or follicular patch test reactions as allergic responses.[27] Such reactions are not uncommon and should be considered nonspecific, primary irritant type of response.

Although some authorities use petrolatum as a vehicle for patch testing metal salts, in my experience, aqueous solutions of metal salts give more reliable patch test results.

Table 6-4. Patch Test Concentrations for Metal Salts

Nickel sulfate	5%
Potassium dichromate	0.25%
*Mercury bichloride**	0.1%
Cobalt sulfate	2%
Ferric chloride	2%
Zinc chloride	2%
Gold chloride	1%
Copper sulfate	5%
Silver nitrate†	2%
Aluminum chloride	2%
Platinum chloride	10%
Manganese chloride	2%
Sodium arsenate	10%
Zirconium oxide powder‡	As is

* This solution may produce a nonspecific irritant-type reaction, which may be confused with an allergic response. In doubtful cases, the patch test for mercury sensitivity should be controlled by testing with yellow oxide of mercury or 5 per cent ammoniated mercury.

† It is best to test this solution by the open patch test method to avoid primary irritant reaction under occlusion.

‡ Place patch over a scratched area.

NEGATIVE PATCH TEST REACTION IN SUSPECTED METAL DERMATITIS

Whenever an individual is suspected of having a metal hypersensitivity and the patch test response is negative, a careful investigation usually reveals that the patient is free of metal allergy. For example, many women are suspected of having nickel dermatitis because of an eruption in the garter area presumably due to a nickel-plated garter buckle or clasp. In several instances, a negative nickel test result was obtained, and further investigation revealed that the dermatitis was actually due to sensitivity to the rubber of the garter.

Whenever nickel sensitivity is suspected but not confirmed by a positive patch test reaction, one must make certain that some other substance is not the cause of the dermatitis.

Allergic metal dermatitis is always accompanied by positive patch test reaction to proper concentrations of the implicated metal salts

FALSE POSITIVE METAL PATCH TEST RESULTS

On several occasions I have observed that if metal salts are tested close to each other, a strong positive patch test reaction to nickel will be accompanied by false positive patch test reactions to the adjacent metal salts, particularly cobalt and copper. These same cobalt and copper salts often show a negative reaction when tested at least 6 inches from the nickel patch test site. Apparently, a strong positive nickel reaction creates a nonspecific hypersensitivity of the surrounding skin and induces false positive reactions to the other metals.

Metal salts should be tested at least 6 inches apart to avoid induction of false positive reactions adjacent to a strongly positive nickel reaction

INTRADERMAL TESTING WITH METAL SALTS

Intradermal testing with metal salts should be considered an investigative procedure at present, because there is no general agreement about its significance, advantages or disadvantages.

I have not observed individuals with allergic hypersensitivity to a metal or its salts in whom I was not able to obtain a positive patch test reaction. Furthermore, I have not encountered individuals with metal hypersensitivity in whom the intradermal test was positive and the patch test reaction negative.

This form of testing has been advocated by Epstein,[28] who emphasized the possibility of the delayed intradermal reaction in the diagnosis of eczematous allergy. Marcussen[29] compared the diagnostic value of the patch and intradermal tests with particular reference to nickel hypersensitivity and concluded that the intradermal test with nickel sulfate, 1: 10,000, appeared to be more sensitive and more specific than a patch test using 5 per cent nickel sulfate and, that, intradermal testing improves the diagnostic results in nickel allergy by approximately 14 per cent.

Marcussen, however, admitted that with nickel sulfate, 1: 10,000, and patch tests with 5 per cent nickel sulfate, there was a closer conformity than expected. He further stated that 5 nickel-sensitive patients showed a negative patch test and a positive intradermal reaction with nickel sulfate, but upon *retesting* 4 of these patients showed a positive patch test reaction.

Except for testing for sarcoid type of reactions with zirconium salts, intradermal tests with metals have no advantage over patch tests

In my own material, a positive patch test reaction to 5 per cent nickel sulfate solution was invariably strongly positive in individuals with proved allergic hypersensitivity to nickel. In my series of 50 individuals with nickel dermatitis, all showed a strongly positive patch test reaction, and 49 showed positive intradermal reactions. Only once was the intradermal test with nickel superior to the patch test.

Testing for sarcoid type of reactions to zirconium salts may be performed by rubbing the zirconium preparation into a test site prepared by multiple scratches or denuded by a dermal curet. In addition, an intracutaneous test may be performed with a 1: 10,000 solution of sodium zirconium lactate.

NICKEL DERMATITIS

Nickel is a ductile, malleable, silvery white metal that is capable of taking a high polish, which imparts durability and hardness to metal objects, particularly the precious metals and stainless steel.

Both at home and abroad, nickel is one of the most common causes of allergic contact dermatitis, particularly in women. It produces more instances of allergic dermatitis than do all the other metals combined.

Exposure. Modern civilization affords ever-increasing opportunities for the general population and industrial worker to come in contact with nickel. As one leading nickel manufacturer claims: "Nickel is with you and does things for you from the time you get up in the morning until you go to sleep at night."[30] This almost continuous exposure is reflected in the increasing number of patients who are sensitized to nickel.

In the general population, nickel dermatitis appears much more frequently in women because men usually acquire nickel sensitivity from industrial exposure. Nickel dermatitis of the earlobe is common in nickel-sensitive women and is produced by nickel in costume jewelry earrings and in gold finish earrings. Occasionally, however, earring dermatitis is due to sensitivity to gold.

The thighs formerly were a common site of nickel eruptions, but since pantyhose and nylon garter clips have been used, dermatitis of the thighs is less common.

Nickel sensitivity is the most common cause of allergic metal dermatitis, particularly in women. Outside of industry, nickel dermatitis in men is rare

Table 6–5 shows the locations and sources of nickel dermatitis on sensitized individuals in the general population.

Nickel is ubiquitous. The nickel-sensitive individual, particularly the woman, is exposed to nickel from the time she gets up until she retires

Table 6-5. Sites and Sources of Nickel Dermatitis

Location	*Nickel Source Causing Dermatitis*
Scalp	Hairpins, curlers, bobby pins
Eyelids	Eyelash curler
Earlobes	Earrings (earlobe dermatitis almost pathognomonic)
Ear canals	Insertion of metallic objects
Back of ears	Spectacle frames
Sides of nose	Nickel coin (patient rubbed nose with coin)
Sides of face	Bobby pins, curlers, dental instruments
Lips	Metal pins held in mouth, metal lipstick holder
Neck	Clasp of necklace, zipper
Upper chest	Medallions, metal identification tags
Axilla	Zipper (unilateral involvement usually)
Breast	Wire support of bra cup
Thighs	Garter clasps, metal chairs, metal coins in pockets
Palms	Handles of doors, handbags, carriages, umbrellas
Fingers	Thimbles, needles, scissors, coins, pens
Wrists	Watch bands, bracelets
Arms	Bracelets
Antecubital area	Metal handle of handbag (resembles atopic eczema)
Ankle	Bracelet
Dorsum of foot	Metallic eyelets of shoes
Plantar aspect	Metal arch support
Pubic area and vulva	Safety pin on napkin
Bullet wounds	* Nickel alloys in bullets and shrapnel
Postoperative sites	* Screws, bolts, plates in orthopedic implants

* May include alloys other than stainless steel.

Industrial Exposure. The manufacture of metal alloys, electric and telephone wiring, silver work, insecticides and fungicides, and the dyeing industry may bring the worker into contact with nickel or its salts.

Ear-Piercing in the Production of Nickel Dermatitis

Gaul[31] reported that this popular fashion has inadvertently produced an outbreak of earlobe dermatitis. An unknown number of subjects develop a generalized nickel sensitivity that persists indefinitely by having their ears pierced and then wearing nickel-containing jewelry. Injury to the skin from mechanical, physical or chemical agents followed by intimate contact with sensitizing allergens favors the development of allergic eczematous dermatitis.

Goldman[32] uses an 18 gauge needle to pierce the earlobe. Previously sterilized, flexible silver or gold wire is inserted into the bevel and inside the needle. The needle carrier is then pulled back; the wire is left in the ear for at least 10 days. Difficulties with this technique are the entangling of hair in the ends of the wire and the possibility that the silver or gold wire may contain nickel. In addition, even pure gold wire may sensitize the patient to gold.

I prefer to pierce the ears with a stainless steel needle (18 to 20 gauge) and to insert stud earrings of stainless steel, that are negative for a spot test for nickel. These earrings are left in place for 3 weeks until the channel

Many women are becoming sensitized to nickel from ear-piercing. It should be done with needles or instruments that have been negative in spot tests for nickel. For 3 weeks, until epithelialization of the puncture wound is complete, earrings giving a negative nickel spot test reaction should be worn

is completely epithelialized, at which time ordinary earrings may be inserted.

Patented ear-piercing instruments and stainless earrings are available from H & A Enterprises, 143–19 25th Avenue, Whitestone, N.Y. 11357.

The Dimethylglyoxime Spot Test for Detection of Nickel

The dimethylglyoxime (DMG) spot test for nickel was discovered by Fleigl.[33] A few drops of a 1 per cent alcoholic solution of DMG, plus a few drops of ammonia water, added to a metallic object, skin or solution will produce a strawberry red, insoluble salt in the presence of available nickel (as little as 1 : 100,000).[34]

The test enables one to determine whether metallic objects can produce dermatitis in nickel-sensitive individuals. A positive test result is obtained with most metal alloys containing nickel, with the exception of stainless steel, showing the safety of this metal for nickel-sensitive persons.

The DMG may be obtained free of charge from Westwood Pharmaceuticals, Inc., 468 Dewitt Street, Buffalo, N.Y. 14213.

The DMG spot test for nickel has detected the nickel in "gold" and other jewelry when the patient or jeweler was unaware of it. Neither DMG nor ammonia will harm jewelry or watches. The red precipitate is readily washed off with water.

The spot test also gives a positive test in black dermographism produced by a nickel-containing metallic object.

Drs. E. J. Rudner and A. H. Mehregan of the Pinkus Dermatology Laboratory, Monro, Mich., use another technique for the detection of nickel in metal. The metal is sponged with acetone and immersed in 5 ml. of 6N hydrochloric acid. It is then immersed in 5 ml. of 2 per cent dimethylglyoxime for 2 minutes. Next it is placed in 5 ml. of 6N ammonium hydroxide and blotted with filter paper. A pinkish-red color on the filter paper indicates the presence of nickel.

Dimethylglyoxime producing a red color in the presence of nickel serves as a useful clinical guide to spot available nickel in jewelry, other metallic objects and solutions and on the skin, which may produce dermatitis in nickel-sensitive individuals

The Influence of Sweating on Nickel Dermatitis

Sweating has a pronounced effect on dermatitis in nickel-sensitive individuals. In the summer, when one is perspiring freely, costume jewelry causes an itchy, prickly sensation within 15 to 20 minutes and dermatitis may appear within an hour in some women. These same individuals can wear nickel-plated objects for several hours in the winter, or when they were not perspiring, without symptoms or dermatitis. Dermatitis due to nickel-plated objects requires the chloride radical in sweat to dissolve the metallic nickel, permitting the soluble nickel salts to act.

The proof that the chloride in sweat can leach nickel from a metallic object was demonstrated by placing a nickel coin in each of 3 jars. The first contained a solution resembling sweat (0.5 per cent sodium chloride, 0.5 per cent urea and 0.17 per cent lactic acid). The second jar contained distilled water, and the third jar contained alcohol. The nickel coins were allowed to remain in the jars for 2 hours. A spot test with dimethylglyoxime was then done with the solutions remaining after the nickels were removed. Only the first jar gave a positive test for nickel.

Talcum or other absorbent powder placed under a nickel-plated object may prevent dermatitis in nickel-sensitive individuals for a short time. The powder acts both as a mechanical barrier, preventing contact of the nickel object with the skin, and as a sponge, absorbing perspiration that ordinarily would

Perspiration, pressure and friction affect the severity of nickel dermatitis in sensitized individuals

Plate 5. The Dimethylglyoxime Test for "Available" Nickel

1. Nickel in Solution

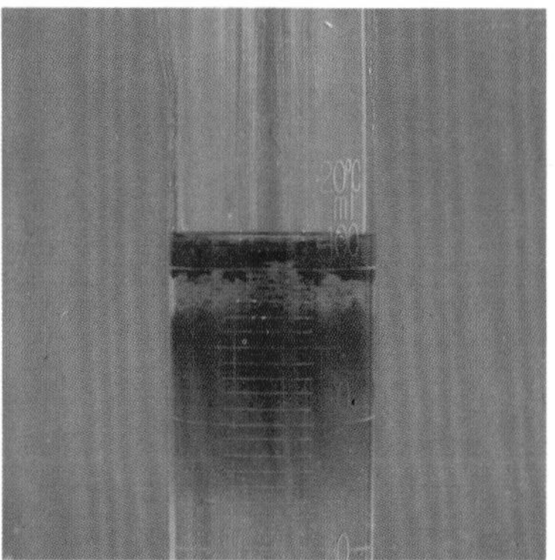

Nickel Sulfate 1 : 1000 Solution

2. Nickel in Coins

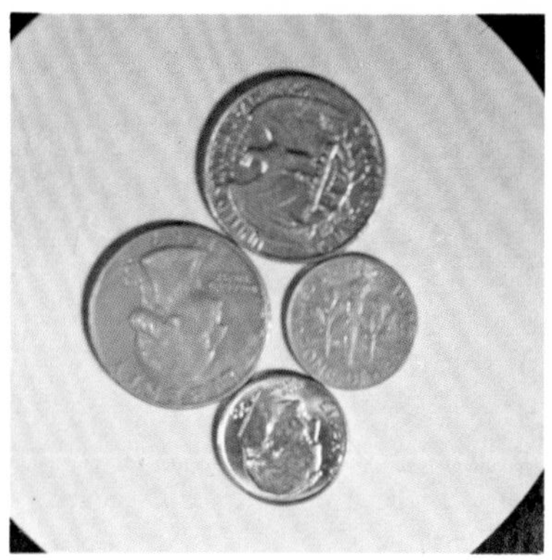

Positive in all Coins Except Pennies

3. Black Dermographism

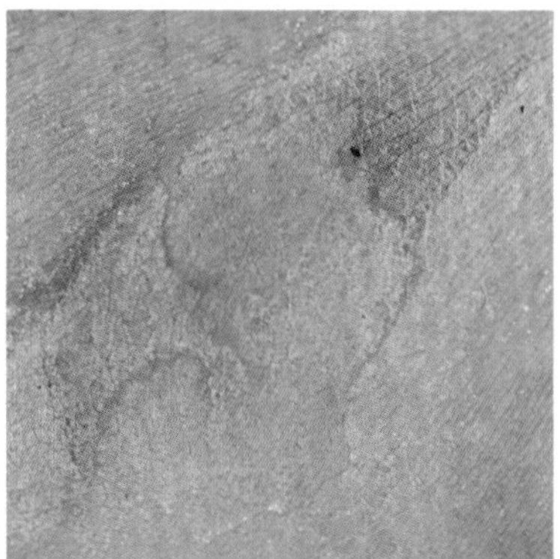

Positive if Produced by a Nickel-plated Object

4. Nickel Patch Test Site

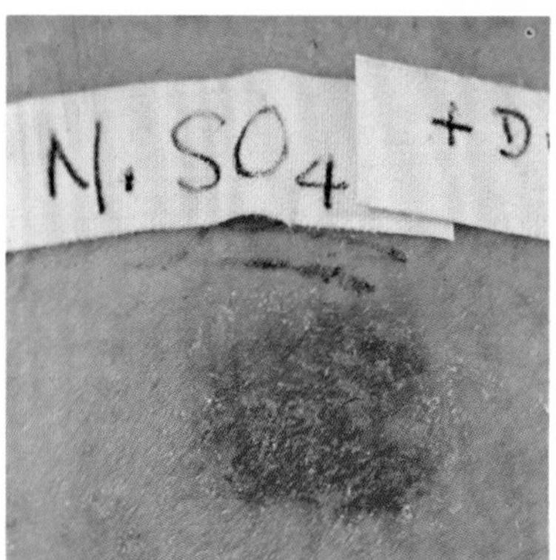

Positive After 1 Week after Removal of Patch

5. Stainless Steel Watch with Nickel-plated Back

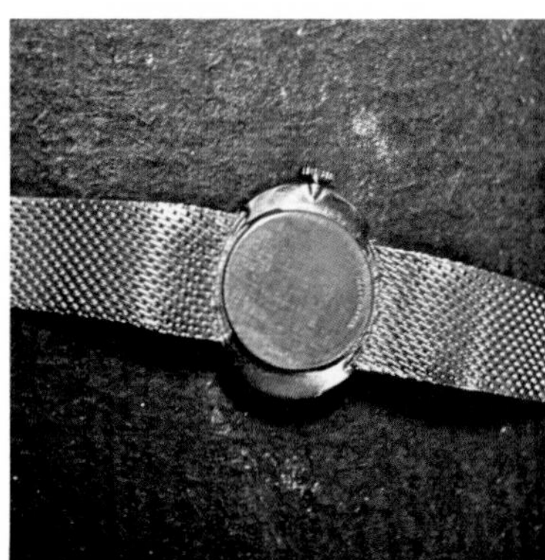

Positive to Nickel-plated Back; Negative to Stainless Steel

→ Produced

6. Nickel Wrist Dermatitis

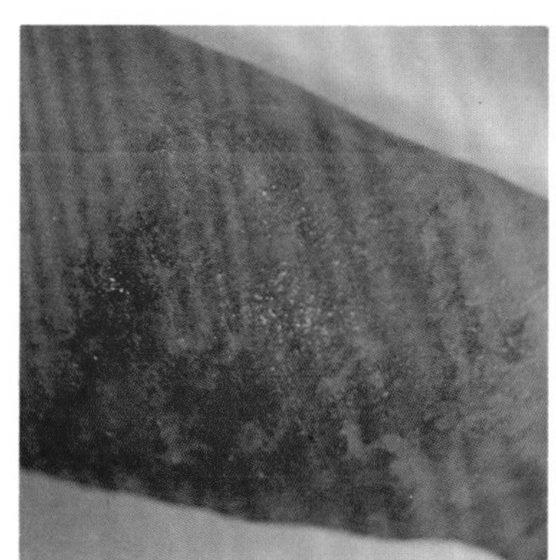

From Nickel-plated Portion of Watch

dissolve and remove soluble nickel salts from the metallic objects.

Pressure in Nickel Dermatitis

Many nickel-sensitive individuals have observed that wearing nickel-containing objects in a loose fashion prevents or minimizes nickel dermatitis. Loss of weight and avoidance of leg-crossing with resultant lessening of pressure on garter clasps may prevent dermatitis of the thighs.

Protective Measures and Substitutes in Nickel-Sensitive Patients

Nickel-sensitive individuals resort to many schemes to avoid contact with nickel. Nickel-sensitive women may substitute gold or silver jewelry for the nickel-plated variety. Many patients coat their offending earrings with clear nail lacquer. Unfortunately, sensitization to the clear lacquer occurs frequently. Some people cover the nickel-plated portion of jewelry with adhesive or cellophane tape, but in warm weather, the adhesive tends to slip off and cause a sticky mess.

Many women cover metallic garter clasps with cloth. Certain undergarments have clasps covered with a plastic paint that do not produce dermatitis unless the paint chips off. I instruct nickel-sensitive women to purchase garter clasps made of nylon (Delrin), such as Trolley Garter Grips.

To prevent dermatitis from metallic eyeglass frames, plastic sleeves have proved satisfactory. Spectacle frames made of plastic materials are readily available; most are made of cellulose acetate or nitrate and rarely cause dermatitis.

Polyurethane coating of metallic objects has been used to prevent nickel dermatitis.[35] This technique requires abrasion of shiny metallic surfaces. The Flecto Company, Inc., Oakland, Calif., supplied the polyurethane coating material (Varathane) for this study.

Prophylactic Corticosteroid Aerosol Sprays in Nickel-Sensitive Individuals

Nickel-sensitive people may obtain protection by use of Decadron Topical Aerosol or Kenalog Aerosol Sprays, which contain corticosteroids as active ingredients. The inactive ingredients include, respectively, isopropyl myristate and isopropyl palmitate, which are synthetic fatty alcohols that form residual films when the Freon in the spray has evaporated. These films are an important protective factor, because only corticosteroid sprays that contain the myristate or the palmitate prevent nickel dermatitis in sensitized individuals.[36]

To prevent an allergic contact nickel dermatitis from earrings, the patient may spray the earlobe and metallic part of the earring twice, at 5-minute intervals, with Decadron or Kenalog Spray. This enables the nickel-sensitive woman to wear her favorite jewelry for several hours in cool weather without acquiring dermatitis. In warm humid weather, the procedure should be repeated every 4 hours. This technique will protect the nickel-sensitive patient from dermatitis due to nickel-plated costume jewelry, garter clips, zippers and many other objects, including batteries in hearing aids.

Optimal Concentration of Nickel Sulfate for Skin Testing

A 5 per cent nickel sulfate solution indicates sensitivity to nickel. Sulzberger[37] stated that a 2 to 5 per cent nickel sulfate solution causes no reaction in normal skin and no positive eczematous response unless the patient is sensitive to nickel. This was borne out by testing 10 patients who were sensitive to nickel and 10 control patients with 5 per cent nickel sulfate. All 10 of the sensitive patients reacted strongly to 5 per cent nickel sulfate. Eight reacted moderately to 2 per cent and even 1 per cent nickel sulfate solution, not only with positive patch test reactions, but also with flare-ups at the site of previous manifestations of nickel dermatitis. Two of these 10 patients, however, reacted so mildly to 2 per cent nickel sulfate solution that one could not be certain of the reaction.

This impression tends to confirm that of Lowenthal,[38] who stated that nickel-sensitive skin appears to react to 2 to 5 per cent nickel sulfate but to no weaker solutions. I recommend the use of 5 per cent nickel sulfate solution for routine testing.*

Morgan[39] found that 8 British patients with positive reactions to nickel sulfate reacted severely to simultaneous patch testing with English "silver" coins that contained an alloy of cupronickel. Similarly, 10 patients who were sensitive to nickel showed a true allergic eczematous reaction to contact with American nickel coins, which are also essentially a cupronickel alloy.

I found that patch testing with nickel coins is a reliable method of ascertaining sensitivity to nickel, provided the World War II nickels are not used, and that nonspecific pressure effects and papular, pustular reactions are not confused with true allergic eczematous reactions. Testing with coins often results in inflammatory spot reaction because of irregularity and spurs, especially along the borders of the coins. In addition, one must not confuse nonspecific follicular, miliaria-type reaction to a coin. A true allergic reaction is invariably accompanied by itching, erythema, papules and small vesicles.

Patch testing with nickel coins, however, is not only a convenient and reliable method of detecting sensitivity to nickel but also of considerable educational value to the patient.

Nickel coins can be used for patch test purposes, provided "nickel-free" World War II nickels are not employed

I patch tested 20 nickel-sensitive individuals with nickel coins in the usual fashion and left them in place for 48 hours. All patients developed erythema, edema and fine vesiculation and complained of severe itching. This was in contrast to effects of a control metal disc that was free of nickel. Coins and discs may produce pressure effects and occlusive lesions resembling miliaria, which are nonspecific and do not itch.

During World War II, some nickels were made of silver, copper and manganese instead of nickel. Patch testing with such nickels, of course, would have no significance as far as sensitivity to nickel is concerned. These coins were not minted after December 31, 1945.

Nickel dermatitis of the hands from normal handling of nickel coins rarely occurs because of inadequate exposure and the protection of the thick horny layer of the palm. I have observed two patients, however, with nickel dermatitis of the fingers due to unusual circumstances. One patient habitually carried coins in the finger portion of her glove; the other rubbed her nose with coins, producing dermatitis not only of the fingers but also of the side of the nose that resembled seborrheic eczema. Both sites cleared promptly when contact with nickel coins was avoided. In none of the other cases of hand dermatitis in nickel-sensitive patients were nickel coins implicated.

Adequate exposure to coins containing nickel can cause dermatitis of hands in sensitized individuals

The thick, horny layer of the palmar aspect of the hands and fingers undoubtedly prevents many cases of dermatitis due to nickel coins at these sites. Prolonged contact, however, with pressure, such as pushing a baby carriage with a nickel-plated handle bar, can produce nickel dermatitis in sensitized women. Experimentally, when nickel coins were kept on the palms under occlusion for 24 hours, allergic dermatitis did occur in 2 nickel-sensitive individuals that I tested.

Nickel Alloys

Metallic nickel encountered by the general public is usually combined with other metals, such as iron, brass, bronze, aluminum, molybdenum, cobalt, titanium, chromium and gold. Even 18 karat gold may contain as much as 20 per cent nickel.

* It is recommended that nickel sulfate solution *certified* to be free of cobalt and other metals be used for patch tests. (Actually, even the "certified cobalt-free" nickel solution contains traces of cobalt.)

Although many investigators use nickel in petrolatum for patch test purposes, it has been my experience that an aqueous solution of nickel is more reliable.

Nickel alloys, with the exception of the stainless steel variety, can produce dermatitis in nickel-sensitive individuals

Table 6–6 is a list of nickel-containing alloys. With the exception of stainless steel, all of them can cause nickel dermatitis in sensitized persons.

Table 6-6. Nickel-Containing Alloys

Allegheny metal
Alnico
Chromel
Coin alloys
Constantan
Duralumin
Enduro metal
German silver (contains copper, zinc and nickel, but no silver)
Hastelloy (a type of stainless steel)
Illium
Invar (a type of stainless steel)
Manganin
Monel metal
Nichrome
Nobilium
Permalloy
Platenite
Stainless steel
Ticonium
Vitallium

Nickel is present in many alloys, including white and yellow gold. Dimethylglyoxime readily spots alloys that can produce nickel dermatitis

Cross-Reactions Between Nickel and Other Metals

This is a controversial subject. Hilt[40] stated that observations of cross-sensitization between chromium and nickel seem to indicate hypersensitivity to a chemical family. Gaul[41] cited 8 patients who were sensitive to chromate and also to nickel and other metals. All *commercial* nickel contains cobalt as a contaminant, because these metals cannot be completely separated at a reasonable cost.[42]

In my series, none of the 40 patients who were sensitive to nickel reacted to either 0.25 per cent potassium dichromate or 5 per cent copper sulfate solution, and only 2 reacted to cobalt. In other words, my nickel-sensitive patients showed a consistent specificity and cross-reacted only rarely with any other metal. In addition to testing my 40 patients with 2 per cent cobaltous sulfate that was certified to be *free from nickel*, I tested 10 of them with pure cobalt metallic powder. All results were negative. Furthermore, neither of the 2 patients who were sensitive to cobalt was sensitive to 5 per cent nickel sulfate solution.

Pirila and Forstrom[43] agree that there is no true cross-sensitivity between cobalt and nickel. They stated that the once common combined sensitivity to cobalt and nickel was due to two independent primary sensitivities possibly due to the cobalt salts that previously were added as brighteners for nickel-plating. Now cobalt has been replaced by argaine brighteners.

Recent investigations confirm that nickel as a rule does not cross-react with other metals, not even with cobalt

Spread of Nickel Dermatitis

Calnan[44] has referred to puzzling features of nickel dermatitis and has classified it into 3 groups: primary—areas in direct contact with the metal; secondary—selective symmetrical areas that are involved when the dermatitis spreads; and associated—areas of dermatitis that appear to have no relationship to the nickel sensitivity.

The secondary eruption behaves like an autosensitization hematogenous spread similar to an id phenomenon. It is usually symmetrical and is related to the activity of the primary site. The secondary site may be the elbow flexure, eyelids, sides of the neck and face. Sometimes the eruption becomes generalized, and at other times it may be manifested as a noneczematous dermatitis, such as erythema multiforme, urticaria or prurigo.

In my opinion, however, the spread of nickel dermatitis to distant areas without contact with nickel may be more apparent than real. A careful history or testing with dimethylglyoxime may reveal that nickel *did* contact all the affected areas.

Dimethylglyoxime proves the presence of nickel in black dermographism, on perspiring fingers and during the initial phases of nickel dermatitis. Use dimethylglyoxime with caution in acute dermatitis because the ammonia stings

Nickel-plated objects in wearing apparel may have a wide range of excursion on the skin. Bracelets and other nickel-plated trinkets may move from wrist to elbow and contact the chest and abdomen if not removed when the patient undresses or bathes. Moreover, wandering, perspiring fingers may convey nickel in solution from metallic objects to distant sites.

So-called secondary areas of nickel dermatitis, which apparently appear without contact with nickel, often actually have been exposed to nickel by wandering nickel objects or perspiring fingers contaminated with nickel

Both Epstein[28] and Calnan[44] have stated that nickel dermatitis is peculiar in that it does not necessarily appear at all sites of contact, but I do not think this is necessarily peculiar. Since certain areas of the skin may perspire more than others, not all areas contacting metal will necessarily dissolve out nickel salt in the same concentrations. Nickel-plated objects contacting relatively dry areas of skin may not produce dermatitis in nickel-sensitive individuals.

Adequate pressure and friction are also necessary to produce nickel dermatitis, because it develops in areas in most intimate contact with nickel. When pressure is avoided, dermatitis may not occur, even in patients with marked hypersensitivity to nickel.

Stoddart[45] has suggested that the infinitesimal amount of nickel dissolved from an infusion needle or a nickel-plated filter may cause transfusion reactions. Such an occurrence could theoretically be caused by nickel-plated needles but not by the usual stainless steel variety. One patient was reported to have developed dermatitis of the hands, asthma and Loeffler's syndrome associated with the inhalation of the vapors of nickel carbonyl.[46]

Management of Nickel Dermatitis

Once allergic hypersensitivity to nickel has been established, it usually lasts for many years. Attempts at desensitization with multiple graduated doses of injections with nickel salts have failed.

Certain European detergents contain sufficient amounts of nickel to maintain nickel dermatitis in sensitized individuals.[18–20] I am not aware of similar reports concerning detergents in the United States.

Patients must be taught how to avoid contact with nickel objects either through the use of proper substitutes or by means of topical Aerosol Decadron or Kenalog Spray.[36] The control of hyperhidrosis, obesity and pressure may help minimize the lesion.[47]

Nickel dermatitis tends to become readily lichenified and secondarily infected. Corticosteroid topical medication combined with an antibiotic preparation is often indicated. Thickened, persistent patches of nickel dermatitis usually respond to intralesional corticosteroid therapy.

Investigations are in progress to determine whether chelating agents, such as the salts of ethylenediamine tetraacetic acid (EDTA), can prevent nickel dermatitis. One drawback is that such salts are sensitizers that cross-react with ethylenediamine.

Chelating agents such as EDTA are being investigated for use in prevention of nickel dermatitis

Valisone Spray is efficient for the treatment of nickel dermatitis.

CHROMIUM DERMATITIS

Chromium is ubiquitous. It ranks sixth of the materials in the earth's crust. Widespread exposure to chromium compounds is therefore not surprising.

The Chemical Test for Chromates. The object is placed in hot water to extract any chromium present. The solution is acidified with diluted hydrochloric acid. Then a 1 per cent alcoholic solution of diphenyl carbazide is added. The development of a persistent red color is specific for hexavalent chromium salts. The test is sensitive to 10 parts per million.

Exposure to Chromates. Chromium compounds have been long recognized for their primary irritant corrosive effects on the skin, and for their potent skin-sensitizing properties and ability to produce allergic contact dermatitis.[48] In industrial exposure, both effects are common, but in the general population, the allergic type of dermatitis is seen almost exclusively.[49]

The public is exposed to chromate in the handling of: detergents and bleaching agents, shaving creams and lotions, chrome-tanned leather articles (particularly shoes), matchheads, certain yellow and orange paints, hide glue and chromated catgut.

Chrome-Tanned Leather Articles. Chrome tanning is used particularly for light, flexible leathers, such as shoe uppers, and leather for other wearing apparel. The chromates are the principal cause of allergic dermatitis from leather articles.

Chromates in Bleaching Agents. Javelle water (*eau de javelle*), a disinfecting and bleaching agent, is essentially a solution of sodium hypochlorite and sodium chloride. Sufficient potassium dichromate may be added as a coloring and stabilizing agent to cause dermatitis in dichromate-sensitive individuals.[50]

Chromates in Matches. Both here and abroad, some matchheads contain chromates.[51] Perspiring fingers touching unlit matches may readily dissolve chromates from matchheads. In addition, the flame and fumes from a lit match may contain considerable amounts of the chemical. After the flame has been extinguished, the charred matchhead still contains traces of chromates, and when placed in pockets, the linings may become contaminated with chromates. Book matches may similarly contaminate pockets.[52] Otitis externa may be caused by cleansing or scratching the ear canal with matches in sensitized individuals.[53]

Samitz extracted matchheads with sulfuric acid and tested the filtrate for hexavalent chromium with alcoholic diphenyl carbazide. Positive results in paper book matches were found in four out of seven domestic brands. Wood stick matches in three samples from Italy, Japan and Sweden gave positive results for the presence of dichromates.[54]

Although Samitz did not encounter any instances of chromate dermatitis from matches, it would seem advisable that individuals with allergic hypersensitivity to chromates should avoid direct contact with matches and have clothes with pockets contaminated with chromates thoroughly washed.

Hide Glues Containing Chrome. Morris has cited several instances of allergic eczematous dermatitis in chrome-sensitive individuals caused by contact with hide glues.[55] Such glues are made by detanning chrome-tanned leather scraps in acids or in lime.

Chrome Alloys. The names and ingredients of chrome alloys are listed in Table 6-7.

Table 6-7. Alloys Containing Chrome

Allegheny metal, Enduro metal	Nobilium
Chromel	Stainless steel (iron, chromium, nickel)
Duralumin	Stellite
Illium	Vitallium

Chromate dermatitis may occur in the manufacture of chrome alloys. Dermatitis that occurs from contact with the finished alloy, however, is usually due to metals other than chrome, particularly nickel.

Metallic chrome, chrome alloys and chrome-plated objects do not produce allergic dermatitis in chromate-sensitive individuals

Chromates in Detergents. Phosphate-containing detergents contain chromium salts, which may produce dermatitis in chrome-sensitive individuals.[20,21]

Brushless Shaving Cream. This is essentially a vanishing cream to which a lubricant has been added, forming an oil-in-water emulsion. Chromic acid or chromates may be added to prevent rusting of razor blades. To date I am unaware of dermatitis from this source of chromate exposure.

Chromated Catgut. Tritsch and his colleagues[56] reported an experiment with 5 chrome-sensitive individuals on whom implanted threads of chromic plain catgut produced a granulomatous inflammation with secondary involvement of the epidermis.

The general population is exposed to chromates in leather, matches, glue, paint, detergents, chromic catgut, bleaches and cement

Chrome-Plated Materials. These metallic objects have not been shown to cause allergic dermatitis, probably because of insolubility in sweat. This is in sharp contrast to nickel-plated objects, which are a common cause of allergic contact dermatitis. As a rule, when the metallic chromium in chrome-plated objects is suspected as the cause of allergic contact dermatitis, further investigation usually reveals that the nickel in the chrome-plated object is the culprit.

Fregert[53] suggests that chromate-sensitive patients avoid the use of metal cigarette lighters, which may be chromium-plated. It has been my experience, however, that individuals with even a high degree of hypersensitivity to chromates can handle chrome-plated objects without difficulty. Samitz has never seen allergic contact dermatitis from metallic chrome.

Industrial Exposure to Chromates. Some of the reported types of industrial chromate dermatitis include the following:

1. Automobile industry. Primer paints containing zinc chromate have caused many cases of allergic contact dermatitis among sensitized workers.[57] Hexavalent chromate used as a chromate dip to prevent corrosion of nuts and bolts used in automobile assembly has been reported as another cause.[58] Adequate rinsing of the nuts and bolts decreases the hazard.

2. Welding industry. Gases and fumes from welding, especially those from the welding of chromium steel alloys, may contain large amounts not only of chromium oxide but also of hexavalent chromium.[59] Exposure may produce allergic contact dermatitis in individuals who are sensitized to chromates. Such welders cannot continue welding, but they may undertake another job in the same workshop without subsequent recurrences of dermatitis.

Shelley[60] reported a flare of a chrome dermatitis of the palms due to the inhalation of fumes from acetylene welding by a patient with a markedly positive patch test reaction to a 0.25 per cent aqueous solution of potassium bichromate.

In industry, there is exposure to chromate in paints, welding fumes, cement, spackle compounds and anti-corrosive agents

3. Foundry industry. In addition to cement, foundry sand may be contaminated with chromates, which originate from the addition to the sand of ground, worn, chromium magnesite bricks, which are used as refractory material in the steel furnace.

4. Pulp industry. Fregert et al.[61] report sensitization to chromium and cobalt in the processing of sulfate pulp.

Cement Dermatitis and the Chromates

Cement dermatitis refers to dermatitis produced by Portland cement, which is named after the natural limestone found on the Isle of Portland, England.[62] Not only construction workers but also artists and do-it-yourself homebuilders are exposed to cement and the hazards of cement dermatitis.[63–65]

The main sensitizers in cement are the dichromates, but other metals, such as nickel and cobalt, may be present. Reports constantly appear from various countries indicating that cement continues to produce many cases of chromate dermatitis.[66] Soluble chromates have been identified in most of 25 samples of British cement.

Cement is essentially a mixture of lime and clay and may occur naturally in certain parts of the world. The best commercial cement, however, is manufactured. Calnan[67] believes that cement may be contaminated with chromium compounds during its manufacture. Soluble hexavalent chromium is apparently present in all cements and originates in the kiln by oxidation from trivalent chromium present in the cement slurry and raw materials.[68] Traces of chromates may also get into cement from the wear of machine parts. In some factories, huge chromium balls are used for crushing stones to be used in cement.

Many workers, including masons, tile setters and cement workers who develop cement dermatitis show positive patch test reactions to potassium dichromate. Not infrequently such dermatitis is persistent and tends to become widespread.

In addition to specific dichromate dermatitis, cement may cause a primary irritant type of dermatitis. Cement is hygroscopic and may cause dryness and fissuring of the skin. In addition, the high alkaline content may cause a caustic action. Finally, grains of silica in cement may mechanically irritate the skin and cause dermatitis.

The varieties of cement dermatitis include allergic contact dichromate sensitivity, irritation because of hygroscopic properties, alkaline-medium injury from rough silica particles and chrome ulcers

There is great likelihood that the irritant effect and the alkaline content of cement interfere with the skin's defenses, permitting sensitization to the dichromates in cement to take place more readily.

The incidence of cement dermatitis is highest among workers handling wet cement on small building jobs. In cement factories and on large-scale building jobs, the filling of cement and the mixing and placing of the concrete are usually done mechanically, eliminating contact with cement by the workers.

Cement dermatitis is often a primary irritant dermatitis complicated by a secondary allergic contact sensitivity to hexavalent chromates. Not infrequently individuals develop cement dermatitis after having worked with cement for many years without difficulty.

Cement as ordinarily used is a primary irritant under a patch test. When diluted enough to avoid a primary irritant effect, the chromium concentration may be so reduced that a positive patch test reaction will not be obtained, even if the patient has been sensitized to chromates. It therefore seems advisable to test with dichromate directly when chromate sensitivity is suspected in an individual handling cement.

In addition to chromium, Finnish cement has been reported as containing *cobalt* and *nickel*.[69] Hypersensitivity to cobalt and nickel may produce cement eczema under such circumstances.[70] Patch tests, therefore, should be performed in suspected cement dermatitis not only with dichromate but also with nickel and cobalt.

Protective clothing and a no-touch technique should be valuable in preventing future attacks of cement dermatitis in cement workers.

Sertoli and his colleagues[71] reported the successful use of a combination of barium hydrate, nitrate and chloride with lead acetate to inactivate and precipitate hexavalent chromium salts in cement.

Allergic cement dermatitis is usually due to the dichromate content. Rarely, nickel or cobalt is implicated

Chromium Dermatitis from Galvanized Sheets. Chromium dermatitis has been reported from chromates used on the surface of galvanized sheets (iron sheets galvanized with zinc) to prevent rusting.[72]

Railroad Industry. Sodium dichromate is added to diesel locomotive radiator fluids as an antioxidant to prevent rusting of radiators and pipelines. Since many workers acquired dichromate dermatitis from this source in the past, various substitute antioxidants, such as borates and nitrates, have been unsuccessfully tried. The chromates, therefore, continue to be added to diesel oil in the United States.[73]

Building Repair Industry. Spackle compounds, which are plaster-like mixtures used to repair defects in walls, contain chromates.[73]

Chromates in Corundum. Corundum used in glass polishing may contain chromates, which are capable of producing dermatitis in sensitized individuals.[74]

In men, the chromates are the most frequent industrial sensitizers, the commonest source being cement in the building industry

Other Industrial Exposures. The occupations in which workers are exposed to chromium compounds are listed in Table 6–8.

Clinical Features of Allergic Eruptions Due to Chromates. Such eruptions tend to be insidious and persistent and have a tendency to relapse. Although the eruption may at times be acute and show oozing, there is a greater tendency to dryness, fissuring and lichenification. Chromate eruptions may mimic nummular eczema, atopic dermatitis, neurodermatitis, dry forms of dermatophytosis, and primary irritant reactions. Widespread chromate dermatitis may resemble ragweed dermatitis. When there is much lichenification, lymphoblastomas of the skin may have to be differentiated from chromate dermatitis.

Once chromate sensitivity has been established, the dermatitis tends to become more severe, more extensive and takes longer to clear with each exposure, even when there is prompt removal from contact with the chemical.

Chrome Ulcers

Chromates may have a corrosive, necrotizing effect on living tissue with the formation of ulcers, or "chromeholes."[75] Chrome ulcers on the skin and the perforation of the nasal septum are still common in workers exposed to strong chromate solutions in tanning, electroplating and chrome-producing plants.[76] Chrome ulcers generally occur on exposed areas of the body, chiefly on the hands, forearms and feet, and they develop readily at the site of insect bites and other injuries. In the presence of chrome dust or vapors, ulceration of the nasal septum often occurs.

The typical chrome ulcer is a crusted, painless lesion. Removal of the adherent crust

Table 6-8. Occupational Exposures to Chromates

Acetylene workers	Enamelers	Photoengravers
Aniline workers	Explosives (ammonia and pyroxylin) workers	Photographic workers
Artificial flower makers	Frosters (glass and pottery)	Photogravure workers
Battery (dry) makers	Furniture polishers	Pottery workers
Bleachers	Glass colorers	Railroad employees (diesel locomotives)
Blueprint makers	Glaze workers (pottery)	Stainless steel and other chrome alloy makers
Candle (colored) makers	Ink makers	Tannery (chrome) workers
Carbon printers (photography)	Linoleum workers	Textile printers
Cement makers	Lithographers	Vulcanizers
Chrome workers	Match-factory workers	Wallpaper printers
Chromium platers	Mixers (rubber)	Waterproofers (paper and textiles)
Color makers	Mordanters	Wax ornament workers
Colorers (marble)	Paint makers	Welders
Compounders (rubber)	Painters	Woodworkers (handling wood impregnated with chromated zinc chloride)
Crayon (colored) makers	Paper hangers	
Dye makers	Paper makers	
Dyers	Paper money makers	
Electroplaters	Pencil (colored) makers	
Enamel makers		

reveals a punched-out ulcer, 2 to 5 mm. in diameter, with a thickened, indurated, undermined border and a base that is covered with exudate. Ulcers of the nasal septum may be painless, but with continued exposure or trauma, the lesions may extend to the underlying tissues and become painful. These lesions usually heal with an atrophic scar in several weeks if further chrome exposure is carefully avoided. No known therapy accelerates the process.

Chrome ulcers are produced by hexavalent salts and are independent of an allergic reaction

Samitz[77] recommended that 10 per cent *ascorbic acid* in an ointment be applied to the nasal septum for the prevention of chrome ulcers in exposed individuals. In addition, he stated that prompt washing of the exposed skin with an "anti-chrome solution," such as sodium pyrosulfite, or simply with water helps to diminish the degree of ulceration.

Hexavalent chrome is ulcerogenic, but trivalent chrome is not.[50] Apparently the oxidizing properties of hexavalent chromium compounds cause denaturation of the proteins of the skin. This process continues until all the hexavalent chromium is reduced to the tivalent state.

The corrosive, necrotizing action of the chromate ion on living tissue is independent of its sensitizing properties. Perforation of the nasal septum and chrome ulcers of the skin occur in individuals who are not necessarily hypersensitive to the chromates.

Cross-Reaction Between Chromium and Other Metals

Some dichromate-sensitive individuals with cement dermatitis show reactions not only to chromium, but also to cobalt and nickel.[78] It is my opinion that these are not true cross-reactions between chromium, cobalt and nickel, but represent coincidental sensitization to these metals, all of which may be present in European cement.[69]

Patch Testing With Potassium Dichromate

The patch test should be performed with a 0.25 per cent aqueous solution of potassium dichromate. A concentration as low as 0.5 per cent may act as a primary irritant. Gaul[79] has emphasized that even a 0.25 per cent solution may give nonspecific reactions, such as a bright red or even an urticarial elevation, on irritated or recently eczematized skin. These false positive reactions usually fade in a few hours. The significant specific patch test reactions to dichromates have the following features:

1. The patch test site itches rather than burns.
2. The reaction is papulovesicular.
3. The reaction persists for at least three days.
4. The reaction tends to spread beyond the borders of the original patch test site.

Skog and Wahlberg,[80] comparing the threshold of sensitivity to chromium in distilled water, in alkaline buffer solution (pH 12) and in petrolatum, found more absorption from patch testing with chromium in alkaline solution than in the two other vehicles.

Routine patch testing for chromium dermatitis is performed with a 0.25 per cent aqueous solution of potassium dichromate. Testing with trivalent chromium and intradermal testing should be considered investigative

Role of Valence in Chromium Hypersensitivity. Chromium is bivalent, trivalent and hexavalent. Patients with hypersensitivity to chromium will react to an epicutaneous test with hexavalent chromium, e.g., potassium dichromate. In addition, many will react to intradermal trivalent chromium, e.g., chromium chloride.[62] A current explanation for the mechanisms of hypersensitivity to chromium is as follows:

1. Hexavalent chromium, a weak protein binder, readily penetrates the epidermis, whereas trivalent chromium, a strong pro-

tein binder, combines with the protein of the stratum corneum and cannot penetrate.

2. Skin reduces hexavalent chromium to trivalent chromium.
3. The reduced form of chromium then binds the skin proteins to form a complete antigen.[81]
4. The complete antigen is then processed by immunologically competent lymphocytes with the subsequent development of delayed hypersensitivity.

Jansen and Berrens[82] pointed out that hypersensitivity to bichromate (hexavalent chromium, Cr^{6+}) has been generally accepted, but not to trivalent chromium (Cr^{3+}) compounds.

The patch test is usually carried out with $K_2Cr_2O_7$ (0.05 to 1 per cent in water), and sometimes it is tested intracutaneously at dilutions of 1: 10,000 to 1: 100,000 in water.

In calculating test concentrations, some authors may have failed to take into account the large amount of water of crystallization present in certain chromium compounds; therefore, they may have tested with much lower concentrations than they thought. In addition, there may be some essential difference in the form of the Cr^{3+} ion in solutions of different chromium salts. It seems unlikely on the basis of theoretical and experimental data that the Cr^{6+} could serve as a sensitizer, because at a physiologic pH it is not bound with protein. Transformation from Cr^{6+} to Cr^{3+} takes place in the skin. The Cr^{6+}, however, is the better sensitizer because it penetrates the skin better, but once there, it may be transformed into Cr^{3+}, which apparently is bound by skin proteins to become the complete antigen.

Animal tests reflect the conflicting data. It is, therefore, of the greatest importance at this stage in the investigation to standardize the testing methods.

Management of Chromate Dermatitis

Early diagnosis of chromate dermatitis and avoidance of chromium salts are imperative if prolonged disability is to be avoided. Dermatitis due to chromium compounds has a great tendency to chronicity. One cannot depend on hardening or hyposensitization to occur.

Samitz and colleagues[73] have shown that hand towels used by workers in the printing industry, even after washing, contain enough chromates to give a positive spot test reaction. This indicates that disposable towels should be used by workers in the chromate industry.

Workers should be impressed with the importance of reporting for examination at the first appearance of an eruption. If the clinical impression of chromate sensitivity is confirmed by a positive patch test reaction, special precautionary measures, such as proper hygiene and protective clothing, are mandatory to prevent an intractable dermatitis.[83]

Patients with allergic chromate dermatitis should be cautioned to avoid contact with zinc chromate paint, cement, antirust solutions, matches, chrome glue and blueprints and should be investigated for sensitivity to items such as chrome-tanned leather shoes and gloves.[62,63]

Shelley[60] and Fregert and co-workers[61] cautioned patients to avoid chromium-plated metal objects, such as faucets, car accessories, zippers and cigarette lighters. Unless the patient is also sensitized to nickel, however, I do not feel that contact with chrome-plated objects need be avoided. I have never been able to obtain a positive patch test reaction with metallic chrome objects in chromate-sensitive individuals. Sweat apparently is unable to leach chromium salts from chrome-plated objects as it can from leather, or as it can remove soluble nickel salts from metallic nickel objects.

Patients with persistent dichromate eruptions should be checked for systemic effects, although proper precautions usually prevent involvement of internal organs.

The presenting chromate eruption is treated as any other contact type dermatitis. Since there is a great tendency to dryness, fissuring and secondary infection, a broad-spectrum topical antibiotic preparation (preferably not neomycin) often has to be employed in conjunction with antieczematous corticosteroid preparations.

Samitz[83] reported that a 10 per cent aqueous ascorbic acid solution protects chromate-sensitive workers in the printing and lithographing industry, and that the impregnation of ascorbic acid into the filters of respirators enhances protection against inhalation of chromic acid dust. The 10 per cent ascorbic acid solution significantly shortened the time required for healing of skin ulcers produced by potassium chromate in guinea pigs.

Inactivation of hexavalent chromium by ascorbic acid involves reduction to trivalent chromium and subsequent complex formation of the trivalent species.

Chromate dermatitis tends to be lichenified, fissured and persistent

MERCURIAL DERMATITIS, PIGMENTATION AND DEPIGMENTATION

Mercury is one of the oldest metals known. An unusual cutaneous side effect caused by mercury led to the origin of patch testing. In 1895, Jadassohn described a patient with acute eczematous dermatitis confined to the sites to which a gray mercurial ointment had been previously applied for treatment of pediculosis pubis. Subsequent application of the gray ointment to unaffected sites produced eczematous reactions. These observations were the first to show that contact sensitization can be induced by the simple application of a suspected substance to unaffected skin.[84]

There is widespread exposure to mercurial compounds in industry, in weed fungicidal sprays and in medications, preservatives and disinfectants. Sensitization to these compounds is not rare, and the mercuric salts, particularly, are powerful skin irritants.

Relationship of Organic and Inorganic Mercury Compounds. The organic mercurials are used as antiseptics and include Merthiolate (thimerosal), Mercurochrome (merbromin), Metaphen (nitromersol) and Mercresin (mercrocresol). The inorganic mercurials include metallic mercury, ammoniated mercury, yellow oxide of mercury and the phenylmercuric salts (acetate, nitrate, bromide and borate). Cross-reactions between metallic mercury and the organic and inorganic mercurial compounds may occur.

Metallic mercury can produce severe allergic reactions, such as dermatitis, stomatitis, encephalitis and even death. Such cases have been reported from contact with droplets of mercury from a broken thermometer.[85]

Topical sensitization to mercurials brings with it the hazard of "systemic" flares from Mercuhydrin, calomel, mercury amalgam fillings and injuries to red (cinnabar) portions of tattoos

Spilled mercury droplets can be picked up with a clean (shiny) piece of copper. A mixture of sulfur, calcium and water can also fix mercury droplets, as can an aerosol hair spray.

Systemic Mercurial Contact Dermatitis

An allergic eczematous dermatitis due to external sensitization by a mercurial compound may undergo exacerbation or be reproduced through the *systemic* administration of medication containing mercury, such as Mercuhydrin, in sensitized individuals. Such eruptions may become generalized, disabling and occasionally lead to exfoliative dermatitis.[86]

I have reported the case of a woman who had an allergic contact dermatitis of the face due to ammoniated mercury that had been applied for seborrheic dermatitis.[87] Patch testing revealed positive reactions to ammoniated mercury, Merthiolate and Mercurochrome. The patient avoided mercurials and remained well for 2 years. After ingestion of *calomel* (*mercurous chloride*) for an intestinal condition, an eczematous eruption began on the face, became markedly edematous and then became widespread. On the trunk and extremities, the eruption showed an urticarial element. In this instance, there was a cross-sensitivity reaction between several mercurials. The original sensitization had been initiated by topical application of a mercurial, and an allergic eczematous contact type of dermatitis was produced by the ingestion of a mercurial.

Flare-ups in patients sensitized to mercury can occur from unexpected sources, such as a mercury amalgam tooth filling.[88] The red areas of tattoos contain cinnabar (mercuric sulfide), and direct injury, such as a minor laceration, can produce eczematization of these areas.[12] Areas once sensitized, as from cinnabar, may be quiescent for many years, but after a sensitization reaction has been produced by a substance containing a small amount of mercury (e.g., a preservative), the tattooed site will flare.[89]

Industry uses mercury in making batteries, energy cells, flashlights, toys and radios. It appears in mercury vapor lamps for street lights and for fluorescent, germicidal and photocopying lamps

Phenylmercuric Salts (Acetate, Nitrate, Bromide and Borate)

These salts are used mainly as components of vaginal antiseptics, topical contraceptives and preservatives for biological products and cosmetics. Phenylmercuric salts are present in the following agents used for treatment of infection of the vagina and cervix: Aquacort Supprettes (Webster), Trisert Tablets (Ulmer), Nylmerate Solution and Jelly (Holland-Rantos).

Morris[90] pointed out that *phenylmercuric* salts may be used as weed killers, agricultural fungicides and industrial germicides. He stated that sensitivity to phenylmercuric salts must be considered when individuals develop eruptions of the hands or legs after spreading weed or crab-grass killers.

Merthiolate (Thimerosal)

This compound, which is *sodium ethylmercurithiosalicylate*, is used as an antiseptic and preservative in topical medicaments and vaccines. Hypersensitivity reactions may be due to either the mercurial or the thiosalicylate portion of the compound.[91,92] Furthermore, Merthiolate contains ethylenediamine, which is a potent sensitizer.[89]

Merthiolate, widely used as an antiseptic and preservative, contains not only a mercurial, but also thiosalicylic acid. Some preparations contain ethylenediamine. Patch tests should be done with all three in cases of Merthiolate sensitivity

Epstein[93] reported that 5 Merthiolate-sensitive individuals gave positive delayed tuberculin type reactions from intradermal testing with diluting fluid containing Merthiolate as a preservative. Three patients also gave positive patch test reactions to Merthiolate. These findings indicate the need for using controls whenever tests are performed with antigens that have been diluted with fluids containing preservatives.[94]

Consideration should also be given to the possibility that so-called inert ingredients of testing solutions and medications may produce anaphylactic reactions or systemic eczematous contact eruptions in sensitized patients.

Mercury Amalgams

Mercury, without being heated, unites with many metals to form combinations known as amalgams. Dermatitis from amalgams may be caused by metallic mercury or the mercury compound. Amalgams composed of zinc, tin and mercury are used as dental cements. In addition, amalgams of mercury with gold, silver or copper are used as fillings for teeth.

Fernstrom[95] reported that a woman with a strong patch test reaction to mercuric chloride and a silver mercury amalgam filling developed an eczematous reaction on two separate occasions when mercury amalgam fillings were placed in her teeth. Other investigators feel that mercury amalgam fillings can cause a sensitization of the skin.[96]

Gaul[97] investigated three individuals with epidermal sensitivity to mercury in whom silver amalgam dental fillings containing 50 per cent metallic mercury caused neither mucosal irritation nor allergic reaction.

Pigmentation and Depigmentation from Mercurials

Ammoniated mercury has been used for many years as a bleaching agent. This skin lightening substance has been marketed in many compounds. Besides contact sensitization, these medications also can cause grayish brown pigmentation, which is most prominent about the eyelids and chin. Goeckerman reported two cases 50 years ago. The reaction was described as resembling dirty skin. The pigmentation may be diffuse on the face, but the oral mucosa and gums are not involved.

Isotope studies have shown that mercury is absorbed and retained in normal skin, but to an even greater extent in eczematous skin. Electron microscopic studies show the material to be located intracellularly in nuclei, mitochondria, tonofibrils, and with membrane-bound inclusions of epidermal cells.[98]

The slate-gray or brown hyperpigmentation produced by mercury is limited to the sites of application, especially the eyelids and skin creases. Mercurial ophthalmologic ointments may cause the effects on the eyelids and orbits. Histological sections show an upper dermal pigment resembling a tattoo without inflammatory response. The deposition of mercury granules in the dermis is not the only cause of the increased pigmentation; increased melanin production is also stimulated by mercurials. The skin lightening from mercury may be due to inhibition of the enzyme system of the melanocyte.[99]

Mercury in Cosmetics

By official U.S. Government regulation, mercuric chloride and bichloride of mercury may not exceed formulation in excess of 5 and 0.2 per cent, respectively, and adequate warning must be placed on the labels of bleaching creams. Many over-the-counter cosmetic preparations still contain ammoniated mercury in concentration of 3 to 4 per cent, which can produce contact dermatitis and pigmentary changes.[100]

The mercury content of depigmentation medications for topical use is as follows:

Esoterica—3%
Stillman's Freckle Cream—4%
Nadinola Bleach Cream—4%
Peacock's Imperial Cream—3%
Golden Peacock Bleach Cream—3%
Mercolized Cream—3%
Blue Ointment—25% in petrolatum

The numerous allergic reactions and pigmentary changes caused by mercury compounds have prompted a plea for abandonment of mercury therapy.[101]

Irritating Combinations of Mercury with Iodine, Sulfur and Salicylic Acid

Ammoniated mercury and other topical mercury compounds should not be used concurrently with iodine or sulfur since strong primary irritants, such as mercury iodide or mercury sulfide, may be formed.

The combined use of ammoniated mercury and salicylic acid is usually well tolerated on the scalp, but it may irritate the glabrous skin. Irritating mercury salicylate compounds may be formed, particularly in vehicles that contain water and are not promptly used.

Patch Testing for Mercury Sensitivity

Many standard or screening patch test trays include mercuric chloride in a 0.1 per cent aqueous solution, but even this dilution may produce a mild primary irritant reaction in many individuals. Mild erythema and pustular patch test reactions are not of clinical significance. Patients with allergic reactions to bichloride of mercury also show reactions to organic and metallic mercury. Doubtful reactions to bichloride of mercury should be checked by testing with 5 per cent ammoniated mercury or 2 per cent yellow oxide of mercury. Metallic mercury may be tested 0.5 per cent in petrolatum. The phenylmercuric salts may be tested 0.05 per cent in petrolatum.

Persistence of Mercury Sensitivity

Epstein[102] reported a 30-year follow-up study of a 6-year-old girl with an explosive idiosyncrasy to mercury. The sensitivity persisted during the entire 30 years. Although her reactivity to metallic mercury, mercury amalgams, Merthiolate and Metaphen disappeared, the hypersensitivity to ammoniated mercury and to red oxide of mercury persisted. This change of sensitivity was demonstrated both clinically and on patch testing studies.

COBALT DERMATITIS

Cobalt is a silver gray, magnetic, brittle metal, which is widely used in alloys to produce blue color in porcelain, glass pottery and enamels. Probably the most common source of exposure is nickel-plated objects, which practically always contain cobalt. Nickel and cobalt are chemically so similar that it is not possible to separate these metals completely at a reasonable cost. Another source of exposure may be vitamin B_{12}.

Cobalt may be detected (in the presence of 1000 times as much nickel) by using a 1 per cent aqueous solution of 2-nitroso-1-naphthol-4-sulfonic acid at pH 7 to 8, which produces a red coloration.

Allergic cobalt dermatitis is much more common in Europe than in the United States, possibly because of the presence of cobalt in European detergents and of sufficient amounts in European cement to sensitize construction workers and those who work with clay and pottery.

Cobalt dermatitis is apparently much more common in Europe than in the United States, possibly because of the presence of cobalt in European detergents and cement

Occurrence in the General Population

In the past, some American investigators felt that cobalt approached nickel in importance as a producer of allergic contact dermatitis.[103] I recently surveyed our patch test results at the New York Skin and Cancer Unit, however, and found that positive reactions to cobalt are rare and cannot always be related to the presenting dermatitis.

One positive patch test reaction to cobalt was correlated with an allergic reaction to vitamin B_{12} in injectable Berubigen (Upjohn). (One ml. of Berubigen contains 43.4 mcg. of cobalt.) This cobalt-sensitive patient gave a positive patch reaction to 2 per cent aqueous solution of cobalt chloride and to the vitamin B solutions in the strengths of 100 and 1000 mcg. per milliliter. In addition, there were positive delayed scratch and intradermal reactions to the vitamin B_{12} solutions. The patient noted that, following each injection of vitamin B_{12}, the injected area had become red, tender and pruritic, but not eczematous. Oral ingestion of vitamin B_{12} produced similar flares in the sites of previous injections. She also has an intractable hand eczema. Although this patient initially showed no patch test reactions to nickel, the third patch test apparently sensitized her and she now shows strongly positive patch test reactions to it.

Cobalt may be employed as a food additive. The ingestion of food containing cobalt has not been reported as causing any reactions in cobalt-sensitive individuals.

Vitamin B_{12} may be a source of cobalt sensitization. Injection or ingestion of the vitamin may produce flares of dermatitis in sensitized individuals

In one reported case[104] there was a delayed tuberculin type of reaction to intradermal injection, but not to subcutaneous and intramuscular injections, of vitamin B_{12} (Cobione), a cobalt-containing compound.

Kalensky and Schwank[105] described hypersensitivity to cobalt in a cream (Perilacin) used for hyperhidrosis. Patch tests were positive to cobalt, and in one patient, vitamin B_{12} produced positive epicutaneous and intradermal test reactions.

Marcussen[106] described a cobalt-sensitive patient with a dermatitis resembling that produced by nickel. Many of his cobalt-sensitive patients did not show a hypersensitivity to nickel. He felt that cobalt hypersensitivity may be responsible for a typical clinical picture hitherto described as nickel dermatitis. Marcussen concluded that nickel and cobalt are always found together in alloys and salts and that both are sensitizers. Diagnostic patch tests, therefore, should always include *both* nickel and cobalt.

Bandmann and his co-workers[107] also felt that cobalt is not a rare allergen and that one should perform patch tests with cobalt in persons who handle cement, detergents, oils, printing ink and metals. Cobalt-sensitized individuals are primarily masons, tile workers, stonemasons, construction workers, dentists, printers, mechanics, machinists, and workers in the galvanizing industry. These investigators stated that cobalt sulfate should be included among the allergens when testing persons with eczema caused by garters.

Cobalt chloride is an ingredient of the adhesive mixture used for some flypapers and hair dyes.[108]

Cobalt in Hair Dyes. Cobalt is used with a developer to produce light brown shades of hair. First featured by Broux of Paris, cobalt nitrate is used either alone or in mixtures with silver and ammonium compounds. The developer is pyrogallol with or without other phenolic compounds and iron salts.

Nurnberger and Arnold[109] reported Quincke's edema as a manifestation of a cobalt allergy due to sensitization by cobaltous shell splinters in the arm. Injection of a cobalt-iron preparation was followed by a refractory bilateral periorbital edema. Patch testing showed a "monovalent" allergy to cobalt.

Cobalt dermatitis may result from exposure to substances containing the metal, such as hair dyes, flypaper, shell splinters, antiperspirant creams, crayons and fertilizers

Industrial Exposure. Some of the more recently described industrial exposures to cobalt include the following:

1. Industries using hard metals.[110] Cobalt is employed as a binding agent to make hard metal, which consists of metal carbides and a binding agent that are presented and sintered into plates. Wolfram carbide (a tungsten compound) and the carbides of titanium, nobilium and tantalum are frequently used.

Hard metal is characterized by a high degree wear resistance. Consequently, it is used for rock drills, cutting tools, drawing, pressing and stamping tools and also for mechanical parts exposed to heavy strain.

Hard metal may produce primary irritant dermatitis with folliculitis or a chronic lichenified eczema. In addition, allergic eczematous contact dermatitis may develop, which in most instances is due to the cobalt.

2. Polyester resin industry. Cobalt naphthenate is commonly used in the manufacture of polyester resin. Several instances of allergic contact dermatitis were encountered in Great Britain that were attributed to workers handling cobalt naphthenate in polyester synthesis.[111]

3. Paint industry. Cobalt siccatives or driers, which are present in certain paints, have been reported as producing allergic contact sensitivity in paint factory workers.[112] These are organic cobalt-naphthenate or cobalt-resinate based on linseed oil.

4. Cement industry. Although the cobalt content of cements may be low (less than 0.01 per cent), cement workers in Holland have become sensitized to cobalt.[113]

Industrial exposure to cobalt includes hard metals, polyester resins, paints, cements, pottery, ceramics, pigments, glass alloys and lubricating oils

Marcussen[106] also found two patients with cobalt hypersensitivity with coincident hypersensitivity to dichromate. Both of these cement workers had typical cement dermatitis characterized by dry, lichenified eczema of the hands, arms and feet. Since these patients had positive patch test reactions to both dichromate and cobalt, it would be difficult to determine what role the cobalt hypersensitivity played in the production of the cement dermatitis.

Camarasa[114] found that a high percentage of bricklayers in Barcelona showed hypersensitivity to both chromium and cobalt, but he noted that hypersensitivity to cobalt does not appear in patients allergic to chromium and working in other occupations. DeFonseca[115] concluded that cobalt has a higher hypersensitizing power than nickel and that sensitization to chromium augments sensitivity to cobalt.

Mueller and Breucker[116] found that in most of their 79 cobalt-sensitive patients, the most frequent cause of dermatitis was cement (29 per cent), and that when these patients showed reactions to chromium and nickel, the sensitization was due to simultaneous exposure to the three metals and not to cross-reactions.

Combined reactions to cobalt, nickel and chromium are not uncommon and do not represent cross-reactions but simultaneous, distinct and specific sensitizations

5. Carbide industry. McDermott[117] reported that cobalt is a common binding component in all grades of carbide. Pneumoconiosis and allergic sensitization from such cobalt-carbide compounds can occur.

6. Pottery workers. Dermatitis from exposure to *wet* clay containing cobalt may occur.[118] Cobalt dermatitis from *dry* clay or finished wares is relatively rare. Cobalt may be added to clay to neutralize the yellow color produced by impurities.

7. Manufacture of alloys containing cobalt. Alloys containing cobalt include: *Alnico*, *Duralumin*, *Nobilium*, *Permalloy*, *Stellite*, *Ticonium* and *Vitallium*. Allergic dermatitis in workers making alloys of cobalt has been shown by patch tests to be due in some instances to the dust of metallic cobalt.[119] The dust also has been reported as causing asthma. It is believed that a dusty atmosphere containing metallic cobalt particles favors a sensitization to cobalt.

8. Miscellaneous industries employing cobalt. Currently, cobalt is used extensively in the carbide, glass, ceramic, enamel, electrical and pigment industries.

Cross-Reactions Between Nickel and Cobalt

Birmingham[120] reported that results of patch tests with nickel and cobalt are confusing, because it is extremely difficult, if not impossible, to obtain cobalt-free nickel and nickel-free cobalt. Reports of cross-reactions between cobalt and nickel, therefore, may be attributable to tests with impure metal.

Cross-reaction between nickel and cobalt are not very frequent. In my material, patch tests revealed that most patients with allergic contact nickel sensitivity do not cross-react with the available cobalt solutions. Furthermore, several patients had strong patch test reactions to cobalt, but did not react to patch tests with a 5 per cent nickel sulfate solution. Patch testing of cobalt-sensitive patients with nickel may induce sensitization to the nickel, proving that the metals do not originally cross-react. Beikko and Forstreom[121] concluded that there is a "pseudo-cross sensitivity" between cobalt and nickel.

Intradermal Testing with Cobalt

Marcussen[122] pointed out that impure cobalt solutions complicate the interpretation of intradermal tests with cobalt chloride and that cobalt chloride, even in high dilutions, may produce nonspecific tuberculin-type reactions. Marcussen found that, in normal persons, immediate wheal reactions to cobalt chloride may be seen, and in many cases a bright red flare, sometimes flat, and sometimes papular, develops immediately or in a few hours and disappears after varying lengths of time. The pathogenesis of these immediate reactions is unknown, but he feels that a papular response to cobalt chloride 10^{-4} when read 48 to 96 hours after the injection appears to be a reliable test for cobalt allergy. Individuals with hypersensitivity to nickel give a somewhat longer reaction than do controls to the slightly impure cobalt. It is suggested that the reliability of the test would be enhanced if the cobalt chloride were 10 times purer.

It is maintained that intradermal testing with cobalt is necessary because cobalt is a potent sensitizer in very low concentrations and sensitization may be engendered, and eczematous reactions maintained, by trace elements in the patient's environment. It is claimed that hypersensitivity to cobalt may not be regularly demonstrable by the classic patch test procedure and that intradermal testing is more reliable.

The concept of dermatitis due to trace elements may explain paradoxical results, such as false negative reactions in patients with metal dermatitis, the persistence of the dermatitis when the allergen had been removed, and so-called cross-reactivity between various metals.[123]

The concept that trace elements of metals may produce allergic contact dermatitis is difficult to reconcile, however, with the fact that individuals with proved nickel dermatitis show a positive patch test reaction to a nickel coin or to a 5 per cent sulfate solution but may show a negative patch test reaction to a 1 or even a 2 per cent nickel sulfate solution.

Moreover, as Camarasa[114] noted, atopic individuals may show false positive intracutaneous reactions to metal salts. In these patients, a positive intracutaneous test with cobalt should be controlled with a patch test to the metal.

In the present state of our knowledge, a diagnosis of allergic cobalt dermatitis is justified if the patient was actually exposed to cobalt, a patch test to 2 per cent cobalt chloride is positive and an intracutaneous test with 1: 1000 cobalt chloride gives a delayed tuberculin reaction in a nonatopic person.

COPPER DERMATITIS

Copper, a common component of alloys and plating materials, may rarely be the offending agent in patients with metal dermatitis, particularly when patch testing excludes commonly involved metals, such as nickel, chromium, mercury or cobalt.[124]

The rating of allergic reactions to copper seems to be borne out because in the past decade in the Allergy Department of the New York Skin and Cancer Unit we have been able to authenticate only 3 cases of allergic reactions to metallic copper or its salts. We recently studied a patient with a combined allergic reaction to gold and copper. We agree with Epstein[125] that multiple metal allergies in one individual are due to separate and simultaneously induced sensitivities by each offending metal.

In the past, when copper salts were being used for iontophoresis for fungous infections on severely eczematized feet, no instances of dermatitis due to these salts were encountered, proving how rarely sensitization to copper occurs.

Exposure to copper salts may take place from contact with insecticides, fungicides, food processing procedures, fertilizers and mordants used in fur dyeing.[126]

D'Alibour's solution contains copper sulfate, zinc sulfate and camphor water. Concentrated solutions of copper sulfate are caustic and produce primary irritation. Copper and copper alloy in silver metallic jewelry corrode readily on the skin, and in the presence of adequate concentration of salt, a primary irritation is produced.

Copper in dental alloy has been implicated as a possible cause of oral lesions of lichen planus.[24]

Copper is ubiquitous in all United States coinage except the zinc coated steel pennies of 1943. In Saltzer's case of copper sensitivity, a penny, a nickel and a dime provoked erythema and vesiculation at the patch test site within 24 hours.[124]

Allergic reactions to copper are rare. In the presence of salt, copper corrodes readily on the skin to form a primary irritant dermatitis. Patients with marked copper hypersensitivity may react positively to a penny, nickel or dime, all of which contain copper

So-called copper itch, which is caused by a dust of copper precipitate, is probably due to the presence of arsenic in the mixture.[127]

Barranco[128] reported the case of a woman with copper sensitivity who had a persistent papulourticarial eruption until an intrauterine contraceptive device containing copper, polyethylene and barium was recovered.

DERMATITIS AND DISCOLORATION FROM GOLD

A sharp distinction should be made between metallic gold and gold salts, such as gold chloride, as far as ability to sensitize and produce allergic contact dermatitis is concerned. Kligman[129] found gold chloride to be a strong sensitizer in humans. Soluble gold salts can cause occupational dermatitis, and when gold salts were used for systemic therapy, there were frequent allergic reactions.

The statement that "Gold in jewelry is nonsensitizing,"[130] is not borne out by personal experience and by reports in the literature.[131–133] Considering the great number of individuals who are exposed to gold jewelry, however, the number of proved cases of gold sensitivity is very low, probably because of the insolubility of gold in bodily secretions.

Comaish[134] reported a case of allergic dermatitis due to gold in a ring with positive patch test reaction to gold chloride.

Exposure to gold salts may take place in porcelain, gold-plating, gilding glass and photography. Recently, gold leaf has been added to eye shadows.

Bowyer[135] emphasized that an allergic eczematous patch test reaction to gold may develop into a persistent dermal infiltrate. Shelley and Epstein[132] reported that allergic gold dermatitis may be manifested as a chronic papular eruption.

Elgart and Higdon[133] cited a case of gold sensitivity with stomatitis from a gold crown and a flare of dermatitis at sites contacted by gold jewelry.

Metallic gold in jewelry and dental appliances can readily produce allergic dermatitis and stomatitis

Allergic gold dermatitis may become papular and persistent. Patch tests for gold allergy should include gold salts because gold leaf, metallic gold, or gold scrapings may yield false negative reactions in gold-sensitive patients. Sweat, pressure and friction may be required to produce a reaction from metallic gold

Forster and Dickey[136] described a patient with a contact gold sensitivity due to a 14 karat gold ball prosthesis implanted after enucleation of an eye. For 5 years a dermatitis persisted until the prosthesis was removed. The patient had a positive patch test to copper sulfate, gold sodium thiosulfate, the gold ball and gold leaf.

Malten and Mali[137] observed 4 patients with gold contact dermatitis who showed positive patch test reactions to a 2 per cent aqueous gold trichloride solution and who recovered rapidly when gold contact was avoided. These authors theorized that, since metallic gold is corroded only by substances such as halogens or alkaline cyanides that are not present in the body, gold dermatitis is probably not based on an ordinary allergic mechanism, but on "an enzymatic interference in a biochemically deviant individual" as described by Rostenberg.[131]

Gold Ring Dermatitis

In most instances, dermatitis from a ring is due to a primary irritation from trauma, accumulated detergents or the corrosive action of salt on the ring. Allergic gold ring dermatitis does occur rarely.

A white gold ring actually contains about 58 per cent gold, 5 to 17 per cent nickel, 2 per cent zinc and the balance copper. The whiter the gold the greater the nickel content. Palladium may be present in expensive white gold. Yellow or greenish yellow gold is usually free of nickel.

The dimethylglyoxime test[33] readily detects the presence of nickel in metallic jewelry. Whenever allergic dermatitis from a gold ring is suspected, a dimethylglyoxime test, and patch tests with gold chloride, copper sulfate and nickel sulfate should be performed to determine which metal is the culprit.

White gold may contain palladium, nickel, zinc, copper or silver. The dimethylglyoxime spot test readily detects nickel in a gold ring

Gomaish's[134] case of allergic gold ring dermatitis showed that both the dermatitis and the positive gold patch reaction persisted for several months after exposure to the gold had ceased. Repeated patch tests with scrapings from the ring (18 karat) and pure gold leaf were negative at 48 and 72 hours. Patch testing with gold chloride (chloroauric acid, 2 per cent) showed a strongly positive eczematous response at 48 hours, and redness and infiltrated papules persisted at the site for over 2 months but were fading at 3 months.

Lack of reaction to ring scrapings and gold foil indicates the importance of testing with gold solutions in gold allergy.

Discoloration from Gold Rings

Black dermographism from cosmetics or dentifrices is the most common discoloration under a ring. Another source of discoloration may be skin secretions and perspiration, which contain sulfides and chlorides. These chemicals combine with the molecules of silver and copper that are usually present in a gold alloy to form black salts, such as silver chloride and copper sulfate. This reaction sometimes occurs only when a woman is pregnant, apparently because of changes in body chemistry.

In some maritime, semitropical climates the chlorides from the sea may combine with normal skin secretions to form corrosive chemicals.

Workers in rubber factories may be exposed to sulfides, which may tarnish rings. Heavy industrial smog often is thick with sulfides from the burning of low-grade, sulfur-laden coal and fuel oil or with other corrosive chemicals, such as phosphates. These air pollutants can attack gold alloys directly, even when jewelry is not being worn. When the tarnishing ring is slipped back on the finger, or a bracelet onto the arm, the thin film of tarnish rubs off in a black smudge.

Smudging or discoloration of the skin may be due to black dermographism or to chlorides and sulfides in the atmosphere or in sweat

Patch Testing for Allergic Gold Hypersensitivity

Gold foil, gold metal objects or scrapings from them may give false negative patch test reactions, but a gold salt, such as a 1 per cent aqueous solution of gold chloride, is reliable. Gold chloride, like other metal salts, may produce a pustular patch test reaction, which is not significant for an allergic response. Incidentally, gold chloride may produce gold dermatitis in photographers who use it in their work.

A 1 per cent gold trichloride or a 0.5 per cent gold sodium thiosulfate solution may also be used to test for gold sensitivity.

Testing with gold leaf gives diverse results; some gold-sensitive individuals give positive reactions, while others do not. Some patients react with gold leaf only when they perspire freely.

A positive patch test reaction to gold may persist for several months

PLATINUM DERMATITIS

In industry, soluble platinum salts, liquid platinum sprays and splashes of platinum salts have been reported as causing dermatitis and asthma.[138,139]

Metallic platinum, as used in jewelry, photography, dentistry and the chemical and electrical industries, rarely causes contact dermatitis, although dermatitis due to a platinum ring has been reported.[140] Rhodium is often used to plate white gold and platinum, and in this instance, the platinum dermatitis occurred when the rhodium plating wore off. Sometimes, if the ring is replated with rhodium, the platinum-sensitized individual can again wear the ring without difficulty. Most jewelry made of platinum is either pure platinum or 90 per cent platinum and 10 per cent iridium.

Platinosis[141] is a disease caused, not by metallic platinum, but usually by its complex salts, primarily chloroplatinates, and affects mainly workmen in platinum refining workshops. The cutaneous manifestations include pruritus, erythema, eczema and urticaria, which are usually seen on the parts of the body exposed during work.

Patch tests for platinum sensitivity may be performed with a 1 per cent chloroplatinic acid solution.

Platinum salts can produce urticaria on contact

Complex salts of platinum are not readily soluble in distilled water but solubility is improved if physiologic saline is used. These compounds dissolve in dilute hydrochloric acid, but such solutions are probably not suitable for patch testing.

PALLADIUM SENSITIVITY

Use of palladium is increasing, and it may be encountered in jewelry (in white gold alloys[140] and as a substitute for platinum) and in brazing and industrial alloys (particularly gold alloys). Palladium is also used in industrial catalysts, electrical contacts and electroplated deposits.

Munro-Ashman et al.[142] described a case of palladium sensitivity in a research worker investigating precious metals. Tests with nickel-free palladium, 0.1 and 1 per cent, were strongly positive, and a patch test with nickel sulfate was negative.

ARSENICAL CONTACT DERMATITIS

Contact dermatitis due to arsenic is rare in the general population, but not in industry. The roasting of lead, copper, gold and cobalt ores that contain arsenic exposes the worker to arsenic trioxide (white arsenic). Arsenic exposure may also take place in the manufacture of insecticides, fungicides, weed killers, poisons used for baits, glasses, enamels and alloys.

Irritant and allergic contact dermatitis may be produced. Folliculitis with secondary pyoderma and furunculosis is not uncommon. So-called "*smelters itch*," due to *arsenic trioxide*, is not uncommon among smelt workers, who may develop eczematous eruptions, folliculitis, furunculosis and ulcerative lesions on the extremities and nasal septum. Birmingham[143] described similar lesions in children exposed to arsenic trioxide in a mining community. The presence of sweat, excoriations or wounds facilitates the formation of arsenical ulcers.

A 10 per cent aqueous solution of sodium arsenate or 5 per cent arsenic trioxide in starch may be used for patch testing. Arsenic not infrequently produces nonspecific pustular patch test reactions.

CONTACT DERMATITIS DUE TO ALUMINUM SALTS

Allergic reactions to these salts appear to be extremely rare. Irritant follicular reaction from aluminum salts in antiperspirants, however, is common. Steinegeer[144] attributed unusual and transient skin lesions, which were grayish brown and blue, to air pollution from an aluminum factory.

DISCOLORATION AND DERMATITIS DUE TO IRON SALTS

Allergic contact dermatitis due to iron is apparently extremely rare. Nater[145] reported an instance of epidermal hypersensitivity to iron, but the patch test reaction may have been the nonspecific pustular variety. Baer[146] cited a metal worker with an allergic reaction to iron who had a positive (eczematous) patch test reaction.

For many years, I have used Monsel's solution, which contains ferric chloride, without encountering any allergic reactions.

Stainless steel is essentially an iron-chrome alloy.

The ferroxyl test may be used to show the presence of free iron in corroded metallic objects. The metallic article is immersed in a gel containing 1 per cent sodium chloride and 0.2 per cent ferricyanide. A positive reaction is indicated by a blue growth that resembles seaweed from the corroded metal.

ANTIMONY IRRITATION

Antimony and its compounds are used in alloys, type metal, batteries, foil, ceramics, safety matches, ant paste, textiles and medicinals (such as tartar emetic, Fuadin and antimony sulfide).

Antimony is strongly irritating to tissues, including mucous membranes. Chronic antimony poisoning is similar to chronic arsenic poisoning with symptoms of itchy skin, pustules, stomatitis and conjunctivitis.

Antimony may produce "antimony spots," an irritant folliculitis in freely perspiring workers exposed to antimony trioxide dust,[147] which is due to penetration of the dust into the sweat follicles. In addition, lichenoid and eczematous eruptions resembling atopic dermatitis may occur.[148]

Antimony trioxide may be present in fireproof packaging, and antimony pentasulfides are used in fireworks and matches.

BERYLLIUM DERMATITIS AND GRANULOMAS

Beryllium is a light metal that forms the oxide and several soluble and insoluble solutions. It is employed in the manufacture of alloys for electrical equipment and ceramics, and it is present in some phosphors used in cathode ray tubes and a few fluorescent lights. Soluble beryllium salts are easily hydrolyzed, with the formation of the free acid, causing severe irritations of the skin with papulovesicular eczematoid, weeping and itchy lesions. When particles penetrate the skin, ulcers and necrosis may occur.

Skin granulomas and ulcers should be excised surgically. Beryllium dermatitis should be treated with wet dressings and parenteral or oral antibiotics to prevent infections. Steroid therapy (adrenocorticotropic hormone [ACTH] or cortisone) is helpful in decreasing the hypersensitive reaction to beryllium and as an anti-inflammatory agent in the treatment of the chemical pneumonitis.

Curtis[149] reported 13 cases of beryllium dermatitis among workers in 2 beryllium extraction plants near Cleveland. The criteria for establishing the dermatitis as an allergic eczematous type were fulfilled. Pure beryllium metal is insoluble with respect to the skin and sweat and cannot be used per se for patch testing. Consequently, anions, acidity and primary irritancy of the soluble beryllium compounds were eliminated as direct factors in causing clinical dermatitis. Beryllium fluoride sensitizes the skin to a high degree, which accounts for the high incidence of dermatitis among these workers in the fluoride process of beryllium extraction. Beryllium sulfate and beryllium chloride have less capacity to sensitize the skin, and beryllium nitrate has little or none, according to these experiments.

For patch tests, a 1 or 2 per cent unbuffered solution of beryllium fluoride, beryllium sulfate, beryllium chloride, beryllium nitrate, beryllium ammonium fluoride, or beryllium benzenesulfonate is suitable.

When beryllium phosphors were widely used in fluorescent tubes, many instances of beryllium granulomas occurred after people had received cuts from the broken tubes.[150–152]

Surgical excision was the only cure for beryllium granuloma before ACTH or corticosteroid was found to bring about improvement.[153,154]

I reported the complete resolution of a beryllium granuloma following injury with a fluorescent tube by the use of 5 per cent cortisone in Aquaphor.[155]

In Europe, as late as 1967, fluorescent tubes were still reported as producing beryllium granuloma.[156] In this report, a young man had cut his right ring finger on a broken fluorescent tube. Patch tests with beryllium sulfate 2 per cent and beryllium nitrate 0.38, 0.19 and 0.019 per cent gave positive results. A total dosage of nearly 2000 mg. of prednisone induced regression of the granuloma, but no sooner was the drug discontinued than a deterioration set in. The granuloma was therefore extirpated. Five years later the patch test reaction became positive again. Nevertheless, the operation had favorable clinical and functional results.

It seems likely that repeated tests with beryllium salts in order to follow the evolution of the disease may cause sensitization, and, in some instances, excision of the granuloma seems preferable to corticosteroid therapy.

Some beryllium granulomas may respond to corticosteroid therapy, but often surgical excision becomes necessary

ZIRCONIUM GRANULOMAS

These granulomas of the skin, originally seen following the use of zirconium sodium lactate as a deodorant,[157,158] continue to occur following the use of zirconium oxide for the treatment of rhus plant dermatitis.

In the deodorants that produced granulomas, soluble salts were used. In the topical preparations for rhus dermatitis, mostly insoluble salts are employed. Table 6–9 is a list of the products containing zirconium that are currently available for prophylaxis and treatment of plant dermatitis.

Table 6-9. Rhus Plant Medications Containing Zirconium

Trade Name	*Zirconium Salt*	*Zirconium Content*
Antivy (CIBA)	Zirconium oxide	4%
Rhulicream, Rhulihist, Rhulispray (Lederle)	Zirconium oxide	1%
Ziradryl Cream (Parke, Davis)	Zirconium oxide	4%
Ziradryl Lotion (Parke, Davis)	Zirconium oxide (also 1% Benadryl hydrochloride and camphor)	2%
Zircobarb Lotion (Vogel)	Carbonated hydrous zirconium	5%
Zirnox (Bristol)	Zirconium oxide	4%

Palmer and Welton[159] reported a case of lupus miliaris disseminatus faciei in an individual who was exposed to a zirconium oven in a metal alloy factory.

Zirconium, like beryllium, can produce sarcoid granulomas.[160]

Clinical Appearance. The lesions usually appear four to six weeks following initial use of the zirconium preparation and are limited to the sites of contact. They appear as persistent, firm, shiny, erythematous, flesh or apple-jelly colored papules, which are solitary, grouped or coalescent. Eczematous changes are also usually present. Pruritus is minimal or absent.[161,162]

Zirconium salts used in deodorants and rhus plant dermatitis may produce sarcoid granulomas in sensitized individuals

Histological Appearance. The epidermis is normal. In the dermis, large aggregates or tubercles of distinctive epithelioid and Langhans' giant cells are present. A minimal inflammatory reaction is occasionally present. Foreign body material is not detected by polarized light microscopy. Differentiation from sarcoidosis is not possible histologically.[163,164]

Mechanism of Production of Zirconium Granuloma. Zirconium granulomas may be produced by either soluble or insoluble salts, but they must first be introduced *into* the skin. The granulomas then develop in individuals who have acquired an allergic hypersensitivity to zirconium. Any defect in the protective layer of the skin enhances the development of hypersensitivity.

In the axillae, minute abrasions from shaving, as well as excess friction and sweating, enhance the penetration of the zirconium salts of the *deodorants*. The preparations containing zirconium salts used for treatment of rhus dermatitis readily penetrate through the acutely inflamed skin and through denuded areas, vesicles and bullae.

The zirconium granulomas composed of epithelioid cells represent an acquired allergic reaction of the delayed type due to the reaction of zirconium in sensitized individuals.

Tests for Zirconium Hypersensitivity. Either patch or intracutaneous testing may be employed to determine allergic hypersensitivity to zirconium salts.

In patch testing, the zirconium preparation may be rubbed into a test site that has been prepared by multiple scratches or denuded by a dermal curet. The site is then covered with an occlusive dressing for two days. In sensitized individuals, a positive reaction consists of the development of reddish brown papules in about four weeks. Such papules show a sarcoid granulomatous infiltrate histologically.

In intracutaneous testing, a small wheal is made by injecting a 1:10,000 dilution of sodium zirconium lactate. A positive reaction consists of a discrete papule, which appears in 8 to 14 days. In about a month, the papule clinically and histologically has the appearance of a sarcoid lesion. It may persist for 6 to 24 months.

Prognosis. Axillary granulomas produced by the soluble zirconium lactate in deodorants usually disappear within a few months. Lesions produced by the insoluble zirconium oxide preparations used for rhus plant therapy usually remain unchanged for several months to years and are refractory to therapy. Temporary improvement is obtained by the use of corticosteroids either systemically or intralesionally.[165]

Since zirconium compounds used for poison ivy dermatitis can produce intractable granulomas and are of questionable value, consideration should be given to discontinuing their use

ZINC DERMATITIS AND DISCOLORATIONS

Zinc chloride is a strong primary irritant, and can produce ulcerations resembling those produced by chromic acid. Allergic reactions to this caustic zinc salt are extremely rare. Sources of exposure are dental fillings, preservation and fireproofing of timber, solder flux, and Moh's chemosurgery for skin cancer.

Although *zinc oxide* is completely inert allergenically, it is probably the most common cause of black dermographism produced by jewelry. Zinc oxide present in cosmetics, lotions and dentifrices is much harder than most metals in jewelry and coins. *Zinc stearate* is so soft that it cannot cause black dermographism.

D'Alibour solution, which contains zinc sulfate, copper sulfate and camphorated water, is sometimes used as a wet dressing, but it has not been reported as a cause of allergic dermatitis.

Zinc pyrethione is present in a 1 per cent concentration in Head and Shoulders Shampoo. For patch testing, a 0.5 per cent concentration in petrolatum may be used.

REFERENCES

1. Marcussen, P. V.: Eczematous Allergy to Metals. Acta Allerg., *17*, 311, 1962.
2. Gaul, L. E.: Incidence of Sensitivity to Chromium, Nickel, Gold, Silver and Copper Compared to Reactions to Their Aqueous Salts, Including Cobalt Sulfate. Ann. Allergy, *12*, 429, 1954.
3. Marcussen, P. V.: Clinical and Pathogenic Aspects of Cutaneous Reactions to Metals. Proc. Int. Cong. Derm., *2*, 1067, 1962.
4. Fonesca, A.: Findings on Hypersensitivity to Groups of Metals. Dermatologia Intertionale, *8*, 44, 1969.
5. Foussereau, F., and Languier, P.: Allergic Eczema from Metallic Foreign Bodies. Trans. St. John Hosp. Derm. Soc., *52*, 220, 1966.
6. Wilkinson, J. V.: Some Metallurgical Aspects of Orthodontic Stainless Steel. Amer. J. Orthodont., *48*, 192, 1962.
7. Brettle, J.: A Survey of the Literature on Metallic Surgical Implants. Injury, *2*, 26, 1970.
8. Josephson, B. M.: Allergy to Coins. Letter to the Editor. J.A.M.A., *23*, 348, 1965.
9. Schroeder, H. A., and Nason, A. P.: Trace Metals in Human Hair. J. Invest. Derm., *53*, 71, 1969.
10. Leider, M.: On the Mechanical Pathogenesis of Some Dermatologic Appearances. Arch. Derm., *76*, 501, 1957.
11. Sulzberger, M. B., and Tolmach, J. A.: Allergic Flare-Up Reactions in Red Tattooing: Observations on Development and Subsidence of Mercurial Sensitivity and on Allergic Granulomatous and Sarcoid Reactions. Hautarzt, *10*, 110, 1959.
12. Biro, L., and Klein, W. P.: Unusual Complications of Mercurial (Cinnabar) Tattoo. Arch. Derm., *96*, 2, 1967.
13. Lowenthal, L. J. A.: Reactions in Green Tattoos. Arch. Derm., *82*, 237, 1960.
14. Bjoernber, A.: Allergic Reaction to Cobalt in Light Blue Tattoo Markings. Acta Dermatovener., *41*, 259, 1961.
15. Bjoernber, A.: Reactions to Light in Yellow Tattoos from Cadmium Sulfide. Arch. Derm., *88*, 267, 1963.
16. Goldstein, N.: Mercury-Cadmium Sensitivity in Tattoos: Photoallergic Reaction in Red Pigment. Ann. Intern. Med., *67*, 948, 1967.
17. Shelley, W. B., et al.: Intradermal Tests with Metals and Other Inorganic Elements in Sarcoidosis and Anthroco-Silicosis. J. Invest. Derm., *31*, 301, 1958.
18. Malten, K. E., et al.: Nickel Sensitization and Detergents. Acta Dermatovener., *49*, 10, 1969.
19. Malten, K. E., and Spruit, D.: The Relative Importance of Various Environmental Exposures to Nickel in Causing Contact

Hypersensitivity. Acta Dermatovener., *49*, 14, 1969.
20. Quinones, P. A., and Garcia Munox, C. M.: Contact Allergy Due to Nickel and Chrome. Presence of These Compounds in Detergents Used in the Household. Ann. Derm. Syph., *92*, 383, 1965.
21. Feuerman, E. J.: Housewives' Eczema and the Role of Chromates. Acta Dermatovener., *49*, 288, 1969.
22. Professional Services Division, Proctor and Gamble Co., Personal Communication.
23. Frykholm, K. O.: On Mercury from Dental Amalgam: Its Toxic and Allergic Effects and Some Comments on Occupational Hygiene. Acta Odont. Scand., *15*(Suppl. 22), 1957.
24. Frykholm, K. O., et al.: Allergy to Copper Derived from Dental Alloys as a Possible Cause of Oral Lesions of Lichen Planus. Acta Dermatovener., *49*, 268, 1969.
25. Gaul, L. E.: Ring Dermatitis: Primary Irritation from Action of Salt on Jewelry Alloys. Arch. Derm., *77*, 526, 1958.
26. Buckley, W. R., and Lewis, C. E.: The "Ruster" in Industry. J. Occup. Med., *2*, 23, 1960.
27. Fisher, A. A., et al.: Pustular Patch Test Reactions. Arch. Derm., *80*, 742, 1959.
28. Epstein, S.: Contact Dermatitis Due to Nickel and Chromate Observation on Dermal Delayed (Tuberculin-Type) Sensitivity. Arch. Derm., *73*, 236, 1956.
29. Marcussen, P. V.: Comparison of Intradermal Test and Patch Test Using Nickel Sulphate and Formaldehyde. J. Invest. Derm., *40*, 263, 1963.

Nickel

30. *The Romance of Nickel.* New York, New York International Nickel Co., Inc., 1960.
31. Gaul, L. E.: Development of Allergic Nickel Dermatitis from Earrings. J.A.M.A., *200*, 176, 1967.
32. Goldman, L., and Kitzmiller, K. W.: Earlobe Piercing with Needles and Wire. Arch. Derm., *92*, 305, 1965.
33. Fleigl, F.: *Spot Testing, Inorganic Applications*, (Vol. 1). New York, Elsevier, p. 149.
34. Samitz, M. H., and Pomerantz, H.: Studies of the Effects on the Skin of Nickel and Chromium Salts. A.M.A. Arch. Ind. Health, *18*, 473, 1958.
35. Moseley, J. C., and Allen, H. J.: Polyurethane Coating in the Prevention of Nickel Dermatitis. Arch. Derm., *103*, 58, 1971.
36. Fisher, A. A.: Steroid Aerosol Spray in Contact Dermatitis. Arch. Derm., *89*, 841, 1964.
37. Sulzberger, M. B.: Dermatitis Eczematous (Contact-Type) Due to Nickel. Soc. Trans. Arch. Derm., *41*, 815, 1940.
38. Lowenthal, J. J. A.: *Eczemas: A Symposium by Ten Authors.* Baltimore, Williams and Williams Co., 1954, p. 37.
39. Morgan, J. F.: Observations on Persistence of Skin Sensitivity with Reference to Nickel Eczema. Brit. J. Derm., *65*, 84, 1953.
40. Hilt, G.: Hexavalent Chromate Dermatitis in the Group of Eczematous Dermatitis Caused by Sensitization to Metals. Dermatologica, *109*, 143, 1954.
41. Gaul, L. E.: Incidence of Sensitivity to Chromium, Nickel, Gold, Silver, and Copper Compared to Reactions to Their Aqueous Salts Including Cobalt Sulfate. Ann. Allergy, *12*, 429, 1954.
42. Rostenberg, A., Jr., and Perkins, A. J.: Nickel and Cobalt Dermatitis. J. Allergy, *22*, 466, 1951.
43. Pirila, V., and Forstrom, L.: Pseudo-Cross Sensitivity Between Cobalt and Nickel. Acta Dermatovener., *46*, 40, 1966.
44. Calnan, C. D.: Nickel Sensitivity in Women. Int. Arch. Allergy, *11*, 73, 1957.
45. Stoddart, J. C.: Nickel Sensitivity as a Cause of Infusion Reactions. Lancet, *2*, 741, 1960.
46. Sunderman, F. W., and Sunderman, F. W., Jr.: Loeffler's Syndrome Associated with Nickel Sensitivity. Arch. Intern. Med., *107*, 3, 1961.
47. Fisher, A. A., and Shapiro, A.: Allergic Eczematous Contact Dermatitis Due to Metallic Nickel. J.A.M.A., *161*, 717, 1956.

Chromates

48. Epstein, S.: Contact Dermatitis Due to Nickel and Chromate. Arch. Derm., *73*, 236, 1956.
49. Walsh, E. N.: Chromate Hazards in Industry. Council on Industrial Health. J.A.M.A., *153*, 1305, 1953.
50. Nater, J. P.: Possible Causes of Chromate Eczema. Dermatologica, *126*, 160, 1963.
51. Fregert, S.: Book Matches as a Source of Chromate. Arch. Derm., *88*, 546, 1963.
52. Fregert, S.: Chromate Eczema and Matches. Acta Dermatovener., *42*, 473, 1962.
53. Fregert, S.: Otitis Externa Due to Chromate of Matches. Acta Dermatovener., *42*, 473, 1962.
54. Samitz, M. H.: Personal Communication.
55. Morris, G. E.: Chromate Dermatitis from Chrome Glue and Other Aspects of the Chrome Problem. A.M.A. Arch. Industr. Health, *11*, 368, 1955.

56. Tritsch, H., Orfanos, C., and Luckerath, I.: Experiments on the Allergic Skin Reaction to Chromated Catgut. Hautarzt, *18*, 355, 1967.
57. Engel, H. O., and Calnan, C. D.: Chromate Dermatitis from Paint. Brit. J. Industr. Med., *20*, 192, 1963.
58. Newhouse, M. L.: A Cause of Chromate Dermatitis Among Assemblers in an Automobile Factory. Brit. J. Industr. Med., *20*, 199, 1963.
59. Fregert, S.: Chromate in Welding Fumes with Special Reference to Contact Dermatitis. Acta Dermatovener., *43*, 119, 1963.
60. Shelley, W. G.: Chromium in Welding Fumes as a Cause of Eczematous Hand Eruption. J.A.M.A., *189*, 772, 1964.
61. Fregert, S., Gruyberger, B., and Heijer, A.: Sensitization to Chromium and Cobalt in Processing of Sulphate Pulp. Acta Dermatovener., *52*, 221, 1972.
62. Possick, P. A.: Cement Dermatitis. Cutis, *5*, 103, 1969.
63. Siedlecki, J. T.: Potential Health Hazards of Materials Used by Artists and Sculptors. J.A.M.A., *204*, 1178, 1968.
64. Kleinman, G. D.: *Occupational Health of Construction Workers in California*. Berkeley, California Department of Public Health, 1967, p. 4.
65. Neuman, Y. B.: *Contact Dermatitis in Cement Workers and Their Rehabilitation*. Jerusalem, Israel, Seminar on Research in Rehabilitation, 1968.
66. Anderson, F. E.: Cement and Oil Dermatitis: The Part Played by Chrome Sensitivity. Brit. J. Derm., *72*, 108, 1960.
67. Calnan, C. D.: Cement Dermatitis. J. Occup. Med., *2*, 15, 1960.
68. Jaeger, H., and Pelloni, E.: Epicutaneous Tests to Dichromates, Positive in Cement Eczemas. Dermatologica, *100*, 207, 1950.
69. Pirila, V., and Kajanne, H.: Sensitization to Cobalt and Nickel in Cement Eczema. Acta Dermatovener., *45*, 9, 1965.
70. Pirila, V.: On the Role of Chrome and Other Trace Elements in Cement Eczema. Acta Dermatovener., *34*, 136, 1954.
71. Sertoli, A., Venturi, W., and Fabbri, P.: The Inactivation of the Eczematogenous Power of Cement by Means of Barium Salts. Clin. Derm., *21*, 390, 1968.
72. Fregert, S., Gruyberger, B., and Heijer, A.: Chromium Dermatitis from Galvanized Sheets. Berufsdermatosen, *18*, 254, 1970.
73. Samitz, M. H., Shrager, J., and Katz, S.: Studies on the Prevention of Injurious Effects of Chromates in Industry. Industr. Med. Surg., *31*, 427, 1962.
74. Richter, G., and Heidelbach, U.: Chromate Eczema After Glass Polishing with Corundum. Berufsdermatosen, *17*, 8, 1969.
75. Samitz, M. H., and Epstein, E.: Experimental Cutaneous Chrome Ulcers in Guinea Pigs. Arch. Environ. Health, *5*, 463, 1962.
76. Edmundson, W. F.: Chrome Ulcers of the Skin and Nasal Septum and Their Relationship to Patch Testing. J. Invest. Derm., *17*, 17, 1951.
77. Samitz, M. H.: Some Dermatologic Aspects of the Chromate Problem. Arch. Industr. Health, *11*, 361, 1955.
78. Meneghini, C. L.: Cointributo allo studio delle dermatosi professionali da cemento e calce. G. Ital. Derm., *93*, 303, 1952.
79. Gaul, L. E.: Chromate Sensitivity of Specific and Nonspecific Positive Patch Tests. Ann. Allergy, *16*, 435, 1958.
80. Skog, E., and Wahlberg, J. E.: Patch Testing with Potassium Dichromates in Different Vehicles. Arch. Derm., *99*, 697, 1969.
81. Samitz, M. H., et al.: Chromium Protein Interactions. Acta Dermatovener., *49*, 142, 1969.
82. Jansen, L. H., and Berrens, L.: Hypersensitivity to Chromium Compounds. Dermatologica, *137*, 65, 1968.
83. Samitz, M. H.: Ascorbic Acid in the Prevention and Treatment of Toxic Effects from Chromates. Acta Dermatovener., *50*, 64, 1970.

Mercury

84. Sulzberger, M. B.: *Dermatologic Allergy*. Springfield, Ill., Charles C Thomas, 1940, pp. 60–61.
85. Frykholm, K. O., and Wahlgren, F.: A Fatal Case of Mercurial Dermatitis with Complication. Acta Derm. Syph., *44*, 362, 1964.
86. Miedler, L. H., and Forbes, J. D.: Allergic Contact Dermatitis Due to Metallic Mercury. Arch. Environ. Health, *17*, 960, 1964.
87. Fisher, A. A.: Recent Developments in the Diagnosis and Management of Drug Eruptions. Med. Clin. N. Amer., *43*, 791, 1959.
88. Juhlin, L., and Sven, O.: Allergic Reactions to Mercury and Red Tattoos and Mucosa Adjacent to Amalgam Fillings. Acta Dermatovener., *48*, 103, 1968.
89. Fisher, A. A., Pascher, F., and Kanof, N. B.: Allergic Contact Dermatitis due to the Ingredients of Vehicles. Arch. Derm., *104*, 286, 1971.
90. Morris, G. E.: Dermatoses from Phenylmercuric Salts. Arch. Environ. Health, *1*, 53, 1960.

91. Ellis, F. A.: The Sensitizing Factor in Merthiolate. J. Allergy, *18*, 212, 1947.
92. Gaul, L. E.: Sensitizing Component in Thiosalicylic Acid. J. Invest. Derm., *31*, 91, 1958.
93. Epstein, S.: Sensitivity to Merthiolate: A Cause of False Delayed Intradermal Reactions. J. Allergy, *34*, 225, 1963.
94. Reisman, R. E.: Delayed Hypersensitivity to Merthiolate Preservative. J. Allergy, *43*, 245, 1969.
95. Fernstrom, A. I. B., Frykholm, K. O., and Huldt, S.: Mercury Allergy with Eczematous Dermatitis Due to Silver-Amalgam Fillings. Brit. Dent. J., *113*, 206, 1962.
96. Gotz, H., and Fortmann, I.: Can Amalgam Fillings Cause a Mercury Sensitization of the Skin? Z. Haut. Geschlechtskr., *26*, 34, 1959.
97. Gaul, L. E.: Immunity of the Oral Mucosa in Epidermal Sensitization to Mercury. Arch. Derm., *93*, 45, 1966.
98. Burge, K. M., and Winkelmann, R. K.: Mercury Pigmentation. An Electron Microscopic Study. Arch. Derm., *102*, 51, 1970.
99. Lamar, L. M., and Bliss, B. O.: Localized Pigmentation of the Skin Due to Topical Mercury. Arch. Derm., *93*, 450, 1966.
100. Kern, A. B.: Mercurial Pigmentation. J.A.M.A., *99*, 129, 1969.
101. Kahn, G.: Three Thousand Years of Mercury—A Plea for Abandonment of a Dangerous, Unproven Therapy. Cutis, *6*, 537, 1970.
102. Epstein, E.: Explosive Idiosyncrasy to Mercury. A 30-year Follow-Up Study. Cutis, 7, 65, 1971.

Cobalt

103. Rostenberg, A., Jr., and Perkins, A. J.: Nickel and Cobalt Dermatitis. J. Allergy, *22*, 467, 1951.
104. Young, W. C., Ulrich, C. W., and Fouts, P. J.: Sensitivity to Vitamin B_{12} Concentrate. J.A.M.A., *143*, 893, 1950.
105. Kalensky, J., and Schwank, R.: Hypersensitivity to Cobalt Caused by an Antihydrotic Cream. Cesk. Derm., *43*, 423, 1962.
106. Marcussen, P. V.: Cobalt Dermatitis. Clinical Picture. Acta Dermatovener., *43*, 231, 1963.
107. Bandmann, H. J., and Fuchs, G.: Cobalt Contact Allergy. Its Relationships to Dichromate and Nickel Contact Allergy and its Occupational Dermatological Importance. Hautarzt, *14*, 207, 1963.
108. Zelger, J.: Cobalt Allergy. Derm. Wschr., *146*, 425, 1962.
109. Nurnberger, F., and Arnold, W.: Quincke's Edema as a Manifestation of a Cobalt Allergy Due to a Sensitization by Cobaltous Shell Splinters. Berufsdermatosen, *17*, 21, 1969.
110. Skog, E.: Skin Affections Caused by Hard Metal Dust. Industr. Med. Surg., *32*, 266, 1963.
111. Bourne, L. B., and Milner, F. J. M.: Polyester Resin Hazards. Brit. J. Industr. Med., *200*, 100, 1963.
112. Pirila, V.: On Occupational Diseases of Skin Among Paint Factory Workers, Painters, Polishers and Varnishers in Finland: Clinical and Experimental Study. Acta Dermatovener., *27*(Suppl. 16), 1, 1947.
113. Nater, J. P.: Cement Eczema. Nederl. T. Geneesk., *102*, 250, 1958.
114. Camarasa, G. J. M.: Cobalt Contact Dermatitis. Acta Dermatovener., *47*, 287, 1967.
115. DeFonseca, A.: Joint Sensitization with Chromium, Cobalt and Nickel in Cement Eczema. Acta Derm. Sifilgiogr., *61*, 151, 1970.
116. Mueller, R., and Breucker, G.: Cobalt as as Work-Dependent Eczematogen and as Co-Allergen with Chromium and Nickel. Derm. Wschr., *154*, 276, 1968.
117. McDermott, F. T.: Dust in the Cemented Carbide Industry. J. Amer. Ind. Hyg. Assoc., *32*, 188, 1971.
118. Pirila, V.: Sensitization to Cobalt in Pottery Workers. Acta Dermatovener., *33*, 193, 1953.
119. Schwartz, L., et al.: Allergic Dermatitis Due to Metallic Cobalt. J. Allergy, *16*, 51, 1945.
120. Birmingham, D.: Nickel and Cobalt Hypersensitivity. Trans. Arch. Derm., *68*, 740, 1953.
121. Beikko, P., and Forstreom, L.: Pseudo-Cross Sensitivity Between Cobalt and Nickel. Acta Dermatovener., *46*, 40, 1966.
122. Marcussen, P. V.: Intradermal Test Using Cobalt Chloride. Acta Dermatovener., *43*, 472, 1963.
123. Everall, J., Truter, M. R., and Truter, E. V.: Epidermal Sensitivity to Chromium, Cobalt, and Nickel. Acta Dermatovener., *34*, 447, 1954.

Copper

124. Saltzer, E. I.: Allergic Contact Dermatitis Due to Copper. Arch. Derm., *98*, 37, 1968.
125. Epstein, S.: Cross-Sensitivity Between Nickel and Copper. J. Invest. Derm., *25*, 269, 1965.
126. Foussereau, J., et al.: Allergy to Copper Gas. Med. France, *76*, 4489, 1969.
127. Schwartz, L., Tulipan, L., and Birmingham, D. J.: *Occupational Diseases of the Skin* (Ed. 3). Philadelphia, Lea & Febiger, 1957, p. 265.

128. Barranco, V. P.: Eczematous Dermatitis Caused by Internal Exposure to Copper. Arch. Derm., *106*, 386, 1972.

Gold

129. Kligman, A.: The Identification of Contact Allergies by Human Assay. J. Invest. Derm., *47*, 393, 1966.
130. Fregert, S., and Hjorth, N.: In A. J. Rook et al. (eds.): *Textbook of Dermatology*. Oxford, Blackwell Scientific Publications, 1968, p. 1883.
131. Fox, J. M., Kennedy, R., and Rostenberg, A., Jr.: Eczematous Contact-Sensitivity to Gold. Arch. Derm., *83*, 956, 1961.
132. Shelley, W. B., and Epstein, E.: Contact-Sensitivity to Gold as a Chronic Papular Eruption. Arch. Derm., *87*, 388, 1963.
133. Elgart, M. L., and Higdon, R. S.: Allergic Contact Dermatitis to Gold. Arch. Derm., *103*, 649, 1971.
134. Comaish, S.: A Case of Contact Hypersensitivity to Metallic Gold. Arch. Derm., *99*, 720, 1969.
135. Bowyer, A.: Epidermal Reactions and Prolonged Dermal Reactions to Patch Testing with Gold Salts. Acta Dermatovener., *47*, 9, 1967.
136. Forster, H. W., and Dickey, R. F.: A Case of Sensitivity to Gold Ball Orbital Implant. Amer. J. Ophthal., *32*, 659, 1949.
137. Malten, K. E., and Mali, J.: Contact Eczema Due to Gold. Allergie Asthma, *12*, 31, 1966.

Platinum

138. Marshall, J.: Toxicity of Platinum. S. Afr. Med. J., *26*, 8, 1952.
139. Roberts, A. E.: Platinosis. Arch. Industr. Hyg., *4*, 549, 1951.
140. Sheard, C., Jr.: Contact Dermatitis from Platinum and Related Metals: Report of Case. Arch. Derm., *71*, 357, 1955.
141. Parrot, J. L.: Platinum and Platinosis. Arch. Environ. Health, *19*, 685, 1969.

Palladium

142. Munro-Ashman, D., Munro, D. D., and Hughes, T. H.: Contact Dermatitis from Palladium. Trans. St. John Hosp. Derm. Soc., *55*, 196, 1969.

Arsenic

143. Birmingham, D., and Key, M. M.: An Outbreak of Arsenical Dermatitis in a Mining Community. Arch. Derm., *91*, 457, 1965.

Aluminum

144. Steinegeer, S.: Endemic Skin Lesions Near an Aluminum Factory. Fluoride Quart. Rept., *2*, 37, 1969.

Iron

145. Nater, J. P.: Epidermal Hypersensitivity to Iron. Hautarzt, *11*, 223, 1960.
146. Baer, R.: Allergic Contact Sensitization to Iron. J. Allergy Immunol., in press.

Antimony

147. Stevenson, C. J.: Antimony Spots. Trans. St. John Hosp. Derm. Soc., *51*, 40, 1965.
148. Paschoud, J.: Occupational Arsenic and Antimony Contact Eczema. Dermatologica, *129*, 410, 1964.

Beryllium

149. Curtis, C. H.: Cutaneous Hypersensitivity to Beryllium. Arch. Derm., *64*, 470, 1951.
150. Nichol, A. D., and Dominiquez, R.: Cutaneous Granuloma from Accidental Contamination with Beryllium Phosphorus. J.A.M.A., *140*, 855, 1949.
151. Davis, C., Cooper, M. M., and Grimes, O. F.: Skin Granuloma following Laceration by a Fluorescent Lamp. Calif. Med., *71*, 203, 1951.
152. Helwig, E. B.: Chemical Granuloma (Beryllium) of Skin. Milit. Surg., *109*, 540, 1951.
153. Kennedy, B. F.: Effect of Adrenocorticotropic Hormone (ACTH) on Beryllium Granulomatosis and Silicosis. Amer. J. Med., *10*, 134, 1951.
154. Dobson, R. L.: General Discussion on the Treatment of Chronic Beryllium Poisoning with ACTH and Cortisone. A.M.A. Arch. Indus. Hyg., *3*, 543, 1951.
155. Fisher, A. A.: Nonsurgical Treatment of Cutaneous Beryllium Granuloma. A.M.A. Arch. Derm., *68*, 214, 1953.
156. Folesky, H.: Some Aspects of Beryllium Granuloma. Berufsdermatosen, *15*, 93, 1967.

Zirconium

157. Shelley, W. B., et al.: Intradermal Tests with Metals and Other Inorganic Elements in Sarcoidosis and Anthraco-Silicosis. J. Invest. Derm., *31*, 301, 1958.
158. Sheard, C.: Granulomatous Reactions Due to Deodorant Sticks. J.A.M.A., *164*, 1085, 1957.
159. Palmer, L., and Welton, W.: Lupus Miliaris Disseminatus Faciei. Zirconium Hypersensitivity as Possible Cause. Cutis, *7*, 74, 1967.

160. Rublin, L.: Granulomas of Axillae Caused by Deodorants. J.A.M.A., *162*, 953, 1956.
161. Williams, R. M., and Skipworth, G. B.: Zirconium Granulomas of Glabrous Skin Following Treatment of Rhus Dermatitis. A.M.A. Arch. Derm., *80*, 273, 1959.
162. Epstein, W. L., and Allen, J. R.: Granulomatous Hypersensitivity After Use of Zirconium-Containing Poison Oak Lotions. J.A.M.A., *190*, 162, 1964.
163. Baler, G. R.: Granulomas from Topical Zirconium in Poison Ivy Dermatitis. Arch. Derm., *91*, 145, 1965.
164. Shelley, W. B., and Hurley, H. J.: Allergic Origin of Zirconium Deodorant Granulomas. Brit. J. Derm., *70*, 75, 1958.
165. LoPresti, P. J., and Hambril, G. W.: Zirconium Granuloma Following Treatment of Rhus Dermatitis. Arch. Derm., *92*, 188, 1965.

7

Contact Dermatitis in Childhood

Both allergic and irritant varieties occur during childhood and infancy.[1] The reactivity of the skin to potent contact sensitizers in early infancy is less than later in life. The irritant type of dermatitis readily takes place in individuals of all ages, including the newborn. Allergic dermatitis due to poison ivy oleoresin and to certain topical medications is by no means rare in early life.[2] Dermatitis due to wearing apparel, particularly wool, and to sensitizers in shoes is frequent.

Irritant and allergic contact dermatitis from topical medications readily occurs in infancy

Certain topical medications that produce sensitization in adults, including mercury, benzocaine and antihistamines, also produce dermatitis in children. Also, concentrations of medications that are not irritating to adults may produce dermatitis in children. In general, it is best to prescribe topical medications such as Vioform, precipitated sulfur, mercury, resorcin and salicylic acid in one third the concentration prescribed for adults. Antibiotic ointments may be prescribed in the same strength as for adults. Children are also susceptible to photosensitizing reactions from tar preparations used for topical medication and to the essential oils of perfumes.

Children may acquire severe irritant dermatitis and burns from accidental contact with a host of potentially harmful household products, including caustics.

Caustic Burns. So many caustic substances are used that inevitably children will suffer caustic burns. Proper treatment depends on whether the burn was caused by an acidic or alkaline substance. The burn should be touched with the pH portion of a urine dipstick. Alkali burns may be treated with orange juice or vinegar; acid burns are treated with bicarbonate paste or Milk of Magnesia.

Other household irritants include polishes, waxes, solvents, detergents, bleaching agents, disinfectants and insecticides. Widespread dermatitis may be produced by baby oils containing antiseptics, such as oxyquinoline sulfate. The eruptions may resemble prickly heat.

Highly perfumed oils, toilet soaps and dusting powders may also cause infantile dermatitis. These preparations may accumulate in the folds of the skin, particularly in the axillary and inguinal folds, where staphylococcal infections may become superimposed on the dermatitis. In general, the infant's skin tolerates lotions better than oils.

The use of nonperfumed oils, powders, and soaps free of antiseptics is recommended for infants. When the infant begins to crawl about, dermatitis of the legs, knees and elbows may be produced by floor polish, floor wax, rough fabrics used in rugs and carpets, and oily dust on furniture. The wearing of cotton coveralls prevents such dermatitis.

Dermatitis may occur from exposure to irritants and sensitizers while participating in activities such as fingerpainting, shop work and chemistry experiments. Crayons may also produce dermatitis.

SOAP AND DETERGENT DERMATITIS

"Detergent hands" may occur in young girls who wash doll clothes. Honigman[3] showed that a subacute primary irritant dermatitis is usually brought about by prolonged bubble baths, bathing too frequently, using excessive amounts of the bubble bath concentrate or a combination of these factors. Children with atopic eczema, who normally tend to have xerotic skin, are often severely affected.

Asteatosis and primary irritations are the inevitable results of overindulgence in bathing. Bubble bath assuredly can contribute to this problem.

Bubble baths are available as powders, liquids and aerosol foams. They are often packaged in containers appropriately shaped for subsequent use as a toy when empty. The attractive container, ease of bathing the child and the preference for a bubble bath account for the popularity with both parent and child.

DIAPER DERMATITIS

Diaper dermatitis (napkin dermatitis, erythema of Jacquet), the most common form of contact dermatitis in infancy, is produced by prolonged contact with urine or feces or both, or by residual antiseptics, soaps and detergents in the diapers.

The most common cause of diaper dermatitis is ammonia. Less commonly, acid urine and stools or soaps, detergents and antiseptics in diapers are causative factors

In most instances, dermatitis is caused by the irritative effect of ammonia in the urine. The ammonia is produced by the splitting of urea contained in the urine by the ammoniagenes bacillus present in the stool. Urine containing ammonia is alkaline and slimy and has a pungent odor.

Brown and Wilson[4] stated that the urea-splitting *B. proteus* occurs much more frequently than *B. ammoniagenes* in some cases of diaper dermatitis. Montes et al.[5] isolated *Candida albicans* from lesions of 27 patients with diaper dermatitis but from the skin of only 5 controls. Its frequency decreased following cure of the rash. *Escherichia coli* and *Staphylococcus aureus* were found in many lesions of diaper dermatitis, but they were also frequent in normal skin. A synergistic action between these bacteria and *C. albicans* is possible. In many infants, regardless of the presence of dermatitis, the microbial population of the diaper region was very high.

The Role of Diet

It appears that high protein foods (other than milk) may be responsible for acid stools and urine which, when left in contact with the skin, produce "acid scald."

Clinical Picture of Ammoniacal Dermatitis

The dermatitis is present over the external genitalia and buttocks, usually sparing the creases. The eruption may spread to include the entire lower half of the abdomen, and even the skin of the feet, coming in contact with ammoniacal urine, may become involved.

In mild cases, only a slight erythema confined to the diaper area is found. When neglected, the affected skin becomes scalded and edematous. Vesicles and bullae may supervene. Eroded bullae may become eczematous and pyodermic lesions may appear. Herpetiform ulcers are not uncommon.

In male infants, diaper dermatitis may appear as ulcers of the meatus of the glans; the ulcers may become covered with a diphtheritic type of membrane. Urination is painful and the infant may become restless.

Moderate and severe cases of diaper dermatitis are accompanied by the unmistakable odor of ammonia upon removal of the diaper or underpants. The odor is not usually present in freshly voided urine, but it may become apparent after the child has slept all night without a change of diaper. When occlusive coverings are used over the diaper, the ammoniacal odor becomes accentuated.

Management of Ammoniacal Dermatitis

The management of ammoniacal diaper dermatitis consists of the proper care of the diapers, the prevention of the formation of ammonia, and the treatment of existing dermatitis.

Proper Diaper Changing. In many instances, this is the most badly performed duty in infant hygiene when the soiled diaper is removed and the apparently unsoiled part is used to wipe the baby. As a result, fecal material containing millions of microorganisms is spread over the child's skin, and without additional cleansing, a clean diaper is put on. When next the child urinates, these organisms are supplied with nutriment, urea and warmth, resulting in the rapid multiplication of urease-liberating microorganisms and the enzyme production of ammonia.

Not infrequently the ammonia causes dermatitis with subsequent infection. If babies were carefully washed with warm water and a mild soap after each bowel movement, there would be a marked decrease in dermatitis and infections due to secondary invading microorganisms.

Care of Diapers. Diapers should be removed as soon as soiled. When frequent changes are not feasible, maintaining the infant in the prone position tends to reduce the incidence of diaper dermatitis, because there is less tendency for the feces and urine to become compressed under the gluteal area. The acidification of diapers with vinegar helps prevent the formation of ammonia in the excreted urine. When diapers are washed at home, following the last rinse of the diapers in the washing machine, 1 cupful of vinegar is added to the tub, and the machine is filled halfway. The diapers are then spun dry without further rinsing and dried by air or in a dryer. When diaper service is utilized, the cleaned diapers are soaked in a solution of 1 oz. of vinegar per gallon of water for 10 minutes and then dried.

Products such as Diaperine, which is a complex benzyl ammonium chloride compound, and Diaper-safe, which is o-benzyl-p-chlorphenol (OBPC), have been advocated as germicides for soaking diaper material. These compounds are more expensive than vinegar, but not necessarily more efficient. They destroy the ammoniagenes bacillus and prevent the interaction of the bacillus with urea of the urine. The formation of ammonia is thereby inhibited.

When diaper dermatitis is present, occlusive materials over the diaper area should be avoided. Recently available special diapers, such as Babycare (Riegel) and Bobaby (Lee-Colbert), have inner linings of synthetic cloths containing hydrophobic fibers, which allow passage of the urine to the outer cotton layers, keeping the skin relatively dry and preventing diaper dermatitis.

An acid urine and diaper prevent ammoniacal dermatitis

Specialized diaper laundering services are available.

Acidification of the Urine. Since ammonia is found only in alkaline urine, acidification of the urine helps prevent the formation of this irritant. The oral administration of sodium acid phosphate (sodium biphosphate, N.F.; NaH_2PO_4) is a safe, practical method of rendering the urine acid. This salt should not be confused with phosphate of soda (Na_2HPO_4), which is a laxative and renders the urine alkaline.

Sodium acid phosphate may be administered in powder form in milk to infants according to the following schedule and dosage:

Under 6 months: 5 grains 3 times daily
Six to 12 months: 10 grains 3 times daily
Over 1 year: 15 grains 3 times daily

It is best to administer the sodium acid phosphate in individual packets. Acidifying the diaper with vinegar and the urine with sodium acid phosphate may eliminate ammonia in the urine within 24 to 48 hours.

Role of Position in Diaper Dermatitis. Newborn infants kept in the prone (belly) position have less diaper rash and self-inflicted excoriations than infants kept in the supine position.

Usually an eruption that is concentrated over the genital area is due to urine, whereas one that is concentrated over the anal region is more often associated with diarrhea.

Treatment of Existing Dermatitis. In severe cases of diaper dermatitis the following adherent paste should be applied to the affected areas:

Burow's solution	5.0 ml.
Anhydrous lanolin	20.0 grams
Plain Lassar's paste	up to 60.0 grams

When the diaper area is severely inflamed, the skin should be cleansed with mineral or olive oil rather than with soap and water.

In the presence of eczematization, 1 per cent Vioform may be added to the paste. When secondary infection and ulceration have taken place, the involved area should be painted with 1 part Castellani's carbolfuchsin paint to 6 parts water before the paste is applied. This dye preparation is also effective for superimposed moniliasis.

In males, ammoniacal ulcers of the meatus and the glans penis should be coated with a thick layer of boric acid ointment in addition to elimination of the ammonia from the urine.

Absorbent and adherent pastes are preferable to creams and ointments in the diaper area

Psoriasiform Napkin Dermatitis

This syndrome has been variously interpreted as an early manifestation of psoriasis, a seborrheic dermatitis, a candida infection and a disease su generis. Fergusson et al.[6] stated that treatment with antimonilial dyes in the napkin area is superior to therapy with steroid creams. Finally, the clinical appearance of the napkin eruption, the predominant incidence in the warmer months, and the fact that all the infants were hospital born were all thought to support a monilial etiology.

Psoriasiform napkin dermatitis in several of my patients cleared up with the use of equal parts of a corticosteroid cream and Lassar's paste. This combination adheres well to the diaper area and is more efficacious than a corticosteroid cream or ointment alone.[7]

PERIANAL DERMATITIS

Frequent soft or liquid stools and undigested food particles or their split products in feces may produce perianal dermatitis. Coating the area with zinc oxide ointment is protective and healing in such instances. Mercurial, formaldehyde or strong detergent disinfectants on a thermometer may produce contact dermatitis in the perianal area.

Superinfection with monilia is often a complication. The application of Castellani's carbolfuchsin paint diluted with 6 parts water twice daily is effective for moniliasis.

Toilet seat dermatitis may be produced by strong detergents used to cleanse the seat. In addition, lacquer or paint covering the seat may cause a clearly defined pattern of dermatitis on the posterior aspect of the thighs and buttocks.

CLOTHING DERMATITIS

Contact dermatitis in childhood is not uncommonly due to woolen clothing. Rough cuffs and collars, particularly when wet, readily irritate the skin, especially in children with atopic dermatitis.

Residues of soap and detergent in laundered clothes can also be irritating. Highly starched garments may initiate a dermatitis. Clothing dyes rarely cause dermatitis in infancy. New clothing and bed linens should be washed before coming in contact with the inflamed skin of chidren. Clothing that has been dry cleaned or contaminated with moth preventatives or insecticides should be thoroughly aired before being worn by the child.

Children's flame-retardant night clothing, which contains formaldehyde resins and other resins, may produce dermatitis.

Rough-textured and woolen clothing and occlusive footwear frequently cause dermatitis in children

DERMATITIS OF THE FEET

Dermatitis Due to Shoes

This type of dermatitis in children may be due to allergic sensitization to ingredients in shoes, particularly rubber. Frequently a nonspecific dermatitis is produced by the friction and irritation of an ill-fitting shoe. The dorsal aspect of the first toe may be involved in both the allergic and the irritant type of shoe dermatitis. It is not rare for friction of tight-fitting shoes to localize atopic dermatitis to this site. It may be necessary to perform patch tests with shoe ingredients in order to differentiate such atopic dermatitis from allergic contact dermatitis due to shoes.

Dermatitis Due to Hyperhidrosis and Occlusive Footwear

Children whose feet perspire excessively and who wear socks containing synthetic fibers, sneakers, rubbers or rubber-soled shoes for prolonged periods may suffer from sweaty sock dermatitis, an eruption of the toes and interweb areas due to maceration by unabsorbed sweat.[8] These areas readily become eczematous and infected. Paronychial infections and dystrophic nail changes in neglected cases are not uncommon.

This syndrome must be distinguished from tinea pedis, contact dermatitis from shoes and atopic dermatitis. Scrapings and cultures for tinea may be necessary in the differential diagnosis. Allergic contact dermatitis due to shoes usually spares the interdigital areas. Patch tests may be necessary to rule out sensitization to chemicals in footwear. Sweaty sock dermatitis is often confused with atopic dermatitis of the feet, particularly if hyperhidrosis also causes dermatitis of the antecubital fossae.

Control of Hyperhidrosis. Children with hyperhidrosis of the feet should wear all-cotton hose and, whenever feasible, shoes with perforated uppers, or sandals. Prolonged wearing of rubbers, boots, sneakers or other occlusive footwear should be avoided. Foot baths of potassium permanganate made by dissolving a 5-grain tablet in 2 quarts of water should be used nightly for 20 minutes. Each morning, ZeaSORB Powder (Stiefel) should be dusted onto the feet and into hose and footwear.

In many instances the following dusting powder is most effective in controlling hyperhidrosis and bromhidrosis:

Fluffy tannic acid powder
Bentonite
Purified talc
aa q.s. ad. 60.0
Dispense in sifter top box

Sweaty sock dermatitis should be combatted by use of nonocclusive footwear, permanganate baths and dusting powder

Treatment of Contact Dermatitis of the Feet

In the acute phase, the use of foot baths with cool Burow's solution, 1 part to 20 parts water, for 20 minutes twice daily reduces inflammation and edema. In the presence of secondary infection, dilute potassium permanganate baths, made by dissolving a 2-grain tablet of potassium permanganate in 2 quarts of water, should be employed twice daily. After the foot baths, zinc oxide ointment or plain Lassar's paste may be applied. If the dermatitis is oozing, an absorbent paste should be applied:

Burow's solution	10.0 ml.
Anhydrous lanolin	20.0 grams
Plain Lassar's paste	up to 60.0 grams

In the presence of fissuring the following ointment should be used:

Tincture of benzoin	2.0 ml.
Zinc oxide ointment	up to 20.0 grams

When secondary infection is present, the feet should be rested for several days and antibiotic preparations such as Ilotycin, Terramycin or Aureomycin ointments should be applied. Systemic antibiotic therapy is indicated in severe infections, particularly when lymphangitis and lymphadenitis supervene.

Contact Cheilitis and Perioral Dermatitis

In children, the lips and adjacent skin are commonly irritated. Children with a habit of licking often have an inflammation of this area. In addition, saliva that is trapped between the thumb and the mouth of a thumb-sucking child may produce a dermatitis of the lips and cheeks. Similarly, children who are salivating because of teething may suffer from a facial dermatitis. The constant chewing of bubble gum can produce dermatitis of the face and cheilitis because of the macerating effect of the moist gum and the irritation of essential oils.

Children whose eating habits permit foods such as spinach, carrots and citrus fruit to remain on the cheeks may suffer from dermatitis due to the irritation of food juices. The facial dermatitis produced by saliva or food juices may closely resemble atopic eczema.

Regurgitation of food particles may cause a contact dermatitis around the mouth and on the neck and chin.

Rubber-sensitive children may acquire a perioral dermatitis resembling perlèche from chewing rubber pencil erasers or rubber bands.

The dermatitis produced by saliva and food juices often does not respond to creams and ointments. Adherent, protective pastes, such as plain Lassar's paste, give better results. When the infant's skin is constantly bathed by saliva or irritating fluids, the application of the following absorbent and protective paste is advisable:

Burow's solution	5.0 ml.
Anhydrous lanolin	10.0 grams
Talc U.S.P.	10.0 grams
Zinc oxide ointment	up to 60.0 grams

PLANT DERMATITIS

Poison ivy, poison sumac and poison oak are the most common causes of allergic eczematous contact dermatitis in children. Contact with resins of trees may also produce allergic dermatitis. Anemones and buttercups contain a blister-producing lactone that can cause vesiculation in children who crush or chew the plants.

Although allergic rhinitis due to ragweed protein is common throughout childhood, ragweed oil dermatitis is extremely rare during this period.

Vick's Vaporub contains several plant substances, including oil of turpentine, oil of eucalyptus and oil of cedar, which may irritate or sensitize the child's skin. In addition, this nostrum contains camphor, menthol, oil of nutmeg and thymol.

Poison Ivy (Rhus) Dermatitis

Although poison ivy dermatitis is essentially a summer disease, it may occur whenever children come into contact with the dried oleoresin on the twigs of the dormant plant. Not infrequently, pets, particularly long-haired dogs, contact poison ivy plants and transmit the oleoresin to children. Ingestion of Rhus plants may produce systemic symptoms, such as vomiting, diarrhea, fever, convulsions and stupor. Acute nephritis may accompany ingestion or marked cutaneous involvement.

There is no difficulty in sensitizing newborn infants to poison ivy oleoresin.[2] Although clinically one may see many severe cases of poison ivy dermatitis in children, experimental evidence seems to indicate that poison ivy reactions are more intense in adults and that the reactivity does not reach its zenith for several years. It is likely that most children become sensitized before adolescence.

COSMETIC DERMATITIS

Infants and children may acquire cosmetic dermatitis by contact with cosmetics worn by the mother and other attendants or applied in play.

The cheeks and forehead of an infant may be affected by the mother's perfume, face powder, lipstick or hair lacquer. Dermatitis may occur if an attendant handles a child before her nail polish is dry. Berloque dermatitis in children, resulting in patchy pigmentation, may be seen from the photosensitizing effect of perfumes and toilet waters. Occasionally, children use irritating or sensitizing eye make-up.

ATOPIC DERMATITIS DUE TO CONTACT WITH PROTEINS

Rarely, atopic infants, particularly those allergic to eggs or fish, acquire marked edema of the skin or oral mucosa from contact with the foods to which they are allergic. In addition, contact with egg white, in susceptible infants, may produce the clinical picture of atopic dermatitis. Usually the eruption from contact with proteins is urticarial rather than eczematous.

Protein allergens, such as wool and silk, are said to produce wheals by contact with infantile skin.[9] Atopic dermatitis may also be produced. Theoretically, such eruptions may be due to transepidermal penetration of protein allergens into the corium.

Contact urticaria may occur in atopic individuals from exposure to a dog's saliva.

PATCH TESTING

Patch testing in childhood has not been standardized. Children from infancy to the eighth year may have nonspecific patch test reactions to 5 per cent nickel sulfate and 5 per cent formaldehyde solutions, which usually are not primary irritants in adults.[10] Such false positive reactions are usually follicular and quickly fade after the patch is removed, in contradistinction to significant specific patch test reactions, which persist for several days and often spread.

Patch test reactions in childhood have to be interpreted with great care, because standard concentrations of chemicals for testing adults may produce nonspecific irritant reactions in early life. Until materials used for patch tests in children are restandardized, reactions should be checked on 3 young controls.

Patch test results with a shoe tray indicate that potassium dichromate often gives nonspecific reactions in childhood, whereas rubber chemicals appear to give more reliable results.

TREATMENT OF CONTACT DERMATITIS

In the acute phase of contact dermatitis, cold, wet dressings of Burow's solution, diluted 1 to 20 for infants and younger children and 1 to 10 for older children, are generally useful.

Corticosteroid and antibiotic topical medications may be employed in the same strength as for adults, provided the dermatitis is localized. In widespread eruptions, one third the adult strength should be employed.

Vioform, tar, ammoniated mercury or salicylic acid should be used in one fourth the adult strength.

In severe, widespread contact dermatitis, systemic corticosteroid therapy is indicated in children. Initially, Kenacort Syrup (Squibb), which contains 4 mg. triamcinolone per milliliter ($\frac{1}{2}$ teaspoonful 3 times daily), or Aristocort Syrup (Lederle), which contains 2 mg. triamcinolone per milliliter (1 teaspoonful 3 times daily), is given for younger children. It is less expensive to prescribe prednisone tablets, which may be crushed and given with fruit juice. Young children may be given one half of a 5-mg. prednisone tablet 3 times daily.

The initial doses of corticosteroid therapy are given for 3 days and then gradually reduced over 2 weeks to avoid a rebound effect.

For control of pruritus, Temaril Syrup (Smith, Kline & French) or Atarax Syrup (Roerig) may be given ($\frac{1}{2}$ teaspoonful 3 times daily) to young children.

For children who are restless and unable to sleep because of dermatitis, 2 teaspoonfuls of Benadryl Elixir (Parke, Davis) may be administered at bedtime.

REFERENCES

1. Waldbott, G. L.: Contact Dermatitis in Children. Int. Arch. Allergy, *12*, 273, 1958.
2. Epstein, W. L.: Contact-Type Delayed Hypersensitivity in Infants and Children: Induction of Rhus Sensitivity. Pediatrics, *27*, 51, 1961.
3. Honigman, J.: Bubble Bath Dermatitis in Children. Cutis, *2*, 406, 1966.
4. Brown, C. P., and Wilson, F. H.: Diaper Region Irritations. Pertinent Facts and Methods of Prevention. Clin. Pediat., *3*, 409, 1964.
5. Montes, L. F., et al.: Microbial Flora of Infant's Skin. Arch. Derm., *103*, 640, 1971.
6. Fergusson, N. G., et al.: Napkin Dermatitis with Psoriasiform "Ide." Brit. J. Derm., *78*, 289, 1966.
7. Andersen, S., et al.: Psoriasiform Napkin Dermatitis. Brit. J. Derm., *84*, 316, 1971.
8. Gibson, W. B.: Sweaty Sock Dermatitis. Clin. Pediat., *2*, 175, 1963.
9. Sulzberger, M. B., and Baer, R. L.: Whealing Capacity of the Skin of New-Born or Young Infants. Arch. Derm., *41*, 1029, 1940.
10. Marcussen, P. V.: Primary Irritant Patch-Test Reactions in Children. Arch. Derm., *87*, 378, 1963.

8

Dermatitis from Clothing

Clothing may produce irritant and allergic reactions, which may result in eczematous, petechial, urticarial or pigmented eruptions. The allergic reactions are usually due to dyes or synthetic resin finishes.

Clothing may produce irritant, eczematous, petechial, pigmented and urticarial reactions

WOOL IN CLOTHING

Wool is the natural, highly crimped fiber from sheep. Minute scales on the fiber allow interlocking to form felt cloth and mill-finished worsteds. These scales may be harsh enough to cause mechanical irritation in many individuals.

Friction with woolen garments, particularly in association with sweating and atopic dermatitis, may produce a nonspecific pruritus and dermatitis.

Allergic dermatitis due to the natural, unprocessed wool fiber is extremely rare. True allergic hypersensitivity to processed wool fibers does occur rarely and may be due to dyes, bleaches, oils and other chemicals added to the fiber.

Purpuric Eruptions from Wool. Petechial and purpuric eruptions due to woolen garments have been described.[1] So-called pigmented purpuric eruptions of the lower extremities, including Schamberg's disease, often occur in areas exposed to woolen underwear, but the role of these garments is unclear.

In addition, a water-soluble formaldehyde urea finish applied to woolen khaki shirts worn by British soldiers has been implicated as the cause of a purpuric eruption. The sedatives Sedormid and Carbromal, both of which are capable of producing purpuric dermatitis medicamentosa, are also urea compounds.[2]

Wool and Atopic Dermatitis. Wool has been reported as producing contact atopic dermatitis.[3] There is no doubt that the wearing of woolen clothing by atopic individuals may prolong and even precipitate recurrences. These patients often complain of severe pruritus from contact with woolen garments. Contact atopic dermatitis of the ankles, wrists and neck due to woolen snowsuits is common.

Wool atopic dermatitis is usually due to a nonspecific irritating effect. In addition, wool may be an inhalant allergen.[4]

As an irritant or allergen, wool is usually not tolerated by those suffering from atopic dermatitis. They should avoid contact with woolen garments and wear smooth, non-woolen clothing close to the skin. Linen, cotton, poplin, gabardine, suede, chamois and synthetic fibers (Orlon or nylon) are permissible. When woolen clothing must be worn, the skin should be separated from it by a cotton undergarment or scarf.

Woolen garments can produce a nonspecific dermatitis, particularly in atopic skin. Allergic reactions to preshrunk wool containing formaldehyde resins may occur

Shrinkproof woolen fibers may contain formaldehyde resins, which can produce allergic reactions.

IRRITATION DUE TO MOHAIR

Mohair is the resilient hair fiber obtained from the Angora goat. It provides a crisp, firm and slightly scratchy feel to fabrics even when used in low percentage blends with other fibers. Its addition to clothing produces itching and discomfort in many individuals, but allergic sensitivity has not been reported.

ROLE OF SILK IN WEARING APPAREL DERMATITIS

Silk is extensively employed for clothing and is sold under a wide variety of names, including satin, foulard, faille, crepe, chiffon, pongee, taffeta, jersey and mousseline de soie.

Dermatitis from silk is rare and may take unusual forms, such as a contact urticaria. It may resemble a dry atopic dermatitis rather than an eczematous reaction.[5]

The nature of the silk allergen is in dispute.[6] Three possibilities are the silk fiber, the gum or glue (sericin) in raw silk, and the silkworm protein. Silk used as a filter for biological products may cause anaphylaxis.[7]

COTTON WEARING APPAREL

Cotton fibers are made from cellulose. The wash and wear or crease resistant cotton fibers usually contain formaldehyde resins. Cotton clothes processed without formaldehyde resins are available under the trade names of Aileen, I to I, and Red Eye. In personal communications, Drs. W. Schorr and W. P. Jordan have informed me that there are traces of formaldehyde in these cotton clothes. It is, however, not certain whether formaldehyde-sensitive individuals would react to clothing made from such fabrics.

In addition, cotton fibers may be subjected to mechanical and chemical processes such as the following:

1. *Sanforizing.* This is an antishrink finish for cotton in which no chemicals are used and from which there is no skin hazard. Sanforizing is a controlled shrinkage process in which the yarns are mechanically rearranged and shortened the amount they would be if laundered.

2. *Mercerization.* This finishing process consists essentially of impregnating the material with a cold, strong, sodium hydroxide solution, which increases the strength and affinity for dyes and, if done under tension, increases the luster of the fiber. The sodium hydroxide is removed so that there is no hazard to the wearer.

3. *Sizing.* This consists of the application of starch, glues, vegetable gums, rosins or shellac to impart a stiff, polished or glazed surface. Sized cotton cloth includes organdy, piqué, costume cambrics, sheeting and mosquito netting.

The starch, which may not be removed by laundering, can cause dermatitis. Traces of glues and rosins in sized cotton cloth may produce dermatitis in sensitized individuals.[8]

LINEN (FLAX)

This soft fiber is obtained from the inner bark of the flax plant. Linen clothes rarely produce dermatitis.

SYNTHETIC OR MAN-MADE FIBERS USED IN CLOTHING

Synthetic fibers are used more and more in clothing. The unprocessed synthetic fibers are free from irritating and sensitizing properties, but the dyes and finishes that are added may produce allergic contact dermatitis. Synthetic fibers include the following:[9]

Acetate	Nylon	Rubber
Acrylic	Olefin	Saran
Metallic yarns	Polyester	Spandex
Modacrylic	Rayon	Triacetate
		Vinyon

Table 8–1 is a list of popular synthetic fibers, with their trademarks and producers.

Rayon. One of the first synthetic fibers was rayon (viscose). It is made from modified cellulose obtained from wool, pulp or cotton linters.

Spun rayon, rayon-acetate blends and rayon-polyester blends may contain formaldehyde resins. Unprocessed rayon does not cause dermatitis. Rayon has at least 90 trade names from Avril to Zantrel. (For other brands, see Table 8–1.)

Table 8-1. Synthetic Textile Fibers

Type	*Trademark*	*Producer*
Polyester	Dacron	DuPont
	Fortrel	Fiber Industries (Celanese)
	Kodel	Tennessee Eastman
	Mylar	DuPont
	Terital	Societya Montecatini, Italy
	Terylene	I.C.I., Ltd., Great Britain
	Vycron	Beaunit Mills
Acrylic	Acrylan	Chemstrand
	Creslan	American Cyanamid
	Orlon	DuPont
	Zefran	Dow Chemical
Modacrylic	Dynel	Union Carbide
	Verel	Tennessee Eastman
Rayon	Bemberg	American Bemberg
	Coloray	Courtaulds
	Colorspun	American Viscose
	Corval	Courtaulds
	Cupioni	American Bemberg
	Fortisan	Celanese Fibers
	Jetspun	American Enka
	Ondelette	DuPont
	Spun-Lo	Industrial Rayon
	Topel	Courtaulds
Acetate	Acele	DuPont
	Arnel (triacetate)	Celanese Fibers
	Avisco Acetate	American Viscose
	Celaperm	Celanese Fibers
	Chromspun	Tennessee Eastman
	Estron	Tennessee Eastman
Nytril	Darvan	Celanese Fibers
Nylon	Antron	DuPont
	Blanc de Blancs	Enka
	Cadon	Chemstrand
	Caprolan	Allied Chemical
	Cumuloft	Chemstrand
	Enkaloft	Enka
	Enkalure	Enka
	Nomex	DuPont
	Nylex	Polymers
	Nyloft	Firestone
	Nypel	Nypel
	Poliafil	Poliafil
	Sparkling	DuPont
	Speckelon	Chemstrand
	Tynex	DuPont

Many celluloses, such as cotton and rayon, are finished with formaldehyde resins

Acetate. One of the oldest synthetic fibers, acetate is made of wool pulp or cotton linters with a catalyst, acetic anhydride and acetic acid. Reactions from the undyed and unprocessed fibers have not been reported.

Acrylic. Acrylic fibers are made of water, petroleum, natural gas, limestone, ammonia and acrylonitrile.

The completely polymerized fibers are practically inert chemically and have not been known to cause allergic reactions. Acrylic finishes on nylon stockings and other clothing have not been reported as producing dermatitis.

Metallic Yarns. In one type, aluminum foil is bonded or laminated between two clear layers of film. In the other type, there is a vacuum deposition of aluminum on the surface of Mylar, a polyester film, which in turn is bonded between two clear layers of film. To add strength to the metallic yarn the fibers may be wrapped with nylon or Fortisan, a rayon fiber. For colors other than silver, pigments are added to the bonding adhesive.

Most metallic yarns are so fine that their incorporation into clothing produces no mechanical irritation. Allergic contact dermatitis has not been reported.

Modacrylic. These fibers contain less acrylonitrile than do acrylic fibers. Modacrylic fibers, particularly Dynel, are used in the production of synthetic fur, chemical and fire resistant work clothing, and crease-resistant fabric for men's and boys' slacks. Dermatitis from such fibers has not been reported.

Nylon. This synthetic fiber is used alone or in combination with other fibers. It is hexamethylene diamine condensate of adipic acid and is made of coal, air, water and petroleum. The names under which it is marketed are given in Table 8–1.

Dermatitis due to unprocessed nylon has been reported,[10,11] but it is apparently rare. Indeed, even dermatitis produced by the dyes and finishes in nylon clothing is becoming less common.

So-called nylon stocking dermatitis, formerly fairly common, was actually due to azo and aniline dyes and not to nylon.[12] Individuals who reacted to these dyes sometimes showed cross-reactions to paraphenylenediamine. At present, this type of dermatitis is rare because of improved dyeing processes.[13,14] Since an aqueous emulsion of completely polymerized methyl methacrylate has been used as a finish on certain nylon hosiery, dermatitis from this finish has not been reported. So-called nylon hair-net dermatitis is due to either the dye in the nylon or the rubber band.[15]

Nylon clothing may occasionally produce nonspecific dermatitis. Since nylon fabrics are not readily absorbent, freely perspiring individuals may complain of pruritus and dermatitis from the maceration and irritation of unabsorbed sweat when wearing nylon garments. In addition, since nylon is a lipophilic fiber, it is conceivable that an accumulation of sebum in the garment may create a condition favoring eczema.[16]

Plastic Gloves and Films from Olefin Fibers. The olefin fibers include polyethylene and polypropylene.[17] These are paraffin-based fibers. Polyethylene is nondyeable, but polypropylene fibers that are dyeable have been introduced. The use of these fibers in clothing is negligible, although disposable polyethylene gloves for use in physical examination have become available. Dermatitis from these gloves has not been reported.

The finished polyethylene products are of two types—a low density and a high density product, depending on the amount and types of low polymers employed. The manufacturer of the film states that polyethylene will not cause dermatitis, but the additives "may exude to the surface of the resin in time" and produce dermatitis.

In clothing, the polyester fibers, particularly Dacron, are largely responsible for the wash and wear properties. They have not been shown to be sensitizers or irritants.

Saran and Other Vinyl Plastics. Saran, the generic name for certain polyvinylidene resins, may be used in belts, suspenders and raincoats. Saran Wrap is used for occlusive dressings and may produce miliaria and maceration, particularly in patients with atopic dermatitis. Dermatitis due to Saran Wrap has been reported.[18]

Plastics closely related to Saran include the following polyvinyl resins:

Flamenol	Koroseal
Kogene	Vinylite Q
Korogel	Elastiglass

There have been reports of contact dermatitis caused by watchbands, garters and suspenders made of Elastiglass, which is a vinyl acetate and chloride polymerization product. The dermatitis in these cases was ascribed to traces of the plasticizer or stabilizer (dibutyl tin maleate or dibutyl sebacate), which was not properly removed during the production of Elastiglass.[19] I have seen dermatitis due to vinyl identification wristbands.

Plastic mittens and tablecloths made of vinyl plastic produce allergic contact dermatitis.[20] Allergic skin reactions to epoxy resins used as plasticizers and stabilizers in polyvinyl chloride films also have been reported.[21]

Spandex. This is the generic name for nonrubber stretchable fibers manufactured from polyurethane elastomers. These fibers are being used increasingly in stretchable garments, including surgical support hose and bandages.

Allergic contact dermatitis due to mercaptobenzothiazole in the fibers of spandex girdles and bras has been reported from abroad.[22]

In the United States, the following spandex fibers are manufactured without mercaptobenzothiazole and are nonsensitizing:

Lycra (DuPont)
Blue "C" (Chemstrand)
Vyrene (U. S. Rubber)
Numa (American Cyanamid)

Many rubber-sensitive individuals substitute apparel made of such American spandex provided the garments are free of rubber edges. Vanity Fair and Warner manufacture rubber-free girdles and bras in which Lycra spandex is the only elastomer.

Vinyon. Originally, vinyon was a trademark for vinyl chloride and acrylonitrile filaments, but it is now generic and includes a copolymer of polyvinyl chloride and polyvinyl acetate.

Vinyon has been used in the manufacture of work clothes. There have been no reports of dermatitis caused by it.

DERMATITIS DUE TO CLOTHING DYES

In view of the fact that textiles dyed with synthetic colors have been worn on a vast scale for nearly a century, and frequently in direct contact with the skin, the instances of irritation or dermatitis attributed to them are remarkably few.

The term *aniline dye* generally refers to all types of synthetic colors regardless of whether they are derived from aniline. In the U.S. Tariff Commission Report, 30 to 40 per cent of the azo dyes are classified as aniline dyes.

Vat dyes are a class of water-soluble colors generally used on cellulose materials. These colors are dyed by solubilizing them through reduction, applying them to the material in the reduced state and then re-oxidizing them to the final shade on the fabric.

Disperse dyes, which may include azo and anthraquinone types, are insoluble in water but are suspended by dispersing agents so that they may be applied to synthetic fabrics, such as cellulose acetate, nylon, polyamids and polyesters.

Most dyes, especially the common water-soluble and pigment types (vat dyes), do not appear to cause dermatitis. A few dispersed and miscellaneous dyes have been reported to be the cause of dermatitis in hypersensitive or sensitized individuals. The picture is often confused because of the wide range of dyeing assistants and finishing agents, many of which can cause contact or allergic dermatitis if not inactivated or removed during textile processing.

The disperse dyes (both azo and anthraquinone) used on synthetics can produce textile dye dermatitis. These dyes are not used on cotton, linen, wool and viscose rayon, which may be used in dye-sensitive patients

It is almost impossible to tell which dyes are most used for dark colored materials because the type of dye used depends upon the fabric. Cottons and rayons are generally dyed with direct, azo, sulfurs and vat colors, depending upon the desired fastness and end use requirements. Premetallized and after-treated acid dyes are used on wool and nylon. Dispersed colors are used on other synthetic fabrics.

Anthraquinone Dyes in Clothing

Anthraquinone dyes are a large class of compounds containing or derived from anthraquinone or its derivatives or homologues. They include acid, disperse, vat, pigment and solvent dyes, the chemical structures of which are described in Volume 3 of the *Colour Index*, Society of Dyers and Colorers, 3rd Ed., Yorkshire, England, 1971.

The term *aniline dyes* is obsolete and a misnomer because the dyes may or may not be derived from aniline and the term has no toxicological significance.

Anthraquinone dyes are used extensively in the United States. The acid dyes are used largely on wool and nylon; the disperse types are used on synthetic hydrophobic fibers, such as acetates and polyester. The vat types are used on cotton and rayon, and the pigments can be used on any fiber.

Several anthraquinone dyes are related chemically to paraphenylenediamine, e.g., Disperse Violet 8, Disperse Blue 5, Disperse Violet 1, and acid blue 27. Individuals with paraphenylenediamine sensitivity might have a cross-sensitivity to such dyes.

Anthraquinone dyes may cross-react with paraphenylenediamine

Cronin[23] concluded that a standard dye screening series is not feasible because of the large number of dyes used. Each patient tends to have an individual pattern of dye sensitivity and will not necessarily cross-react to other dyes. The only way to establish or refute a diagnosis is to patch test with the suspected piece of material. It is usually not necessary to extract dyes from clothing for testing as suggested by Fregert.[24]

Patch tests for dye sensitivity should be performed with the suspected material rather than individual dyes in a test series

It is impossible to tell by inspection whether a fabric contains a particular dye. Tracing the sensitizing dye may be of great value, however, since patients sensitized to a disperse dye may have to avoid synthetic materials and resort to wearing rayon, cotton, linen or wool.

Unfortunately, it is often difficult to identify the particular dye producing a dermatitis, because dyes may have many code names and are constantly being modified.

Wilson and Cronin[25] reported 5 instances of contact dermatitis from a green anthraquinone dye in the blue uniforms of 5 nursing sisters. Since this dye had been used for many years, it is possible that the uniforms were not dyed in the accustomed way and leached out onto the skin of the wearer, causing sensitization.

Clinical Picture of Garment Dye Dermatitis

Dye dermatitis due to blouses, sweaters or dresses affects the part of the trunk not protected by a slip, usually the axillae, neck and arms. Long-sleeved garments may affect the antecubital fossae. If a slip is the offending garment, the waist is usually affected. Bra dermatitis affects the breasts and waist. Dermatitis due to men's trousers may affect the anterior part of thighs and the popliteal fossae.

Garment dye dermatitis usually affects the neck, axillae and arms in women. Areas covered by a slip are usually spared

Nylon Stocking Dermatitis

Cronin[26] stated that nylon stocking dye dermatitis still occurs occasionally. Of 35 recently studied patients, 33 reacted on patch testing to yellow azo dye, Disperse Yellow 3. Four men, while working in a stocking factory, developed dermatitis from the same yellow dye. Two thirds of these patients also reacted to paraphenylenediamine.

Nylon stocking dye dermatitis is usually symmetrical and commonly affects the popliteal fossae, the inside of the thighs and the dorsal aspect of the feet. Sometimes only one of these sites is affected, and if the feet only are involved, a shoe dermatitis is often suspected.

Sometimes the patient who reacts to darker shades of nylon stockings may be able to wear stockings of lighter shades without difficulty.

Foussereau et al.[27] reported women and men with nylon hosiery dermatitis from sensitivity to Disperse Yellow 3 (4′-acetamido-2-hydroxy-4-methylazobenzene). Disperse Yellow 3 may show cross-reactions to paraphenylenediamine, the rubber antioxidants (diphenyl-n′-isopropyl paraphenylenediamine and n-phenyl-n′-isopropyl paraphenylenediamine), sulfanilamide and derivatives of para-aminobenzoic acid, such as benzocaine, Novocaine and para-aminosalicylic acid.[28]

Disperse Yellow 3, an azo dye causing nylon stocking dye dermatitis, may cross-react with paraphenylenediamine and derivatives of para-aminobenzoic acid

The diagnosis is established by testing a fragment of stocking and by testing 2 per cent Disperse Yellow 3 in petrolatum. Occasionally disperse dyes (Disperse Red 1, Disperse Blacks or anthraquinone) may produce stocking dye dermatitis.

Dermatitis due to formaldehyde resins in hosiery, rubber antioxidants, accelerators and tanning agents in shoes may have to be ruled out as the cause of dermatitis when the feet alone are involved.

Sidi and Arouete[29] suggested that the steam heating of stockings before applying pieces as patch tests may convert a negative or doubtful test into a positive one. Occasionally nylon dyes may be extracted from textiles by immersing in hot alcohol for 30 to 60 minutes.[30]

Paraphenylenediamine and Textile Dermatitis

This substance is used to dye only furs and very inexpensive fabrics.

Nevertheless, allergic sensitization to paraphenylenediamine may be significant in the production of dermatitis due to aniline and azo dyes.[28] These dyes are rarely the cause of primary sensitization. In many instances, an existing sensitization to chemical substances of the "para" group is reactivated. Thus, the primary sensitization engendered by paraphenylenediamine crosses over to azo and aniline dyes. The mechanism is explained by the liberation of paraphenylenediamine or another derivative of the "para" group owing to the splitting of the azo double bond. Persons who are allergic to paraphenylenediamine are not necessarily hypersensitive to all azo dyes, and sensitization to one azo dye does not necessarily imply allergy to others.

In clinical practice, many individuals with allergic hypersensitivity to paraphenylenediamine show cross-reactions with many aniline and azo dyes. In the past, many women with nylon stocking dye dermatitis showed positive patch test reactions to paraphenylenediamine, although it was not used to dye hosiery. The incidence of paraphenylenediamine hypersensitivity has remained high, but nylon stocking dye dermatitis has become rare because the dyeing processes have been improved so that the aniline dyes no longer bleed from the nylon fibers.

About one half of the patients with azo or anthraquinone dye dermatitis from clothing or stockings show cross-reactions with paraphenylenediamine

Significance of the Bleeding of Dyes

The incidence of textile dermatitis is greatly enhanced if the dye bleeds readily from the fabric, but this rarely occurs, and then only in patients with marked hyperhidrosis. The fastness of modern dyeing enables many individuals with allergic hypersensitivity to aniline dyes to wear dyed clothing without difficulty.

Role of Perspiration in Dye Dermatitis

The hydrogen ion concentration of human sweat varies from pH 4.2 to 7.5. It is more acid after exercise and in warm weather. Some dyes are more readily dissolved by acid than by alkaline perspiration. The variation in the pH of sweat on different areas of the body, therefore, may determine the site of dye dermatitis. In addition, a high fat content of perspiration may readily dissolve fat-soluble dyes, producing dermatitis. Perspiration from areas where there is little admixture of sebum will not solubilize such dyes, and dye dermatitis will not become established in sensitized individuals.[29]

Certain individuals tolerate light colors in clothing but acquire dermatitis from dark clothes, particularly those dyed black and dark blue. As a rule, the concentration of dyes in dark clothing is much higher than in light-colored clothing. Dark dyes bleed more readily than do dyes of a lighter hue.

Most popular dyes for black materials are sulfur dyestuffs, vat black dyestuffs, aniline black, indocarbon black and direct blacks.

Often dyes are implicated as causing textile dermatitis, when, in reality, the dermatitis is produced by dye intermediates or chemical agents such as acids or swellers, which are used as adjuvants in the dyeing process. The dye intermediates are more likely to cause dermatitis than the finished dyes, and under certain conditions, such as the heat of ironing, some dyes break down into their intermediates.

In rare instances, a chemical irritant may remain in the fabric and cause dermatitis. For example, if excess oxidizing bichromate is not removed in vat or mordant dyeing, dermatitis may occur in those handling or wearing the fabric.

Testing for Dye Sensitivity in Clothing

Patients should be patch tested with small pieces of material from clothing they have worn in direct contact with affected areas. These pieces may be taken from a seam or similar areas so that the garment will not be mutilated. In the sensitized patient, this method usually produces a definite patch test reaction.

Management of Clothing Dye Dermatitis

Patch testing reveals the clothes to which the patient is sensitive. Sometimes only one or two garments have to be discarded.

Whenever possible, an attempt should be made to trace the dye to which the patient is sensitive. This is difficult, because even if the manufacturer reveals the commercial names of the dyes, they must be translated into official names, identified and tested.

As Cronin[23] emphasized, most patients with dye dermatitis are sensitized to disperse dyes, which are used almost entirely in synthetic fibers (nylon, polyester, acrylics and acetate rayon) and seldom in viscose rayon, cotton, linen or wool.

The disperse dyes used in synthetic fibers, which are the most common cause of dye dermatitis, may be tested as 1 per cent in petrolatum or aqueous solution

Role of Dyes in Fur Dermatitis

Paraphenylenediamine, the main fur dye, is rarely used for dyeing textiles. Occasionally other oxidizing dyes, such as aniline black and o-aminophenol, are also employed in the dyeing of furs. Because of the careful oxidation of the dye and the thorough removal of excess or unoxidized dyes, fur dye dermatitis is a rarity. Paraphenylenediamine is now so well fixed to most furs that even individuals with strong allergic hypersensitivity to it can wear furs without risking dermatitis.

In extremely rare instances, the hair of the fur is the cause of dermatitis. Individuals who are allergic to cat hair may not be able to tolerate fur coats made of wildcat, ocelot or leopard. Many individuals who do not tolerate wool can wear Persian lamb coats.

Patch Tests with Fur Dyes. The dyes used in fur should be tested in the following concentrations:

Paraphenylenediamine (2% in petrolatum)
Aniline black (10% in oil, or the pure powder)
Para-aminophenol (10% in petrolatum)
Pontamine black (pure powder)

Clinical Picture of Fur Dermatitis. This type of dermatitis usually begins about the neck, chin, face and wrist, and in severe cases may spread to other parts of the body. Furs are more apt to cause allergic dermatitis of the eyelids than are other articles of apparel. Fur dye dermatitis may occur only after a poorly processed fur has become wet by rain, water or perspiration, causing the dyes to bleed.

Occasionally a dermatitis occurs from the mechanical friction of coarse, stiff hairs of certain furs against the neck and wrists. The lining usually protects the wearer from the chemicals used for tanning and dressing the hide.

DERMATITIS FROM CHEMICAL FINISHES APPLIED TO CLOTHING

Finishes are used in fabrics for the following reasons:[9]

To improve drape
To soften or stiffen fabric
To increase durability
To control shrinkage
To impart crease resistance
To provide water repellency
To provide oil repellency
To impart wash and wear properties
To fix color
To reduce pilling
To impart germicidal properties
To impart flame resistance
To impart antistatic properties
To increase or decrease luster
To impart a better feel
To prevent runs and unraveling

Starches and sulfonated castor oil were the first finishes used and were applied to enhance the appearance and feel of the fabric. Highly starched uniforms and collars may cause irritant dermatitis.

In recent years, numerous antiwrinkle and creaseholding finishes have been applied to fabrics, including the following resins:

Formaldehyde resins
Ester gums
Acrylates
Methacrylate
Polystyrene
Vinyl resins
Glycol resins
Alkyd resins
Ketone resins
Coumarins and indene polymers
Phthalic and maleic anhydride
Rosin

Mixtures of these resins also may be used. Resin finishes may cause dermatitis particularly when the resin is not completely polymerized or cured. In such cases there may be enough free monomers or uncured resins remaining in the fabric to produce dermatitis in sensitized individuals. Certain resins may also undergo decomposition while on the fabric and generate irritant decomposition products or offensive odors. Completely cured resins rarely cause dermatitis.

Permanent Press Finishes

Most textiles manufactured for apparel contain a mixture of cotton and rayon and a synthetic fiber, such as nylon or polyester.

Approximately 80 per cent of fabrics contain cotton or rayon treated with a formaldehyde cross-linking resin to stabilize shrinkage in washing and impart resistance to wrinkling. Permanent press clothing contains twice as much formaldehyde as does clothing without this type of finish.

Table 8–2 is a list of fibers containing permanent press resins.

Table 8-3 is a list of fabrics that are supposed to be free of formaldehyde resins, providing they are composed entirely of such fibers.

Federal law requires designation of exact fiber content by generic name on the neck of a garment.

The urea and melamine formaldehyde resins formerly used in textiles are now being

Table 8-2. Fibers Containing Formaldehyde Resins

Spun rayons
Rayon-acetate blends
Cotton labeled as durable press, "wash and wear" or wrinkle resistant
Shrinkproof woolens
Polyester blends with rayon or cotton

Table 8-3. Fibers Free of Formaldehyde Resins

Cellulose acetate
Wool
Nylon
Polyester (Dacron, Fortrel, Avlin, Quintesse, Trevera)
Acrylic (Orlon, Creslan, Zephran)
Modacrylic
Regular pure finish cotton

Table 8-4. Recently Introduced Crease Resistant Resins

Dimethylol dihydroxyethylene urea
Dimethylol urea
Dimethylol alkyl carbamates

replaced by others that cause less discoloration on laundering (E. Cronin, personal communication, 1971). These newer formaldehyde resins are listed in Table 8–4.

Dr. W. Jordan (personal communication, 1971) stated that dimethylol dihydroxyethylene urea and dimethylol alkyl carbamates are the leading crease resistant finishes in the United States. Formaldehyde is used in their synthesis, and it is the source of the methylol group for cross-linking cellulose fibers. These compounds contain excess formaldehyde to assure complete methylolation of the cyclic urea or carbamate, and approximately 0.1 per cent free formaldehyde remains on the treated fibers. It is possible that free formaldehyde may be regenerated by hydrolysis of the cross-links by acids and human sweat.

The newer dimethylol crease resistant and drip dry resins leave about 0.1 per cent free formaldehyde on the treated fibers

These resins may cause dermatitis not only from wearing apparel but also from no-iron sheets and pillowcases (S. Fregert and E. Tegver, personal communication, 1971).

Patch Testing for Sensitivity to Permanent Press Finishes

Patients suspected of having dermatitis from clothing treated with these finishes should be tested with the following substances:

Formalin (2% in water)
Urea formaldehyde (5% in petrolatum)
Melamine formaldehyde (5% in petrolatum)
Dimethylol dihydroxyethylene urea (10% in petrolatum)
Dimethylol urea (10% in petrolatum)
Dimethylol alkyl carbamates (5% in petrolatum)
Pieces of the fabric (which has been worn by the patient)
Water in which the fabric sample was incubated for 5 minutes at 60° C

In practice, it is not uncommon to encounter allergic eczematous contact dermatitis in a distribution highly suggestive of drip dry or wrinkle resistant clothing dermatitis, yet it is often difficult to obtain a positive patch test reaction with the fabric. Formaldehyde resin dermatitis in some instances may not be reproduced by patch testing because contributory factors, such as prolonged contact, sweating and friction, are absent in the testing procedure.

Indeed, it also is possible that sweat or sebum and friction could break the cross-links in formaldehyde resins and release free formaldehyde. Results of testing with a piece of unworn fabric, therefore, may differ from testing with a piece of worn fabric.[30]

Patch tests should be performed with fabrics that have been worn and subjected to sweat, sebum and friction

Relationship of Free Formaldehyde and Crease Resistant Finishes

Crease resistant fabrics are treated and cured before leaving the finishing plant, but enough formaldehyde may be liberated subsequently to produce eye, nose and throat irritation and dermatitis among garment workers and sales clerks.[31,32] Allergic formaldehyde dermatitis in the consumer is fairly common in Scandinavia,[33,34] and latent sensitivity is increasing in the United States.[35] Some cases of dermatitis may also be caused by intermediate products (dimethylol urea) in the incompletely cured resin.[36] Washing the garments either at the textile plant or by home laundering (alkaline wash) may remove most of the formaldehyde.[37]

A large proportion of resin-treated cloth is delivered to the garment maker in the uncured condition, The resins are cured at the time of pressing, but long storage at high temperature, 90 to 120 °F, and high humidity may reverse the curing reaction. After being pressed, the garments are usually washed before they are packaged, thereby lessening future release of formaldehyde.

Dr. W. P. Jordan (personal communication) found that the methylolated resins have between 1 and 3 per cent excess formaldehyde. He feels that current tests for formaldehyde are not relevant when done directly on treated fabric, since these tests break cross-links, generating formaldehyde that did not exist in the fabric. He found that the Schiff formaldehyde test can be performed on water in which the fabric sample was incubated for 5 minutes at 60 °C. Such indirect testing may be more relevant than direct tests because he has not seen a fabric that gave a negative result by the indirect method and a positive result by patch testing the patient.

Drs. E. Keran and W. F. Schorr (personal communication) analyzed 112 fabrics and found *none* that was completely free of formaldehyde. The 100 per cent polyester knit and Orlon acrylic fabrics consistently had the least amount of formaldehyde.

Quantitative chemical testing for formaldehyde with many fabrics said to be free of formaldehyde resins may show a positive reaction for formaldehyde in a low concentration, which may not be clinically significant.

Clinical Appearance of Dermatitis Due to Formaldehyde Resin

Women with hyperhidrosis are most commonly affected with an eczematous eruption beginning in the axillae. The sides of the neck, antecubital fossae and inguinal areas may also become involved. Lichenification readily takes place.[38]

Women are affected about 5 times as frequently as men, perhaps because they wear clothes closer to the skin, providing greater opportunity for sweat to leach formalin resins and initiate the reaction. It is also likely that women's clothes are more universally treated with formaldehyde resins than are those of men. When the dermatitis is caused by trousers, the inner thighs, gluteal folds and backs of the knees are most characteristically affected.[39]

Management of Dermatitis Due to Clothing Resins

Once it is determined that clothing dermatitis is produced by formaldehyde or its resins, any new clothing should receive several machine washings. Garments made of 100 per cent polyester, acrylic or cotton are usually well tolerated.

Patients with formaldehyde or formaldehyde resin sensitivity usually tolerate clothing made of 100 per cent synthetic fibers (nylon, polyester and acrylic) or cotton

The constant wearing of a formalin-free blouse as a protective undergarment may prevent recurrences of clothing dermatitis in formaldehyde-sensitive individuals.

Once the dermatitis has healed, some formalin-sensitive persons can resume wearing drip dry and crease resistant clothes in cool weather, when they do not sweat too profusely and when the garments fit loosely.

The linings of coats and dresses worn by formaldehyde-sensitive individuals should be tested for free formaldehyde. Such linings may have been treated with this chemical so that perspiration and hot pressing will not cause lining dyes to bleed.

Formaldehyde-containing linings should be removed and replaced. Sometimes the old linings can be reused after they have been thoroughly washed and rinsed.

Role of Free Formaldehyde in Clothing Dermatitis

Free formaldehyde is often used to aftertreat fabrics to make them fast to perspiration and steam pressing. Cellulose fibers have been strengthened by treatment with formaldehyde since the turn of the century.

Formaldehyde gas liquefies at 21 °C and is usually available as formalin, which is a concentrated aqueous solution containing 37 to 40 per cent formaldehyde. Free formaldehyde is readily removed by washing clothing, but appreciable amounts of formaldehyde resin remain in garments even after prolonged and repeated boiling in strong detergent solutions. Free formaldehyde is always found in finished fabrics that have been treated with formaldehyde resins.[40,41]

Allergic hypersensitivity to formaldehyde does not necessarily imply hypersensitivity to formaldehyde resins. The presence of significant amounts of free formaldehyde in clothing is mainly due to incomplete condensation of the resins or inadequate washing. There is no general agreement as to the permissible amount of free formaldehyde in the finished product. Dr. W. F. Schorr (personal communication) states, "It would be reasonable to allow formaldehyde sensitive patients to wear clothing with a formaldehyde content *below* 0.075%. The fact that the odor of formaldehyde can be detected in a textile when in storage or when the fabric is subjected to ironing is not necessarily of clinical significance."

Employees handling wearing apparel containing formaldehyde resin finishes often complain of the odor of formaldehyde and a burning sensation of the eyes when new stocks of summer clothes are received. Although the odor is easily detected (usually at a concentration of 1 to 2 parts per million), apparently it is not sufficient to cause contact dermatitis. Under conditions of storage and the absence of free circulation of air, it would be noticed even when the amount was far below a clinically significant concentration. Adequate ventilation soon dissipates the odor.

Formaldehyde Reactors and Clothing Dermatitis

Some patients with strongly positive patch test reactions to formaldehyde can wear garments that show positive chemical reactions for free formaldehyde. Many cases of clothing dermatitis due to formaldehyde reported from abroad may be due to excessive free formaldehyde in the finished fabric. In Europe, extensive use of formaldehyde as an antiperspirant may have sensitized many individuals. In areas of the United States where formaldehyde is used as an anhidrotic, dermatitis from formaldehyde in clothing also occurs.[42]

Qualitative Test for Formaldehyde in Clothing

To determine the presence of free formaldehyde in a fabric, a small sample of the material is added to 5 ml. of 1 per cent sulfuric acid solution. The mixture is brought to the boiling point and allowed to stand for 5 minutes. One drop of this heated solution is added to 2 ml. of 72 per cent sulfuric acid, and a few grains of chromotropic acid are added. The mixture is then heated over an open flame. An intense reddish purple color demonstrates not only free formaldehyde, but also easily depolymerizable formaldehyde resins.

Although free formaldehyde can be detected by testing a sample of clothing, it does not necessarily mean that the concentration is sufficient to cause clinical dermatitis, even in individuals who have shown a positive patch test reaction to 2 per cent formaldehyde.

Diagnosis of Clothing Dermatitis Due to Formaldehyde

In order to establish the diagnosis of clothing dermatitis due to free formaldehyde, the criteria in Table 8–5 should be fulfilled.[43]

Table 8-5. Criteria for Formaldehyde Clothing Dermatitis

1. The suspected fabric should show the presence of free formaldehyde.
2. The patient should show a positive patch test reaction to 2 per cent formaldehyde.
3. A positive patch test reaction should be obtained with the formaldehyde resin-impregnated materials.
4. Wearing of the fabric should produce clinical dermatitis.

Antimicrobial Agents in Textiles

Dr. S. Fregert (personal communication, 1971) pointed out that the following antimicrobial agents present in textiles may be sensitizers: methyl-p-hydroxybenzoate, organic mercury compounds, dimethyldithiocarbamate, sulphonamide (anionic), dichlorodihydroxy-diphenyl-methane, dibromosalicylanilide, tribromosalicylanilide, salicylanilide, 3,4,4′-trichlorocarbanilide, pentachloro-phenol-laurate, o-phenyl-phenol, tertiary butyl-m-cresol, p-chloro-m-cresol, p-chloro-m-xylenol, o-benzyl-p-chloro-phenol, 2,2′-methylene-bis-(3,4,6-trichlorophenol), DDT and dieldrin.

Scotchgard

This stain-repellent finish can cause clothing dermatitis.[44]

Use of Special Solvents for Extraction and Patch Testing of Clothing Finishes

Routine patch tests with a moistened piece of a garment may fail to produce a positive patch test reaction because the procedure does not duplicate clinical conditions. In use, sensitizing finishes in clothing may be leached out and concentrated by sweat. Furthermore, the friction produced when the garment is worn insures intimate contact of the finish with the skin.

It has been suggested that more positive reactions would be obtained if finishes were extracted from fabrics by use of solvents, such as the following:

2-Propanone (acetone diethyl ketone)
2-Butanone (methyl-ethyl ketone)
Ethanol (ethyl alcohol)
4-Methoxy-4-methyl pentanol (pentoxol, Me-6-G)

The dissolved finishes could then be concentrated and used for patch testing.[24]

I have found that Butyrolactone (General Aniline and Film Corp.) may be substituted for any of these solvents. My studies indicate that it is neither a sensitizer nor an irritant and may, therefore, be safely used as a solvent for patch test purposes.

Table 8-6. Most Commonly Used Dry Cleaning Materials and Concentrations for Patch Testing

Perchlorethylene (25% in olive oil). This halogenated hydrocarbon is employed extensively throughout the dry cleaning industry
Chloroform (as is)
Acetone (as is)
Alcohol (70% aqueous or as is)
Benzene (25% in olive oil)
Naphtha (25% in olive oil)
Turpentine (10% in olive oil)
Carbon tetrachloride (25% in olive oil)
Gasoline (25% in olive oil)
Kerosene (25% in olive oil)
Ether (as is)

DERMATITIS FROM DRY CLEANING PREPARATIONS

Some individuals acquire dermatitis on coming into contact with recently dry cleaned clothing, furs or blankets. When the history indicates that garments produced dermatitis after being dry cleaned, patch tests with the cleansers listed in Table 8–6 may be helpful in pinpointing the cause.

In evaluating patch test reactions to dry cleaning fluids, one must always perform control tests to rule out primary irritant reactions.

A great variety of chemicals are used to remove specific stains, such as rust, blood, albumin, silver nitrate, coffee, soft drinks, inks, paints and dyes. Many of these spot removers are powerful skin irritants, including hydrofluoric acid, glacial acetic acid, carbolic acid, nitrobenzene and strong alkalies. Workers in the dry cleaning industry are more likely to acquire dermatitis from such chemicals than are people who wear the cleaned garments, but if all traces of such cleansers are not removed, dermatitis may be produced.

When properly used, dry cleaning agents and stain removers are completely removed and are not permitted to come in contact with the skin. Patients with dermatitis or with easily irritated skin, however, should avoid contact with recently dry cleaned material until the garments have been thoroughly aired for several days.

DERMATITIS DUE TO LEATHER APPAREL

Dermatitis may occur from wearing leather shoes, jackets, wristwatch straps, hat bands, gloves and trusses. Tanning agents, dyes and finishing oils are the main sensitizers in leather garments.[45,46]

DERMATITIS FROM CONTAMINATED CLOTHING

Poison ivy oleoresin may cling to clothing and retain its dermatitis-producing potential for several days. Residual detergents, especially enzyme detergents, can also produce dermatitis.

In India, allergic dermatitis (dhobi itch) may be produced by laundry markings made with the oleoresin of the India marking nut tree.

Hosiery can be contaminated by chemicals and dyes leached out of shoes. Hosiery dermatitis may, therefore, actually be due to the chemicals in shoes.

Clothes may be contaminated by oil, grease, cements, insect sprays and other agents that are handled in work or hobbies.

When fiber glass curtains are washed with clothes, broken particles of fiber glass may be transferred to the clothing. Entire families may suffer from a petechial or scabies type of eruption due to such contamination.[47,48]

Workers in the fiber glass industry may bring home particles on their skin or clothing, which may be conveyed to other members of the family and produce an "epidemic" irritant dermatitis.

DERMATITIS DUE TO MECHANICAL PRESSURE OF CLOTHING

Stretch garment dermatitis[49] is a syndrome caused by pressure or tension on the skin from the wearing of tight-fitting stretch garments, such as bras, girdles and socks. The condition is not due to chemical sensitization but is mechanical.

Two principal forms of stretch garment dermatitis are: (1) a nondescript, erythematous and eczematous eruption, usually nonexudative, confined to the area covered by the garment and most severe where it binds most closely; and (2) an exaggeration of an already existing dermatosis in the areas covered by the garment.

Stretch garment dermatitis is an etiologic rather than a morphologic entity, and undoubtedly is a variant of Koebner's isomorphic phenomenon. Similar outbreaks of dermatitis may result from wearing garments that are not made of stretch material but are so tight-fitting that they produce friction and pressure (e.g., narrow-cut, short-rise trousers).

BLOUSING GARTER DERMATITIS

Minkin[50] and Gibbs[51] have described a syndrome of pigmentation of the ankles and dorsa of the feet in soldiers who wear either blousing garters or boot laces around their legs to keep fatigues neatly in place. The resultant mild edema and subsequent deposition of hemosiderin and melanin resemble changes of the lower extremities in patients with stasis dermatitis secondary to varicose veins. If the constriction is prolonged, one would assume hemosiderin deposits would occur as in the pigmented purpuric eruptions. The cutaneous changes occur distal to the site of constriction.

Edema of Lower Extremities. Women wearing tight panty girdles and other constricting clothing may develop edema of the lower extremities.[52]

Constrictive clothing may produce edema, mechanical irritation, Koebner's isomorphic phenomenon and purpuric eruptions

DERMATITIS AND PURPURA FROM RUBBER CLOTHING

Rubber or elasticized underwear may produce an allergic contact eczematous dermatitis associated with a secondary eruption resembling lichenoid pigmented dermatitis, eczematoid purpura or a variant of pigmented purpuric dermatitis.[53] Positive reactions in 23 patients were obtained with rubber antioxidants and accelerators, particularly n-phenyl-n-isopropyl-paraphenylenediamine.

DERMATITIS FROM FLAME RESISTANT CLOTHING

Flame proofed sleepwear has been reported as causing dermatitis in England.[54] Flameproofing is accomplished by either a Pyrovetex or a Roxelle process involving formaldehyde resins and THPC (tetra-BIS(hydroxymethyl)phosphonium chloride). Treated clothing is being introduced in the United States.[55]

Flame resistant clothing may contain formaldehyde resins

PARASITES AND CLOTHING

Parasites may contaminate clothing and produce dermatitis. Arthropods, such as lice and scabies mites, may infest clothing. The body louse, *Pediculus humanus* var. *corporis*, is rarely seen on the patient's skin, because it lays its eggs in and infests the seams of undergarments. It leaves the underclothing only to feed. The dermatitis produced by these blood-sucking lice is most marked in areas that are in most intimate contact with the clothing, such as the upper portion of the back and buttocks.

The scabies mite and the louse are most likely to infest hairy or woolen garments.

BEES AND CLOTHING

White or light-colored clothing with a smooth, hard finish is less likely to incite bees to sting than are dark, rough or wooly materials. Leather, possibly because of its odor, seems to be an attractant. It has been recommended that women wear a head covering, such as a silk scarf, when bees are present in order to prevent one from accidentally becoming caught in the hair. Clothing having a strong odor from perspiration, as well as perfume and scented hair dressings, may attract bees.

CLOTHING ACCESSORY DERMATITIS

The many accessories used on clothing, particularly nickel-plated or rubber objects, may produce sharply localized areas of dermatitis. Nickel-plated zippers, clips, buckles and pins, therefore, may produce dermatitis in nickel-sensitive individuals. Rubber shoulder pads, dress shields and collars and the rubber portion of girdles and bras can produce dermatitis in sensitized individuals. Other accessories such as studs and buttons, dyed dress labels, clothing marked with inks and articles carried in pockets may produce dermatitis.

Some garments contain inlaid patches of different colors and materials, such as gloves with leather inlays and socks with stripes of different colors, which may produce circumscribed areas of dermatitis.

FACTORS AFFECTING CLOTHING DERMATITIS

Friction, heat, humidity and particularly excessive perspiration play important roles in the production of clothing dermatitis. Tight-fitting clothing can produce dermatitis, which may not recur when the patient wears a larger garment or loses weight. The patient may acquire dermatitis from a particular article in the summer, but not in cooler weather or in drier climates. Hyperhidrosis, particularly when clothing is nonabsorbent, readily produces miliaria. The change of pH in sweat when evaporation is hindered may be a factor in producing dermatitis. Sweat also leaches dyes and finishes from clothing, which may produce dermatitis in sensitized patients. Control of excessive perspiration enables some patients to wear clothing which would otherwise produce dermatitis.

GENERAL MEASURES FOR MANAGEMENT OF CLOTHING DERMATITIS

When clothing is suspected of producing or aggravating an existing dermatitis, the following procedures should be employed.

Washing of Clothes. Whenever washable garments are suspected of causing dermatitis, such clothes, particularly socks, stockings, shirts and undergarments, should be washed to remove irritants and sensitizers before being worn again. All undergarments should be carefully washed and rinsed to remove all detergents, sebum and sweat.

Handling of Dry Cleaned Clothes. Clothing

that has been dry cleaned should be removed from the plastic bag and thoroughly aired before being worn to allow complete evaporation of solvents and irritants used in the dry cleaning process.

Weight Reduction. Weight loss in obese individuals, with a resulting lessening of friction and maceration, may permit them to wear garments that previously produced dermatitis.

Control of Hyperhidrosis. Attempts to control hyperhidrosis with antiperspirants and mild sedation, and avoidance of hot drinks and an overheated environment, may aid in the prevention of clothing dermatitis.

Use of Protective Garments. When sleeveless dresses are not feasible, white nylon slips with sleeves may protect hypersensitive skin from irritation of rough woolen and tweed dresses. Similarly, a white cotton shirt may protect the skin from contact with irritating garments. White cotton scarves are useful to protect the neck from friction of furs and of collars of coats or blouses.

Dark undergarments, particularly those colored with black, blue or brown dyes, should be avoided until the dermatitis clears up.

Use of Protective Sprays. Some individuals have found that spraying the axillae and other skin folds with a topical aerosol spray, such as Decadron (Merck, Sharp & Dohme), may help prevent clothing dermatitis, because the product forms a protective film of isopropyl myristate and corticosteroid.

Spray on Shield (Kleinert) and Serene (Sheffield) are commercially available sprays containing silicones in solution to act as barriers and protect clothing from perspiration, thereby preventing the leaching of dyes and finishes.

Avoidance of the Panty Girdle Syndrome. Women with lower abdominal and inguinal dermatitis should avoid wearing a panty girdle, because it has a closed crotch, which prevents evaporation of perspiration or secretions. These girdles also increase the humidity and temperature in the genitocrural area. The tight fit may cause a mechanical irritation, especially in obese women.[56] The intimate contact of the perspiring skin with the girdle may produce dermatitis from dyes, finishes and detergents used for cleansing the garment.

Another panty girdle syndrome is caused by the tourniquet effect of a tight-legged girdle, which constricts the venous and lymphatic return from the legs, with resultant edema and stasis dermatitis.[49] A regular girdle, with loosely fitting panties, prevents occlusion and constriction.

Management of Dermatitis from Linings. Dermatitis may occur from the presence of formaldehyde used to make linings perspiration-fast. Formaldehyde-lining dermatitis may often be successfully managed by removing the lining, thoroughly washing and rinsing it, and then replacing it. In extremely sensitive individuals, formaldehyde-free linings should be used.

Dermatitis from inexpensive lining material may be due to the presence of dyes that are not light-fast, because these compounds tend to bleed more readily than do dyes used on fabrics exposed to light. Replacement with a lining material of better quality, particularly of a light hue, has enabled several individuals to wear dresses and coats that previously produced dermatitis.

REFERENCES

1. Greenwood, K.: Dermatitis with Capillary Fragility. Arch. Derm., *81*, 947, 1960.
2. Hellier, F. F.: Dermatitis Purpurea After Contact with Textiles. Hautarzt, *11*, 173, 1960.
3. Hill, L. W.: Wool as Cause of Eczema in Children. New Engl. J. Med., *245*, 407, 1951.
4. Osborne, E. D., and Murray, P. F.: Atopic Dermatitis: Study of Its Natural Course and of Wool as Dominant Allergenic Factor. Arch. Derm., *68*, 619, 1953.
5. Sheldon, J. M., Lovell, R. G., and Mathews, K. P.: *A Manual of Clinical Allergy*. Philadelphia, W. B. Saunders Co., 1953, p. 33.
6. Urbach, E., and Gottlieb, P. M.: *Allergy*. New York, Grune & Stratton, 1946, p. 245.
7. Brown, S. F., and Coleman, M.: Severe Immediate Reactions to Biologicals Caused by Silk Allergy. J.A.M.A., *165*, 2178, 1957.
8. Braitman, M.: Dermatitis and Fabrics. J. Med. Soc. New Jersey, *52*, 757, 1955.
9. *Textile Fibers and Their Properties*. Technical Bulletin, Burlington Industries, Inc., New York, 1963.
10. Morris, G. E.: Nylon Dermatitis. New Engl. J. Med., *263*, 30, 1960.
11. Prassa, M. N.: Bullous Dermatitis of Feet Caused by Pure Nylon. Bull. Soc. Franc. Derm. Syph., *62*, 508, 1955.

12. Dobkevitch, S., and Baer, R. L.: Eczematous Cross-Hypersensitivity to Azo Dyes in Nylon Stockings and to Paraphenylenediamine. J. Invest. Derm., *9*, 203, 1947.
13. Fleming, A. J.: The Provocative Test for Assaying the Dermatitis Hazards of Dyes and Finishes Used on Nylon. J. Invest. Derm., *10*, 281, 1948.
14. Calnan, C. D., and Wilson, H. T. H.: Nylon Stocking Dermatitis. Brit. Med. J., *1*, 147, 1956.
15. Calnan, C. D., Marten, R. H., and Wilson, H. T. H.: Nylon Hair-Net Dermatitis. Brit. Med. J., *3*, 544, 1958.
16. Sonneck, H.: The Significance of Correct Care of Perlon Linen for the Prevention of Skin Diseases. Z. Haut. Geschlechtskr., *25*, 227, 1958.
17. Harris, D. K.: Some Hazards in the Manufacture and Use of Plastics. Brit. J. Industr. Med., *16*, 233, 1959.
18. Osbourn, R. A.: Contact Dermatitis Caused by Saran Wrap. J.A.M.A., *188*, 1159, 1964.
19. Morris, G. E.: Vinyl Plastics: Their Dermatological and Clinical Aspects. A.M.A. Arch. Industr. Hyg., *8*, 535, 1953.
20. Templeton, H. J.: Contact Dermatitis from Plastic Mittens. Arch. Derm., *61*, 854, 1950.
21. Fregert, S., and Rorsman, H.: Hypersensitivity to Epoxy Resins used as Plasticizers and Stabilizers in Polyvinyl Chloride Resins. Acta Dermatovener., *43*, 10, 1963.
22. Munro-Ashman, D.: Contact Dermatitis from Spandex Thread. Case Report. Trans. St. John Hosp. Derm. Soc., *52*, 131, 1966.
23. Cronin, E.: Studies in Contact Dermatitis. XVIII. Dyes in Clothing. Trans. St. John Hosp. Derm. Soc., *54*, 156, 1968.
24. Fregert, S.: Extraction of Allergens for Patch Testing. Acta Dermatovener., *44*, 107, 1964.
25. Wilson, H. T. H., and Cronin, E.: Dermatitis from Dyed Uniforms. Brit. J. Derm., *85*, 67, 1971.
26. Cronin, E.: Studies in Contact Dermatitis. XIX. Nylon Stocking Dermatitis., Trans. St. John Hosp. Derm. Soc., *54*, 165, 1968.
27. Foussereau, J., et al.: Allergic Eczema from Disperse Yellow 3 in Nylon Stockings and Socks. Trans. St. John Hosp. Derm. Soc., *58*, 15, 1972.
28. Hautklin, D. H.: Chronic Eczemata Caused by Dyes and Other Products Used in the Manufacturing of Textiles. Z. Haut. Geschlechtskr., *26*, 4, 1959.
29. Sidi, E., and Arouete, J.: Sensitization to Azo Dyes and to the Para Group. Presse Med., *67*, 55, 1959.
30. Wilkinson, D. S.: Ancillary Aids in Elucidation of Causes of Contact Dermatitis. Brit. J. Derm., *86*, 445, 1972.
31. Bourne, H. G., Jr., and Seferian, S.: Formaldehyde in Wrinkle-Proof Apparel Produces Tears for Milady. Industr. Med. Surg., *28*, 232, 1959.
32. Bourret, J., et al.: Occupational Dermatoses Produced by Formaldehyde and its Industrial Derivatives. Arch. Mal. Prof., *19*, 611, 1958.
33. Hovding, G.: Contact Eczema Due to Formaldehyde in Resin Finished Textiles. Acta Dermatovener., *41*, 194, 1961.
34. Berrens, L., Young, E., and Jansen, L. H.: Free Formaldehyde in Textiles in Relation to Formalin Contact Sensitivity. Brit. J. Derm., *76*, 110, 1964.
35. Baer, R. L., et al.: Changing Patterns of Sensitivity to Common Contact Allergens. Arch. Derm., *89*, 3, 1964.
36. Andrup, O.: "Creaseless-Treated" Textiles as a Cause of Eczema. T. Norske Laegeforen., *77*, 679, 1957.
37. Malten, K. E.: Textile Finish Contact Hypersensitivity. Arch. Derm., *89*, 215, 1964.
38. Skog, M.: Axillary Eczema in Women, A Syndrome. Acta Dermatovener., *39*, 369, 1959.
39. Cronin, E.: Formalin Textile Dermatitis. Brit. J. Derm., *75*, 267, 1963.
40. Fisher, A. A., Kanof, N. B., and Biondi, E. M.: Free Formaldehyde in Textiles and Paper: Clinical Significance. Arch. Derm., *86*, 753, 1962.
41. Hovding, G.: Free Formaldehyde in Textiles: Cause of Contact Eczema. Acta Dermatovener., *39*, 357, 1959.
42. Quinn, S. E., and Kennedy, C. B.: Contact Dermatitis Due to Formaldehyde in Clothing Textiles. J.A.M.A., *194*, 123, 1965.
43. Marcussen, P. V.: Contact Dermatitis Due to Formaldehyde in Textiles. 1934–1958: Preliminary Report. Acta Dermatovener., *39*, 348, 1959.
44. Eskelson, Y. D., and Goodman, L. S.: Contact Dermatitis from "Scotchgard," Stain Repellent for Fabrics: Report of Case. J.A.M.A., *183*, 136, 1963.
45. Morris, G. E.: Cross-Sensitization of the Feet and Hands Due to Chrome-Tanned Leather Shoes and Gloves. New Engl. J. Med., *257*, 567, 1957.
46. Jacobs, P. H.: Contact Dermatitis Due to Flight Gloves. Aerospace Med., *35*, 70, 1964.
47. Abel, R. R.: Fiberglass: Washing Machine and Fiberglass. Arch. Derm., *93*, 78, 1966.
48. Fisher, B. K., and Warentin, J. D.: Fiberglass Dermatitis. Arch. Derm., *99*, 717, 1969.

49. Mihan, R., and Ayres, J.: Stretch Garment Dermatitis. California Med., *108*, 109, 1968.
50. Minkin, W.: Military Aspects of Dermatology. Cutis, *8*, 961, 1968.
51. Gibbs, R. C.: Blousing Garter Dermatitis. Dermatologica Internat., *8*, 83, 1969.
52. Ribaudo, C. A., and Formato, A. A.: Panty Girdle Syndrome. N.Y. J. Med., *65*, 456, 1965.
53. Batschvarov, B., and Minkou, D. M.: Dermatitis and Purpura from Rubber Clothing. Trans. St. John Hosp. Derm. Soc., *54*, 178, 1968.
54. Martin-Scott, I.: Contact Textile Dermatitis (With Special Reference to Fireproof Fabrics). Brit. J. Derm., *78*, 632, 1966.
55. Taylor, J. S.: Public Health Service. Personal communication.
56. Curth, H. O., and Williamson, S. W.: Skin Brevities. The Panty Girdle as a Cause of Genital Irritation. Skin, *3*, 182, 1964.

Plate 6. Sensitizers in Wearing Apparel

1. Leather Hat Band

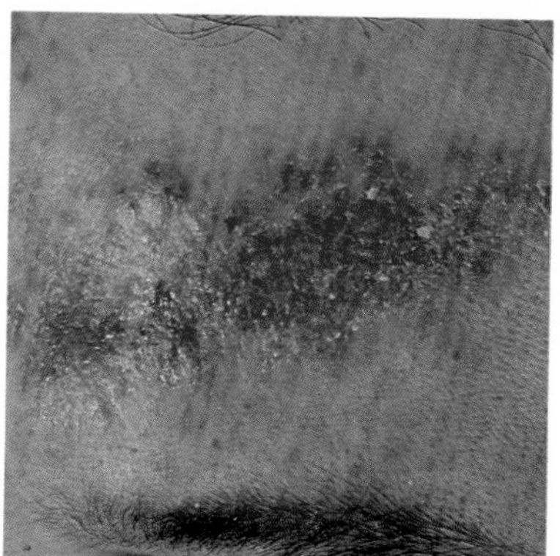

Formaldehyde

2. Shoe Buckle

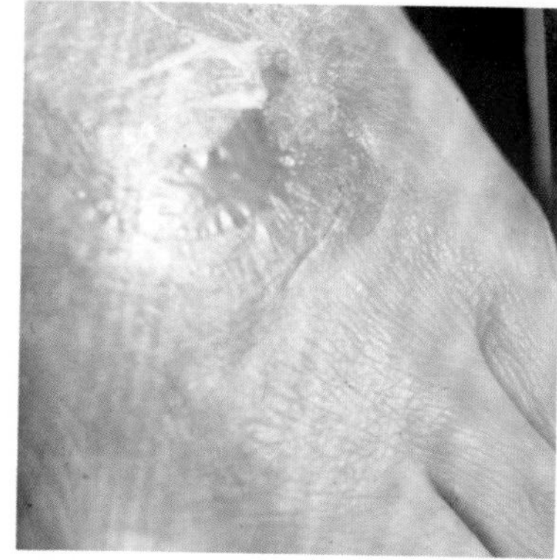

Nickel

3. Shoe Tanning Agent

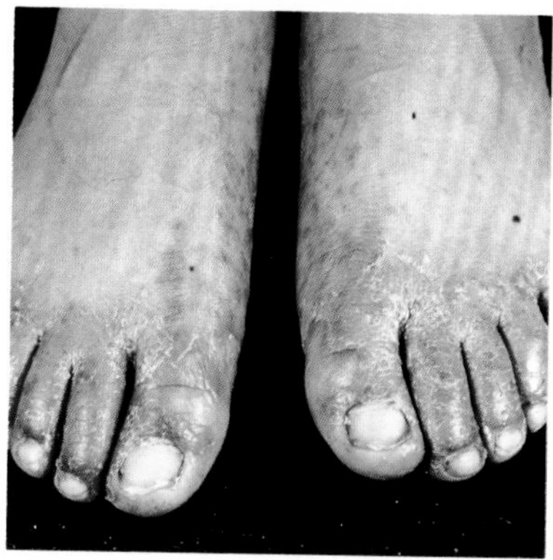

Potassium Dichromate

4. Shoe Glue

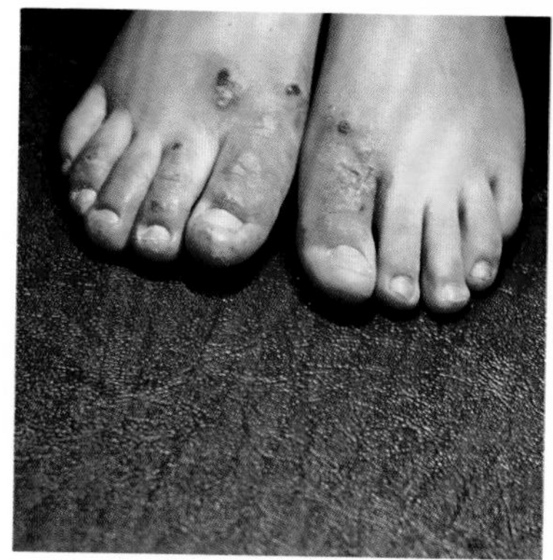

Phenolformaldehyde

5. Black Dress Dye

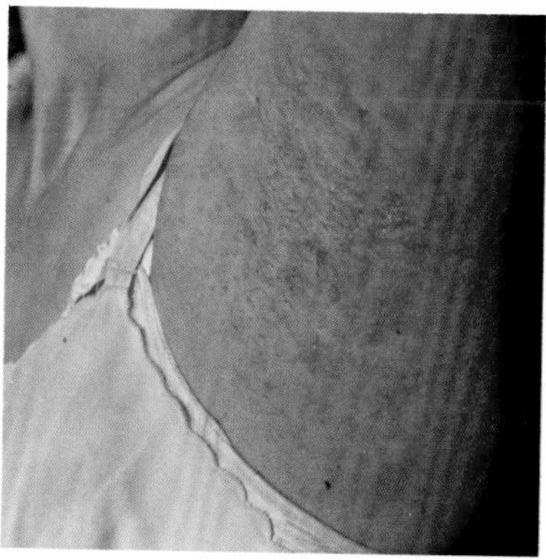

Azo Dye

6. Rubber Waist Band

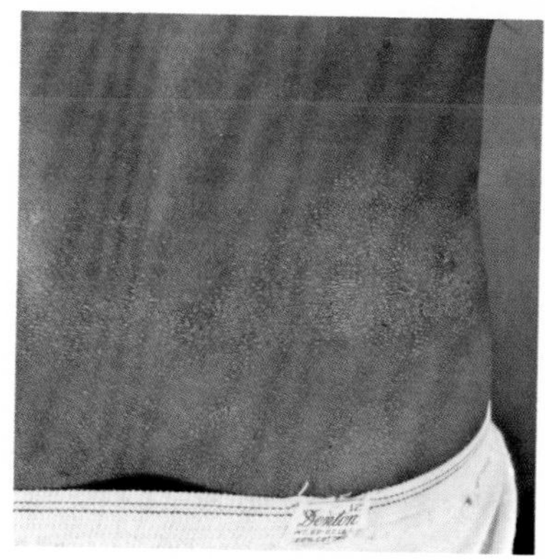

Mercaptobenzothiazole

9

Shoe Dermatitis

Shoe dermatitis may be divided into two categories: (1) *mechanical* or *irritative* and (2) *allergic*.

SHOE DERMATITIS DUE TO MECHANICAL FACTORS

Ill-fitting shoes and anatomical foot abnormalities may cause excessive friction and wearing away of protective linings and thus allow more intimate contact of shoe sensitizers with the skin. Orthopedic correction of deformities or orthopedic shoes may be necessary to correct this type of dermatitis.[1]

Particularly in children, it is not rare for friction of tight-fitting shoes to localize atopic dermatitis to the dorsal aspect of the big toes. Shoes that are too large also may produce irritating folds in the leather.

Hack[2] pointed out that since shoes soaked by perspiration tend to become brittle, leading to breakdown of the linings and uppers and warping of innersoles, moisture-absorbing wooden shoe trees should be inserted into the shoes as soon as they are removed from the feet and left in until the next wearing, which ideally should not be for at least 36 hours. This means that the patient should have at least two pairs of "everyday" shoes.

Ill-fitting shoes, wet shoes, rough, overfull, worn or uneven linings, may produce a mechanical irritative shoe dermatitis

Overfull linings that become soaked by water or perspiration tend to dry in hard ridges if trees are not put in the shoes.

Mechanical irritation may result from innersoles that tear or crack, exposing the soles to tacks or the rough edges of tack holes. Innersoles may develop irritating ridges or concavities at points of excessive weight-bearing.

Drying wet shoes by high heat, such as in ovens or on radiators, may make leather lining brittle and uneven.

Wooden shoe trees absorb sweat and moisture and keep shoes and linings in shape, thereby preventing shoe dermatitis in some cases

ALLERGIC SHOE DERMATITIS

Common causes of allergic shoe dermatitis include the following:

Rubber box toes
Rubber cements
Tanning agents—chrome, vegetable, formaldehyde, glutaraldehyde
Dyes
Nickel-plated shoe accessories
Synthetic leather

The diagnosis of allergic shoe dermatitis depends on the history, the clinical picture, positive patch test reactions to the ingredients of shoe materials and the patient's ability to wear proper substitute shoes without acquiring dermatitis. The management of a case of shoe dermatitis is not completed with the diagnosis and the treatment of an existing dermatitis. The patient must be informed how he can obtain acceptable shoes free from the specific materials to which he is allergic. Otherwise he is doomed to frequent recurrences or to the wearing of poor substitutes, such as sandals.

Rubber box toes, rubber cements and tanning agents are common causes of shoe dermatitis

CLINICAL PICTURE OF SHOE DERMATITIS

Most frequently, shoe dermatitis begins on the dorsal aspect of the big toe with eventual extension to the other toes and onto the feet. Often patients give a history of recurrent eruptions of the feet for many years. The webs and soles usually are free of involvement. Straps, webbings and thongs, particularly on sandals, may produce an eruption at sites where they contact the skin.

Id eruptions of the hands, especially during acute exacerbation of shoe dermatitis, are common. Contact dermatitis of the feet becomes readily infected and eczematous. Often, injudicious treatment of a shoe dermatitis with irritants and sensitizers produces widespread and even generalized eruptions. It is surprising how often patients with shoe dermatitis eventually become hospitalized for a severe, disabling dermatitis due to improper treatment of the original condition.

Eruptions produced by shoes are frequently misdiagnosed as ringworm, eczema or psoriasis.

Usually the dorsum of the foot is involved in shoe dermatitis. Occasionally the volar aspect or the toe webs may also become involved

PATCH TESTS FOR SHOE DERMATITIS

Whenever possible, patch testing should be performed with pieces of material from the suspected shoe. A positive reaction should be followed by testing with a shoe screening patch test tray to determine, if possible, the sensitizer, so that advice can be given about how to obtain shoes free of the causative agent.

Testing with Shoe Material. Pieces of the shoe and the shoe lining should be obtained from portions of the shoe contacting the main sites of dermatitis.[3] This material may be obtained by means of scalpel or skin biopsy punch. Dr. Silas O'Quinn suggests the use of a mastoid curet. The lining is separated from the leather and then applied with the sticky inner surface under a patch.[4]

The Use of a Shoe Screening Patch Test Tray

When a positive patch test reaction is obtained with material from shoes or when an eruption strongly suggests a shoe dermatitis but testing with material from the suspected shoes is negative, testing should be performed with materials and chemicals listed in Table 9-1.

Table 9-1. Shoe Diagnostic Screening Patch Test Series

Rubber box toe material (as is)
1% Monobenzyl ether of hydroquinone in petrolatum (antioxidant)
1% Mercaptobenzothiazole in petrolatum (accelerator)
1% Tetramethylthiuram monosulfide in petrolatum (accelerator)
1% Hexamethylenetetramine in petrolatum (accelerator)
1% Phenyl beta-naphthylamine in petrolatum (antioxidant)
0.25% Potassium dichromate in aqueous solution (tanning agent)
5% Formaldehyde in aqueous solution (tanning agent for white shoes)
2% Paraphenylenediamine in petrolatum (may cross-react with shoe dyes and n-isopropyl-n-paraphenylenediamine, a rubber antioxidant)
5% Nickel sulfate in aqueous solution (eyelet, buckles and tips of shoelaces)

ROLE OF RUBBER IN SHOE DERMATITIS

Rubber, rubber box toes, rubber cements and constituents of rubber compounds (e.g., oxidizers, accelerators, fixers and thinners) may be present in shoes. Rubber cements are used widely in joining shoe uppers, the outer leather and the linings and also for temporarily holding facings and bindings in place. Heel pads and sock linings are affixed by rubber cements.

Fiber innersoles (and counters) are frequently found, particularly in high styled women's shoes and in more expensive shoes generally. *Fiber* is a term that usually indicates cellulose fibers bound together with latex cements.

Rubber cements are a common cause of shoe dermatitis.[5–7] The monobenzyl ether of hydroquinone can produce not only dermatitis, but also depigmentation.

In addition, reports from abroad[8,9] implicate reactive phenolic resins added to neoprene adhesives as the etiologic agents of shoe dermatitis in some cases.

Antioxidants and accelerators in rubber box toes and cement are common sensitizers

RUBBER AND NONRUBBER BOX TOES

Rubber box toes, which are usually soft, are made from natural rubber, synthetic rubber or a combination of both and fixed into position by rubber cements. They are found in most of the less expensive oxford-type shoes and are the most common causes of shoe dermatitis. The sensitizers are usually the rubber accelerators and antioxidants listed in Table 9–1.

Whenever the dermatitis is confined to the dorsal aspect of the toes or feet, an effort should be made to obtain nonrubber box toe shoes, which are made of polystyrene, polyvinyl acetate, pyroxylin or acrylic resins. These are rarely sensitizers, but shoes containing such box toes are difficult to identify and obtain.

ROLE OF ADHESIVES IN SHOE DERMATITIS

Fish glues, gutta percha, pyroxylin, cellulose acetate and cellulose nitrate cements, polyvinyl acetate, polyisobutylene, phenol-formaldehyde and rubber adhesives are used in shoes. The wearing away of linings allows exposure of the feet to these compounds. Rubber cements and phenolic resins are common causes of shoe dermatitis.

When the rubber cement in a worn heel pad causes dermatitis, the use of LePage fish glue as a substitute adhesive usually proves satisfactory. Felt or fabric innersoles can be utilized to prevent contact of the plantar surface with rubber in midsoles.

While the role of the rubber box toe and cements is being evaluated, the patient may wear unlined moccasin sandals or unlined cloth or plastic shoes before special or expensive shoes are ordered.

PRESENCE OF RUBBER IN NONRUBBER SHOES

Leather shoes may contain rubber in the box toes or in adhesives. In my material, about 75 per cent of all cases of leather shoe dermatitis were due to rubber in the shoes. A positive reaction to one or more of the rubber chemicals in the diagnostic shoe tray should alert one of the possibility that rubber may be the cause of the dermatitis.

SHOE LEATHER TANNING AGENTS

The chrome salts, aldehydes and vegetable tannins are the principal compounds used for leather tanning, the process that changes the collagen of the leather into a stable compound that resists wear, water, putrefaction and heat changes.[10]

Chrome Tanning. Leather chemists emphasize that *hexavalent* chromates are not used to tan leather and should not be present in any finished products. Trivalent hydrated basic chromium sulfates, which are used to tan shoe *uppers* and *lining leather*, polymerize and react with the hide protein. *Sole leathers* are usually tanned commercially with vegetable extracts.

Although Morris[11] and Fregert[12] showed that chromium dermatitis from shoes is due to trivalent chromium, patch tests are often performed with potassium dichromate, because sensitization to trivalent chromium is often detected by testing with hexavalent chromate.

Patch tests with hexavalent dichromates may detect shoe dermatitis due to chrome sensitivity, although the trivalent salts are used in the tanning process

Sodium dichromate may be used in dyeing brown, yellow and dark red leather, and chromates may be employed in the dyeing of nonleather synthetic uppers.

Cronin[13] has emphasized that *vegetable*-tanned leather, free of chromates, can produce shoe dermatitis.

Scutt[14] reported many cases of sandal dermatitis due to chrome sensitivity and concluded that contact with chrome-tanned shoe leather is a major cause of atopic eczema.

It has been my experience that only dichromate-sensitive patients whose feet perspire profusely acquire shoe dermatitis, indicating the importance of the control of sweating. Perspiration can leach the chrome from chrome-tanned leather.[15]

Chrome is gradually removed from the collagen of leather by the action of sweat acids

Vegetable Tanning. This ancient method of tanning leather is still extensively employed for processing hides to make heavy leather for soles, harnesses and industrial belting. Trees and plants from all over the world, such as cutch from Borneo, and our own native chestnut, spruce and oak trees, are sources. Vegetable tanning involves the long maceration of the hide in a progressively stronger infusion of the tanning material.

The following plant substances may be used as vegetable tanning agents:

Wood of chestnut tree
Bark from mangrove tree
Pods from caesalpiniaceous tree
Leaves and twigs from Malayan rubiaceous vine
Bark from hemlock tree
Nuts from Terminalia chebula tree
Bark from chestnut oak tree
Wood of quebracho tree
Cups from acorn of Turkish oak
Leaves from sumac tree
Bark from acacia tree

Cronin[13] reported that many individuals are allergic to vegetable-tanned leather. In the United States, aside from imported India sandals, allergic reactions to vegetable-tanned shoes is rarely reported.

In requesting vegetable-tanned shoes, it must be emphasized that the inner leather lining, if any, must also be vegetable-tanned. It has been my experience that some vegetable-tanned shoes have chrome-tanned linings.

Leather insoles may be of purely vegetable tannage, chrome tannage or a chrome retan of vegetable tannage.

Leather lining is generally a chrome retan. It is therefore necessary to use vegetable-tanned upper leather for quarter linings in the presence of chrome sensitivity.

Aldehyde Tanning. This is most commonly used in white skins, such as nu-bucks, elk and white kid. Formaldehyde is one of the aldehydes used for this type of tanning. The aldehydes are usually so firmly bound to the leather that dermatitis from this source is rare. Sometimes phenolic-hydroxylcarboxyl compounds called syntans are used in the processing of white leather. These compounds include resorcinol and xylenol and have not been reported as producing dermatitis.

A positive patch test reaction to formaldehyde in a patient with dermatitis of the feet should suggest possibility of a shoe dermatitis, particularly if white shoes have been worn.

Glutaraldehyde. Hides may be tanned with glutaraldehyde to yield soft, glove leathers, which are being evaluated as components of commercial footwear. Glutaraldehyde has been shown to be a sensitizer.[16]

Role of Dye Sensitivity in Shoe Dermatitis

Leather dyeing is done principally with the azo-aniline group of dyes. The specific dyes used in shoes are usually a trade secret and are not readily made available to physicians for testing, but this is rarely necessary because these dyes are usually so well fixed to the leather that dermatitis is extremely rare.

When the patient has shoes redyed, the possibility of dermatitis is increased, because the dye in the redyed shoes is not likely to be as fast as the original dye. Some dyes used in leather, with the vehicles and concentrations for patch testing, include the following:

Bismarck brown—pure
Amido-azobenzol—10% in olive oil
Amido-azotoluene hydrochloride—1% aqueous
Chrysoidine brown—pure powder

Although paraphenylenediamine is not used as a shoe dye, it often cross-reacts with the dye used in shoes. The addition of paraphenylenediamine to the diagnostic tray has proved helpful in alerting one to the possibility of shoe dye dermatitis. A positive reaction to paraphenylenediamine in a patient with shoe dermatitis, however, does not necessarily mean that the dermatitis is due to dyes unless a positive reaction to a specific shoe dye also is obtained. Two of 3 patients whom I treated with redyed shoe dermatitis showed cross-reactions between the shoe dye and paraphenylenediamine.

Although primary dye dermatitis in leather shoes is rare, it is encountered more frequently in fabric and plastic shoes. I have studied several patients with shoe dermatitis due to dyes that bled readily from fabric shoes. Most of these patients also reacted to paraphenylenediamine. The area of dermatitis from shoe dyes may assume the shape of shoe uppers.

Traces of paraphenylenediamine found in vegetable-tanned and chrome-tanned shoes are usually completely oxidized and not capable of producing dermatitis.

Paraphenylenediamine may also show cross-reactions to rubber additives that are chemically related to the dye.

Paraphenylenediamine is not used to dye shoes, but it cross-reacts with shoe dyes and certain rubber antioxidants

MISCELLANEOUS TYPES OF SHOE DERMATITIS

"*Japanese Hot Foot.*" Japanese shoes with plastic uppers and imitations of the ripple sole produced a number of cases described by Kauth[17] as "Japanese hot foot." Shellow[18] and Weiner[19] reported that the occlusive action of the footwear produced the dermatitis.

"*Flip-Flop*" *Dermatitis.* Asymmetrical dermatitis of the feet due to Japanese-made rubber flip-flop shoes first appears on the dorsa in a V pattern.[20]

"*Vamp Disease.*" Shapiro and Gibbs[21] reported 7 women who developed inflammatory swellings on the dorsal aspect of the base of the hallux secondary to irritation from the edge of the vamp of a shoe. The swelling is characterized by a horn-filled sinus, resembling a clavus, on the surface. The process may extend deeply to involve the extensor hallucis longus tendon. Avoiding the ill-fitting shoes is probably the most important therapeutic measure, but incision and drainage during the subacute state and possible excision of any residuum may be necessary at a later date.

ROLE OF CONTAMINATED SHOE LININGS IN SHOE DERMATITIS

Rarely, stocking dyes bleed onto the lining of shoes. Patch testing with such contaminated shoe linings may be misleading, because the sensitizing dye originally came from stockings. Even when there is a change to stockings without sensitizing dyes, shoe dermatitis may persist for several months if the patient continues to wear the contaminated shoes. This is a type of secondary shoe dermatitis, the primary cause being the stocking dyes.

In my experience, colored cloth linings in leather shoes have not caused dermatitis. Positive patch test reactions with cotton shoe linings have to be carefully evaluated, because the sensitizing substance may have come from the stockings or deeper portions of the shoe. Dyes, chromates and rubber chemicals may be leached out of shoes onto such linings. Cotton fabric linings may be impregnated with antimildew agents, which rarely cause dermatitis.

Chrome-tanned leather linings may produce dermatitis in chromate-sensitive individuals.

ROLE OF NICKEL SENSITIVITY IN SHOE DERMATITIS

Nickel-plated objects in or on shoes play a relatively minor role in the production of shoe dermatitis. Dermatitis of the instep may be caused by nickel-plated lace eyelets. The metal tips of shoelaces, especially if tucked inside the shoe, may produce dermatitis. Contact of the foot with buckles or other nickel-plated shoe ornaments may be responsible for shoe dermatitis in individuals sensitive to nickel. Nickel-plated arch supports may produce dermatitis of the soles in patients hypersensitive to nickel.[22]

INDIAN SANDAL DERMATITIS

In sensitized individuals, Indian and thong sandals produce a dermatitis matching the areas contacted by the straps and thong.

Minkin et al.[23] reported a patient sensitized by buffalo-hide sandals made in East India who later developed a contact dermatitis to the leather lining of an American-made shoe. This leather lining also originated in India. The offending agent was probably a vegetable tannin.

In view of the current number of allergic reactions to East Indian sandals and the apparent presence of similarly tanned leather products in American-made shoes, vegetable-tanned leather may become a much more prevalent cause of shoe dermatitis in the United States.[24,25]

Vegetable-tanned sandals from India have produced many instances of dermatitis

LEATHER FUNGICIDES

Numerous antimildew agents, including chlorinated phenols (G-4), chlorinated salicylanilides, thirams and mercaptobenzothiazole, are used in the manufacturing of shoes. Although these antiseptics have been reported as causing allergic dermatitis when employed in products such as soaps and weed killers, and in rubber additives, their use as antimildew agents in leather rarely causes shoe dermatitis.

From time to time, new antimildew agents are introduced that produce dermatitis but are soon eliminated by the manufacturer. At present, the antimildew agents in the finished leather products and shoes are rarely implicated in dermatitis.

SHOES MADE FROM ARTIFICIAL LEATHER

Synthetic resins may be formulated to resemble leather. Vinyl, acrylic and latex can be used to impregnate cotton and other fabrics for such purposes. Real leather can often be distinguished from the artificial variety by tearing the material. Leather tears with a ragged edge from which extruding fibers may be seen. Dermatitis may occur from artificial leather shoes. The dyes, vinyl and unpolymerized acrylic resins, formaldehyde, antioxidants and plasticizers used in plastic shoes may produce dermatitis, The diagnosis usually is not difficult, because the patient readily correlates the onset of the dermatitis with the wearing of such shoes.

Shoes made of Corfam are no longer as readily available as in the past. Such shoes did not absorb perspiration readily and certain colored Corfam leather contained chromates. Only white Corfam is definitely free of chromates.

Chromates may be present in colored Corfam shoes. Only white Corfam is free of chromates

CONTROL OF HYPERHIDROSIS

Perspiration can leach chromates, rubber additives and dyes from shoes and cause contact of these potential sensitizers with the skin. The control of hyperhidrosis, therefore, often prevents or minimizes shoe dermatitis.[26] I recommend use of a non-caking dusting powder, such as the following:

Fluffy Tannic Acid Powder (Merck and Co.)
Bentonite
Talc
Equal parts—up to 2 oz.
Dispense in sifter box. Dust onto feet and into hosiery and shoes

This powder tans and toughens the skin and helps control hyperhidrosis.

ZeaSORB Powder (Stiefel), dusted freely into shoes and hosiery, tends to lessen perspiration and may act as a mechanical barrier to allergens. Theoretically, there would be no allergic contact shoe dermatitis without perspiration or moisture. Some individuals can wear shoes containing chemicals to which they are allergic provided the weather is cool and they do not perspire freely or their feet are protected with a drying powder.

Individuals who perspire freely often cannot tolerate shoes made of plastics or other materials that do not absorb sweat and do not "breathe" unless they use an absorbent dusting power. The sweaty foot syndrome due to occlusive footwear, unlike allergic dermatitis from shoe ingredients, often involves the soles and interweb areas.

Some patients acquire shoe dermatitis only when their shoes get wet or their feet perspire excessively

ROLE OF MECHANICAL PROTECTION IN SHOE DERMATITIS

Mechanical protection against shoe sensitizers has been afforded in the past by wearing Saran Wrap, waxed paper, oiled silk, plastic paper or aluminum foil inside shoes. These agents have proved to be generally uncomfortable and unsatisfactory because they are occlusive.

Some patients obtain protection by wearing cotton cloths, muslin, Surgitube or Kleenex inside their shoes. Women and girls who perspire freely and wish to wear nylon stockings might find useful the cotton foot, seamless nylon stockings termed "Heavenly Soles," which are manufactured by Sedgfield Knitting Mills, P. O. Box 4064, Reading, Pa. 19606. These are suitable for wear only with oxfords, because the cotton foot shows with other types of shoes.

For children, square toe socks (Tru Last, J. W. Landenberger and Co., 3800 Castor Av., Philadelphia, Pa. 19124) may be helpful in minimizing shoe dermatitis.

THE PURCHASE OF SHOES FREE OF SPECIFIC SENSITIZERS

Manufacturers, wholesalers and retailers are not always cooperative in transmitting information that will enable patients to obtain specific types of shoes. When it is realized that several hundred manufacturers sell 130 types of footwear under more than 2500 brand names, one realizes the difficulty in obtaining accurate information about a specific pair of shoes.

The purchase of shoes free of certain allergens is expedited if the patient has a written statement of his requirements to show to the manager of the shoe store rather than to a sales person who may not be familiar with all the types of shoes in stock.

SHOES MADE TO ORDER

The Foot-So-Port Shoe Company, a subsidiary of Musebeck Shoe Co. Inc., Oconomowoc, Wis. 53066, will make shoes eliminating rubber cements and other material to which the patient shows a positive patch test reaction. This company supplies the following for patch test purposes: Corfam, Vulcatex, bark, tanned cowhide, insole split leather, Texon Insole material, brown Cretan calf, black Cretan calf, wool tongue felt, twill, and Elmer's All-Purpose Glue. (Dr. Silas O'Quinn recommended this company.)

The patient is tested with a shoe screening patch test tray and with the samples of materials used in the manufacture of the Foot-So-Port shoe. The results of the patch survey, plus a prescription specifying the materials to be omitted in shoe construction, such as rubber cements and chrome-tanned leathers, are given to the patient. He takes them to a Foot-So-Port dealer who determines the proper size and helps the patient choose a suitable style. The patch test survey records along with the prescription are sent to the

Musebeck Shoe Company with the shoe order, which is usually filled within about 5 weeks.

Julius Altschul, Inc., 117–125 Grattan Street, Brooklyn, N. Y. 11237, upon special request from a retailer will provide children shoes up to size 13 and girls shoes up to size 10 made with nonrubber cements.

READY-MADE SHOES FREE OF DICHROMATES AND RUBBER CEMENT

Men's Shoes. The Alden Shoe Company, Taunton Street, Middleborough, Mass. 02346, manufactures Derma-Pedic shoes, which are not only vegetable-tanned, but also free of rubber adhesives. This company distributes the Derma-Pedic shoe throughout the United States and, upon request, will give the names of retailers who can supply such shoes. I have found the Derma-Pedic shoes virtually nonallergic for men.

Boys' Shoes. The Alden Shoe Company also manufactures the Sable shoe for boys, which is identical to the Derma-Pedic shoe for men.

Children's Shoes. The Walk-In Shoe Company, Parkway and Columbia Streets, Schuylkill Haven, Pa. 17972, manufactures vegetable-tanned shoes which are free of rubber cements. This company makes both regular and orthopedic shoes.

Women's Shoes. Women with dichromate hypersensitivity often satisfactorily wear shoes with nonleather uppers, such as vinyl plastics, nylon mesh or raffia (straw), which are obtainable in most retail shops.

SHOES FREE OF RUBBER BOX TOES

The Bixby Box Toe Co., Inc., of Haverhill, Mass. 01830, makes box toes in women's shoes involving the print-on technique in which resins in the nylon family are used, and the box toe is apparently free of rubber cement. Some women's shoes sold under the "Palizzio," "Mr. Seymour" and "I. Miller" labels do not have rubber based box toes, but other parts of the shoes may contain rubber cements.

Beckwith-Arden, Inc., Wakefield Industrial Center, P. O. Box 328, Wakefield, Mass. 01880, sells polystyrene, pyroxylin or nonrubber box toes to Knapp Shoes, Tom McAn, M. T. Shaw, Allen Edmonds, Weyenberg-International, Craddock-Terry Green Shoe and G. R. Kinney.

The Miller Shoe Co., 4015 Cherry Street, Cincinnati, Ohio 45223, makes orthopedic shoes for women. Shoes with heels up to 1-inch high have rubber box toes, but a number of patterns in higher heels have nonrubber toe boxes.

SHOES FREE OF RUBBER CEMENTS

The American Footwear Manufacturers Association, 4575 Prudential Tower, Boston, Mass. 02199, states that the following companies can supply shoes free of rubber adhesives:

For Children: Vo-Gal Shoe Companv
Appelton Street
Lawrence, Mass.

For Women: American Footwear
Altoona, Pa.

For Men: Siboney Shoe Company
Division of Suave Shoe Company
Miami, Fla.

NONLEATHER VINYL SHOES

Injection Molded Vinyl Shoes. These shoes have been manufactured in Japan and Taiwan over the past decade and are virtually nonallergenic. They may be purchased in large discount department stores and cost about $5 a pair.

Sears, Roebuck and Company carries these vinyl shoes for children. They were previously available for *women* who apparently did not purchase them readily. For men, Sears Roebuck has shoes with vinyl uppers and composition soles that are cemented to the uppers. I have been unable to find out the nature of this cement, but several patients with rubber sensitivity were able to wear these shoes without difficulty.

GENERAL TREATMENT OF SHOE DERMATITIS

In the presence of an acute dermatitis of the feet, strong antiseptics, such as iodine, or sensitizers, such as benzocaine and topical antihistamine medications, should be avoided because the skin of the feet is readily irritated and sensitized. Widespread, crippling dermatitis requiring hospitalization has resulted from the injudicious treatment of shoe dermatitis.[27]

Potassium permanganate or silver nitrate wet dressings are poorly tolerated in acute allergic shoe dermatitis, because they produce excessive dryness and cracking of the skin. Wet dressings of Burow's solution or boric acid are better tolerated.

In the management of chronic shoe dermatitis, the wearing of shoes free of specific sensitizers and the use of bland medication will not necessarily cure the dermatitis. Friction, sweating and scratching may prolong it. Frequently, a superimposed neurodermatitis has to be treated. Prolonged treatment with corticosteroid medication, tar or Vioform may be necessary. A short course of systematic corticosteroid therapy may hasten healing.

SHOE POLISH DERMATITIS

Shoe polish contains waxes, solvents, dyes and turpentine. In one instance,[28] a perfume in shoe polish produced a contact dermatitis. *Shoemakers* may be exposed to the following sensitizers:

Adhesives (phenolic resins and rubber-base adhesives)
Leather (bichromates)
Polishes (nigrosine, pine oil, formalin)
Rubber (accelerators and antioxidants)
Solvents (turpentine)

REFERENCES

1. Fisher, A. A.: Some Practical Aspects of the Diagnosis and Management of Shoe Dermatitis. A.M.A. Arch. Derm., *79*, 267, 1959.
2. Hack, M.: Chemical and Mechanical Etiology of Shoe Dermatitis. Cutis, *6*, 529, 1970.
3. Epstein, E.: Shoe Contact Dermatitis. J.A.M.A., *209*, 1487, 1969.
4. Samitz, M. H., and Dana, A. S.: *Cutaneous Lesions of the Lower Extremities.* Philadelphia, J. B. Lippincott Co., 1971, p. 125.
5. Shatin, H., and Reisch, M.: Dermatitis of the Feet Due to Shoes. A.M.A. Arch. Derm., *69*, 651, 1954.
6. Blank, I. H., and Miller, O. G.: A Study of Rubber Adhesives in Shoes as the Cause of Dermatitis of the Feet. J.A.M.A., *149*, 1371, 1952.
7. Gaul, L. E.: Results of Patch Testing with Rubber Antioxidants and Accelerators. J. Invest. Derm., *29*, 105, 1957.
8. De Vries, H. R.: Allergic Dermatitis Due to Shoes. Dermatologica, *128*, 68, 1964.
9. Suurmond, D., and Verspyck Mijnssen, G. A. W.: Allergic Dermatitis Due to Shoes and a Leather Prosthesis. Dermatologica, *134*, 371, 1967.
10. Walsh, E. N.: Council on Industrial Health, Chromate Hazards in Industry. J.A.M.A., *153*, 1305, 1953.
11. Morris, G. E.: Cross-Sensitization of the Feet and Hands Due to Chrome-Tanned Leather Shoes and Gloves. New Engl. J. Med., *257*, 567, 1957.
12. Fregert, S., and Rorsman, H.: Allergy to Trivalent Chromium. Arch. Derm. (Sweden), *90*, 1, 1964.
13. Cronin, E.: Shoe Dermatitis. Brit. J. Derm., *78*, 617, 1966.
14. Scutt, R. W. B.: Chrome Sensitivity Associated with Tropical Footwear in the Royal Navy. Brit. J. Derm., *78*, 337, 1966.
15. Wilson, J. A.: *Viewing Leather Through the Eyes of Science.* Boston, The Shoe Trade Publishing Co., 1924.
16. Jordan, W. P. et al.: Contact Dermatitis from Glutaraldehyde. Arch. Derm., *105*, 95, 1972.
17. Kauth, B.: Japanese Hot Foot Ailment Spreads. Utica, N.Y., Observer-Dispatch, June 18, 1939.
18. Shellow, H.: Dermatitis from Japanese Rubber-Thong Slippers. Family Phys., *1*, 44, 1961.
19. Weiner, E.: Dermatitis of the Feet Due to Wearing of Impermeable Shoes. J. Amer. Podiat. Assoc., *50*, 545, 1960.
20. Griffin, J. N.: Flip Flop Dermatitis. Brit. Med. J., *2*, 1431, 1965.
21. Shapiro, L., and Gibbs, R. C.: Vamp Disease: Inflammation of the Great Toe Due to Pressure from Women's Shoes. Arch. Derm., *102*, 661, 1970.
22. Fisher, A. A., and Shapiro, A.: Allergic Eczematous Contact Dermatitis Due to Metallic Nickel. J.A.M.A., *161*, 717, 1956.
23. Minkin, W., Cohen, H. J., and Frank, S. B.: Contact Dermatitis to East Indian Leather. Arch. Derm., *103*, 522, 1971.
24. Rothenborg, H. W., and Hjorth, N.: Indian Sandal Dermatitis. Ugeskr. Laeg., *133*, 802, 1971.
25. Lynch, P. J., and Rudolph, A. J.: Indian Sandal Strap Dermatitis. Letter to the Editor. J.A.M.A., *209*, 1209, 1969.

26. Gaul, L. E., and Underwood, G. B.: Failure of Modern Footwear to Meet Body Requirements for Psychic and Thermal Sweating. Arch. Derm., *62*, 33, 1950.
27. Calnan, C. D., and Sarkany, I.: Studies in Contact Dermatitis. IX. Shoe Dermatitis. Trans. St. John Hosp. Derm. Soc., *43*, 8, 1959.
28. Broughton, R. H.: An Unusual Case of Shoe Polish Contact Dermatitis. J. Roy. Nav. Med. Serv., *55*, 54, 1969.

10

Dermatitis from Rubber, Adhesives and Gums

This group of compounds not infrequently produces contact dermatitis. Natural rubber latex is rarely a sensitizer, but synthetic rubber with or without a mixture of natural rubber is a common sensitizer. In general, fully cured or polymerized synthetic plastics are allergenically inert, whereas fully cured rubber products often cause allergic contact dermatitis.[1]

In the United States, rubber fibers are marketed under the following names:

- Buthane (B. F. Goodrich)
- Contro (Firestone)
- Darleen (Darlington Fabrics)
- Filatex (Filatex)
- Hi-Flex (B. F. Goodrich)
- Lactron (U.S. Rubber)
- Lastex (U.S. Rubber)
- Laton (U.S. Rubber)
- Revere (U.S. Rubber)

Completely cured synthetic plastics rarely cause dermatitis; fully cured rubber products and garments, however, often produce allergic dermatitis

So-called rubber itch or rubber poisoning may be due to any one of a dozen primary irritants or allergens that workers encounter in the rubber industry,[2] including the following chemicals:

12

- Accelerators
- Antioxidants
- Colors (azo dyes)
- Phenolformaldehyde resins
- Plasticizers
- Rosin
- Soap and detergents
- Solvents (turpentine)
- Acids and alkalies
- Bleaches
- Oils
- Tar
- Tricresyl phosphate
- Polyester resins

Rubber Accelerators. Organic sulfur compounds and other chemicals are used to speed up vulcanization of rubber. Many are potent sensitizers that can produce dermatitis in sensitized individuals using the finished rubber product.

Table 10–1 is a list of the chemicals and trade names of primary accelerators in use in the rubber industry as compiled by W. E. McCormick, Manager of the Environmental Control Department of the B. F. Goodrich Company.

Secondary rubber accelerators, which are usually of a nonsulfur nature, are listed in Table 10–2.

Of the numerous accelerators listed in Tables 10–1 and 10–2 those named in Table 10–3 appear to produce most cases of rubber dermatitis.

Rubber Antioxidants. These chemicals are used to keep rubber from drying and cracking by preventing oxidation. Of the numerous

Table 10-1. Primary Rubber Accelerators

Chemical Name	*Trade Name*
Activated dithiocarbamate	Butyl eight
Ammonia-acetaldehyde condensation product	Aldehyde-ammonia
2-Benzothiazyl-n,n-diethylthiocarbamyl sulfide	Ethylac
Benzothiazyl disulfide	Altax, MBTS, Thiofide
1,3-bis(2-Benzothiazyl mercaptomethyl) urea	El Sixty
Bismuth dimethyldithiocarbamate	Bismata
Butyraldehyde acetaldehyde-aniline reaction product	Accelerator 100
Butyraldehyde-aniline condensation product (tributylidene aniline)	Beutene Accelerator 808, A-32
Butyraldehyde-monobutylamine condensation product	Accelerator 833
Cadmium diethyl dithiocarbamate	Ethyl Cadmate
Copper dimethyl dithiocarbamate	Cumate
n-Cyclohexyl-2-benzothiazile sulfenamide	Santocure, Conac S, Delac S, Cydac accelerator
1-3 Dibutyl thiourea	Penzone B
Dibutyl xanthogendisulfide	C-P-B
1, 3-Diethyl thiourea	Pennzone E, Linde molecular sieve CW-3120
2-(2, 6-dimethyl-4-morpholinothio) benzothiazole sulfenamide	Santocure-26
2, 4-Dinitrophenyl dimethyldithiocarbamate	Safex
Dipentamethylenethiuram tetrasulfide	Tetrone A, Sulfads
Heptaldehyde aniline condensation products	Hepteen base
Lead dimethyldithiocarbamate	Ledate
Lead dithiocarbamates (from mixed amines)	SPDX and SPDX-A
2-Mercaptobenzothiazole	MBT, Captax, Thiotax (or Mertax, Rotax)
2-Mercaptoimidazoline (ethylene thiourea)	NA-22
2-Mercaptothiazoline	2-MT
2-(Morpholinothio) benzothiazole sulfenamide	Santocure MOR
Nickel dibutyldithiocarbamate	BTN
N-Tert-butyl-2-benzothiazole	Santocure NS
N,N-Diisopropyl benzothiazole-2-sulfenamide	DIBS, Dipac
N-N-Dimethyl cyclohexylamine salt of dibutyl dithiocarbamic acid	RE-50A RE-50B
N-Oxydiethylene-2-mercaptothiozyl sulfenamide (N-oxydiethylene-2-benzothiazole sulfenamide)	Amax, NOBS, Special
p-Nitrosodimethylaniline	Accelerator I
Piperidinium pentamethylene dithiocarbamate	Pip Pip, Accelerator, 552
Poly-p-dinitrosobenzene	Polyac
Potassium pentamethylenedithiocarbamate	Accelerator 89

Table 10-1. Primary Rubber Accelerators *(Continued)*

Chemical Name	*Trade Name*
Selenium diethyl dithiocarbamate	Ethyl Selenac, Selazate, Ethyl Seleram
Selenium dimethyldithiocarbamate	Methyl, Seleram
Tellurium diethyldithiocarbamate	Tellurac
Tetrabutylthiuram monosulfide	Pentex
Tetraethylthiuram disulfide	Ethyl Tuads, Thiuram E, Ethyl Thiuram, Ethyl Tuex, Aceto TETD
Tetramethylthiuram disulfide	Vulcacure TMD, Thiurad, Methyl Tuads, Thiuram M, Tuex, Methyl Thiuram, TMT-Henley, Cyuram DS, Aceto TMTD
Tetramethylthiuram monosulfide	Thionex, Unads, Mono-thiurad, TMTM-Henley, Monex, Cyuram MS, Aceto TMTM
Thiocarbanilide (or N,N′-diphenylthiourea)	A-1
Thiohydropyrimidine	Thiate
Trimethyl thiourea	Thiate E
Zinc butylxanthate	ZBX
Zinc dibenzyldithiocarbamate	Arazate
Zinc dibutyldithiocarbamate	Butyl Zimate, Butasan, Butazate, Butyl Ziram
Zinc diethyldithiocarbamate	Ethyl Zimate, Ethasan, Ethazate, Ethyl Ziram, Aceto ZDED
Zinc dimethyldithiocarbamate	Methyl Zimate, Methasan, Methazate, Methyl Ziram, Aceto ZDMD, Ziram
Zinc pentamethylene dithiocarbamate	ZPP
Zinc salt of 2-mercaptobenzothiazole	Zenite, Zetox, ZMBT, Bantox, Pennac ZT OXAF, Vulcacura ZT

Table 10-2. Secondary Rubber Accelerators

Chemical Name	*Trade Name*
Di-n-butyl amine	Linde molecular sieve CW1115
Diorthotolylguanidine	DOTG
Diorthotolylguanidine salt of dicatechol borate	Permulux
Diphenylguanidine	DPG
Diphenylguanidine phthalate	Delac P, Guantal
2-Ethyl-β-propylacrolein-aniline product	Phenex
Formaldehyde monoethylamine condensation product	Trimene base
Hexamethylene tetramine	Hexamethylene tetramine, Hexa
Methylene-p-toluidine (anhydro formaldehyde-p-toluidine)	A-17, Accelerator No. 8
n,n′,n″-Triphenylguanidine	Triphenylguanidine
Piperidine	Linde molecular sieve CW-1015

Table 10-3. Accelerators Producing Most Cases of Rubber Dermatitis

Mercaptobenzothiazole
Tetramethylthiuram monosulfide
Diphenylguanidine
Hexamethylenetetramine (methenamine)

Table 10-4. Antioxidants Causing Most Cases of Rubber Dermatitis

Monobenzylether of hydroquinone
Phenyl-beta-naphthylamine
n-Isopropyl-n-phenylparaphenylenediamine (IPPDA)
4, 4′-diaminodiphenyl methane

antioxidants used in industry, those listed in Table 10–4 are probably the most sensitizing.

Rubber Peptizers. Certain organic sulfur compounds, such as thio-beta-naphthol, are added in the manufacture of products such as soft rubber tubing because of the softening effect. Such peptizers occasionally produce allergic dermatitis from contact with the finished rubber product.[3]

For patch test purposes, most rubber accelerators and antioxidants are tested 1 per cent in petrolatum, except n-isopropyl-n-paraphenylenediamine, which is tested 0.1 per cent in petrolatum

The North American Contact Dermatitis Group is evaluating the use of the following mixtures of rubber chemicals to expedite patch test procedures.

Mercapto mix 1%
- Mercaptobenzothiazole (MBT) 1%
- n-Cyclohexylbenzothiazylsulphenamide (CBS) 1%
- Dibenzothiazyldisulfide (MBTS) 1%
- Morpholinylmercaptobenzothiazole (MDR) 1%
- 0.25% each

Thiuram mix 1%
- Tetramethylthiuram disulfide (TMTD) 1%
- Tetramethylthiurammonosulfide (TMTM) 1%
- Tetraethylthiuramdisulfide (TETD) 1%
- Dipentamethylenethiuramdisulfide (PTD) 1%
- 0.25% each

PPD mix 0.60%
- Phenylcyclohexyl-p-phenylenediamine (CPPD) 1%
- Isopropylaminodiphenylamine identical with phenylisopropyl-p-phenylenediamine (IPPD) 0.1%
- Diphenyl-p-phenylenediamine (DPPD) 1%
- 0.25% + 0.10% + 0 25%

Naphthyl mix 1%
- Phenyl-beta-naphthylamine (PBN) 1%
- Di-beta-naphthyl-p-phenylenediamine (DBNPD) 1%
- 0.5% each

Table 10–5 is a list compiled by Fregert (personal communication, 1971) of chemicals that are used in *both* rubber and plastics and should be taken into consideration in the investigation of suspected rubber and plastic contact dermatitis.

Monobenzylether of Hydroquinone (*Agerite Alba*). This rubber antioxidant is not only a sensitizer but can also cause depigmentation, apparently independent of its sensitizing quality. Depigmentation often occurs in the absence of preceding inflammation or dermatitis.

Table 10-5. Chemicals Used in Both Rubber and Plastics

Phenyl-alpha-naphthylamine
Phenyl-beta-naphthylamine
p-Hydroxyphenyl-beta-naphthylamine
Aldol-alpha-naphthylamine
n-Isopropyl-n′-phenyl-p-phenylenediamine
Mercaptobenzimidazole
2,6-Di-tertiary butyl-4-methylphenol
2,6-Di(methylbenzyl)4-methylphenol
Bis(5-methyl-3-tertiary butyl-2-hydroxyphenyl)-monosulfide
2, 5-Di-tertiary butylhydroquinone
2,5-Di-tertiary amylhydroquinone
Tri(p-nonylphenyl)phosphite

Great care should be exercised when monobenzylether of hydroquinone is used to treat hyperpigmentation. Treatment should be begun on a small trial area to determine whether sensitization develops and to make certain that the depigmenting action is not excessive.

The rubber antioxidant monobenzylether of hydroquinone (agerite alba), present in rubber and cement, is a sensitizer and depigmenting agent

At present, careful handling of the monobenzylether of hydroquinone has reduced the number of cases of depigmentation in the rubber industry.

The compound 4-tertiary butyl catechol, an antioxidant used in rubber and plastics, may also cause leukoderma.

Wilson[4] in a recent study showed that a formidable number of chemical additives are used in the rubber industry and many are potential skin sensitizers. In this series, however, sensitivity was attributed to a thiuram accelerator or mercaptobenzothiazole in all but 2 cases.

Tetraethyl and Tetramethyl Thiuram Disulfides. Both ethyl and methyl compounds of this series are popular accelerators for vulcanization of rubber.

The ethyl compound, known as disulfiram, may have the following commercial designations:[5]

Disulfide, bis(diethylthiocarbamyl)	Ethyl Thiurad
Tetraethylthiuram disulfide	Antabuse
TTD	Etabuse
Cronetal	Abstinyl
Abstensil	Thiuranide
Stopetyl	Esperal
Contralin	Tetradine
Antadix	Noxal
Antietanol	Tetraetil
Exhorran	Tetraethyl-X

The methyl analogue, called thiram, has the following commercial names:

Tetramethylthiuram disulfide	Pernasan
Disulfide bis(dimethylthiocarbamyl)	Puralin
TMTDS	Nomersan
TMTD	Pomasol
Thiurad	Pomarsol
Thiosan	Tersan
Thylate	Tuads
Tiuramyl	Tulisan
Thiuramyl	Arasan

Both disulfiram and thiram are sensitizers and can be leached from finished rubber products by moisture and sweat, thereby producing dermatitis in sensitized individuals. Sensitized workers exposed to these chemicals in the rubber industry can also readily acquire allergic contact dermatitis. In addition, the combination of exposure to these rubber accelerators and ingestion of alcohol or paraldehyde can cause marked erythema and sometimes urticaria and itching. This reaction is the basis for the use of disulfiram in the form of Antabuse tablets to produce an intolerance to alcohol in alcoholics.[6]

The combination of exposure to the accelerators disulfiram and thiram and the ingestion of alcohol or paraldehyde can produce erythema, itching and urticaria

Not only ingestion of disulfiram, but also topical exposure to thiram, will produce an alcohol-sensitization effect. Erythema, urticaria and itching resulting from combined ingestion of alcohol and exposure to these compounds are nonallergic and occur in all individuals so exposed.[7]

Aside from its use as a rubber accelerator, thiram is used extensively as a germicide, fungicide, pesticide and insecticide under the commercial designations Arasan, Naguets, Panoram and Tersan. Carbamates closely related to thiram used for similar purposes include Ferbam, Ziram, Sineb, Nabam, Vapam and Extam.

These products are used extensively on gardens, lawns, golf courses, fruits and plants. The general population, as well as the rubber worker, the chemist and the farmer, therefore is exposed to thiram and its analogues. Allergic eczematous contact dermatitis may occur in sensitized individuals from these exposures. In addition, individuals ingesting alcohol may experience erythema, urticaria and itching when in contact with these chemicals.

Van Ketal[8] suggests that patients in whom ingestion of alcohol aggravates their dermatitis should be patch tested with thiuramdisulfide (TMTD).

Patients who complain that alcohol makes their dermatitis worse should have patch tests with TMTD

Mercaptobenzothiazole (MBT). This is one of the most common causes of dermatitis due to rubber. Fregert[9] studied 12 patients with hand dermatitis from rubber gloves and contact allergy to mercaptobenzothiazole (MBT) with a view to elucidating cross-sensitivity patterns.

The molecular requirements for cross-sensitivity were found to be a combination of a benzene and a thiazole ring as well as a thiol group in 2-position.

4-Isopropyl-Aminodiphenylamine (IPPDA). This rubber antioxidant, also known as n-isopropyl-n-phenyl-paraphenylene, is chiefly used in rubber tires, heavy duty rubber goods and rubber boots. Dermatitis from this chemical has been reported abroad[10] and in the United States.[11] Most rubber antioxidants may be tested in a 1 per cent concentration in petrolatum, but this compound is such a powerful sensitizer that it should be tested in a 0.1 per cent concentration. Cross-reactions may occur with the hair dye para-aminodiphenylamine.[12]

The antioxidant 4-isopropyl-aminodiphenylamine, used particularly in heavy rubber goods and some plastics, is a powerful sensitizer. Cross-reactions may occur with oxidation-type hair dyes

Substituted Paraphenylenediamines in Rubber. The n,n′-disubstituted paraphenylenediamines used in the rubber industry range from the symmetrical dialkyl of 6 or more carbon atoms each to the N,N′-diphenyl and the unsymmetrical n-alkyl-n′-phenyl of 3 to 8 carbon atoms. Skin sensitization decreases with increasing molecular weight, but so does antiozonant activity. Test subjects who are already sensitive to one substituted paraphenylenediamine are cross-sensitized to another. There has been a trend toward using similar compounds having a larger alkyl group in place of the isopropyl group.

These rubber substituted paraphenylenediamines are capable of producing lichenoid purpuric eruptions (see chapter on non-eczematous contact dermatitis).

RUBBER SUBSTITUTES

The problem of rubber additives is difficult because most are reactive chemicals and capable of inducing sensitization. Nevertheless, continuous efforts should be made to find the least sensitizing ones. The problem of contact dermatitis from rubber may sometimes be solved by replacement with plastics, especially when rubber products are used in prolonged contact with the skin, as in clothing, gloves and shoes. Rubber gloves may be replaced by polyvinyl chloride or other materials. A high proportion of cases of shoe dermatitis are due to rubber additives, and could be reduced by the wider use of plastic shoes, which are worn extensively in Japan. The rubber tabs of women's stocking suspenders (garters) can be replaced by hard nylon or similar material.

DERMATITIS FROM RUBBER GLOVES, WEARING APPAREL AND OTHER RUBBER ARTICLES[13]

Rubber Gloves. In sensitized individuals, hand dermatitis may be initiated or made worse by rubber gloves.[14] Rubber glove dermatitis should be suspected when a hand dermatitis stops abruptly above the wrist. The eruption may mimic a photodermatitis.[15] Even when the patient is not allergic to rubber, the rubber gloves may make an existing hand dermatitis worse owing to an occlusive, macerating effect. In the presence of dermatitis of the hands, cotton-lined rubber gloves, into which cornstarch has been sprinkled, should be used. The cotton liners and powders can absorb sweat and minimize maceration.

Polyvinyl dermal gloves worn inside cotton-lined rubber gloves may also be helpful in controlling dermatitis.

Surgeons and others who are allergic to rubber gloves should be informed that the Pioneer Rubber Company of Willard, Ohio, makes a neoprene glove containing less accelerator and antioxidant than do gloves made with a mixture of natural rubber. In addition, the B. F. Goodrich Industrial Products Co., Sundries Sales Department, Akron, Ohio, can provide a Eudermic surgical glove, which can be tolerated by many rubber-sensitive individuals. Recently, Seamless, a Division of Dart Industries, New Haven, Conn. 06503, has provided "Original Brown Milled Surgeons' Gloves," which are also free from the usual sensitizers in rubber gloves.

Polyvinyl or silicone gloves may also be substitutes for rubber gloves. Surgeons and others who are allergic to acrylic monomer should be aware that this monomer may penetrate through rubber gloves.[16]

Acrylic monomer can pass through rubber gloves

Rubber Sponges. Contact with rubber sponges can produce dermatitis in rubber-sensitive individuals.[17] For example, women may acquire facial dermatitis from rubber sponges used for application of cosmetics. The eyelids often show marked involvement in such cases. Rubber sponge dermatitis mimics eruptions due to cosmetics. In an attempt to correct the situation, the patient often applies so-called nonallergic cosmetics with her dermatitis-producing rubber sponge. Cellulose sponges, cloth pads or brushes can be used as substitutes for rubber cosmetic sponges.

Girdles, Bras and Other Undergarments Containing Rubber. Individuals with rubber hypersensitivity may substitute rubber undergarments with those made of spandex (Lycra, Vyrene, Blue C), which is free of mercaptobenzothiazole. Rubber-sensitive patients must also be certain to obtain all-Lycra spandex garments in which the edges or "narrows" do not contain rubber (Warner's and Vanity Fair). Not only mercaptobenzothiazole[18] but also 4-isopropyl-aminodiphenylamine[19] has been implicated in spandex dermatitis.

Allergic clothing dermatitis due to elasticized underwear with a secondary eczematous purpuric eruption has been reported.[20] Most of these patients showed a positive patch test reaction to 4-isopropyl-aminodiphenylamine.

A purpuric eruption from elasticized underwear associated with sensitivity to 4-isopropyl-aminodiphenylamine may occur

Dress Shields. The rubber padding in dress shields may produce axillary dermatitis, which must be differentiated from dermatitis due to dresses or antiperspirants.[21] Nonrubber dress shields (Kleinert's) are available for persons hypersensitive to rubber.

Elastic in Hairnets. Dermatitis due to elastic in hairnets may closely simulate seborrheic dermatitis. In such instances, wrap-around hairnets without elastic may be substituted. Some individuals use hair ribbons as a substitute.

Rubber Panties. In many instances rubber panties produce an occlusive, macerating and irritating type of dermatitis in the diaper area. Occasionally, such garments produce an allergic dermatitis. Plastic panties may be used when there is a specific sensitivity to rubber.

Rubber Dental Plates. Although rubber dentures are not in vogue at present, such dentures occasionally cause stomatitis. The more widely used acrylic dentures are readily available substitutes.

Rubber Edge on Eyelash Curler. Dermatitis on the eyelids may mimic nail polish dermatitis. Plastic eyelash curlers without rubber edges are available as substitutes in rubber-sensitive individuals.

Rubber Kneeling Pad. I have seen 2 rubber-sensitive individuals acquire dermatitis in the prepatellar area that simulated neurodermatitis and was caused by contact with rubber kneeling pads. Covering the pad with cloth or plastic enabled these patients to use the pads without acquiring dermatitis. Nonrubber, sponge pads are available as substitutes.

Rubber Support Pessary and Contraceptive Diaphragms. Vaginitis and vulvitis may be produced by such rubber articles in rubber-sensitive individuals. Plastic devices are now available as substitutes.

Rubber Dental Sheeting. In certain dental procedures, fine rubber sheeting is stretched across the face to isolate the work area. In one patient, who had developed facial dermatitis on two occasions from rubber dental sheeting, spraying of the cheeks with Decadron Aerosol Spray before application of the sheeting prevented dermatitis from occurring.

Rubber Headrest. Women with rubber sensitivity may acquire an eruption resembling nuchal neurodermatitis from contact with the rubber kidney-shaped headrest attached to the shampoo tray in beauty parlors. Placing a plastic sheet or a towel over the rubber headrest prevents dermatitis.

Condoms. Rubber dermatitis from condoms is not rare.[22] In two instances I found that a preservative powder that had been dusted on the condom was the cause of dermatitis. In such cases, removal of the powder by washing enabled the patients to use the condom without acquiring dermatitis. In one instance, the powder contained 10 per cent monobenzylether of hydroquinone. Several rubber-sensitive individuals found by trial and error that only certain brands produced dermatitis.

Nonrubber condoms, Fourex (Schmidt) and Lambskin (Youngs Rubber), made of processed sheep's intestine are available for individuals who cannot tolerate rubber contraceptives. Such preparations are popularly called "fishskins."

Dermatitis of Hands from Rubber Articles. Aside from rubber gloves, rubber dermatitis may be encountered on the hands and wrists from rubber bands, rubber finger guards, art gum erasers, stethoscopes, rubber hand grips of vibrators and rubber in cuffs.

Many Swedish post office workers who wear rubber protectors on their fingers develop a rubber dermatitis[23] due to a rubber accelerator.

Dermatitis from Miscellaneous Rubber Articles. Rubber aprons and mammary prostheses may also cause dermatitis. Rubber goggles may produce circumorbital dermatitis.

Rubber Dermatitis in Childhood. Aside from dermatitis due to rubber panties, dermatitis from rubber is rarely encountered in children, although rubber toys and balloons have caused dermatitis in several children. In these, the eruption was most marked on the face and resembled atopic dermatitis.

Certain substances that resemble putty and are used as toys have produced dermatitis. These products are composed of partially polymerized butadiene and mineral oil, with small amounts of polymerization catalysts and antioxidants. These products are easily moldable into any shape, and their resiliency enables them to be used as bouncing toys. So many instances of dermatitis were produced by such products (Flubber, Roobly-Rubber and Plubber) that they have been withdrawn by the manufacturer.[24]

Rubber in Footwear. The role of rubber in the production of dermatitis from shoes is discussed in the chapter on shoe dermatitis.

Juhlin and Penten[25] reported that small rubber particles in footwear that are pressed into sweat pores during exercise may produce "black heel," which may simulate malignant melanoma.

Dr. Scholl's Air Pillo insoles contain rubber latex with mercaptobenzothiazole as the accelerator.

Rubber in Adhesive Tape. Until recently the adhesive mass in most adhesive tape contained rubber in the form of either natural latex or synthetic elastomers. Most such adhesive tapes also contained zinc oxide and substances derived from coniferous resins, such as turpentine, balsams and rosin. In addition, antioxidants, to provide resistance to deterioration, and plasticizers, to facilitate spreading of the adhesive mass on cloth, are the ingredients in many adhesive tapes and plasters.[26]

Traumatic Irritant Adhesive Tape Dermatitis. Most skin reactions related to adhesive tape are mechanical. One type of traumatic adhesive tape reaction results from the shear-

Plate 7. Allergic Rubber Dermatitis Caused by Mercaptobenzothiazole

1. Perlèche-like Dermatitis

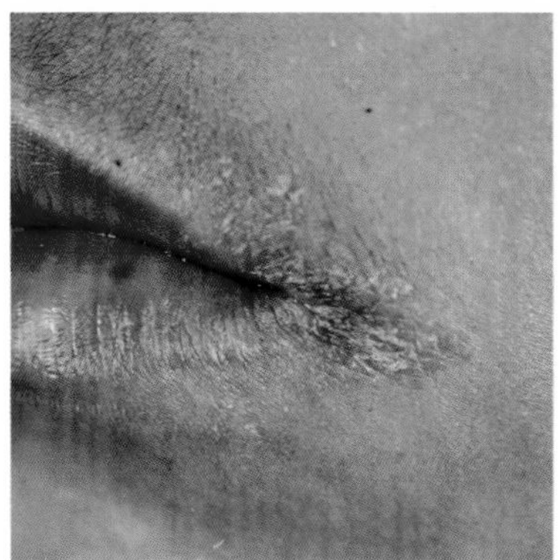

Chewing of Pencil Eraser (N.Y. Skin and Cancer)

2. Penile Dermatitis

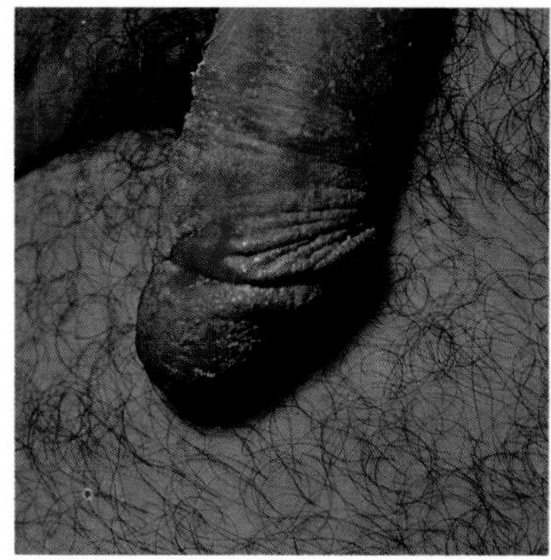

Rubber Condom

3. Dermatitis of Trunk

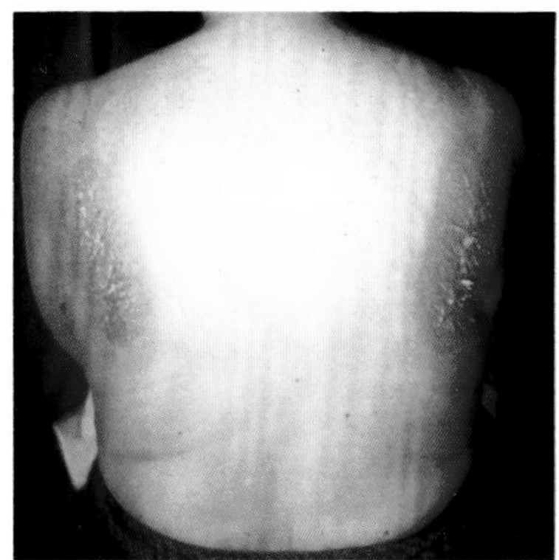

Rubber Girdle

4. Thigh Dermatitis

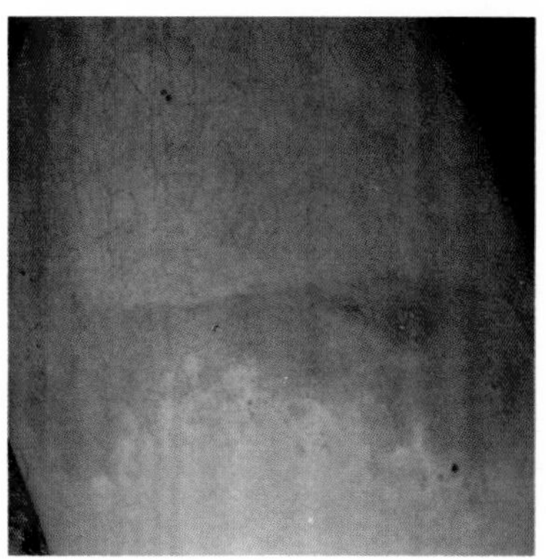

Garter Belt (N.Y. Skin and Cancer)

5. Foot Dermatitis

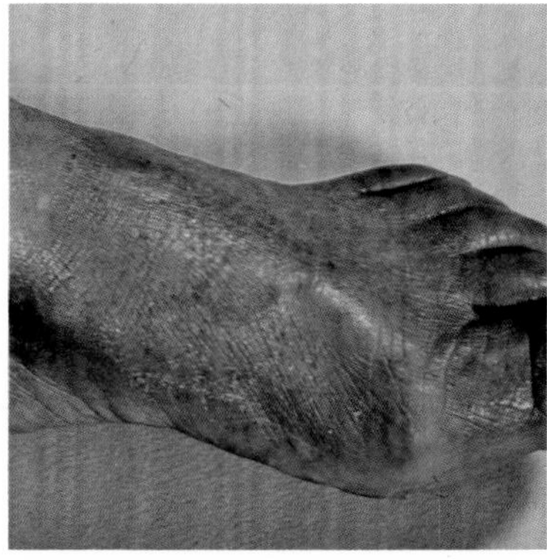

Rubber Slippers

6. Psoriasiform Knee Dermatitis

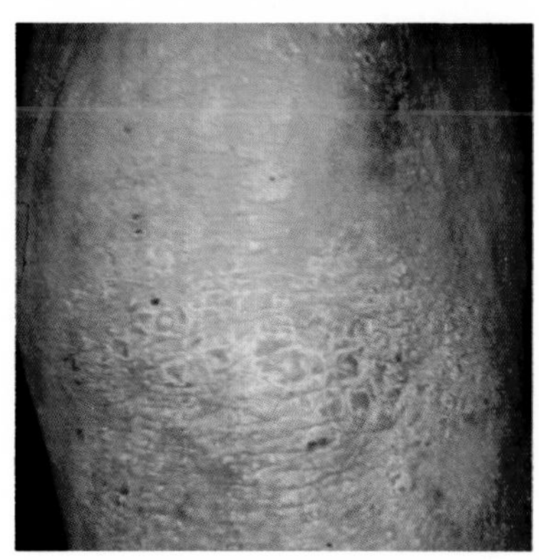

Rubber Kneeling Pad

ing stresses at the tape-skin interface and is most frequently encountered when tape is applied with tension that exceeds the physiological tolerance of skin.

Narumi[27] has shown that adhesive plaster applied with tension readily can produce erythema and even blistering.

The other type of irritant adhesive tape reaction involves the mechanical plugging of the follicular and sweat ostia, producing a follicular rash resembling prickly heat.

Traumatic or irritant adhesive tape dermatitis usually remains localized to the site of contact, but the allergic reactions tend to spread.

Allergic Rubber Mass Adhesive Tape Dermatitis. Allergic reactions may be due to the rubber compounds incorporated with the adhesive mass. Rubber accelerators or antioxidants usually are the causes, although resins and turpentine added to rubber masses may produce allergic dermatitis. Patients with allergic reactions to rubber mass adhesive tape may also react to Scotch Tape.[28]

Allergic dermatitis from adhesive tape is usually due to its rubber content. Nonrubber tape, which is nonirritating and nonsensitizing, is now available

Band-Aid Patches. Occasionally, the vinyl film backing of Band-Aids may produce an allergic contact dermatitis because of plasticizers and stabilizers in the film.

DUO Brand Surgical Adhesive (Thayer Co.). This crepe latex rubber compound is free from the usual antioxidants and accelerators used in rubber cements. Many women use this adhesive to apply false eyelashes. No instance of dermatitis has come to my attention from such use. This adhesive may be used on the scalp for toupees and around ileostomy wounds when other rubber cements irritate the skin or cause allergic reactions.

Self-Adhering Adhesive. Gauztex (General Bandages, Inc.) which is made of gum rubber, does not contain any rubber additives, such as accelerators or antioxidants, In addition, its manufacturer makes an oil-resistant tape that does not contain rubber but is made from plasticized styrene. Gauztex contains mercuric chloride as a preservative.

Nonrubber Acrylate Mass Adhesive Tape. Such adhesive tape does not contain rubber. Instead, a synthetic acrylate polymer is used as the adhesive mass. I have encountered no instances of allergic dermatitis due to the acrylate adhesive mass.

Acrylate mass adhesive tape is available as Dermicel (Johnson & Johnson) and Steri-Strip and Microspore Surgical Tape (3M), which may be safely used by those who are allergic to the older rubber mass tapes. In addition, nonspecific, mechanical and traumatic adhesive dermatitis is less likely to occur with these tapes.[29]

RUBBER ADHESIVES IN GENERAL USE

Such adhesives are of three general types, although, in many proprietary glues, they may be mixed with other resins and adhesives.

1. *Nonvulcanizing rubber solutions.* These contain natural or synthetic rubber in a petroleum solvent, such as naphtha, benzene, petrol or xylol, with wood rosin, ester gum or shellac for tackiness. They are used in the shoe industry, for surgical tape and for automobile trimmings. Dermatitis is mainly caused by the solvent or the resins.

2. *Vulcanizing solutions or cements.* These contain compounded natural or synthetic rubber with fillers, adhesive agents and vulcanization accelerators (e.g., zinc dithiocarbamate, zinc isopropyl xanthate or mercaptobenzothiazole). They may be supplied as two solutions for mixing together before use. Curing takes place in several hours. They are used for joining rubber and mending punctures. Sensitization dermatitis may occur from the compounding rubber chemicals.

3. *Latex cements.* These are made of latex rubber with or without solvent naphtha, and with wetting agents, glue, ester gum and disinfectants. They are used in the shoe and textile trades.

NONRUBBER SYNTHETIC RESIN ADHESIVES

Resins based on formaldehyde, polyester isocyanates, silicon, acrylic and epoxies may be used for adhesion or lamination.

Formaldehyde resin adhesives are available as solids, aqueous syrups and alcoholic solutions for use in laminating wood and paper and bonding metal, wood, plastics and rubber. Cotton and other fabrics may be impregnated with them. Most formaldehyde resin adhesives contain free formaldehyde, which may cause allergic dermatitis in exposed, sensitized individual.

Gaul,[30] however, found that the failure of formaldehyde to react in the presence of phenol-formaldehyde resin dermatitis and the failure of co-hydroxybenzyl alcohol (saligenin) to react in the presence of formaldehyde sensitivity appear to indicate that, in phenol-formaldehyde resin dermatitis, the sensitizing agent is the resin and not the phenol and formaldehyde components.

Malten[31] described occupational eczema in shoemakers caused by the adhesive used to glue the soles to the shoes. On the basis of positive patch tests, the phenol-formaldehyde synthetic resin CKR 1634 was the allergen. Of 10 patients tested, all reacted to the para-tertiary butylphenol component of this artificial resin, while 2 of them also reacted to formaldehyde.

Calnan and his co-workers[32,33] also implicated para-tertiary butylphenol as the sensitizer in phenol-formaldehyde resin dermatitis.

Foussereau (personal communication, 1970) described dermatitis from glues containing para-tertiary butylphenol-formaldehyde used in watch straps, in the leather industry and in shoemaking.

In many instances, para-tertiary butylphenol is the sensitizer in phenol-formaldehyde resin dermatitis

Silicon rubber is composed of higher chain silicon polymers and forms a substance resembling rubber. There is a single report of cross-reaction to an organic silicon compound in individuals who were allergic to Bisphenol A, an epoxy resin component.[34]

Gloves made of silicon are becoming available for those who are allergic to rubber gloves.

Silicon sprays are nonallergic. They can be used for waterproofing adhesive tape so that patients can bathe or swim. Such sprays can also be used to prevent runs or tears in nylon stockings.

Silicon adhesives are used for bonding silicon elastomer (silastic medical adhesive) to itself or other implantable synthetics, such as Dacron, Teflon and acrylic. A silicon adhesive has been implicated as a cause of dermatitis associated with an implanted cardiac pacemaker.[35]

Glues and adhesives were formerly based on animal skin, bone, fish, gelatin or starch. Gelatin glues derived from boiling animal hoofs in water are not sensitizers. Glues derived from leather hides may contain chromates and cause allergic dermatitis. Fish glues, still used in the shoe industry, are not sensitizers. The alkaline effect of casein glues may produce irritant dermatitis. Some glues contain preservatives, such as formaldehyde or pentachlorophenol, which may be sensitizers. Epoxy glues are prepared in separate containers. Dermatitis may occur before polymerization takes place. Glues and cements made from cotton, such as cellulose acetate and nitrate, usually are not sensitizers. Cotton treated with nitric and sulfuric acid forms pyroxylin, which, when dissolved in ethyl oxide and alcohol, forms collodion, which is not a sensitizer.

VEGETABLE GUMS

These gums are resinous plant exudates. Karaya, acacia and tragacanth are probably the most common sensitizers among them.[36] These gums may be used "as is" for patch tests.

Karaya is an ingredient in many cosmetics, particularly hair-waving lotions. It is used in toothpastes, powders, adhesives and cement substances to make ileostomy and colostomy bags adhere to the skin. Fasteeth, a denture adhesive, contains karaya gum, sodium borate and peppermint flavoring.

Acacia (*gum arabic*) is used in cosmetics and in offset sprays in the printing industry.

Gum tragacanth, an insoluble vegetable gum, absorbs water to form a jelly and may cross-react with acacia. Tragacanth is used in cosmetics particularly gum-based hair dressings, and in troches, toothpastes, depilatories and other topical medications. Exposure may take place from contact with textile finishes and sizing papers or in printing operations or enameling.

Rosin (*colophony*), a natural resin, is used in many adhesive tape formulations. It is the residue left after distilling the volatile oils from certain southern pine trees. Two main types of rosins are gum rosin, which is derived from turpentine by steam inhalation, and wood rosin, which is derived from pine and spruce stumps by solvent extraction and steam distillation. Both gum and wood rosins contain abietic acid, which may be a sensitizer. Traces of turpentine in gum rosin may also be a sensitizer. Cross-reactions between rosin and balsam of Peru can occur. Before use in adhesives, rosins may be esterified with glycerin or alcohol, which probably make them less allergenic. Table 10-6 is a list of sources of exposure to rosin.

Damar, a natural resin obtained from trees in the East Indies and Malaya, is used in varnishes.

Copal, a fossil resin, is used in varnishes and obtained in Africa and the Philippines.

Gum resins are naturally occurring mixtures of gum, oil and resin. There is probably wider exposure to gum benzoin than to other gum resins.

Benzoin is present in tincture of benzoin (10 per cent in alcohol). Compound benzoin tincture contains benzoin with Styrax, balsam of Tolu, aloe and ethyl alcohol. Arning's tincture contains tincture of benzoin, ammonium tumenol, anthrarobin and ether.

Tincture of benzoin may also be present in adhesives, nail polish, perfumes, cuticle removers and inks. Benzoinated lard, water-repellent barrier creams, lozenges and cosmetics also contain benzoin. It may cross-react with balsam of Peru, benzyl cinnamate, benzyl alcohol, eugenol, vanilla and alpha-pinene.[37] It may be tested in a concentration of 10 per cent in alcohol, painted on the skin and left uncovered.

Table 10-6. Sources of Exposures to Rosin

Adhesive tape
Sticky flypaper
Epilating hair pullwax
Brown soap
Brilliantine
Baseball rosin bag
Bowlers' rosin
Furniture polish
Coating for price labels
Varnishes
Glue
Printer's ink
Printing paper surface
Automobile and engineering industry
Car and floor wax

REFERENCES

1. Herrmann, W. B., and Schultz, K. H.: Substances in the Rubber Industry As a Cause of Eczema. Dermatologica, *120*, 127, 1960.
2. Wilson, R. H., Planek, E. H., and McCormick, W. E.: Allergy in the Rubber Industry. Industr. Med., *28*, 209, 1959.
3. Gaul, E. I.: Results of Patch Testing with Rubber Antioxidants and Accelerators. J. Invest. Derm., *29*, 108, 1957.
4. Wilson, H. T. H.: Rubber Dermatitis—An Investigation of 106 Cases of Contact Dermatitis Caused by Rubber. Brit. J. Derm., *81*, 175, 1969.
5. Shelley, W. B.: Golf-Course Dermatitis Due to Thiram Fungicide. J.A.M.A., *188*, 415, 1964.
6. Martensen-Larsen, O.: Five Years' Experience with Disulfiram in Treatment of Alcoholics. Quart. J. Stud. Alcohol., *14*, 406, 1953.
7. Wilson, H.: Side Effects of Disulfiram. Brit. Med. J., *2*, 1610, 1962.
8. Van Ketal, W. G.: Rubber, Alcohol and Eczema. Med. T. Geneesk., *112*, 406, 1968.
9. Fregert, S.: Cross-Sensitivity Pattern of 2-Mercaptobenzothiazole (MBT). Acta Dermatovener., *49*, 45, 1969.
10. Vollum, D. I., and Marten, R. H.: Contact Dermatitis from 4-Isopropyl-amino-diphenylamine. Trans. St. John Hosp. Derm. Soc., *54*, 73, 1968.
11. Jordan, W. P.: Contact Dermatitis from N-Isopropyl-N-Phenylparaphenylenediamine. Arch. Derm., *103*, 85, 1971.
12. Schonning, L., and Hjorth, N.: Cross Sensitization between Hair Dyes and Rubber Chemicals. Berufsdermatosen, *17*, 100, 1969.
13. Fisher, A. A.: Practical Management of Allergic Contact Dermatitis Due to Rubber in Manufactured Articles. Derm. Digest, *2*, 23, 1963.

14. Sidi, E., and Hincky, M.: Rubber Glove Dermatitis. Presse Med., *62*, 1305, 1954.
15. Wilson, H. T. H.: Rubber Glove Dermatitis. Brit. J. Med., *2*, 21, 1960.
16. Pegum, J. S., and Medhurst, F. A.: Contact Dermatitis from Penetration of Rubber Gloves by Acrylic Monomer. Brit. Med. J., *2*, 141, 1971.
17. Furman, D., Fisher, A., and Leider, M.: Allergic Eczematous Contact-Type Dermatitis Caused by Rubber Sponges Used for the Application of Cosmetics. J. Invest. Derm., *15*, 223, 1950.
18. Joseph, H. L., and Maibach, H. I.: Contact Dermatitis from Spandex Brassieres. J.A.M.A., *201*, 202, 1967.
19. Van Dijk, E.: Contact Dermatitis Due to Spandex. Acta Dermatovener., *48*, 589, 1968.
20. Batschvarov, B., and Minkov, D. M.: Dermatitis and Purpura from Rubber in Clothing. Trans. St. John Hosp. Derm. Soc., *54*, 178, 1968.
21. Schultz, K. H., and Hermann, W. P.: Dress-Shield Eczema: Dod (4:4-Dioxypiphenyl) As a Cause. Derm. Wschr., *141*, 124, 1960.
22. Hindson, T. C.: Contact Dermatitis: Contraceptives. Trans. St. John Hosp. Derm. Soc., *52*, 1, 1966.
23. Eriksson, G., and Ostlund, E.: Rubber Bank Note Counters as the Cause of Eczema Among Employees at the Swedish Post Giro Office. Acta Dermatovener., *48*, 212, 1968.
24. Jacobziner, H., and Raybein, H. W.: The Rise and Decline of "Flubberitis." New York J. Med., *63*, 2562, 1963.
25. Juhlin, L., and Penten, B.: Plantar Pseudochromhidrosis Simulating Malignant Melanoma. Acta Dermatovener., *47*, 255, 1967.
26. Sidi, E., and Hincky, M.: Allergic Sensitization to Adhesive Tape: Experimental Study with a Hypoallergenic Adhesive Tape. J. Invest. Derm., *29*, 81, 1957.
27. Narumi, J.: Friction Dermatitis Due to Adhesive Plaster. Jap. J. Clin. Derm., *24*, 1185, 1970.
28. Murphy, J. C., Reit, A. E., and January, H. L.: Cutaneous Hypersensitivity to Adhesive and Scotch Tapes. J. Invest. Derm., *31*, 45, 1958.
29. Hodgson, M. B. E.: The Effects on the Skin of Some New Adhesives and Laminating Materials. Brit. J. Derm., *72*, 102, 1960.
30. Gaul, L. E.: Absence of Formaldehyde Sensitivity in Phenol-Formaldehyde Resin Dermatitis. J. Invest. Derm., *48*, 485, 1967.
31. Malten, K. E.: Occupational Eczema due to Para-Tertiary Butylphenol in a Shoe Adhesive. Dermatologica, *117*, 103, 1958.
32. Engel, H. O., and Calnan, C. D.: Resin Dermatitis in a Car Factory. Brit. J. Industr. Med., *23*, 62, 1966.
33. Calnan, C. D., and Harman, R. R. M.: Studies in Contact Dermatitis. X. Sensitivity to Para-Tertiary Butylphenol. Trans. St. John Hosp. Derm. Soc., *43*, 27, 1959.
34. Fregert, S., and Rorsman, H.: Allergy to a Carbon-Functional Organic Silicon Compound, Dimethylid-(4-hydroxyphenyl)-silane. Nature, *192*, 989, 1961.
35. Raque, C., and Goldschmidt, H.: Dermatitis Associated with an Implanted Cardiac Pacemaker. Arch. Derm., *102*, 647, 1970.
36. Nilsson, D. C.: Sources of Allergenic Gums. Ann. Allergy, *18*, 518, 1960.
37. Hjorth, N.: *Eczematous Allergy to Balsams.* Copenhagen, Munksgaard, 1961, p. 126.

11

Industrial Dermatitis With Particular Reference to the Role of Patch Testing*

Dermatitis is by far the most frequently reported occupational disease, and patch testing with the standard and vehicle series reveals a substantial number of relevant causes. In addition, of course, special test series may have to be performed in workers exposed to diverse contactants.

The International Contact Dermatitis Group[1] in a study of occupational dermatitis in 5 European dermatologic departments found that, of 20 standard substances, chromates and rubber chemicals gave a higher percentage of positive reactions in patients with occupational dermatitis than in nonoccupational dermatitis. Topical medicaments, nickel and benzocaine were more equally divided between both groups of patients.

This study emphasized that 10 per cent of occupational dermatitis cases are not immediately recognized as such on clinical grounds alone. Patch tests may help reveal the cause in many such cases.

Dermatitis is the most common industrial disease. Patch testing is valuable in revealing cases due to allergic contactants

In industry, as elsewhere, patch testing is indicated only in the diagnosis of allergic eczematous contact dermatitis. Aside from investigative procedures, patch tests are of no value in the primary irritant type of contact dermatitis. The diagnosis of industrial dermatitis depends not only on the patch test results, but also on the history, the clinical picture and proved exposure to the suspected contactant.

The patch test is particularly valuable in ascertaining the cause of outbreaks of isolated cases of allergic contact dermatitis in industry where workers are directly or indirectly exposed to many sensitizing chemicals. Although a careful history and personal investigation of the patient's exposure to contactants often reduce the necessity for routine patch tests, such procedures are often necessary to confirm a diagnosis of allergic contact dermatitis.

Most insurance carriers and industrial boards accept a significant patch test reaction as proof of the etiologic basis of an allergic contact dermatitis. A properly performed and correctly interpreted patch test is scientific proof of the relationship of a specific contactant to a particular dermatitis.

Patch testing may also be of great assistance in differentiating occupational and nonoccupational dermatitis, particularly when an individual with a contact dermatitis is

* This material supplements texts discussed in the following sources: Schwartz, L., Tulipan, L., and Birmingham, D. J.: *Occupational Diseases of the Skin* (Ed. 3). Philadelphia, Lea & Febiger, 1957; Fleming, A. J., D'Alonzo, C. A., and Zapp, J. A.: *Modern Occupational Medicine* (Ed. 2). Philadelphia, Lea & Febiger, 1960; and Adams R. M.: *Occupational Contact Dermatitis*. Philadelphia, J. B. Lippincott, 1969.

exposed to sensitizers not only at work but also at play or in pursuit of hobbies. Properly performed patch tests may quickly and efficiently pinpoint the offending contactant, whereas reliance on history and trial and error may prolong the dermatitis while the offending allergen is being pursued.

PATCH TESTING WITH NEW INDUSTRIAL COMPOUNDS

Particular care must be exercised when new manufacturing processes and compounds are introduced. Under such circumstances, the dermatologic hazards of the new procedures and chemicals must be evaluated properly and as fully as possible before a large number of workers are exposed and sensitized.

Animal studies are of value only when the chemical is a strong primary irritant. Preliminary patch tests for primary irritant effects are useful, but they should be done on volunteer or paid subjects rather than on the workers in order to prevent undue apprehension among them, complaints from labor unions or legal action.

The application of a new compound every day or two for 2 to 3 weeks may simulate working conditions and may prove of value in determining the irritant properties of the substance.

Whenever new chemicals are tested, and the proper concentration for testing has not been established, it is much safer to perform the preliminary patch test by the open method. If the reaction is negative, it is then relatively safe to patch test by the usual, covered method.

Solutions of dyes, paints or liquid resins may be painted on the skin and left uncovered, because they evaporate and adhere to the site. Volatile solvents should be allowed to evaporate before being covered.

If it is suspected that the chemical to be tested is a strong sensitizer, it is wise to observe the patient in the office for an hour or so after the patch has been applied. In the rare event that a reaction occurs within this period, the chemicals should be wiped off, and ice cold compresses may be applied. I have noted patch tests with acrylic monomer, alcohol and certain epoxy resin components to cause a severe allergic reaction within 1 hour.

When the closed patch test technique is used with unknown substances or known potent sensitizers, a reading should be taken after 24 hours. Chemicals of relatively low sensitizing capacity are usually left on the skin for 48 hours before the patch is removed for reading. Some chemicals are sensitizers in low concentrations and primary irritants in higher concentrations.

If the exact concentration for patch testing has not been established, preliminary testing should be done with at least a 1:100 dilution by the open method. If the proper dilution for patch testing has been established, it is more convenient to perform the tests by the covered method, especially with substances that would spread unless sealed on.

INTERPRETATION OF PATCH TEST RESULTS WITH NEW COMPOUNDS

The interpretation of results of patch testing with new compounds is fraught with pitfalls, because it may be difficult to distinguish an allergic from a primary irritant reaction. A neat vesicular eruption consisting of closely set, clear vesicles is probably an allergic response, particularly if the site itches and the reaction persists and spreads.

An erosion or a single bulla covering the entire patch test site and confined almost exactly to the area of application is probably a primary irritant reaction. Less marked primary irritant reactions may consist of minute papules and pustulovesicles irregularly situated at follicular or sweat gland orifices, and follicular crusts and minute superficial etched-out ulcers. Primary irritant reactions tend to disappear rapidly when the covering patch is removed, but allergic reactions often become more intense.

Whenever the results of patch testing with a new compound are doubtful, the chemical should be tested on three normal controls. A primary irritant will usually cause a reaction in 1 or 2 of the controls, but an allergen should not cause a reaction in them.

Another type of irritant or false positive reaction may occur when the skin is hyperirritable or an acute dermatitis is present. In such instances, even testing substances used in nonirritating concentrations may produce reactions that are difficult to distinguish from a true allergic response. In case of doubt, patch tests should be repeated after a week or so when the skin is less irritable or the dermatitis less acute.

PRE-EMPLOYMENT PATCH TESTING

The routine use of pre-employment patch tests should be avoided. Workers who do not have a history of allergic dermatitis or who do not present with a dermatitis that is compatible with an allergic contact dermatitis should not be subjected to pre-employment patch test procedures. Although a properly performed patch test usually does not sensitize those who would not, in all likelihood, have become sensitized by the occupational exposure, workers who react positively may claim that the procedure caused the sensitization.

Routine pre-employment patch testing should be avoided for medicolegal reasons

If the worker gives a history of allergic contact dermatitis or presents with a dermatitis compatible with such a diagnosis, pre-employment patch testing may be indicated. Such testing alerts him to avoid further exposure, in the new occupation, to a specific chemical to which he had become sensitized in the past. For legal reasons, it is preferable that the worker be tested with the chemicals to which he has been exposed rather than chemicals on a standard tray.

A worker who shows a strongly positive patch test reaction to a chemical must avoid not only that particular chemical but also immunochemically related allergens. For example, individuals who demonstrate allergic hypersensitivity to paraphenylenediamine should also avoid azo and aniline dyes. On the other hand, a positive patch test reaction to the dichromates does not preclude exposure to other metals, such as nickel and copper, because cross-reactions between these metals do not usually occur.

It is unfair to exclude a worker from employment merely because he has had an allergic contact dermatitis in the past. As a rule, aside from cross-sensitization reactions, allergic contact hypersensitivity is specific and is restricted to one group of chemicals. It would also be unfair to deny employment to an individual because he has had an allergic contact dermatitis and has an "immunologic" scar or his skin had been damaged in the past.

Although strongly positive patch test reactions usually indicate that the patient will acquire severe contact dermatitis if exposed to the sensitizer, mild positive reactions, such as a 1+ rating, need not necessarily exclude a worker from handling the sensitizing compound.

In many instances in which a highly skilled worker has a minimal dermatitis with a weakly positive patch test reaction to a particular chemical, the dermatitis remains mild in spite of continued exposure to the allergen. I have observed several furriers with mild test reactions to paraphenylenediamine and minimal dermatitis who continued to be exposed to the dye for years without much difficulty. Such instances are not examples of hardening, but of a very low-grade sensitization, which may at any time suddenly become more marked. I have also seen low-grade sensitizations with minimal dermatitis from dichromates and formaldehyde in patients who continued to be exposed without acquiring disabling eruptions.

Great care must be taken to dilute strong sensitizers so that a very strongly positive patch test reaction may be avoided. Such reactions may produce marked itching and discomfort for several weeks and may cause a disgruntled employee to claim that he never had any "skin trouble" until the patch test was performed. Medicolegal complications may result from such severe reactions.

USE OF PATCH TESTS TO DETERMINE HARDENING IN INDUSTRY

The term *hardening* as originally introduced by J. Jadassohn, indicated a condition in which an allergic contact dermatitis in sensitized persons disappeared or failed to reappear on repeated exposure to the sensitizing chemical. This concept of a specific hardening has been broadened to include a nonspecific variety.

Nonspecific hardening refers to instances in which a patient acquires a dermatitis from a primary irritant, such as Fiberglas, and subsequently can handle it without acquiring an eruption. The type of nonspecific hardening is neither proved nor disproved by patch testing.

Hardening may be specific or nonspecific

Specific hardening may be described as a form of natural hyposensitization in which certain individuals suffering from an allergic dermatitis may become hyposensitized to the allergen in spite of continued exposure. The term *hyposensitization* is preferred to *desensitization*, because in many instances the hypersensitivity returns, particularly if there is reexposure after a period of avoidance.

Hardening is said to occur under conditions of diminished but continuous contact with the allergen, and it is more likely to occur if the allergic dermatitis appears after a short exposure than after prolonged contact. It is also claimed that hardening is less likely to occur after a severe dermatitis than after a mild attack. Hardening following allergic sensitization is more likely to occur with certain sensitizing chemicals, for example, tetryl, than with sensitizers such as the dichromates.

It is my opinion that hardening, or hyposensitization, occurs only in rare instances and may be attributed to better hygiene so that contact with the allergen is avoided. In most instances in which hardening is cited in the literature, the impression is "clinical" only. Scientific proof of specific hardening would be established when the following criteria have been satisfied:

1. The patient has had an allergic contact dermatitis due to a specific chemical that caused a *strongly* positive patch test reaction.
2. The allergic contact dermatitis produced by the chemical clears and remains clear in spite of exposure to the chemical that caused the positive patch test reaction.
3. The previously strongly positive patch test reaction to the chemical becomes negative or only weakly positive.

Specific desensitization or hardening is the exception rather than the rule

In my experience, hardening, or desensitization, that fulfills these criteria occurs only in rare instances and usually cannot be relied upon in the management of allergic contact dermatitis due to occupational exposures. A recent study of the persistence of allergic eczematous sensitivity to paraphenylenediamine revealed that such hypersensitivity persisted for 10 to 15 years in over 90 per cent of patients, and strongly positive patch test reactions were obtained in sensitized individuals even when they apparently no longer came in contact with the sensitizer.

Workers who acquire an allergic contact dermatitis from a chemical that produces a strongly positive patch test reaction should not be exposed to the sensitizing compound in the hope that hardening, or desensitization, may take place. This expectation is almost never fulfilled.

Attempts at desensitization by exposing the patient's skin to gradually increasing concentrations of the contact allergen also fail. Therapeutic hardening by feeding or injecting graduated amounts of specific contact allergens has been successful only with poison ivy and ragweed oleoresins.

Nonspecific hardening does frequently take place with continued use of mild or moderate primary irritants because of gradual thickening and pigmentation of the skin.

TESTING WITH RUBBER CHEMICALS

Industrial dermatitis from rubber chemicals and from finished rubber products is common. Table 11-1 is a list of the most common rubber sensitizers in industry.

The rubber antioxidant n-isopropyl-n′-phenyl-p-phenylenediamine (IPPD) is a potent sensitizer and can produce eczematous, purpuric and lichenoid eruptions. Test it in a 0.1 per cent concentration in petrolatum

Plate 8. Occupational Dermatoses

1. Telephone Operator

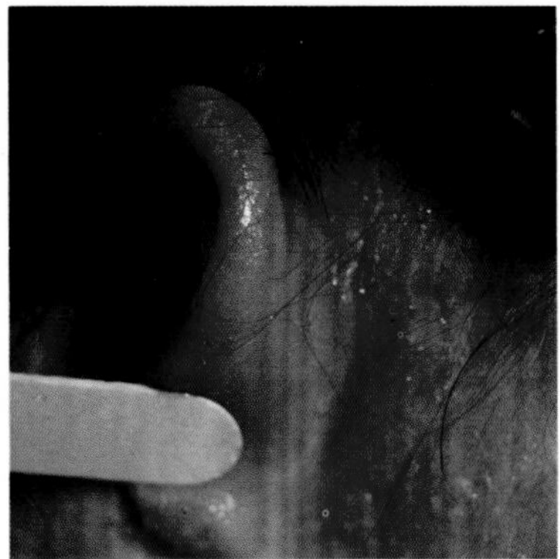

Nickel-plated Head Set

2. Fiberglass Industry

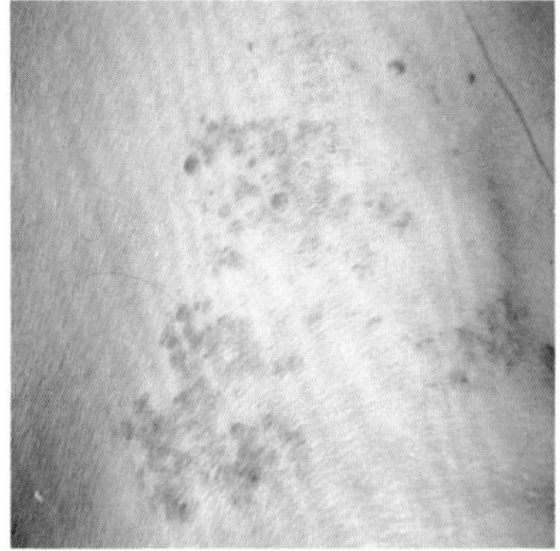

"Mechanical" Purpura

3. Dry Cleaning Industry

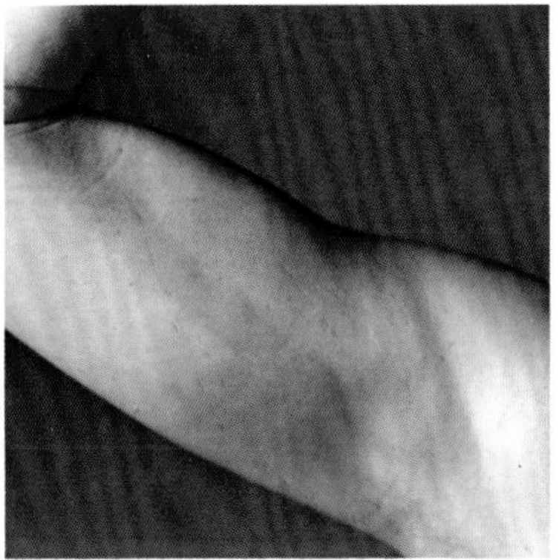

"Chemical" Lymphangitis from Carbon Tetrachloride

4. Chemist

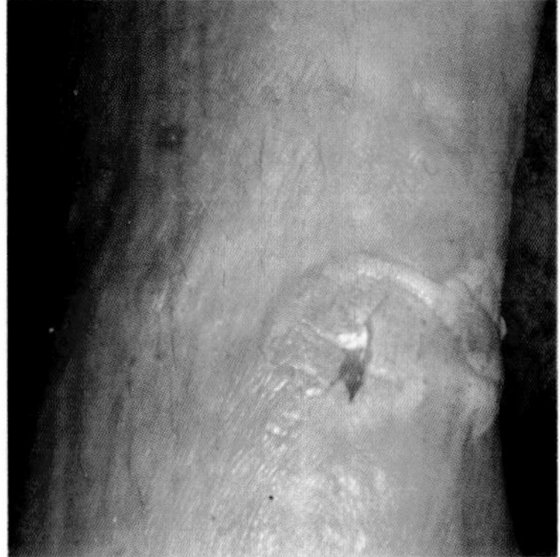

Bullous Reaction to 9-bromoflurene

5. Painter

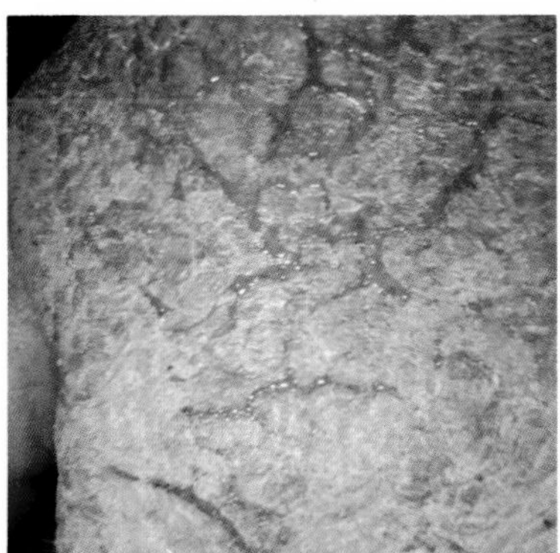

Severe Irritant and Allergic Reactions to Turpentine

6. Glass Worker

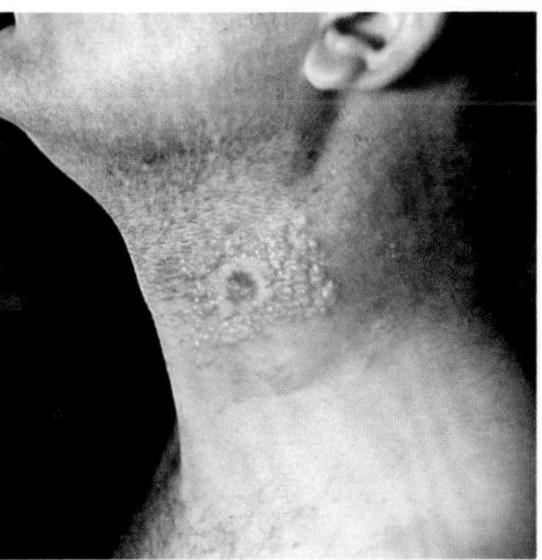

Ammonium Fluoride "Burn"

Table 11-1. Rubber Chemical Patch Test Series*

Accelerators
Mercaptobenzothiazole
Tetramethylthiuram disulfide
Diphenylguanidine
Benzothiazyl disulfide
Zinc dimethyldithiocarbamate
Hexamethylenetetramine
Antioxidants
n-Isopropyl-n′-phenyl-p-phenylenediamine (IPPD)
n-Phenyl-beta-naphthylamine
1,2-Dihydro-2,2,4-trimethyl quinoline
2,2-Methylene-bis-(4-methyl-6-tertiary butyl phenol)
Monobenzyl ether of hydroquinone
Peptizer
Thio-beta-naphtol
Filler
Phenol-formaldehyde resin
Plasticizers
Pine tar, rosin
Solvent
Turpentine

* All may be tested 1 per cent in petrolatum, except IPPD, which is tested in a 0.1 per cent concentration.

n-Isopropyl-n′-phenyl-p-phenylenediamine (*IPPD*) should be tested in a 0.1 per cent concentration, because 1 per cent may sensitize the patient. It is an antizonant (antioxidant) used particularly in tires, truck cushions, belting hose and cables in about 2 per cent strength. It may cause eczematous contact dermatitis[2,3] and a purpuric eruption when used in clothing,[4] and it is a potent sensitizer in the chemical rubber industry.[5,6] It is used and sold in the United States under the following trade names.[17]

Cyzone IP (Cyanamid)
Eastozone 34 (Tennessee Eastman)
Fleezwx (Goodyear)
Flexaone 3C (Naugatuck)
Santoflex 36 (Monsanto)

Abroad, it is known as Nonox-2A. Calnan (personal communication, 1971) has described lichenoid eruptions caused by it.

This compound may cross-react with paraphenylenediamine.[8]

SYNTHETIC RESIN (PLASTIC) DERMATITIS

Plastics are polymerized by the addition of curing agents, stabilizers, plasticizers and catalysts. In addition, accelerators and antioxidants are often added. Any of these chemicals may be irritants or sensitizers.

Plastics Commonly Causing Dermatitis. Epoxy resins and phenolformaldehyde plastics cause allergic and irritant dermatitis. Carbamid-formaldehyde and acrylic plastics cause allergic reactions. Polyester plastics produce irritant and rarely allergic dermatitis.

Plastics Rarely Causing Dermatitis. Polypropylene, polyurethane, Teflon, furene, polycarbonates, silicones, carbonyls, coumarone, cellulose derivatives, polystyrene, polyvinyl chloride (PVC), polypropylene chloride (PPC), polyvinyl acetate (PVA), polybutadiene nitril alkyds and polyethylene are rare causes of dermatitis.

Additives That Are Common Sensitizers. Phthalates (such as dibutyldioctyl), maleates, cobalt-naphthenate, benzoyl peroxide, dimethylaniline and toluenesulfonic acid commonly cause dermatitis. Sensitizers used in both plastics and rubber include naphthylamines, paraphenylenediamine derivatives, mercaptobenzothiazole, phenols and epoxy resin hardeners.

TESTING FOR SYNTHETIC RESIN SENSITIVITY

Synthetic resins in the solid cured or fully polymerized state rarely cause dermatitis.[9,10] The finished product is remarkably free of irritating sensitizing properties. In the manufacture of these synthetic resins, however, there are many opportunities for contact with uncured resins, catalyzers and modifiers, all of which may be skin irritants and sensitizers and readily produce dermatitis unless precautions are taken to protect the worker. In particular, epoxy resin systems have produced many instances of dermatitis.

Solid, completely polymerized resins rarely cause dermatitis. Incompletely cured resins may be irritants and sensitizers

It is possible that the sawing and grinding of completely polymerized resins may cause depolymerization with the release of chemicals that can cause irritation or sensitization. Such synthetic resin dust or grindings should be handled with the same precautions as used with the unpolymerized chemicals.

Outside of industry, dermatitis due to synthetic resins is likely to occur only when the general population is exposed to the resins in the liquid or incompletely cured state, such as epoxy resin glues and adhesives, acrylic monomers employed to make artificial fingernails, and nail lacquer containing formaldehyde resins.

Synthetic resins producing dermatitis in the general population include acrylic artificial nails, acrylic prostheses, nail lacquer, epoxy and formaldehyde resin glues and cements and cellulose ester plastics

Patch Testing With Synthetic Resins.[11,12] Tests with the chemicals involved in the manufacture of these resin systems must be performed with caution to avoid severe reactions. The correct concentrations and the proper vehicles for patch tests are still being evaluated. In the following discussion, suggestions are given for concentrations and for suitable vehicles. The solvents or vehicles should be chosen with care. Many resins can be incorporated in petrolatum for test purposes.

Solvents generally useful include acetone and butyrolactone.

Acetone is a readily available unreactive solvent for the epoxy, polyester and polyurethane monomers and prepolymers. When used as a solvent for urethane prepolymers, the acetone must be reasonably free of moisture. Since it is volatile, fresh solutions must be made for each patch test series.

Butyrolactone is a cyclic ester that is not volatile. It is a nonirritating, nonsensitizing, unreactive solvent suitable for testing many liquid resins and resin components. It is available from Antara Chemicals, a division of General Aniline and Film Corp., 435 Hudson Street, New York, N. Y. 10014.

EPOXY RESINS

The epoxy resins probably cause more instances of occupational dermatitis, both in the United States and abroad,[13] than do any other chemicals introduced in recent years.

The epoxy resins, widely used in industry, produce many cases of occupational dermatitis. Housewives, artists and sculptors may also become sensitized

The versatile epoxy (epoxide or ethoxylene) resins are widely used in manufacturing electrical equipment for enclosing transformers, condensers and other components, in automobile plants for tool and die casting, in paints for surface coating and in aircraft and other industries for adhesive purposes.

Ingredients of Epoxy Resin Systems. In the manufacture and use of epoxy resins, individuals may acquire dermatitis from one or more of the following chemicals, which may be incorporated in the epoxy resin system:[14–16]

Uncured epoxy resin (liquid or solid)
Catalytic agents consisting of amines and anhydrides, which are called converters, hardeners or curing agents
Reactive diluents
Plasticizers
Solvents
Fillers
Pigments
Blends of other resins

Uncured Epoxy Resins. A typical uncured epoxy resin is obtained by the condensation of epichlorhydrin and p,p′-isopropylidenediphenol (Bisphenol A). Other epoxy resins are condensates consisting of a mixture of polyglycidyl ethers. Epoxy resins have little utility in the form in which they are supplied to the market. They must be further polymerized or cured by the addition of curing agents, such as amines, amides, anhydrides or inorganic fluoride compounds. Cured epoxy resins are hard, relatively insoluble materials, which are nonirritating and nonsensitizing.

Bisphenol A cross-reacts with diethylstilbestrol.[17] This hormone may be present in scalp preparations for treatment of alopecia and Aquacort E Jel (Webster), Furestrol Vaginal Suppositories (Eaton) and diethylstilbestrol suppositories (Lilly) for vaginitis. Patients sensitized to Bisphenol A should be informed of the possibility of cross-reactions with diethylstilbestrol.[18,19] Bisphenol A may also cross-react with organic silicone compounds.[20]

The epoxy component Bisphenol A is a sensitizer, which may cross-react with diethylstilbestrol

For patch testing purposes, Bisphenol A may be used in a 1 per cent concentration in petrolatum.

Catalysts and Curing Agents. These chemicals speed the polymerization of epoxy resin.

Liquid epoxy compounds can be cured to form hard, insoluble products by polymerization in the presence of catalysts or by polyaddition with cross-linking agents containing active hydrogen atoms. These curing agents or hardeners may act at either room or elevated temperatures and have been divided into the following four categories:

1. Amine hardeners, e.g., aliphatic polyamines and amino-polyamides
2. Acid hardeners, e.g., polycarboxylic acids and dicarboxylic acid anhydrides
3. Aldehyde-condensation products, e.g., phenol, melamine and urea-formaldehyde resins
4. Inorganic or organic metallic compounds, e.g., boron trifluoride, titanium acid ester and aluminum alcoholate

Of this host of chemicals, amine hardeners appear to be the most potent sensitizers.

Epoxy Amine Hardeners. The amines are used particularly when the epoxy resin is cured, catalyzed or self-hardened at room temperature. These agents are usually aliphatic amines, such as diethylenetriamine, triethylenetetramine and metaphenylenediamine, an aromatic amine hardener. In the uncombined state, they are caustic and can produce severe burns on contact with the skin. In addition, they can cause a severe allergic contact dermatitis characterized by severe redness, edema and itching of the exposed parts. The aliphatic hardeners, diethylenetriamine and triethylenetetramine, are powerful water-soluble skin irritants.[21]

For patch testing purposes, a 0.1 per cent aqueous solution may be used. Even at this low concentration, controls should be employed to make certain that positive results are not due to a primary irritant effect.

The amine epoxy hardeners are powerful irritants and potent sensitizers. In addition, epoxy resin diluents, solvents, modifiers and plasticizers can cause dermatitis

Blends of Other Resins. Epoxy resins may be blended with urea-formaldehyde, phenol-formaldehyde and melamine-formaldehyde resins, all of which are potential sensitizers and irritants.

Nonindustrial Exposure to Epoxy Resins. Epoxy glues are becoming increasingly popular for household use. They are made available in two parts, the hardener and the resin.[22] The labels on the containers state that ingredients contacting the skin should immediately be removed with soap and water. It is claimed that the versatile epoxy glues can cement anything to anything. Artists and sculptors find many uses for these glues and some have acquired epoxy resin dermatitis.

Epoxy resins may be present in household adhesives and glues and be blended with formaldehyde and with polyvinyl resins

Fregert and Rorsman[23,24] have described hypersensitivity to epoxy resins in persons who came in contact with polyvinyl chloride film in which epoxy resins had been used as stabilizers and plasticizers. Such resin films may be used in plastic gloves, adhesive tapes and plastic panties. Handbags and chamber pots made of polyvinyl chloride have caused dermatitis. In addition, dermatitis of the neck occurred from beads that had been treated with polyvinyl chloride. Fregert and Rorsman feel that allergic sensitization to epoxy resins is not uncommon in the general population and have, therefore, included epoxy resins for routine patch testing.[23,24]

POLYESTER RESINS

The finished, completely polymerized polyresins are not dermatologic hazards. Products such as Dacron, polyester fiber and Mylar (polyester film) have not caused dermatitis. Exposure to chemicals in the manufacture of polyresin systems, however, can produce dermatitis, particularly the irritant variety.

Dermatologic Hazards of Components of the Polyester Resin Systems[25,26]

Unsaturated Polyester Resin. This resin rarely irritates or produces allergic contact dermatitis. The polyester resin may be tested in a 10 per cent concentration in acetone.

Styrene (Vinyl Benzene). This chemical, used to modify polyester monomer, is an unsaturated hydrocarbon obtained from storax (styrax) balsam. It may have an irritating, drying and defatting effect on the skin, but it rarely produces allergic dermatitis. Since storax is used in the preparation of compound tincture of benzoin, in perfume and as a fixative for soaps, allergic sensitization to styrene carries with it the possibility of cross-reaction with benzoin compounds and some soaps. Styrene can be removed from the skin with acetone. For patch testing purposes, either 1 per cent styrene in olive oil or 2 per cent styrene in petrolatum can be employed. One per cent styrene in butyrolactone may also be used.

Benzoyl Peroxide. This catalyst, as well as other organic peroxides, is used in compounding polyester resins. It rarely irritates but sometimes sensitizes. Exposure to benzoyl peroxide may occur not only in industry, but also from topical medications in the treatment of acne vulgaris.

Benzoyl peroxide is used in acrylic resin formulation. Dentists and dental technicians may become sensitized to this compound when handling the acrylic monomer.

Aside from its use in resin systems, benzoyl peroxide is used as a flour "improver" in the baking industry and leaves a residue of benzoic acid in the finished product. Bakers who become sensitized to benzoyl peroxide may show cross-reaction with other benzoic acid derivatives and cinnamon.[27]

Benzoyl peroxide is also used as a topical antibacterial agent in the form of benzoyl peroxide ointment, Quinolor Compound Ointment, Vanoxide and Loroxide, Persadox, Benoxyl Lotions and Oxy-5.

Benzoyl peroxide, a polyester catalyst, is also used in acrylic resins, as a flour "improver," in Quinolor Ointment and in Vanoxide, Persadox and Benoxyl Lotion

For patch testing purposes, benzoyl peroxide may be applied in a 0.1 per cent concentration in equal parts of olive oil and styrene, or in a 5 per cent concentration in petrolatum. A 1 per cent concentration in butyrolactone may also be used.

When used as a topical agent, benzoyl peroxide may produce allergic reactions.[28–31]

Organic Peroxide Catalysts. Methylethyl ketone peroxide is frequently used in polyester resin systems. Other peroxides sometimes employed are cumene hydroperoxide, lauroyl, acetyl and cyclohexanone peroxides, all of which are more potent irritants than is benzoyl peroxide. A 0.5 per cent solution of the peroxides in acetone may be employed for patch test purposes.

Cobalt Naphthenate. This accelerator rarely causes irritation but may occasionally produce allergic contact dermatitis. Cobalt naphthenate may be tested in a dilution of 5 per cent alcohol or olive oil.

Dimethylaniline. This accelerator is readily absorbed through the skin and acts as a systemic poison. Primary irritant effects and occasionally sensitization occur from the compound. For patch testing, a 10 per cent concentration in alcohol is recommended.

Hydroquinone. This polyester inhibitor is also widely used in many other synthetic resin formulations. It may cause allergic contact dermatitis and is used as a depigmenting agent in Eldoquin (Elder) and Artra (White). For patch test purposes, 2 per cent concentration in petrolatum may be used.

Tertiary Butyl Catechol. This inhibitor, added to prolong the storage life of polyester resins, may rarely cause allergic sensitization. It may be tested as a 1 per cent solution in acetone.

Tricresyl Phosphate. A plasticizer of vinyl film, this compound may be tested as a 70 per cent solution in alcohol.

Dibutyl Phthalate. This is a plasticizer for synthetic resins. It may be tested "as is."

POLYURETHANES (ISOCYANATE RESINS)

Polyurethanes are used in the manufacture of foams, synthetic rubber, adhesives and coatings. They are made by reacting a diisocyanate with polyols, such as glycols, polyesters and polyethers. The catalyst may be an organotin, cobalt naphthenate or a tertiary amine.[32]

The liquid isocyanate monomer may produce severe irritation of the skin, eyes and respiratory tract. Stringent precautions are usually taken to prevent contact, and few cases of dermatitis have been reported.

In the ultimate processing to form an elastomer, all the remaining isocyanate is consumed, and the final product is neither irritant nor sensitizer.[33,34]

Typical polyurethane resin components include Rigithane 112, Rigithane Catalyst C-112-R2 and Solithane 113.

Rigithane 112 (*Thiokol Chemical Corp.*). For patch testing purposes, a 1 per cent concentration of Rigithane prepolymer in alcohol or acetone should be used. Toluene, xylene, chloroform and methylene chloride are also suitable solvents.

Rigithane Catalyst C-112-R2. This urethane resin catalyst may be tested in a 10 per cent aqueous solution.

Solithane 113 (*Thiokol Chemical Corp.*). The Solithane prepolymer may be patch tested in a 1 per cent concentration in alcohol or acetone.

The Solithane catalysts include the following:

- Solithane Catalyst C-113-300 (tertiary amine catalyst), which may be tested in a 1 per cent alcohol solution
- Diethylethanolamine (tertiary amine catalyst), which may be tested in a 0.5 per cent aqueous solution
- Solithane Catalyst C-113-328 (tertiary amine catalyst), which may be tested in a 10 per cent aqueous solution
- Methyl morpholine (tertiary amine catalyst), which may be tested in a 0.1 per cent aqueous solution
- Triethylenediamine (tertiary amine catalyst), which may be tested in a 0.1 per cent aqueous solution

Skin contaminated with isocyanates and other polyurethane components should be cleansed immediately and thoroughly with isopropyl alcohol

PREVENTION OF IRRITATION FROM LIQUID ISOCYANATES

The liquid monomer can produce a marked inflammatory reaction characterized by edema and redness if it is not immediately removed from the skin. Contaminated skin, therefore, should be washed copiously and thoroughly with water, and the affected area should be treated with 30 per cent isopropyl alcohol and then washed with soap and water.

All contaminated clothing should be removed, preferably in a safety shower.[35,36]

FORMALDEHYDE RESINS

These resins may be tested as a 5 per cent concentration in petrolatum. Formaldehyde sensitivity is not necessarily associated with allergy to the formaldehyde resins.[37]

Malten and VanAerssen[38] demonstrated that *para-tertiary butylphenol* (PTBP) was the sensitizing substance in their patients with phenol-formaldehyde resin dermatitis. It would appear to indicate that the sensitizing agent is the resin and not its phenol and formaldehyde component.

The sensitizing agent in phenol-formaldehyde resin is para-tertiary butylphenol and not the phenol or formaldehyde

Engel and Calnan[39] stated that the para-tertiary butylphenol–formaldehyde resins should be classed with epoxy and polyester resins as potential skin sensitizers and considered in cases of probable adhesive dermatitis.

Para-tertiary butylphenol is also used as an intermediate in the manufacture of varnish and lacquer resins, as a soap antioxidant, as an ingredient in de-emulsifiers for oil field use, in motor oil additives, as a plasticizer for cellulose acetate, as an intermediate for rubber antioxidants and in synthetic oils, insecticides, deodorants and commercial disinfectants. It can also be used in printing inks and in resins to give latex glues an initial adhesive force.

Para-tertiary butylphenol is also a sensitizer and depigmenting agent.[40] The amylphenols and butylphenols may be tested as 1 per cent in petrolatum.

Para-tertiary butylphenol and amylphenol are sensitizers and depigmenting agents

DERMATITIS DUE TO FIBERGLAS (GLASS FIBER, GLASS WOOL)

The finished glass fiber product does not contain uncured resin, and the main hazard is penetration of the skin by small spicules of glass, which cause mechanical irritation. Sensitization to glass fibers apparently does not occur.

Glass fibers are marketed under the following names:

Aerocor (Owens-Corning)
Dolomite (Dolomite Glass Fibers, Inc.)
Famco (American Air Filter Co.)
Fiberfrax (Carborundum Co.)
Fiberglas (Owens-Corning)
Garan (Johns-Manville)
Garanmat (Johns-Manville)
Hi-Mod (House Glsas Corp.)
Modiglass (Modiglass Fibers, Inc.)
Pittsburgh PPG (Pittsburgh Plate Glass Co.)
Ultrastrand (Gustin-Bacon)
Unifab (Ferro Corp.)
Uniformat (Ferro Corp.)
Uniglass (United Merchants)
Unirove (Ferro Corp.)
Unistrand (Gustin-Bacon)
Vitron (Johns-Manville)

The cutaneous irritation from glass fibers varies directly with the diameter of the fibers. A recent development is the production of such small fibers that no discernible cutaneous irritation apparently results.

The handling of glass fibers may cause intense pruritus because fine particles and glass dust may readily penetrate the skin and cause a characteristic miliarial eruption consisting of small erythematous follicular papules. Other skin lesions, including purpura, telangiectasia, folliculitis, urticaria and linear erosions in the skin creases, may also be produced, particularly in fair-complexioned individuals with dry skin. In addition, paronychia may result from the penetration of glass spicules underneath the nailfold.[41]

Glass fiber particles and dust can produce pruritus, folliculitis, erosions, paronychia and mechanical purpura. Hardening often occurs in glass fiber workers

Workers involved in the manufacture of glass fibers may also develop a pustular, follicular acneiform eruption from hydrogenated vegetable oils and coating emulsions. In addition, glass fibers and resins may coat, and interfere with, the porosity of leather footwear, often producing maceration and dermatitis of the feet.

Glass fiber particles may penetrate clothing and underwear, producing a dermatitis on covered portions of the body. Glass particles may be brought home and transferred from the worker's clothes and skin to other members of his family. This type of "contagious" glass fiber dermatitis may be mistaken for scabies.

The washing of glass fiber clothing in a washing machine with the family underwear may produce a family "epidemic" of itching.[42] A precautionary label warning the consumer not to wash glass fiber products with other clothing is needed.[43]

In cases of glass fiber dermatitis, scrapings from the lesions, treated with 20 per cent potassium hydroxide and examined microscopically, may show the presence of glass fibers

Elby and Jetton[44] reported a case of school desk dermatitis due to a primary irritant contact reaction to fiber glass, reinforced plastic chairs and school desks.

ACRYLIC PLASTICS

Acrylic plastics are used in Plexiglas, dental plates, surgical prostheses and contact lenses and for surface treatment of textile fibers. Acrylic plastics have recently come into widespread use and are included in many industrial products.

One of the most commonly used acrylic plastics is methyl methacrylate. In its monomeric form, this ester is liquid, but if it is exposed to light, heat or oxygen, polymerization takes place. The short chain molecules of the monomer join together to form long chains and the liquid becomes a solid. The acrylic plastic also contains additives, such as stabilizers (e.g., hydroquinone, resorcinol and phenol), benzoyl peroxide and dyes. It is nearly always in its monomeric form that acrylic plastic can sensitize, and only in exceptional circumstances does it do so as a finished product.

Dr. S. Fregert (personal communication, 1969) stated that contact allergy to acrylic resins based on esters of acrylic and methacrylic acids is well-known. Methyl methacrylate is usually considered the relevant test substance, but other forms of acrylic resins are common and sensitization to such resins can occur.

Table 11–2 is a list of monomers of acrylic resins that should be taken into consideration at investigation of suspected sensitivity to acrylic resins. These monomers may be tested in a concentration of 0.1 per cent in petrolatum.

Table 11-2. Monomers of Acrylic Resins

Acrylic acid
Acrylates
Methacrylates
2-Chloro-acrylic-methylester
2-Cyano-acrylic methylester
Ethyleneglycol-dimethacrylate
2-Hydroxyethyl-methacrylate
2-Hydroxypropyl-methacrylate
Glycidyl-methacrylate
Aminosubstituted acrylates, e.g.,
  Acryl-amide
  n-Methylol-acrylamide
  Acrylo-nitrile
  Methacrylo-nitrile
  2, 4 Dihydroxy-benzophenone-methacrylate

Dr. S. Fregert, in another personal communication (1969) described a case of allergic contact dermatitis from n-methylol-acrylamide in a painter in the plastic industry. Four acrylic monomers (n-methylol-acrylamide, 2-ethyl-hexylacrylate, butylacrylate and ethylacrylate) were used for processing copolymers with polyvinyl acetate in paints. The four compounds may occur as monomers up to 0.3 per cent in the paints and for patch test purposes may be used as 0.1 per cent in petrolatum. In the painter with the contact dermatitis, a positive patch test was obtained with n-methylol-acrylamide.

Dr. B. R. Balda (personal communication, 1971) observed a case of allergic contact dermatitis to acrylo-nitrile in an acrylic plastic splint (Plexidure) applied for a lacerated finger tendon.

Magnuson and Mobacken[45] described allergic contact dermatitis from acrylate printing plates in a printing plant.

Allergic contact dermatitis due to acrylic plastic occurs mainly among dentists and dental technicians (see chapter on hand dermatitis).

CELLULOSE ESTER PLASTICS

These plastics are used in eyeglass frames, hearing aids, steering wheels, toothbrush and hairbrush handles, tool handles, pens and toys. These products, particularly eyeglass frames, may produce both irritant and allergic reactions.[46]

Industrial sensitization readily develops in workers exposed to the additives used in the manufacture of the cellulose ester plastics. More rarely the finished products can produce allergic contact dermatitis.

Jordan and Dahl[46] found the principal sensitizers in these plastics to include the following:

1. *Resorcinol monobenzoate.* An ultraviolet absorber, which may cross-react with balsam of Peru but not with resorcinol. This chemical is not widely used at present.
2. *Azobenzene dyes.*
3. *Para-tertiary butylphenol.* A sensitizer and depigmenting agent used for heat-stabilizing.
4. *Ethylene glycol monoethyl ether acetate.* A solvent used to weld nosepads to eyeglass frames and laminate plastic sheets.
5. *Plasticizers.* The phthalates are the most common plasticizers in cellulose ester plastics and are very rare sensitizers.

Table 11–3 is a list of the materials that should be used for patch testing individuals suspected of having allergic dermatitis from cellulose ester plastic.

BENZOPHENONE

Ramsey and co-workers[47] reported a case of a black man with a broad-spectrum light sensitivity who simultaneously showed an urticarial and contact sensitivity to a preparation containing 2-hydroxy-4-methoxybenzophenone-5-sulfonic acid (sulisobenzone). Both the benzophenone and the sulfonic acid parts of the molecule were required to elicit the eczematous reaction, while benzophenone alone elicited the urticarial reaction.

A scratch test with 1 per cent 2-hydroxy-4-methoxybenzophenone-5-sulfonic acid gave an immediate wheal and flare response. This is the active ingredient (in 10 per cent concentration) in Sungard. The 1 per cent 2-hydroxy-4-methoxybenzophenone in butyrolactone, which is the same molecule devoid of the sulfonic acid group, also produced a 2+ immediate wheal and flare response. These compounds elicited no response in 4 control subjects.

Benzophenones are often incorporated in textiles and plastics to impart protection from and colorfastness to ultraviolet radiation. They are put into transparent shades

Table 11-3. Patch Tests for Cellulose Ester Plastic Sensitivity[46]

Substance	*Percentage in Vehicle*
Cellulose acetate flakes	As is
Cellulose acetate flakes	10% in methylethyl ketone (MEK)
Cellulose acetate plastic	As is
Cellulose acetate proprionate plastic	As is
Cellulose acetate butyrate plastic	As is
Carbon black	1% in petrolatum album
Black dye mixture	1% in petrolatum album
Solvent yellow 3 (Color Index No. 11160)	1% in petrolatum album
Solvent red 26 (Color Index No. 26102)	1% in petrolatum album
Other colorants of black dye mixture	1% in petrolatum album
Ethylene glycol monoethyl ether acetate	5% in methylethyl ketone
Potassium acid oxalate	0.5% in water
p-Tertiary-butylphenol	2% in petrolatum album
Dimethyl phthalate	As is
Diethyl phthalate	As is
Tricresyl phosphate	5% in petrolatum album
Phenyl salicylate	2% in petrolatum album
Resorcinol monobenzoate	1% in petrolatum album
2,2′-Dihydroxy-4,4′-dimethoxybenzophenone	1% in methylethyl ketone

to protect window displays, plastic lens filters for color photography, aerosol sprays to protect color prints, and many polystyrene, acrylic and rubber products to prevent darkening and loss of strength. They are often included in paints, varnishes and fluorescent lacquers to inhibit degradation of colors. Of particular interest is their use in cosmetics, such as hair sprays, hair dyes, shampoos and detergent bars.

ALUMINUM FLUX DERMATITIS IN CABLE JOINERS

Aluminum conductors have universally replaced expensive copper in power cables. Only one satisfactory flux formula, a red liquid developed by the Aluminum Company of America, has been developed to solder or join aluminum. It is based upon fluoroborate and aminoethylethanolamine. Dermatitis probably occurs in an incidence of 5 to 10 per cent among cable joiners using aluminum, and it is invariably due to sensitization to aminoethylethanolamine.[48,49] So far no sensitivity to fluoroborate has been found, although it may cause nonspecific pustular reactions. Preliminary work suggests that these men are not cross-sensitized to triethanolamine.

Aminoethylethanolamine was used for patch testing as a 1 and 5 per cent aqueous solution. This is hydroxyethyl ethylenediamine and may cross-react with ethylenediamine.

9-BROMOFLUORENE

Chemists or students who prepare 9-bromofluorene in laboratory experiments may acquire a bullous erythema-multiforme type of eruption.[50] This chemical is a powerful irritant and sensitizer.[51,52] Powell[52] obtained a positive patch test reaction in a sensitized individual with a 0.5 per cent solution of 9-bromofluorene in hexane.

DIPHENYLCYCLOPROPANONE

Dr. H. Whittaker (personal communication) described a severe dermatitis caused by diphenylcyclopropanone in a chemistry student. Patch tests were strongly positive with a 0.1 per cent solution in acetone.

ETHYLENE OXIDE

This fumigant vapor is a strong irritant and sensitizer. It is also employed as a solvent and plasticizer in the production of high energy fuels and as a sterilizing agent for surgical instruments and thermolabile materials.

Excessive quantities of ethylene oxide used to sterilize nitrofurazone pads produced dermatitis.[53] Facial irritation from ethylene oxide sterilization of anesthesia facemasks has been reported.[54]

DOWICIDE 32

Dr. R. M. Adams (personal communication, 1972) described a photodermatitis from chlorophenylphenol in Dowicide 32, which is used as an antibacterial agent in disinfectants, adhesives and textiles.

ETHOXYQUIN

Drs. W. S. Wood and R. Fulton (personal communication, 1972) reported allergic contact dermatitis in apple packers from ethoxyquin used with Tide detergent to prevent apple scald, browning of apples that may resemble a fungous infestation.

DINITROCHLORBENZENE

Adams et al.[55] treated 4 air conditioner repairmen who became sensitized to this compound, which was used as an algicide (Nalco 205) in air conditioners. Patch test reactions were positive with dilutions of 1:1000 to 1:1,000,000 in acetone.

Dinitrochlorbenzene is such a potent sensitizer that it has become a standard sensitizing agent in contact dermatitis research. It certainly should not be used industrially.

DIAZONIUM COMPOUNDS

Dr. G. A. W. Verspyck Mijnssen (personal communication, 1967) described a patient who contracted a contact dermatitis to Ozalid photocopy paper. The causative agent was a diazonium compound, 4,n,n′-diethyl aminobenzene diazonium chloride.

This diazonium compound is broken down by ultraviolet irradiation (3600 to 4300 Å) or by daylight. With some chemicals, the diazonium compound forms azo pigments under the influence of ammonia. Molecules with N=N groupings often have sensitizing properties. Patients with a contact dermatitis caused by this brand of copy paper must be patch tested with nonirradiated copy paper to avoid false negative results.

SOLVENTS

The organic solvents are indispensable in modern manufacturing processes. They are used to dissolve and thin lacquers, varnishes and paints and to act as solvents for rubber and natural and synthetic resins. In addition, they are employed in the dry cleaning industry and in the manufacture of organic dyes, artificial silk, glues and cements. They act as extractives for fats, waxes, oils and perfumes.

Dermatitis is frequently caused by contact with the organic solvents used in manufacturing processes and in hand cleansers

Workers are exposed to solvents not only in manufacturing processes, but also in hand cleansers. Usually the employee cleans his hands with solvents that happen to be handy. Painters cleanse with paint thinner, and machinists employ kerosene. Printers, typesetters and lithographers utilize type-wash, which is a petroleum solvent used to clean printing presses. In other industries, the workers use a variety of solvents, e.g., petroleum, coal tar derivatives, chlorinated hydrocarbons, alcohols, ketones and turpentine, to remove materials such as ink, tar, glue, gum, cement and other mucilaginous and viscous substances, grease, oil, stain, lacquer and varnish.

The waterless cleansers, which are essentially products of solvents, are becoming increasingly popular when heavy, tenacious soilage is encountered and water is inadequate. The waterless cleansers are grouped into the following classes:

Class 1—products of the kerosene or Stoddard solvent base (aliphatic solvent oil)
Class 2—products of a mineral oil base
Class 3—products based on solvents of the nonpetroleum oil type, such as glycols, ketones and esters
Class 4—products based entirely on mixtures of surface-active agents

Although these products are called waterless, they do contain water. Some are designed to be used with water; others do not require it. Those that are low in alkali and solvent content cause less dryness and irritation of the skin than do those that are highly alkaline.

Organic solvents dissolve sebum and keratin and penetrate the skin readily. Solvent dermatitis is a common industrial hazard. In addition, the solvents can enter the dermal lymphatics through fissures and lacerations and cause chemical lymphangitis, which is distinguished from the bacterial variety by lack of constitutional symptoms.

Organic solvents can dissolve sebum and keratin, producing dryness, fissuring and dermatitis. They can enter lacerations and produce chemical lymphangitis

The following is a list of the widely used solvents arranged in order of the severity of the primary irritant action on the skin.[56] With the exception of turpentine, these solvents rarely sensitize.

1. *Carbon disulfide*. This compound is used as a laboratory reagent, as a solvent for sulfur and in the manufacture of viscose rayon. It may be tested in a 50 per cent concentration in olive oil.

2. *Petroleum solvents* (*benzine, gasoline*). These aliphatic hydrocarbons are strong skin irritants, particularly if the skin is covered with an impervious material that prevents ready evaporation. They may be tested in a 50 per cent concentration in olive oil.

3. *Coal tar solvents* (*benzol, toluol, xylol*). These aromatic hydrocarbons of the benzene series not only are primary irritants of the skin, but also may cause severe, toxic systemic effects when absorbed through the skin or inhaled. They may be tested in a 50 per cent concentration in olive oil.

Benzine, the petroleum distillate, is also called petroleum benzine, or petroleum ether, and is used as a solvent for fats, resins, rubber and alkaloids. *Benzene* (benzol), a coal tar distillate, also known as phenyl hydride or coal tar naphtha, is widely used as a commercial solvent and in motor fuels.

4. *Turpentine.* This cyclic hydrocarbon is not only a skin irritant, but is also practically the only organic solvent that produces allergic contact dermatitis. Its irritant reaction usually results in drying and fissuring of the skin. The sensitizing effect of oil of turpentine is due to the oxidation products of certain terpenes (Δ^3-carene). The primary irritant effect is dependent on oxidation products of the terpenes. Freshly distilled turpentine containing unoxidized terpenes is less irritating and sensitizing than are older batches.

Turpentine may produce both allergic and irritant reactions, but other organic solvents rarely produce allergic hypersensitivity

For patch testing purposes, a 25 per cent solution of turpentine in olive oil may be employed. Since even this concentration occasionally produces a slightly irritating effect, positive reactions to patch testing with oil of turpentine should be checked with at least 2 normal controls.

5. *Chlorinated hydrocarbon solvents.* The halogenated hydrocarbons include carbon tetrachloride, trichloroethylene and DDT (dichlorodiphenyl trichloroethane, chlorophenothane), which, in addition to their drying and irritating effects on the skin, may produce *chloracne*. Furthermore, DDT in particular has been implicated in the production of porphyria cutanea tarda.

Chlorinated hydrocarbon solvents may degrease the skin, cause chloracne, and, particularly DDT, may produce porphyria cutanea tarda

Carbon tetrachloride is employed as a dry cleaning agent. In addition to irritating the skin, it may produce blood dyscrasias. It may be tested as is, preferably uncovered.

Trichloroethylene is widely used as a dry cleaning agent in compounds such as DuPont Dry Cleaner, Glamorene Rug Cleaner, Tri-Clene Dry Cleaner, Triad Metal Cleaner and Triad Metal Polish. It is also employed to degrease metal, as a solvent for oils, resins, sulfur and phosphorus, and medicinally as a wound cleanser and for relief of angina pectoris. It may be tested in a 50 per cent concentration in olive oil. It may sensitize the patient to alcohol. A combination of alcohol ingestion and trichloroethylene exposure may produce an "aldehyde syndrome," with flushing of the skin, nausea and vomiting.

DDT,* an insecticide, rarely causes allergic dermatitis. When dissolved in kerosene or other organic solvents, it is readily absorbed through the skin and may cause toxic effects. In powder form, suspensions and emulsions, it may safely be applied to the skin. It is tested in a 5 per cent concentration in acetone.

6. *Alcohol* (*methyl*, *ethyl*). Contact allergy due to the lower aliphatic alcohols, such as methanol, ethanol, propanol and butanol, appears to be rare. It is not yet clear whether the pure alcohols or the aldehydes formed from alcohols in the skin are the sensitizers.[57]

Patch testing with alcohol should be done by both closed and open methods. I observed 2 patients with allergic contact sensitivity to alcohol who were tested by rubbing the alcohol onto the skin with a cotton-tipped applicator. In both patients an erythematous reaction appeared at the test site within 10 minutes, persisted for about 1 hour and then slowly faded. Such a reaction might be missed if the usual covered technique had been used. Other observers have noted similar reactions.[58]

The simultaneous ingestion of ethyl alcohol and tetraethylthiuram disulfide (Antabuse) may produce an "aldehyde syndrome" consisting of a vasomotor flush of the skin. This reaction occurs because Antabuse arrests the metabolism of ethyl alcohol at the acetaldehyde level, thus preventing the formation of acetic acid or the free acetyl group. The

* At present, there is a governmental ban of DDT from the commercial and agricultural market.

accumulation of acetaldehyde produces the erythematous flush of the skin.

Ingestion of alcohol and exposure to certain industrial chemicals may produce marked flushing of the skin

Antabuse was used medically after the observation was made that industrial workers exposed to this chemical flushed after they ingested alcohol. In industry, exposure to the following chemicals after ingestion of alcohol has produced a similar reaction: trichloroethylene (an organic solvent),[59] n-butyraldoxime (an antioxidant)[60] and dimethyl formamide (an antifreeze agent).[61] Occasionally an erythematous violaceous, nonpruritic macular eruption of the face, neck and upper trunk may also be produced. The conjunctivae may become congested, and nausea and vomiting may occur.

7. *Glycols.* These aliphatic hydrocarbons have become important as solvents, plasticizers and antifreeze compounds. They are mild skin irritants and rarely sensitize. Since they are soluble in water, they may be patch tested in a 10 per cent aqueous solution.

8. *Esters* (*methyl acetate*, *amyl acetate*). These simple aliphatic esters of organic acids have a low order of toxicity and are extremely rare causes of allergic sensitization. They may be applied directly to the skin for patch testing.

9. *Ketones* (*acetone*, *methylethyl ketone*). These aliphatic ketones have an extremely low order of irritancy and sensitizing potential. They are among the safest solvents employed to dissolve resins and other chemicals for patch testing purposes. They may be applied full strength in patch testing.

10. *Dimethyl sulfoxide* (*DMSO*).* This compound is a versatile and powerful solvent that will dissolve most aromatic and unsaturated hydrocarbons and organic nitrogen compounds. It is miscible with most common organic solvents. It probably alters the permeability of the skin to other substances. Recent reports suggest that it may have therapeutic uses in human and veterinary medicine, in relieving pain, edema and associated manifestations of traumatic and rheumatic disorders when applied to the skin.[62,63]

Approximately 85 per cent of patients experience a typical histamine type of reaction, consisting of transient, mild itching, burning and erythema at the site of application of dimethyl sulfoxide. A fine vesiculation is noted occasionally. Drying, mild to moderate wrinkling and scaling of the skin, as after a mild sunburn, is not uncommon after prolonged administration. Some areas of skin, e.g., the face, neck, axillae and scrotum, are the most sensitive to the irritant properties of dimethyl sulfoxide. Individuals with blond, reddish hair also seem to have more severe reactions than do those with darker hair.

A few cases of generalized dermatitis have occurred following the application of dimethyl sulfoxide. A wheal and histamine type of erythematous reaction may occur at sites *distant* from the areas of application. Rarely, this generalized dermatitis may be severe, and in one case it was associated with laryngeal edema.

Dimethyl sulfoxide (DMSO), an industrial solvent, causes a histamine type of reaction at the site of application

Since this compound is a powerful solvent, it damages clothing, particularly synthetic fabrics. It is a solvent for every plastic material, except Teflon. It does not dissolve cotton or wool.

For patch testing purposes, it may be tested full strength by the open method.

The following instructions and information should be given to patients applying dimethyl sulfoxide:

1. This liquid should not come in contact with nylon or other synthetic fabrics or plastics. It will not harm cotton or wool.
2. Do not get the medicine in the eyes.
3. At the site where the medicine is applied, the skin may become red and small

* This compound has been withdrawn from use as a therapeutic agent.

blisters may form that resemble those due to sunburn.

4. Some people have a garlic odor on their breath after the medicine is rubbed onto the skin.

Patch Testing With Organic Solvents. The covered patch test is not ideal for organic solvents, because many of these compounds are highly volatile and may be primary irritants under a closed patch. Many special devices have been employed for patch testing with the organic solvents.[64]

Aside from 25 per cent turpentine in olive oil and the solvents listed as suitable for testing as 50 per cent in olive oil, I prefer the open test method for solvents. A small amount may be gently rubbed into the forearm. Patients should be observed in the office for about an hour, because with certain solvents, such as alcohol, a true allergic reaction may occur and disappear within this period. If no reaction occurs with an hour, the test site should be inspected in 24 hours.

RELATIONSHIP OF OCCUPATIONAL CONTACTANTS TO DRUG ERUPTIONS

Industrial contact can sensitize individuals to chemicals that are either drugs or immunochemically related to systemically administered drugs. External exposure to the drug usually produces a typical eczematous contact dermatitis in the sensitized individual. Subsequent systemic administration of the drug can produce a distinctive systemic eczematous contact type of dermatitis medicamentosa.[65] It resembles the initial contact dermatitis, except that it is usually more widespread, with the most marked reaction at sites of the original eczematous reaction to occupational exposure.

Table 11–4 is a list of industrial chemicals that may sensitize a patient by external contact and the immunochemically related drugs that may produce an eczematous contact type of dermatitis medicamentosa upon systemic administration.

Ethylenediamine, mercury and formaldehyde have been discussed under standard patch test series.

Hydrazine is the parent chemical of isoniazid (INH, Niconyl, Nydrazine, Rimifon), Apresoline hydrochloride and Nardil (phenelzine sulfate), an antidepressant drug.

In industry, hydrazine is used as a flux in printing, as a stain remover and as an anticorrosive in steam boilers.[66]

A nurse who became sensitive to isoniazid during her work in a tuberculosis ward developed a contact eczema. Although she had never been treated with isoniazid, a dose of 100 mg. caused a severe drug eruption.[67]

PESTICIDES

The most popular insecticides include the following classes:

Chlorinated hydrocarbons

- DDT
- Lindane
- Chlordane
- Aldrin
- Benzene hexachloride
- Dieldrin

Test 1 per cent in petrolatum or acetone

Organic phosphates

- Parathion
- Malathion

Test 0.5 per cent in petrolatum by the closed method or 1 per cent in alcohol by the open method

Table 11-4. Industrial Contactants and Related Drugs

Industrial Contactants	*Immunochemically Related Drugs*
Ethylenediamine hydrochloride	Aminophylline
Hydrazine hydrobromide	Isoniazid, Apresoline, Nardil
Organic and inorganic	Mercurial diuretics
Mercurials	Calomel
Metallic mercury	Protiodide of mercury
Formaldehyde	Urotropin, Mandelamine, Urised

Inorganic insecticides

Arsenic
Fluorides
Paradichlorobenzene
Test 1 per cent in petrolatum

Botanical insecticides

Pyrethrum
Rotenone
Benzyl benzoate
Nicotine
Test full strength in the powder form

The carbamates

Ferbam
Zineb
Carbaryl (Sevin)
Test 1 per cent in petrolatum. May cross-react with accelerators

Many of these pesticides are dispensed in solvents that are irritating to the skin. If possible, the pure active ingredient should be obtained for patch tests. Impurities may cause more trouble than the active pesticides.

INSECT REPELLENTS

Active Preparations. The U.S. Department of Agriculture has tested more than 9000 insect repellents and found that n,n′-diethyl-m-toluamide (commonly known as deet) is the best all-purpose repellent. Other effective agents include ethyl hexanediol, dimethyl phthalate, dimethyl carbate and butopyronoxyl (Indalone).

Over 50 repellent preparations are available commercially. Most of them contain either deet (Off and McKesson Mosquitone) or ethyl hexanediol (6-12 Brand and Skeeto-Go). They are available in a variety of forms, including liquid, foam, pressurized spray, stick, cream and wipe-on tissue. Concentrations of the active ingredient vary with both type of formulation and brand. Preparations in which deet is the only repellent contain from less than 5 per cent (in wipe-on tissues) to more than 40 per cent (in liquids).

Factors Affecting Repellent Action. Some compounds are more effective than others against certain insects; for example, Indalone is better than deet in preventing tick bites. The concentration of the active compound can affect both the range of susceptible insects and the duration of effect.

Cronce and Alden[68] reported a case of flea collar dermatitis. An insecticide (2,2-dichlorovinyl dimethyl phosphate and related compounds) in antiflea dog collars caused primary irritant contact dermatitis in 4 patients who handled dogs wearing these collars. This dermatitis probably will occur with increased frequency and could be confused with mild poison ivy dermatitis or with insect bites.

Shell's No-Pest Strip contains the same insecticides as do flea collars.

Deet may produce a bullous reaction resembling a blistering insect eruption.[69]

Naled, a brominated chemical insecticide, may produce an urticarial maculopapular eruption.[70]

Malathion[71] is occasionally a sensitizer.

Pentachlorophenol is used in a Japanese herbicide that was reported as a cause of dermatitis and death.[72]

OCCUPATIONAL URTICARIA

Occupational urticaria is rare.[73] It is almost always caused by inhalation of an allergenic material. Chemicals occasionally cause generalized urticaria by cutaneous contact and subsequent percutaneous absorption. Occupational urticaria has been caused by exposure to castor bean pomace, complex platinum salts, aliphatic polyamines, spices, penicillin, ammonia, sulfur dioxide, formaldehyde, sodium sulfide, aminothiazole and Lindane. Alcohol and acrylic monomer may occasionally produce it.

In addition to diagnostic inhalation tests for generalized urticaria, a patch test has occasionally been used to reproduce the disease. This unusual use of the patch test is questionable because it is difficult to prevent contamination of the air with the test material, and one does not always know whether absorption occurred by inhalation or through the skin.

Some cases of urticaria now known to be caused by occupational allergens were originally misdiagnosed as psychogenic. Only by suspecting unusual occupational causes, can one correctly diagnose the disease.

PREVENTION OF OCCUPATIONAL DERMATITIS

The ideal individual who has to work with irritants and sensitizers should be nonatopic, free of hyperhidrosis, seborrhea or ichthyosis, and normally pigmented. As Rajka[74] pointed out, for practical and economic reasons such selection is not always feasible.

Birmingham[75] stated that the key to effective prevention is the elimination of skin contact with irritant and sensitizing substances.

Skin Cleansing. It is necessary to provide facilities for cleanliness and to educate and supervise to see that washing is done correctly. Unusual cleaning problems may require special training for employees. Posters such as those available from the Soap and Detergent Association, 295 Madison Avenue, New York, N.Y. 10017, help promote personal hygiene.

In most medium and small industrial plants, protection against skin irritants is heavily dependent upon personal cleanliness. Protective clothing, gloves, sleeves, aprons, boots and face masks are useful and sometimes indispensable, but the time-tested habit of skin cleansing has no substitute.

Barrier Creams. When workmen cannot wear gloves, barrier creams may be beneficial. They also protect the face and neck against chemical and resinous dusts and vapors. To provide worthwhile benefit, however, they should be applied on clean skin at least 3 times each day. In general, barrier creams help protect against irritants, but they do not successfully prevent allergic reactions.

Bjornberg[76] claimed that a plastic film of acrylic polymer protects against potassium hydroxide, phenol, detergents, acids and alcohol. Protection against allergic reaction was shown in patch tests with chromium and plants. Since this is a self-curing acrylic resin, however, sensitization to acrylic may take place.

Birmingham[75] stated that protective barrier creams, industrial cleansers and protective clothing may be obtained from the following sources:

Protective Barrier Creams

Ayerst Laboratories, 685 Third Avenue, New York, N.Y.
Mine Safety Appliances Co., Pittsburgh, Pa.
G. H. Packwood Manufacturing Co., St. Louis, Mo.
West Chemical Products, Inc., Long Island City, N.Y.

Industrial Cleansers

Dameron Enterprises, Inc., Louisville, Ky.
Hammons Products, Inc., Fort Wayne, Ind.
Magnus Chemical Co., Garwood, N.J.
G. H. Packwood Manufacturing Co., St. Louis, Mo.
Sugar Beet Products Co., Saginaw, Mich.
U.S. Borax and Chemical Corp., Los Angeles, Calif.
West Chemical Products, Inc., Long Island City, N.Y.

Protective Clothing Manufacturers

American Optical Co., Southbridge, Mass.
Edmont Manufacturing Co., Coshocton, Ohio
Mine Safety Appliances Co., Pittsburgh, Pa.
Pioneer Rubber Co., Willard, Ohio
Safety Clothing and Equipment Co., Cleveland, Ohio
Standard Safety Equipment Co., Chicago, Ill.
Surety Rubber Co., Carrollton, Ohio
U.S. Safety Service Co., Kansas City, Kan.
West Chemical Products, Inc., Long Island City, N.Y.
Wilson Rubber Co., Division of Bard-Parker Co., Inc., Canton, Ohio

REFERENCES

1. Malten, K. E., et al.: Occupational Dermatitis in 5 European Dermatologic Departments. Berufsdermatosen, *19*, 1, 1971.
2. Jordan, W. B.: Contact Dermatitis from N-Isopropyl-N-PPDA. Arch. Derm., *103*, 85, 1971.
3. Vollum, D. I., and Marten, R. H.: Contact Dermatitis from N-Isopropyl-Amino-Diphenylamine. Trans. St. John Hosp. Derm. Soc., *54*, 73, 1968.
4. Batschvarov, B., and Minkov, D. M.: Dermatitis and Purpura from Rubber Clothing. Trans. St. John Hosp. Derm. Soc., *54*, 178, 1968.
5. Bieber, P., and Foussereau, J.: Role de Deus Amines Aromatiques Dans L'Allergie au Caoutchouc: PBM et 4010 NA, Amines Anti-oxydantes Dans L'Industrie du Pneu. Bull. Soc. Franc. Derm. Syph., *75*, 63, 1968.
6. Munn, A.: Health Hazards in the Chemical Industry. Trans. Soc. Occup. Med., *17*, 8, 1967.

7. U.S. Rubber Company, Medical Department, personal communication.
8. Schonning, L., and Hjorth, N.: Cross Sensitization Between Hair Dyes and Rubber Chemicals. Berufsdermatosen, *17*, 100, 1969.
9. Birmingham, D. J.: New Causes of Occupational Dermatoses. A.M.A. Industr. Health, *20*, 490, 1959.
10. Klauder, J. F.: Actual Causes of Certain Occupational Dermatoses. Arch. Derm., *85*, 441, 1962.
11. Key, M. M., Perove, V. B., and Birmingham, D. J.: Patch Testing in Dermatitis from the Newer Resins. J. Occup. Med., *3*, 361, 1961.
12. Fisher, A. A.: Patch Testing in Industry. Industr. Med. Surg., *36*, 672, 1967.

Epoxy

13. Bourne, L. B., Milner, F. J. M., and Alberman, K. B.: Health Problems of Epoxy Resins and Amine-Curing Agents. Brit. J. Industr. Med., *16*, 81, 1959.
14. Carpenter, C. L., Jr., and Jolly, H. W., Jr.: Contact Dermatitis and Epoxy Resins. J. Louisiana Med. Soc., *117*, 31, 1965.
15. Birmingham, D. J.: Clinical Observations on the Cutaneous Effects Associated with Curing Epoxy Resins. Arch. Industr. Health., *19*, 365, 1959.
16. Tepper, L. B.: Hazards to Health. Epoxy Resins. New Engl. J. Med., *267*, 821, 1962.
17. Gaul, L. E.: Sensitivity to Bisphenol A. Arch. Derm., *82*, 1003, 1960.
18. Fregert, S., and Rorsman, H.: Hypersensitivity to Epoxy Resins with Reference to the Role Played by Bisphenol A. J. Invest. Derm., *39*, 471, 1962.
19. Fregert, S., and Rorsman, H.: Hypersensitivity to Diethylstilbestrol: Cross-Sensitization to Dinestrol, Hexestrol, Bisphenol A, p-Benzyl-Phenol, Hydroquinone-Monobenzylether, and p-Hydroxybenzoic-Benzylester. Acta Dermatovener., *40*, 206, 1960.
20. Fregert, S., and Rorsman, H.: Allergy to a Carbon-Functional Organic Silicon Compound. Dimethyldi-(4-Hydroxy-Phenyl)-Silane. Nature, *192*, 989, 1961.
21. Morris, G. E.: Dermatological Hazards from Epoxy Resins. Clin. Med., *5*, 1219, 1958.
22. Gaul, L. E.: Epoxy Dermatitis from Installing Cathodic Protection. Arch. Derm., *86*, 77, 1962.
23. Fregert, S., and Rorsman, H.: Hypersensitivity to Epoxy Resins Used as Plasticizers and Stabilizers in Polyvinyl Chloride (PVC) Resins. Acta Dermatovener., *43*, 10, 1963.
24. Fregert, S., and Rorsman, H.: Allergens in Epoxy Resins. Acta Allerg., *19*, 296, 1964.

Polyester

25. Harris, D. K.: The Skin Effects of Plastics. Brit. J. Derm., *72*, 105, 1960.
26. Wilson, R. H., and McCormick, W. E.: Plastics: The Toxicology of Synthetic Resins. Arch. Industr. Health, *21*, 536, 1960.
27. Key, M. M., and Discher, D. P.: Polyester Resins—Their Dermatologic Aspects in Industry. Cutis, *2*, 27, 1966.

Benzoyl Peroxide

28. Poole, R. L., Griffith, J. F., and Kilmer MacMillan, F. S.: Experimental Contact Sensitization with Benzoyl Peroxide. Arch. Derm., *102*, 400, 1970.
29. Pace, W. E.: A Benzoyl Peroxide–Sulfur Cream for Acne Vulgaris. Canad. Med. Assoc. J., *93*, 252, 1965.
30. Vasarinsh, P.: Benzoyl Peroxide–Sulfur Lotion: A Histological Study. Arch. Derm., *98*, 183, 1968.
31. Eaglstein, W. H.: Allergic Contact Dermatitis to Benzoyl Peroxide. Arch. Derm., *97*, 527, 1968.

Polyurethanes

32. Simmons, L. F.: *Isocyanate Resins in Modern Plastics*. Bristol, Conn., Breskin Publications, Inc., 1960.
33. Munn, A.: Experiences with Diisocyanates. Trans. Assoc. Industr. Med. Officers, *9*, 134, 1960.
34. Zapp, J. A.: Diisocyanates: Toxicology. A.M.A. Arch. Industr. Health, *19*, 350, 1959.
35. Zapp, J. A.: Hazards of Isocyanates in Polyurethane Foam Plastic Production. A.M.A. Arch. Industr. Health, *15*, 324, 1957.
36. Strayer, S. C.: Safe Use and Safe Handling of Organic Isocyanates. Arch. Industr. Health, *19*, 351, 1959.

Formaldehyde Resins

37. Gaul, L. E.: Absence of Formaldehyde Sensitivity in Phenol Formaldehyde Resin Dermatitis. J. Invest. Derm., *48*, 485, 1967.
38. Malten, K. E., and VanAerssen, R. G. L.: Contact Eczema in Shoemakers and Shoe Wearers Due to Glue Substances. Berufsdermatosen, *10*, 264, 1962.
39. Engle, H. O., and Calnan, C. D.: Resin Dermatitis in a Car Factory. Brit. J. Industr. Med., *23*, 62, 1966.

40. Malten, K. E., et al.: Occupational Vitiligo due to Paratertiary Butylphenol and Homologues. Trans. St. John Hosp. Derm. Soc., *57*, 115, 1971.

Fiberglass

41. Heisel, E. B., and Hunt, F. E.: Further Studies in Cutaneous Reactions to Fiber Glass. Arch. Environ. Health, *17*, 705, 1968.
42. Possick, P. A., Gellin, G. A., and Key, M. M.: Fibrous Glass Dermatitis. Amer. Industr. Hyg. Assoc. J., *31*, 12, 1970.
43. Fisher, B. K., and Warkentin, J. D.: Fiber Glass Dermatitis. Arch. Derm., *99*, 717, 1969.
44. Elby, C. S., and Jetton, R. L.: School Desk Dermatitis. Arch. Derm., *105*, 890, 1972.

Acrylic

45. Magnuson, B., and Mobacken, H.: Allergic Contact Dermatitis from Printing Plates in a Printing Place. Berufsdermatosen, *20*, 138, 1972.

Cellulose Plastics

46. Jordan, W. P., and Dahl, M. V.: Contact Dermatitis from Cellulose Ester Plastics. Arch. Derm., *105*, 880, 1972.

Benzophenone

47. Ramsay, D. L., Cohen, H. J., and Baer, R. L.: Allergic Reaction to Benzophenone. Arch. Derm., *105*, 906, 1972.

Aluminum Flux

48. Crow, K. D., Harman, R., and Hodern, H.: Amine Flux Sensitization Dermatitis in Electricity Cable Joiners. Brit. J. Derm., *80*, 701, 1971.
49. Lane, R. E.: Aluminum Flux Dermatitis. Brit. J. Derm., *81*, 310, 1969.

9-Bromofluorene

50. DeFeo, C. P., Jr.: Erythema Multiforme Bullosum Caused by 9-Bromofluorene. Arch. Derm., *94*, 545, 1966.
51. Keller, F.: Dermatitis Danger from 9-Bromofluorene. Chem. Engin. News, *45*, 8, 1967.
52. Powell, E. W.: Skin Reaction to 9-Bromofluorene. Brit. J. Derm., *80*, 491, 1968.

Ethylene Oxide

53. Hanfin, J. M.: Ethylene Oxide Dermatitis. Letter to the Editor. J.A.M.A., *217*, 213, 1971.

54. La Dage, L. H.: Facial "Irritation" from Ethylene Oxide Sterilization of Anesthesia Face Mask. Plast. Reconstr. Surg., *45*, 179, 1970.

Dinitrochlorbenzene

55. Adams, R. M., et al.: 1-Chloro-2-4-Dinitrobenzene as an Algicide. Report of Four Cases of Contact Dermatitis. Arch. Derm., *103*, 191, 1971.

Solvents

56. Pirila, V.: On the Primary Irritant and Sensitizing Effects of Organic Solvents. Proc. XII Int. Cong. Derm., 1962, p. 463.
57. Fregert, S., et al.: Dermatitis from Alcohols. J. Allergy, *34*, 404, 1963.
58. Drevets, C. C., and Seebohm, P. M.: Dermatitis from Alcohols. J. Allergy, *32*, 277, 1961.
59. Bradodej, Z., and Vyskocil, J.: The Problem of Trichloroethylene in Occupational Medicine. Arch. Industr. Health, *13*, 581, 1956.
60. Lewis, W., and Schwartz, L.: An Occupational Agent (N-Butyraldoxime) Causing Reaction to Alcohol. Med. Ann. D. C., *25*, 485, 1956.
61. U.S. Public Health Service: *Occupational Diseases: A Guide to Their Recognition.* Publication No. 1097. Washington, D.C., Government Printing Office, 1964.
62. Rosenbaum, E. E., and Jacob, S. W.: Dimethyl Sulfoxide (DMSO) in Acute Musculo-skeletal Injuries and Inflammations. I. Dimethyl Sulfoxide in Acute Subdeltoid Bursitis. Northwest Med., *66*, 167, 1964.
63. Feinman, H., Ben, M., and Lenin, R.: The Toxicology of Dimethyl Sulfoxide (DMSO) in Primates. Pharmacologist, *6*, 188, 1964.
64. Blohm, S. G.: A New Technique for Epicutaneous Testing. Acta Dermatovener., *40*, 46, 1960.

Drug Eruption and Occupational Contactants

65. Fisher, A. A.: Relationship of Occupational Contactant to Drug Eruptions. J. Med. Soc. New Jersey, *65*, 493, 1968.
66. Hovding, G.: Occupational Dermatitis from Hydrazine Hydrate Used in Boiler Protection. Acta Dermatovener., *47*, 293, 1967.
67. Herman, W. P., Lischka, G., and Luckerath, L.: Contact Dermatitis and Drug Eruption in Occupational Hypersensitivity to Isonicotinic Acid Hydrazide. Berufsdermatosen, *17*, 13, 1969.

Insecticides

68. Cronce, P. C., and Alden, H. S.: Flea Collar Dermatitis. J.A.M.A., *206*, 1563, 1968.
69. Lamberg, S., and Mulrennan, J. A.: Deet Bullous Eruption Resembling a Blistering Insect Eruption. Arch. Derm., *100*, 582, 1969.
70. Edmundson, W. F., and Davies, J. E.: Occupational Dermatitis from Naled. Arch. Environ. Health, *15*, 89, 1967.
71. Milby, T. H., and Epstein, W. L.: Allergic Contact Sensitivity to Malathion. Arch. Environ. Health, *9*, 434, 1964.
72. Watanabe, S.: Contact Dermatitis Due to the Herbicides PCP and MCPB. Japanese J. Clin. Derm., *24*, 945, 1970.
73. Key, M. M.: Some Unusual Allergic Reactions in Industry. Arch. Derm., *83*, 57, 1961.
74. Rajka, G.: Occupational Choice for Persons with Common Chronic Dermatoses and Pathological Skin Functions. Acta Dermatovener., *47*, 15, 1967.
75. Birmingham, D. J.: Prevention of Occupational Skin Disease. Cutis, *5*, 153, 1969.
76. Bjornberg, A.: Plastic Film as Protection Against Primary Irritants. Acta Dermatovener., *50*, 233, 1970.

12

Contact Photodermatitis*†

Contact photodermatitis, especially the photoallergic variety, is being detected with increasing frequency in the United States and abroad, particularly in Europe and Australia. In recent years, the addition of antibacterial agents to soaps, cleansers and medicated topical preparations has greatly increased the number and severity of cases.[1] There are so many potential photosensitizers in the average household that reports of several thousand cases have been accumulated.[2]

Several thousand cases of photoallergic dermatitis have been reported, some of which have been severe, prolonged and disabling. The relatively recent addition of antibacterial agents to soaps and topical medications has greatly increased the problems of photosensitivity

The chemicals that produce photodermatic reactions are unique in that they produce a contact dermatitis only in the presence of light. Direct sunlight is the usual light source, but diffuse daylight or artificial light may also elicit a photosensitivity reaction.[3]

* This chapter was written in collaboration with Leonard C. Harber, M.D., Professor of Dermatology and Syphilology, New York University School of Medicine.

† This study was supported in part by Grant No. ES00288–07 from the National Institutes of Environmental Health Sciences, National Institutes of Health.

Two broad categories of contact photosensitivity reactions are phototoxic and photoallergic contact dermatitis. It may be difficult to distinguish clinically between them, and indeed, phototoxic substances may also produce photoallergic reactions. Tables 12–1 to 12–4 are lists of chemicals that can produce photocontact dermatitis.

Many hotels and motels supply their guests with so-called *deodorant* antibacterial soaps. Thus many individuals are inadvertently exposed to these photosensitizers even though they do not purchase or request such soaps. Therefore, it is imperative in a suspected case of photodermatitis to inquire whether the patient has recently used soaps supplied by hotels or motels.

The managers of most hotels and motels are not aware that they are providing soaps with potentially dangerous chemicals.

Many individuals are "captive" consumers of photosensitizing soaps which many hotels and motels provide for their guests

Clinical Features of Photodermatitis. Exposed areas, such as the face, V of the neck, back of the hands, uncovered upper extremities and, in women, anterior aspects of the legs, are most frequently the sites of contact photodermatitis. Any skin area receiving sufficient light and photosensitizing chemical, however, may manifest a reaction. The

Table 12-1. Contact Photosensitizers—Antibacterial and Antifungal Agents, Including Halogenated Salicylanilides, Carbanilides and Phenols

Photosensitizer	*Where Encountered**	*Comment*
Dibromosalicylanilide (DBS)	*Old* Lifebuoy, Praise	All of these agents can produce photoallergic reactions. Test 1% in white petrolatum. May be found in deodorant bar soaps, cosmetics, detergents and industrial chemicals
Tribromosalicyanilide (TBS)	Praise, Lifebuoy, Safeguard, Zest	
Tetrachlorosalicylanilide (TCSA, Impregnon)	No longer used in American soaps	
Bithionol	Old soaps and cosmetics. Now off the American market	
Hexachlorophene†	Soaps, detergents, cosmetics, pharmaceuticals†	
Trichlorocarbanilide (TCC)	Zest, Dial, Safeguard	
Multifungin	Australian antimycotic agent	Cross-reacts with TBS
Fenticlor	Australian antimycotic agent	Cross-reacts with bithionol and hexachlorophene
Jadit (buclosamide)	European and Australian antifungal agent	Photoallergic. May cross-react with sulfanilamide

* Most of the severe offenders have been removed from the market, but many remain in possession of consumers.
† The general use of hexachlorophene has been restricted by the FDA.

Table 12-2. Contact Photosensitizers—Plant Substances

Photosensitizer	*Where Encountered*	*Comment*
Furocoumarin (Psoralens)	Cosmetics containing plant extracts, essential oils, colognes, lime, bergamot and sandalwood oil. Direct contact with fennel, parsnip, carrots, angelica, dill, parsley, celery (especially infested with pink rot), atrillal, rue, fig, buttercup, mustard, blind weed, agrimony, yarrow, goose foot, bavachi and St. John's wort	Includes phytophotodermatitis, Berloque dermatitis and meadow grass dermatitis
Methoxysporalen	Trisoralen (Elder) used as a therapeutic agent for vitiligo	
Ragweed(?)	Air-borne pollen and plant	Produces mostly ordinary allergic contact dermatitis, but also possibly a phototoxic reaction from a type of furocoumarin

Table 12-3. Contact Photosensitizers—Therapeutic Agents

Photosensitizer	*Where Encountered*	*Comment*
Chlorpromazine (Thorazine)	Handled by medical and nursing professionals	Photoallergic and phototoxic. Test 1% in white petrolatum
Promethazine (Phenergan)	Topical antihistamine Phenergan cream	Photoallergic
Phenothiazine	Veterinary anthelmintic and commercial insecticide	Photoallergic
Sulfanilamide	Topical antibiotic still used abroad but not in the United States	Photoallergic
Coal tar	Antipsoriatics, cosmetics and hair preparations	Phototoxic and Photoallergic
Fluorouracil	Agent for treatment of actinic keratosis	Phototoxic (?) Affects sun-damaged skin
Chloro-mercapto-dicarboximide (Dangard Shampoo and Vanicide 84)	Sold exclusively by barbers as antiseborrheic shampoo	Photoallergic. Test 0.25% in white petrolatum

Table 12-4. Contact Photosensitizers—Miscellaneous

Photosensitizer	*Where Encountered*	*Comment*
Pitch and petroleum products	Preservative for wood. Industrial use. Contains tar residues	Phototoxic. May produce an intense burning erythema, "smarts" and tar melanosis
Fluorochromes: fluoroscein, eosin and rose bengal	Lipstick and other dyes, and chemical stains. Eosin used in disclosing tablets or solutions to identify dental plaque	Phototoxic
Cadmium sulfide	Yellow tattoo pigment	Phototoxic. May produce papular or nodular swelling in tattoos
Stilbenes (Blankophores)	Textiles, soap, detergents, cosmetics an "whiter than white" preparation	Photoallergic

scalp, and other densely hairy areas, the upper eyelids and the skin immediately under the chin are rarely involved.

When lesions are present on the forearms, the extensor and radial aspects are almost always the most extensively involved. The cubital fossae are frequently spared. There may be sharply demarcated areas of involvement below sleeves. Photodermatitis from sunlight exposure while driving an automobile with a left-hand drive affects the left side of the face and the uncovered left arm and forearm most severely; the right side of the body is most severely involved while driving a foreign car with a right-hand drive. Often such photodermatitis remains unilateral.

Photosensitivity reactions often resemble sunburn and invariably are limited to areas exposed to light. Many types of reaction patterns, however, can occur. The eruption may be eczematous, bullous or fissured, resemble lichen planus or mimic lupus erythematosus. Photodermatitis may disappear promptly when the photocontactant is avoided. Rarely the eruption is persistent. Dermatitis that is limited to, or occurs predominantly on, areas exposed to light should be investigated for the possibility of being a photosensitivity reaction. Dermatitis due to air-borne contactants can closely simulate a photodermatitis.

Air-borne contact dermatitis may closely mimic photodermatitis. Sparing of the skin folds of the neck, the retroauricular, nasolabial and submental areas favors a diagnosis of photodermatitis

PHOTOTOXIC CONTACT DERMATITIS

Phototoxic contact dermatitis occurs in a large percentage of the population upon first exposure and under appropriate conditions, such as sufficient intensity of light and quantity of photosensitizing chemicals. Phototoxic reactions are based on nonimmunologic mechanisms and are often manifested clinically as exaggerated sunburn reactions followed by pigmentation. Occasionally bullae occur on the erythematous areas.

Each compound causing a photocontact dermatitis will absorb only a specific wavelength of light, which is determined by its chemical structure. This wavelength closely corresponds to the absorption peak of the chemical, and because it is usually also the wavelength responsible for the clinical reaction, it is referred to as the action spectrum. Most phototoxic sensitizers have an action spectrum in the ultraviolet band between 2800 and 4300 Å.[3]

Window glass, which usually absorbs most of the ultraviolet, will protect patients from most phototoxic reactions having an action spectrum below 3200 Å, but it does not protect against higher action spectrum photosensitizers, such as tar and the psoralens. The psoralen (furocoumarin) derivatives and certain tars produce most cases of contact phototoxic dermatitis.

Phytophotodermatitis is a plant solar dermatitis produced on skin exposed to plant psoralens (furocoumarins) in the presence of sunlight. Such a dermatitis is followed by marked hyperpigmentation and may occur more readily on wet skin

Phytophotodermatitis Due to Furocoumarins in Plants

When the phototoxic chemical is contacted by exposure to a plant, vegetable or fruit, the resulting photodermatitis is referred to as a phytophotodermatitis. It has long been known that photosensitization dermatitis with residual pigmentation develops in skin that has come into contact with members of the Umbelliferae botanical grouping, such as figs, cow parsnip, wild parsnip, wild carrot, fennel, caraway, anise, coriander, angelica, parsley, parsnip and gas plant.[4] Phytophotodermatitis has also been described in individuals exposed to the oil of Persian limes and in carrot processors and celery pickers.[5] Such phytophotodermatitis, as well as that which follows contact with plants of other species, is probably caused mainly by furocoumarin compounds, which are characteristically present in these plants. These phototoxic substances are lipid-soluble and penetrate into the epidermis with ease. Whether the human skin can be photosensitized by ingestion of furocoumarin-containing foods has not yet been established.

There are two requisites for the initiation of phytophotodermatitis: (1) contact with a sensitizing furocoumarin, and (2) subsequent exposure to ultraviolet radiation of wavelengths greater than 3200 Å (usually sunlight). High humidity increases percutaneous absorption of the psoralens and thus accentuates their phototoxic action.[6,7]

Some of the more potent psoralens have been extracted from plant materials and purified for clinical therapeutic use. Oral administration and topical application have been employed for vitiligo, the leukodermas and other conditions in which potentiation of sunburn, erythema and pigmentation is desired.

The clinical features of psoralen photodermatitis depends upon the intensity of light exposure and the nature of the psoralens. The skin changes range from mild erythema to large bullae with marked hyperpigmentation.

A bullous plant photodermatitis is often mistaken for a poison ivy eruption or bullous reactions from blister beetles or insect bites

Certain clinical manifestations of phytophotodermatitis have been given specific names such as berloque dermatitis and meadow grass dermatitis. Berloque dermatitis is produced at sites exposed to a combination of certain perfumes and sunlight. The streaky erythema of the eruption is followed by pigmentation. Oil of bergamot, containing bergapten (5-methoxy-psoralen), is probably the principal cause of photodermatitis produced by perfumes, such as Shalimar, and toilet waters.[8] The phototoxic action of Shalimar is enhanced by stripped or denuded skin.[9]

Meadow grass dermatitis (dermatitis bullosa striata pratensis), another example of phytophotodermatitis, is produced by contact of the skin with meadow grass and subsequent exposure to sunlight. The eruption is a phototoxic reaction characterized by bizarre, criss-cross linear streaks of erythema and vesicles or bullae, which heal with hyperpigmentation. The photosensitizing agent is not grass, but either the yellow-flowered wild meadow parsnip, which belongs to the carrot family (agrimony) or a common wild yellow-flowered herb of the rose family. The skin of individuals who sunbathe on the meadows may become impregnated with the juices of these weeds or wild flowers containing furocoumarins. Subsequent exposure to sunlight produces the phototoxic dermatitis.

Occasionally, the bites of chiggers or other arthropods infesting grass may produce a pseudo-phytophotodermatitis that may be confused with meadow grass dermatitis. Itching is more intense and pigmentation is less marked in dermatitis produced by arthropods than in meadow grass dermatitis.

The phototoxic contact dermatitis produced by oil of the rind of the Persian lime is another example of phytophotodermatitis. Erythema and pigmentation may occur on the hands of individuals, such as bartenders, exposed to a combination of lime oil and sunshine.

Phototoxic Tar Dermatitis

Coal tar derivatives are among the most commonly encountered photosensitizers. At least 300 compounds have been isolated from coal tar, many of which are used in diverse industries, including the manufacture of drugs, dyes, perfumes, synthetic resins, explosives, insecticides and disinfectants. The known active photosensitizers of coal tar are acridine, anthracene, phenanthrene and pyridene. Wood tars are not photosensitizers and do not contain any of these photosensitizing chemicals. The action spectrum for coal tar contact photosensitivity is in the 3500 to 4000 Å range.

Photodermatitis due to tar may appear as a severe sunburn referred to as "flashes" and "smarts" in workers exposed to tar, pitch or creosote and sunlight. Actual contact with pitch or creosote is not necessary for the production of a photosensitive reaction, since the volatile fumes emanating from these products in the presence of sunlight can produce a photodermatitis. Moderate to marked pigmentation may occur at the sites of tar photodermatitis. The ability of coal tar derivatives to photosensitize the skin is sometimes used as a therapeutic measure in the treatment of psoriasis.

Contact with coal tar or with volatile derivatives, such as pitch or creosote, may produce a photocontact dermatitis and "smarting"

Photodermatitis due to tar and pitch may be accompanied by an intense burning sensation of the skin and conjunctiva. In sensitive individuals, bright, diffuse daylight can also produce smarting. In one series, 70 per cent of white workers exposed to pitch fumes were affected, while Negro workers were not affected.[10] The increased pigmentation of the skin of Negro and Indian workers proved to be a protection against pitch photosensitivity. Smarting and erythema may continue 1 to 3 days after exposure to pitch fumes has been avoided. There may be a latent period of 2 weeks or more between the initial exposure to pitch fumes and the appearance of photosensitivity.

PHOTOALLERGIC CONTACT DERMATITIS

Photoallergic contact dermatitis is a form of delayed allergic hypersensitivity reaction due to a specifically altered state. The concentration of a drug needed to elicit a photoallergic reaction is much lower than that needed to produce a phototoxic reaction. Some photoallergens can also produce ordinary allergic contact dermatitis in the absence of light. As in allergic eczematous contact dermatitis, cross-reactivity may be seen in drug-induced photoallergy. For example, cross-photosensitization between chlorpromazine (Thorazine) and promethazine (Phenergan) may occur.

Although photoallergic contact dermatitis has been shown to be immunologic through the use of passive transfer, lymphocytic stimulation test and macrophage inhibition, it may be difficult to distinguish *clinically* between a phototoxic and a photoallergic reaction. The criteria in Table 12–5 may be helpful in distinguishing between the two types.

Photoallergic Contact Dermatitis Due to Soap Antiseptics

Most of the photosensitizing antiseptics contain halogenated salicylanilides and related compounds, which are some of the most important causes of allergic photodermatitis. Because of changing policies of manufacturers and Food and Drug Administration rulings, it is difficult to give an accurate compilation of preparations that are used as antiseptics and have caused these photoallergic reactions.

Tetrachlorosalicylanilide (*TCSA; Impregnon*). This antiseptic is not now in use in the United States. In Great Britain many instances of photodermatitis have been reported from exposure to soap containing it.[11,12] In a small U.S. test market of a product containing 0.5 per cent tetrachorosalicylanilide, several instances of photosensitization were reported and verified by patch tests.[13] The individuals developed intense itching and erythema in areas exposed to the sun. In some instances, papules and vesicles also appeared.

Tetrachlorosalicylanilide, formerly present in Coleo soap, has been replaced by hexachlorophene, but photoallergic dermatitis from the old Coleo soap is still being reported. The agent TCSA can produce both allergic contact dermatitis and photoallergic contact dermatitis.[14]

Present statutes do not require that all agents incorporated into a non-drug or cosmetic preparation be identified on the package. Some unlisted ingredients may be photosensitizers

Tribromosalicylanilide (*TBS*). This antiseptic, a currently favorite deodorant agent in many soaps and detergents has produced allergic photocontact dermatitis from its presence in Lifebuoy, Safeguard and Praise soaps.

Table 12-5. Comparison of Phototoxic and Photoallergic Reactions*

Reaction	*Phototoxic*	*Photoallergic*
Incidence	Relatively high (theoretically 100%)	Low (but could theoretically reach 100%)
Reaction possible on first exposure	Yes	No
Incubation period necessary after first exposure	No	Yes
Length of incubation period	Often 6 hours after first exposure	5 to 21 days
Chemical alteration of photosensitizers	No	Yes
Clinical changes	Exaggerated sunburn. Sometimes blisters. Pigmentation may be marked	Varied morphology. Usually very little pigmentation
Clinical symptoms	Often burning and smarting. Usually little itching	Itching common and may be severe
"Flares" at distant previously involved sites possible	No	Yes
Recurrence from exposure to ultraviolet alone	No	Sometimes in persistent light reactors
Can persistent light reaction develop?	No	Rarely
Cross-reactions to structurally related agents	Possible	Frequent
Broadening of cross-reactions following repeated photopatch testing	No	Possible
Concentration of drug necessary for reaction	High	Low
Action spectrum	Usually similar to absorption spectrum	Usually higher wavelength than absorption spectrum
Passive transfer	No	Possible
Macrophage inhibition	No	Possible
Lymphocyte stimulation test	No	Possible
Histopathology	Predominantly epidermal	Allergic inflammatory reaction in epidermis or cutis

* From Baer, R. L., and Harber, L. D.: Reactions to Light, Heat, and Trauma. In Samter's *Immunologic Diseases*. (Ed. 2). Boston, Little, Brown and Co., 1971, p. 974.

Table 12-6. Old Stock Preparations Containing Bithionol*

Preparations	*Manufacturer*
Absorbene Medicated Soap	W. F. Young
Acne-Dome Cream	Dome Chemicals
Acne-Dome Medicated Cleanser	Dome Chemicals
Acne Ointment	Vabert
Acnemed Cream	Vitaring
All Clear Medicated Astringent	DuBarry
All Clear Medicated Face Wash	DuBarry
Banish Shampoo	Breck
Bio-Cleanser	Helena Rubinstein
Bio-Shampoo	Helena Rubinstein
Clearasil Soap	Vick Chemical
Enden Cream Shampoo	Helena Curtis
First Aid Cream	Johnson & Johnson
Lip-Eze	Chap Stick
Medicated compressed powder	DuBarry
Medicated make-up	DuBarry
Medicated Make-up	Rexall
Medicated Scrub Soap	Dorothy Gray
Medicated soap	Helena Rubinstein
Nozane	Noxzema
Palmer's Skin-Success Soap	E. T. Browne Drug Co.
Polytar Shampoo	Stiefel Laboratories
Sebb Shampoo	Max Factor
Sulfur 8 Hair and Scalp Conditioner	Pharmaco
Thylox Medicated Soap	Colfax Laboratories, Division of Shulton
Velveteen Shampoo	Dorothy Gray

* Modified from O'Quinn et al.[24]

Dibromsalan (*DBS; 4,5-dibromosalicylanilide* [*DBS*]). This chemical, which was present in Lifebuoy soap, has caused photoallergic contact dermatitis.

Trichlorocarbanilide (*TCC*). This agent, present in Dial, Zest and Safeguard soaps, is a potent photosensitizer.[15]

There are numerous reports in the literature that these halogenated salicylanilides and related chemicals are producing photodermatitis.[15–20]

Bithionol (*Bisphenol,* Actamar*). Bithionol, 2,2′-thiobis(4,6-dichlorophenol) is a bacteriostatic agent related to hexachlorophene. It can produce both ordinary and photoallergic dermatitis.[21–23] Bithionol often shows cross-reactions not only to hexachlorophene but also to the halogenated salicylanilides.

* **Bithionol (Bisphenol) should not be confused with Bisphenol A, which is an epoxy resin component.**

So many instances of photosensitivity occurred from bithionol that Food and Drug Administration regulations now forbid its use. Nevertheless, severe photosensitivity is still being produced from old stock preparations that are still being sold. Table 12–6 is a list of topical medications that originally contained bithionol and still occasionally produce reactions.[24]

Recent FDA regulations have prevented the incorporation of bithionol into new products, but numerous old preparations are still being sold and producing severe photodermatitis

Patients who have applied bithionol preparations may become sensitized not only to ultraviolet light, but also to the visible rays, including that which is transmitted through glass and that which emanates from fluorescent light tubes. The photosensitivity is not necessarily confined to the areas to which bithionol was applied; it may occur over widespread areas and the sensitized individual may become a persistent light reactor.[25]

Hexachlorophene. This widely used halogenated phenol antiseptic very rarely produces ordinary contact allergy. Cross-contact sensitivity and photocontact sensitivity to hexachlorophene have been observed in guinea pigs with primary photosensitivity to tetrachlorosalicylanilide and tribromosalicylanilide.[1] It is not yet certain whether hexachlorophene is a primary photosensitizer, although such photosensitivity has been reported.[17]

Cross-Reaction Between Bithionol, Hexachlorophene and the Halogenated Salicylanilides. Cross-reaction may occur with tetrachlorosalicylanilide and tribromosalicylanilide, and bithionol is apparently a primary photosensitizer engendering cross-sensitivity to both. Reactions to hexachlorophene in patients with contact photodermatitis from bithionol not requiring any light represent cross-sensitivity between a photosensitizer and a simple contact allergen.

Fenticlor (bis[2-hydroxy-5-chlorophenyl]sulfide) and *Multifungin* (5-bromo-4-chlorosalicylanilde). These topical antifungal agents, used in Australia, are photoallergens. Fenticlor, chemically related to bithionol, also cross-reacts with hexachlorophene. Multifungin is chemically related to tribromosalicylanilide with which it cross-reacts.[26,27]

Jadit (chlorosalicylamide). This antifungal agent with the formula 4-chlorohydroxybenzoic acid-n-butilamide, employed in Australia and Europe, can cause a photoallergic reaction that may be persistent.[28] The photosensitizing action is probably related to that of the halogenated salicylanilides.

The halogenated salicylanilides and related chemicals used as antiseptics in deodorant soaps and cosmetics are the causative agents in most patients with allergic contact photodermatitis

Photoallergic Reactions From Phenothiazine and Its Derivatives

Phenothiazine is employed as an insecticide and as an anthelmintic in human and veterinary medicine. It is a parent substance for methylene blue, a dye that is a powerful photosensitizer.[29]

Orchard workers employing phenothiazine as an insecticide against moths exhibited photosensitivity. Since many individuals were involved, it was presumed that the reaction was one of phototoxicity rather than photoallergy.

Chlorpromazine (Thorazine). Allergic photocontact dermatitis occurs principally among medical and nursing personnel who contaminate their hands while injecting the drug.[30,31] Those receiving the drug systemically may acquire a phototoxic dermatitis.

Phenothiazine and its derivatives Thorazine and Phenergan produce allergic contact dermatitis (without light) and photocontact dermatitis

Promethazine hydrochloride (Phenergan). This antihistamine can also produce phototoxic and photoallergic reactions. In France, where Phenergan Cream is used extensively as a topical antipruritic, many instances of photocontact dermatitis occurred. Photosensitivity seems to be induced primarily by *contact* with Phenergan.[32] Systemic administration without topical application does not appear to induce photosensitivity.[33] Cross-photosensitivity may occur between Phenergan and Thorazine.[34]

Many phenothiazine compounds can also produce ordinary allergic contact sensitization. Cross-reactions between the phenothiazine compounds may include *both* the photoallergic and the ordinary allergic variety. Sometimes the cross-reactivity extends only to the photoallergic phenomenon. For example, allergic eczematous contact sensitivity may be present to Phenergan alone, while cross-photoallergic reactions may occur between both Phenergan and Thorazine.[35]

Sulfanilamide

This antibacterial agent can apparently produce both *phototoxic* and *photoallergic re-*

actions.[36] The phototoxic reactions are produced by systemic administration of the drug. Window glass usually protects the individual from such phototoxic reactions. On the other hand, the topical application of sulfanilamide preparations may engender photoallergic contact sensitivity. Fortunately, many topical sulfanilamide preparations are used on covered parts of the body so that photosensitivity reactions are not common.

Topical sulfanilamide compounds are not used extensively at present. Other topically applied sulfonamide compounds, such as sulfacetamide, sulfathiazole and sulfadiazine apparently are not photosensitizers. Hypoglycemic sulfonamides, such as chlorpropamide (Diabinese) and tolbutamide (Orinase), thiazide diuretics, such as chlorothiazide (Diuril) and hydrochlorothiazide (Esidrix, HydroDIURIL, Oretic), and quinethazone (Hydromox), however, may produce photoallergic and cross-photosensitization reactions when administered systemically.[37]

Allergic Photodermatitis From Sunscreening Agents

True sunscreening agents, which absorb erythemal ultraviolet radiation rather than scatter it as do certain opaque powders, can become photosensitizers by virtue of such an absorptive process. The esters of para-aminobenzoic acid (PABA) used in sunscreens can produce a photodermatitis.[38–40]

Digalloyl trioleate may act as a photosensitizer.[41] Sunscreens containing cinnamates have been reported as sources of photoallergy.[42]

Sunscreening agents containing PABA esters, digalloyl trioleate and the cinnamates, instead of providing protection, may paradoxically produce allergic photosensitization

Miscellaneous Photosensitizers

Epstein has reported that ragweed pollen[43] benzocaine[44] and Dangard[45] are photosensitizers.

Dangard, a chloro-mercapto-dicarboximide, is used exclusively by barbers as an antiseborrheic agent in Q.E.D. hair groom and shampoo. Dangard is also a trade name for Vanicide 89 Re, which is used as an antiseptic in cosmetic and pharmaceutical preparations.

Photosensitivity reactions from blankophores (optic brightening agents),[46] cadmium sulfide,[47,48] the yellow pigment in tattoos, fluorouracil[49] and the chromates[50] have been reported.

Photosensitivity reactions have been reported from such diverse substances as benzocaine, ragweed pollen, fluorouracil, blankophores and the chromates

PHOTOPATCH TESTS IN PHOTOCONTACT DERMATITIS

A clinical diagnosis of photosensitivity depends on obtaining a detailed and accurate history of exposure to sunlight and the appearance of the eruption on parts of the body so exposed. When the diagnosis of photosensitivity is in doubt, and proof of its role in the production of an eruption is desired, photopatch testing may be indicated. Such testing is not a simple procedure and is not at present suitable for routine office practice. Epstein[51] has described a simplified procedure, which has value as an office diagnostic aid.

The purpose of photopatch testing is to produce lesions under controlled conditions on normal appearing skin of the lower lumbar area that are identical to lesions occurring clinically on areas exposed to light.

The following has been our experience with the commonly used light sources in phototesting:

1. *Natural sunlight:* Natural sunlight is the best source of light, because it simulates clinical conditions and provides a continuous spectrum. The ideal time to expose the patient is at noon during the summer. Unfortunately, sunlight is not regularly available at any given time under standardized conditions.

2. *Fluorescent tubes:* These tubes afford a continuous spectrum, are inexpensive and can be readily standardized for office use. (Consult General Electric, Sylvania and Westinghouse literature for the emission spectrum of the specific fluorescent tube.) Testing for photo-allergic contact dermatitis requires only the fluorescent black light tubes.
3. *Carbon arc lamps:* These provide continuous sources of irradiation. "Sunshine Carbons" (Union Carbide) are a useful type of carbon arc lamps. Such lamps are cumbersome and difficult to standardize and require filters.
4. *Hot quartz mercury vapor lamp:* These lamps are usually available as therapeutic agents in most dermatologists' offices. In addition, the time required to reach an erythematous dose is short. Filters as described by Epstein should be used.[51] Such mercury lamps have the disadvantage of providing a mercury line spectrum that is discontinuous; the patient, therefore, may not receive the wavelengths of light responsible for the eruption. We recommend this lamp for photopatch testing, however, using the technique described by Epstein.[51]

Table 12–7 summarizes the target skin distance and the time necessary to photopatch test with sunlight and artificial light sources. The dose will vary depending on the patient's pigmentation and the age of the artificial light sources. All equipment should be biologically standardized with caution.

Technique of Photopatch Testing*

Photopatch testing is based on the same principles as testing for ordinary contact dermatitis, but certain variations are crucial.

1. All material to be tested is applied in duplicate.
2. Care must be exercised in preventing stray light from reaching the test site by covering all sites with opaque blotting paper.
3. Between 24 and 28 hours after application of the tests, one of the occlusive patch test coverings is removed, and this site is evaluated as in ordinary patch testing.
4. Radiation of about 3200 Å is then given to this site.
5. Between 24 and 28 hours after irradiation, the site is re-evaluated and compared with the light-produced control site. (This is 56 hours after the patches have been applied.)

* When phototesting with commercial products, such as soap, control studies on at least 10 individuals must be done to rule out primary irritant reactions.

Table 12-7. Radiation Factors Involved in Positive Photopatch Test Reactions (Lumbar or Gluteal Area)

Light Source	*Type*	*Target Skin Distance*	*Time For Test Exposure*
Natural sunlight	June, noon, New York City		20 minutes
Carbon arc	Sunshine carbon (Union Carbide Co.)	50 cm.	5 to 20 minutes with window glass filter
Fluorescent tube	Westinghouse, G.E. or Sylvania black light; bank of 4 tubes	25 cm.	30 to 40 minutes
Hot quartz mercury vapor lamp (with filter)	Hanovia	75 cm.	30 minutes with window glass filter

6. Interpretation: If there is no reaction at either site, there is no ordinary allergic contact or photocontact sensitization. If there is equal reaction of both sites, it is an ordinary allergic contact dermatitis. Photosensitization has taken place if the reaction at the radiation site is more pronounced than at the nonradiated site.

Bithionol, hexachlorophene, the halogenated salicylanilides and related compounds are tested as a 1 per cent concentration in white petrolatum. Cosmetics may be applied as they are available in commercial preparations. Soaps and shampoos are tested in a 1 to 5 per cent concentration in an aqueous solution or in white petrolatum. Other compounds are tested in the same concentration as for ordinary patch testing.

Photopatch tests attempt to reproduce photodermatitis under controlled conditions

Erythema, which may be produced by phototesting normal skin with 2800 to 3150 Å radiation, is assessed in terms of decreased erythema threshold, increased magnitude of response and persistence. The erythema readings are usually obtained immediately after irradiation, after 24 and 72 hours, and 1 week following irradiation. Lesions that may be induced include erythema, wheals, papules, vesicles and plaques. These can be due to solar urticaria, polymorphous light eruption and other photodermatoses.

Whenever it is too cold to expose the lumbar area or it is otherwise inconvenient to perform phototesting at this site, the following procedure may be substituted:

1. The normal skin of the forearm is used as the test site.
2. The suspected photocontactant is applied in duplicate under any patch that blocks out light. One of the patches is removed 24 hours later and irradiated with a 30-minute exposure to natural sunlight at noon.
3. Twenty-four hours after the exposure, the irradiated and nonirradiated sites are compared. It is also strongly advisable to irradiate a site to which no agent has been applied in order to ascertain the erythematous response of the individual's skin to sunlight alone.
4. If any of the phototest sites appear abnormal, further testing may be undertaken to eliminate the possibility of a primary irritant or allergic contact dermatitis.

Photopatch tests with any light source, whether natural or artificial, have drawbacks and may be difficult to interpret

Features of Photopatch Testing with Phenothiazine Derivatives

Certain photosensitizers, such as Phenergan and Thorazine, often produce an allergic eczematous contact sensitivity without light. In such instances, exposure to sunlight produces an increased reaction. The increase in intensity of an ordinary patch test reaction on exposure to light must be carefully interpreted, because it may be a nonspecific irritating effect.

If possible, controls should be used as on other positive patch test reactions. Epstein[52] pointed out that whenever an allergen can produce both photoallergic and ordinary allergic contact hypersensitivity, the photoallergic reaction appears to be more intense. Thus, an allergen capable of producing both photoallergic and ordinary allergic eczematous contact dermatitis will produce a photoallergic reaction in areas exposed to light, while the same concentration of the drug that reaches the skin from within will not produce a contact dermatitis.

Epstein pointed out unique features of photoallergic reactions to the phenothiazines. The wavelengths that produce the photoallergic reactions are not always identical to those absorbed by the phenothiazine drug. These drugs have a maximal absorption in the ultraviolet wavelengths below 3100 Å. Once the patient is photoallergic to them, however, he may also react to longer ultraviolet wavelengths and even visible light.

This is called "widening of the action spectrum."[52]

MANAGEMENT OF PHOTOCONTACT SENSITIVITY

General Treatment

Exposure to the photosensitizing agent must be eliminated, and the patient should minimize exposure to sunlight for at least 2 weeks.[53] It is advisable to give the patient a list of related drugs that produce cross-photosensitivity and that are to be avoided. This list is particularly important when the salicylanilides and phenothiazines are implicated. When topical therapeutic or cosmetic agents are involved, the patient should be given a list of nonsensitizing substitutes.

Individuals with an acute photosensitivity reaction with severe erythema and edema may obtain relief with ice cold compresses of Burow's solution diluted 1:10. It is often beneficial to superimpose these compresses on a thin layer of petrolatum to prevent excessive drying.

In generalized cases, systemic corticosteroid therapy often gives prompt symptomatic relief. The dosage is similar to that for any generalized acute dermatitis.

Protection Against Light

The avoidance of sunlight must often be extended beyond the period of acute dermatitis because excretion of the photosensitizing chemical from the skin may be delayed. In severe cases, confinement of the patient in a darkened room for several days may speed recovery. Window glass usually does not protect against contact phototoxic or contact photoallergic reactions.

Knowledge of the action spectrum of a photosensitizer is often of value, because ordinary window glass (3 mm. thick) usually affords protection against ultraviolet radiation below 3200 Å.[54]

Patients with a photosensitivity dermatitis may obtain protection from adequate clothing. Closely woven brown, orange and red fabrics are best. White shirting becomes much more permeable to erythema-producing radiation when wet with water or perspiration.

Repeated, short exposures to sun have occasionally been of aid in desensitizing individuals. Such desensitization is probably nonimmunologic and is due to increased melanin formation and thickening of the horny layer. Dark-skinned individuals are less apt to have photosensitivity reactions than are fair-skinned people. Birmingham[5] noted that the skin of Mexican and Negro harvesters affords protection against the phototoxic effects of the celery pink rot. Crow et al.[10] noted that dark-skinned workers are protected against photodermatitis from pitch.

Pigmentation of skin, color of clothes and reflection and scattering of sunlight may affect intensity of a photodermatitis

Use of Sunscreening Agents. Sunscreening agents are of two main varieties—chemical and physical. Chemical sunscreens, which can absorb light and are protective in photodermatitis, have an absorption spectrum below 3200 Å and include para-aminobenzoic acid and its esters, the benzophenones, digalloyl trioleate and the cinnamates. These agents may occasionally cause allergic contact photodermatitis and, more rarely, produce ordinary allergic contact dermatitis.

Physical sunscreens form an opaque barrier to solar radiation without absorbing such rays. These agents do not produce allergic or photoallergic reactions but are usually not cosmetically acceptable. They include zinc oxide, talc and titanium dioxide.

Sunlight-absorbing agents contain chemicals that may be sensitizers or photosensitizers. Occasionally lanolin, almond oil and cocoa butter, rather than the light-absorbing agents, are the sensitizing ingredients in preparations.

There are currently a host of sunscreens, and new agents constantly appear. A preparation that is popular one summer may fade into obscurity the next season. Most sunscreens have labels stating the active sunscreening agent. Once a patient has developed allergic hypersensitivity to chemicals used to prevent sunburn, he should be given the names of the chemicals so that he can avoid

Table 12-8. Sunscreening Agents Containing PABA or its Esters

Trade Name	*Ingredients*
Beauty on the Beach (Renauld)	p-Aminobenzoate ester plus imidobenzoate
Block Out (Sea & Ski)	p-Aminobenzoate*
Bronze Lustre Moon Drops Moisturizing Lotion (Revlon)	p-Aminobenzoate*
Bronze Lustre Moon Drops, Regular Formula (Revlon)	p-Aminobenzoate*
California Bronze Suntan Cream (Max Factor)	p-Aminobenzoate*
California Bronze Suntan Oil (Max Factor)	p-Aminobenzoate*
Coppertone Baby Tan (Plough)	p-Aminobenzoate with a salicylate
Expose Suntan Liquid (Walgreen)	Glyceryl aminobenzoate
Filtray Lotion (Carmel)	PABA
Hance Suntan Creme (Hance)	Isobutyl p-aminobenzoate
Negasol (Lydia O'Leary)	Glyceryl p-aminobenzoate
Pabafilm (Owen Laboratories)	PABA
Palm Spring Tanning Cream (Helene Curtis)	p-Aminobenzoate*
Pre-Sun (Westwood)	PABA in alcohol
Sea & Ski Dark Tanning Foam	p-Aminobenzoate*
Sea & Ski Dark Tanning Lotion	Glyceryl p-aminobenzoate
Sea & Ski Dark Tanning Oil	p-Aminobenzoate*
Sea & Ski Suntan Lotion	Glyceryl p-aminobenzoate
Sea and Sunprotectol (Lamond)	Ester of PABA
Skol Regular Lotion (J. B. Williams)	p-Aminobenzoate*
Skolex Sun Cream (J. B. Williams)	p-Aminobenzoate*
Solar Cream (Doak)	PABA
Squaw Tan Lotion (Schram)	Menthyl aminobenzoate
Suave Suntan Lotion (Helene Curtis)	p-Aminobenzoate*
Sunbath Moisturizing Tanning Lotion (Revlon)	Isoamyl aminobenzoate
Suntan Lotion (Norwich)	Ester of PABA
Tanfastic Dark Tanning Lotion (Sea & Ski)	Glyceryl p-aminobenzoate
Tanfastic Suntan Lotion with Cocoa Butter	Glyceryl p-aminobenzoate
Tanfastic Suntan Oil Plus Cocoanut Oil	p-Aminobenzoate*
Tanfastic Tanning Butter with Cocoa Butter	No sunscreen present
Tartan Lotion (McKesson)	Ester of PABA

* p-Aminobenzoate is amyl-p-n-dimethyl aminobenzoate.

them in the future. In addition, he should be advised how to obtain sunscreens that do not contain the specific sensitizer.

Patients with hypersensitivity to hair dyes and procaine or benzocaine should avoid the use of sunscreens containing para-aminobenzoic acid esters because cross-reactions may occur between these groups of chemicals.[38–40]

A recent study by one of us (A.A.F.) of 20 paraphenylenediamine-sensitive individuals revealed that 4 patients cross-reacted to para-aminobenzoic acid esters and 2 reacted to the acid.

Occasionally allergic reactions to sunscreens are confused with hypersensitivity reactions to sunlight or sun poisoning. Indeed, general members of this group of chemical sunscreens may act as allergic photosensitizers.

The efficacy of light-absorbing sunscreens was studied by Pathak and his co-workers,[55] who reported that the chemicals that protect best against actinic injury under laboratory conditions include para-aminobenzoic acid (PABA) the benzophenones, esculin, isoamyl-p-n,n′-dimethylaminobenzoate (Escalol 506) and para-aminosalicylic acid. The most effective agent was 5 per cent para-aminobenzoic acid in ethyl alcohol. The prolonged effectiveness resulted from adsorption of para-aminobenzoic acid by the intact epidermis and partial chemical conjugation with constituents of the horny layer. Only the ethanolic solution at pH 4.5 to 4.8 was effective even after repeated washings with water. In the clinical tests, this was among the most effective preparations, even after exercise and swimming. Also it provided excellent protection against snow-reflected sunlight encountered on ski slopes in the Alps. Escalol 506 was also effective in these studies, but most of the commercial preparations were ineffective.

While Macleod and Frain-Bell[56] agreed that para-aminobenzoic acid is an effective sunscreen, they reported that perspiration, swimming and washing lower the photoprotective factor considerably. These investigators found that a combination of a benzophenone (Mexenone) and a physical sunscreen (zinc oxide, kaolin, titanium dioxide and ferric oxide) give the best photoprotection.

Para-aminobenzoic acid in alcohol, and effective sunscreen, may occasionally produce allergic contact sensitivity. The alcohol may sting and be drying

Para-aminobenzoic acid and its esters in alcohol (Pre-Sun, PABA film and Block Out) often impart a burning or stinging sensation and may be uncomfortably drying, particularly for patients with inflamed or eczematous skin. On rare occasions, para-aminobenzoic acid produces ordinary allergic reactions. Table 12–8 is a list of currently popular sunscreen agents that contain this acid or its esters and may have to be avoided by individuals who are allergic to these compounds.

Anthranilates present in A-Fil (Texas Pharmacal) and in Squaw Tan Lotion (Schram) are ortho-benzoates, which are apparently much less common sensitizers than are para-benzoates.

Digalloyl trioleate is the sunscreen in Sunprotectol (Lamond) and Sunswept Cream (Texas Pharmacal), which was formerly known as Neo-A-Fil, and these preparations must be avoided by those who are photosensitive to digalloyl trioleate.[41]

Cinnamates are sensitizers. Table 12–9 is a list of sunscreening products to be avoided by those with allergic photosensitivity to the cinnamates.[42]

Benzophenones are sunscreens. There is a single case report of allergic contact sensitivity to sulisobenzone (2-hydroxy-4-benzophenone-5-sulfonic acid), which is present in Uval Lotion (Dome) and Sunguard (Miles Laboratories). Solbar (Person & Covey) is a combination of oxybenzone and dioxybenzone.[57] Synonyms for sulisobenzone include Spectra-Sorb UV 284 and Uvinul MS-40.

The salicylates are still widely used in over-the-counter sunscreening products. These are usually menthyl benzyl and phenyl compounds, which are very rare sensitizers. Table 12–10 is a list of sunscreening agents that contain salicylates.

Benzyl salicylate, one of the first documented cosmetic sunscreens used in the United States, is a low grade contact allergen and the allergenicity is potentiated by the

Table 12-9. Sunscreening Agents Containing the Cinnamates

Trade Name	*Ingredients*
Beach Party Tanning Cream (Walgreen)	Cinnamate*
Bronze Lustre Moisturizing Tan Cream (Revlon)	Isobutyl salicyl cinnamate
Bronze Lustre Moisturizing Tan Gelee (Revlon)	Isobutyl salicyl cinnamate
Glamomour Tan Sun Cream (Beauty Counselors)	Cinnamate*
Golden Gaby Suntan Lotion (Gaby)	Cinnamate*
Hypoallergic Suntan Lotion (Almay)	Cinnamate*
Moon Drops Bronze Lustre Moisturizing Tanning Lotion and Gelee (Revlon)	Isobutyl salicyl cinnamate
Rupaque (Elder)	Red Veterinary Petrolatum, zinc oxide and cinnamate
Sundare Lotion (Texas Pharmacal)	Cinnamate*
Sun Foam (Beauty Counselors)	Cinnamate*
Sun Lo (Beauty Counselors)	Cinnamate*
Sunbath Moisturizing Tanning Lotion (Revlon)	Isobutyl salicyl cinnamate
Sunbath Spray with Insect Repellent (Revlon)	Isobutyl salicyl cinnamate
Suntan Gelee (Rexall)	Cinnamic acid derivative

* Cinnamate is 2-ethyoxyethyl p-methoxy cinnamate.

Table 12-10. Sunscreening Agents Containing the Salicylates

Trade Name	*Ingredients*
Coppertone Baby Tan (Plough)	H-Salicylate* and p-aminobenzoate
Coppertone Suntan Lotion (Plough)	H-Salicylate*
Coppertone Suntan Oil (Plough)	H-Salicylate*
Gaby Greaseless Suntan Lotion (Gaby)	Sodium salicylate
Gramercy Suntan Lotion (Fisher Scientific)	Menthyl salicylate
Lip Gloss Stick (Arex)	H-Salicylate*
Lipkote (Coppertone [Plough])	H-Salicylate*
Nolex Lotion (Kahlenberg)	H-Salicylate*
Noskote (Coppertone [Plough])	H-Salicylate*
QT Quick Tanning Lotion (Coppertone [Plough])	H-Salicylate* and dihydroxy acetone
Screenex Lotion (Dermatological Prescription Labs)	Triethanolamine salicylate
Sun and Windproof Cream (Helena Rubinstein)	Glyceryl salicylate
Sunburn Preventative (Almay)	Phenyl salicylate and tannic acid
Sunscreen Lotion (Arex)	H-Salicylate*
Suntanning Lotion (Marcelle)	2-Ethyl hexyl salicylate
Tanya Hawaiian Suntan Lotion and Oil (Tanya)	H-Salicylate,* cocoanut oil and cocoa butter

* H-Salicylate is homomenthyl Salicylate.

phototoxic effects produced by topical application of methoxsalen.[58]

Sunlight scattering agents contain opaque powders, such as titanium oxide, kaolin, zinc oxide or talc. The opacity that these powders impart may not be as acceptable as sunscreens that are invisible, but these powders have the advantage of not being sensitizers.

Products containing titanium dioxide form an opaque barrier between the sun and the skin and are sometimes called sunshades, parasols, or physical sunscreens. Titanium dioxide scatters both ultraviolet and visible light radiation (2900 to 7000 Å) rather than absorbs the rays. Titanium dioxide may occasionally be so occlusive that it produces miliaria.

The use of titanium dioxide in lipsticks may prevent contact photosensitivity from the presence of photosensitizing eosin dyes. More recently introduced refined eosin lipstick dyes are less apt to produce photosensitizing reactions.

The inclusion of titanium dioxide, an effective nonsensitizing sunscreen for all wavelengths of ultraviolet light, with para-aminobenzoic acid may prevent photosensitizing reactions. Solar Cream (Doak) contains 4 per cent para-aminobenzoic acid and 5 per cent titanium dioxide. The opaqueness of titanium dioxide, however, makes a sun screen visible and masklike.

Many lifeguards have found that zinc oxide ointment applied to the nose and lips is an effective sunscreen that sticks to the skin in spite of perspiration and swimming. Red Veterinary Petrolatum (RVP [Elder]) is another type of physical sunscreen, which of course, is greasy.

Table 12–11 is a list of the currently available physical sunscreens.

Physical sunscreens such as zinc oxide, titanium dioxide and RVP are efficient sunscreens but often not acceptable cosmetically

Management of Contact Photodermatitis Due to Specific Photosensitizers

Psoralens. Patients sensitized to the psoralens must be cautioned not only against sunlight but also against intense artificial illumination.

Photosensitivity reactions due to psoralens in perfumes (berloque dermatitis) may be avoided by having patients apply the perfume to covered parts of the body or on their clothing.

Birmingham[5] reported that physical sunscreens protect celery harvesters against phototoxic reactions due to pink rot in celery but chemical sunscreens did not.

Tar. Individuals receiving tar therapy in whom a photosensitivity reaction is to be avoided should apply the tar at night only and carefully remove it in the morning. Patients should be warned that even though the tars have apparently been completely removed from the skin avoidance of exposure to strong sunlight for several days is important, since even traces of the tar may cause phototoxic reactions. Purified or refined tars are less apt to cause photosensitivity reactions. Occasionally it may be desirable to substitute wood tars (e.g., pine tar), which are not photosensitizers.

The Phenothiazines. Medical and nursing personnel and those in the pharmaceutical industry who handle Thorazine, and certain insecticides should be warned of the photosensitizing capacity of the phenothiazines.

Table 12-11. Physical Sunscreens

Trade Name	*Ingredients*
A-Fil Cream (Texas Pharmacal)	Titanium dioxide and menthyl anthranilate
RVP (Elder)	Red Veterinary Petrolatum
RVPlus (Elder)	Red Veterinary Petrolatum, titanium dioxide and mica
Rupaque (Elder)	Red Veterinary Petrolatum, zinc oxide and methoxy cinnamate
Shadow (Beauty Counselors)	Calamine and iron oxide

Even when patients with photosensitivity to Thorazine no longer contact the drug, exposure to sunlight may produce flare-ups of photodermatitis for several months. Thorazine is excreted almost unchanged in the urine, and sensitized nurses and orderlies who handle linens may experience flare-ups of dermatitis.

The phenothiazines can also produce an allergic eczematous contact dermatitis without light. Phenergan Cream produces both contact and photocontact dermatitis. The systemic administration of Phenergan apparently does *not* initiate photosensitization.

PERSISTENCE OF PHOTOSENSITIVITY

Most patients are "transient" light reactors with a normal erythema threshold.[22] In such individuals, photosensitivity eruptions usually rapidly improve upon avoidance of both the photosensitizer and exposure to sunlight. For some reason, however, a few individuals are *persistent light reactors* with a markedly lowered erythema threshold. Photoreactions in such individuals may persist for months to years with continued exposure to light even though there is no contact with photosensitizers.[15]

The mechanism perpetuating the disability is not clear. The adverse photoreactivity in this group is manifested by markedly diminished erythema thresholds in the sunburn range (2900 to 3100 Å) in addition to positive patch test results with long ultraviolet wavelengths (3200 to 4000 Å). Persistent light reactors usually are people who were first known to be photoallergic to bithionol or halogenated salicylanilides. The incidence of people who have persistent light reactivity has been estimated at less than 1 per cent to as high as 30 per cent of the contact photoallergic groups studied at university centers.

This type of reaction has also been reported as an iatrogenic disability following systemic use of chlorpromazine, sulfanilamide or promethazine. Therapy has included administering psoralens or the antimalarial drugs.

Exceedingly short exposures to ultraviolet light will elicit allergic photocontact dermatitis in highly sensitized individuals.[59] Persistent light reactors, therefore, must take extreme precautions to avoid even the slightest exposure to light. The theory has been advanced that persistent light reaction is due to the unsuspected persistence of the responsible chemical in the skin.[60] Such an assumption remains to be proved, however.

Persistent light reactors are severely handicapped individuals who suffer with intense itching. Their skin becomes lichenified, fissured, pigmented and sometimes depigmented. Occasionally a photodermatitis resembling lupus erythematosus develops. Sidi and co-workers[61] emphasized that such lesions may be difficult to reverse unless the patient spends prolonged periods in the dark.

Unfortunately, the therapy in most instances of persistent photosensitivity is unsatisfactory. Some persistent light reactors may improve with the following regimen:

1. Avoid sunlight during the peak hours of solar radiation (i.e., 10:00 A.M. to 3:00 P.M. solar time).
2. Apply a high potency topical steroid preparation, such as 2 per cent Hytone, Synalar-HP or 0.5 per cent Aristocort Cream, in the morning followed by a sunscreen, even if there is to be no sun exposure. Reapply both preparations several times daily.[24]

Patients who perspire freely may apply para-aminobenzoic acid in alcohol (Pre-Sun), the steroid cream and a sunscreen, such as Doak's Solar Cream (para-aminobenzoic acid and titanium dioxide) or Texas Pharmacal's A-Fil (menthyl anthranilate and titanium dioxide). If these pink opaque covers are not acceptable, a benzophenone cream (Solbar, Uval) may be substituted.

3. In some individuals, sunscreens are not photoprotective. Such patients must use protective clothing, wide brimmed hats, long sleeves, gloves and even veils.
4. Persistent light reactors should avoid *all* antibacterial (deodorant) soaps because of the possibility of cross-sensitivity between the halogenated salicylanilides, bithionol and hexachlorophene. Patients with known sensitivity to benzocaine, paraphenylenediamine or the

sulfonamides should avoid para-aminobenzoic acid sunscreens.

5. The persistent light reactor should avoid exposure to artificial lamps with high irradiation, such as movie projector lamps, fluorescent lights, sun lamps and even strong incandescent lights.[62]
6. During acute flare of a persistent photodermatitis, systemic corticosteroids should be given for a week or so. In the presence of infection, a nonsensitizing antibiotic ointment such as Ilotycin should be applied.

Ointments containing local anesthetics, such as benzocaine, or antihistamine topical medications, should be avoided since they are notorious sensitizers.

Persistent light reactors have intractable pruritus, fissuring and lichenification long after the causative photosensitizer is avoided. A combination of a corticosteroid cream and a sunscreen with strict avoidance of sun exposure may be helpful. Systemic steroids and hospitalization may be necessary in severe cases

REFERENCES

1. Harber, L. C., Targouik, S. E., and Baer, R. L.: Studies on Contact Photosensitivity to Hexachlorophene and Trichlorocarbanilide in Guinea Pigs and Man. J. Invest. Derm., *51*, 373, 1968.
2. Harber, L. C., and Levine, G. M.: Photo Sensitivity Dermatitis from Household Products. GP, *39*, 95, 1969.
3. Baer, R. L., and Harber, L. C.: Photosensitivity Induced by Drugs. J.A.M.A., *192*, 989, 1965.
4. Pathak, M. A., Daniels, F., Jr., and Fitzpatrick, T. B.: The Presently Known Distribution of Furocoumarins (Psoralens) in Plants. J. Invest. Derm., *39*, 225, 1962.
5. Birmingham, D. J., et al.: Phototoxic Bullae Among Celery Harvesters. Arch. Derm., *83*, 73, 1961.
6. Baer, R. L., and Harber, L. C.: Effect of Humidity on the Photosensitive Response to 8-Methoxypsoralen. J. Invest. Derm., *44*, 61, 1965.
7. Sommer, R. G., and Jillson, O. F.: Phytophotodermatitis (Solar Dermatitis from Plants) Gas Plant and the Wild Parsnip. New Engl. J. Med., *276*, 1484, 1967.
8. Harber, L. C., et al.: Berloque Dermatitis. Arch. Derm., *90*, 572, 1964.
9. Sams, E. M.: Photodynamic Action of Lime Oil (Citrus Aurautifolia). Arch. Derm., *44*, 571, 1941.
10. Crow, K. D., et al.: Photosensitivity Due to Pitch. Brit. J. Derm., *73*, 220, 1961.
11. Calnan, C., Harman, R., and Wells, G.: Photodermatitis From Soap. Brit. Med. J., *2*, 1266, 1961.
12. Wilkinson, D. S.: Photodermatitis Due to Tetrachlorosalicylanilide. Brit. J. Derm., *73*, 213, 1961.
13. Vinson, L. K., and Flatt, R. S.: Photosensitization by Tetrachlorosalicylanilide. J. Invest. Derm., *38*, 327, 1962.
14. Epstein, S., and Enta, T.: Photoallergic Contact Dermatitis. J.A.M.A., *194*, 1016, 1965.
15. Osmundsen, P. E.: Contact Photodermatitis due to Tribromosalicylanilide. Brit. J. Derm., *81*, 929, 1969.
16. Harber, L. C., Harris, H., and Baer, R. L.: Photoallergic Contact Dermatitis. Arch. Derm., *94*, 255, 1966.
17. Freeman, R. G., and Knox, J. M.: The Action Spectrum of Photocontact Dermatitis: Caused by Halogenated Salicylanilides and Related Compounds. Arch. Derm., *97*, 130, 1968.
18. Epstein, J. H., Woepper, K. D., and Maibach, H. I.: Photocontact Dermatitis to Halogenated Salicylanilides and Related Compounds. Arch. Derm., *97*, 236, 1968.
19. Harber, L. C., Harris, H., and Baer, R. L.: Structural Features of Photoallergy to Salicylanilides and Related Compounds. J. Invest. Derm., *46*, 303, 1966.
20. Auerbach, R., and Pearlstein, H. H.: Photosensitivity and Soap. New York J. Med., *72*, 747, 1971.
21. Gaul, L. E.: Sensitivity to Bithionol. Arch. Derm., *87*, 383, 1963.
22. Jillson, O. F., and Baughman, R. D.: Contact Photodermatitis from Bithionol. Arch. Derm., *88*, 409, 1963.
23. Epstein, J., Rees, W., and Baughman, R. D.: Contact Photodermatitis from Bithionol. Arch. Derm., *90*, 153, 1964.
24. O'Quinn, S. E., Kennedy, B., and Isbell, K. H.: Contact Photodermatitis Due to Bithionol and Related Compounds. J.A.M.A., *199*, 89, 1967.
25. O'Quinn, S. E.: The Sun and Your Skin. Cutis, *4*, 585, 1968.
26. Burry, J. M.: Photoallergies to Fenticlor and Multifungin. Arch. Derm., *95*, 287, 1967.

27. Burry, J. M.: Cross Sensitivity Between Fenticlor and Bithionol. Arch. Derm., *97*, 496, 1968.
28. Burry, J. M., and Hunter, G. A.: Photocontact Dermatitis from Jadit. Brit. J. Derm., *82*, 224, 1970.
29. DeEds, F., Wilson, R. H., and Thomas, J. O.: Photosensitization by Phenothiazine. J.A.M.A., *114*, 2095, 1940.
30. Cahn, M. M., and Levy, E. J.: Ultraviolet Light Factor in Chlorpromazine Dermatitis. Arch. Derm., *75*, 38, 1957.
31. Epstein, J. H., and Brunsting, L. A.: Topical Application of Chlorpromazine: Its Effect on the Erythema Response to Ultraviolet Light. J. Invest. Derm., *30*, 91, 1958.
32. Sidi, E., Hincky, M., and Gervais, A.: Allergic Sensitization and Photosensitization to Phenergan Cream. J. Invest. Derm., *24*, 345, 1955.
33. Newill, R. G. D.: Photosensitivity Caused by Promethazine. Brit. Med. J., *2*, 359, 1960.
34. Epstein, S.: Allergic Photo-Contact Dermatitis from Promethazine (Phenergan). Arch. Derm., *81*, 175, 1960.
35. Epstein, S., and Rowe, R. J.: Photoallergy and Photocross Sensitivity to Phenergan. J. Invest. Derm., *29*, 319, 1957.
36. Epstein, S.: Photoallergy and Primary Photosensitivity to Sulfanilamide. J. Invest. Derm., *2*, 43, 1939.
37. Harber, L. C., Lashinsky, A. M., and Baer, R. L.: Photosensitivity Due to Chlorothiazide and Hydrochlorothiazide. New Engl. J. Med., *261*, 1378, 1959.
38. Satulsky, E. M.: Photosensitization Induced by Monoglycerol Parraminobenzoate. Arch. Derm., *62*, 711, 1950.
39. Meltzer, L., and Baer, R. L.: Sensitization to Monoglycerol Paraaminobenzoate: A Case Report. J. Invest. Derm., *12*, 31, 1949.
40. Goldman, G. C., and Epstein, E.: Contact Photosensitivity from Sun-Protective Agent. Arch. Derm., *100*, 447, 1969.
41. Sams, W.: Contact Photodermatitis. Arch. Derm., *73*, 142, 1956.
42. Goodman, T. F.: Photodermatitis from a Sunscreening Agent. Letters to the Editor. Arch. Derm., *102*, 503, 1970.
43. Epstein, S.: Role of Dermal Sensitivity in Ragweed Contact Dermatitis. Arch. Derm., *82*, 48, 1960.
44. Epstein, S.: Photocontact Dermatitis from Benzocaine. Arch. Derm., *92*, 591, 1965.
45. Epstein, S.: Photoallergic Contact Dermatitis: Report of a Case Due to Dangard. Cutis, *4*, 856, 1968.
46. Burckhardt, W.: Photoallergic Eczema Due to Blankophores (Optic Brightening Agents). Hautarzt, *8*, 486, 1957.
47. Bjoernber, A.: Reactions to Light in Yellow Tattoos from Cadmium Sulfide. Arch. Derm., *88*, 267, 1963.
48. Goldstein, N.: Mercury-Cadmium Sensitivity in Tattoos. A Photoallergic Reaction in Red Pigment. Ann. Intern. Med., *67*, 984, 1967.
49. Sams, W. M.: Untoward Response with Topical Fluorouracil. Arch. Derm., *97*, 14, 1968.
50. Tronnier, H.: Photosensitivity of Eczema Patients (With Particular Reference to Chromate Eczema). Arch. Klin. Exp. Derm., *47*, 494, 1970.
51. Epstein, S.: Simplified Photopatch Testing. Arch. Derm., *93*, 217, 1966.
52. Epstein, S.: Allergic Photo-Contact Dermatitis from Promethazine (Phenergan). Arch. Derm., *81*, 175, 1960.
53. Knox, J. M.: Clinical Aspects and Types of Drug-Induced Photosensitivity. Ann. Allergy, *19*, 749, 1961.
54. Blum, H. F.: Sunburn. In A. Hollander (ed.): *Radiation Biology* (Vol. 2). New York, McGraw-Hill Book Co., 1955.
55. Pathak, M. A., Fitzpatrick, T. B., and Frenke, E.: Evaluation of Topical Agents that Prevent Sunburn: Superiority of Paraaminobenzoic Acid and its Esters in Ethyl Alcohol. New Engl. J. Med., *280*, 1459, 1969.
56. Macleod, T. M., and Frain-Bell, W.: The Study of Some Agents Used for the Protection of the Skin from Exposure to Light. Brit. J. Derm., *84*, 226, 1971.
57. Baer, R. L., and Ramsay, D. N.: Polyvalent Light Sensitivity. Allergic Contact Sensitivity to Sulisobenzone. Arch. Derm., *104*, 446, 1971.
58. Kahn, G.: Intensified Contact Sensitization to Benzyl Salicylate. Arch. Derm., *103*, 497, 1971.
59. Willis, I., and Kligman, A. M.: Photocontact Allergic Reactions: Elicitations by Low Doses of Long Ultraviolet Rays. Arch. Derm., *100*, 535, 1969.
60. Willis, I., and Kligman, A. M.: Mechanism of Persistent Light Reactor. J. Invest. Derm., *51*, 385, 1968.
61. Sidi, E., Hincky, M., and Germaw, A.: Allergic Sensitization and Photosensitization to Phenergan Cream. J. Invest. Derm., *24*, 345, 1955.
62. Willis I.: Sunlight and the Skin. J.A.M.A., *27*, 1088, 1971.

13

Cutaneous Reactions to Cosmetics

According to law, a cosmetic is not intended to affect the structure and any function of the body of man. Kanof[1] ponted out that the legal definition should be in accord with the biological fact that the structure and the function of the skin are affected by environmental influences, including the application of cosmetics.

It is therefore suggested that the term *cosmetic* be defined in law to mean articles to be rubbed, poured, sprinkled or sprayed on, introduced into or otherwise applied to the normal or to previously altered (scar, birthmark) human skin or any part thereof for cleansing, beautifying, promoting attractiveness or altering the appearance, and such articles shall be those that are not intended to alter or to interfere with the physiologic competence of the human skin or body. It is further suggested that the definition of the term *drug* be revised to make clear that the phrase "intended to affect the structure and any function" has no biological application to the definition of the term *cosmetic.*

Texts and articles dealing with cosmetics stress the great care in the selection and compounding of ingredients used in modern cosmetics.[2–8]

A 2 to 4 per cent incidence of positive reactions to cosmetics among patients seen by dermatologists has been recorded. This figure may be high because the dermatologist tests patients who are more susceptible to dermatitis than is the general population.[9]

Although the incidence of cosmetic dermatitis is low, the vigilant dermatologist must nevertheless suspect and test cosmetics for irritancy and allergic reactions

Types of Dermatitis and Damage From Cosmetics. Chemicals in cosmetics may produce primary irritant reactions, allergic dermatitis, photosensitivity and hair and nail breakage.[10] Since most of the obvious irritating compounds are eliminated from products by the manufacturers, the most common type of reaction from cosmetics is allergic sensitization. Certain commonly employed cosmetics, however, may be irritants unless they are carefully applied. One must also consider the rare possible interaction and addition or synergistic effects of two or more cosmetics simultaneously or successively applied to the same area or, in cases of contamination, even to different areas.

Allergic Reaction to Cosmetics. An individual may use a cosmetic product for years without reacting and then suddenly acquire an allergic hypersensitivity to one or more substances in the formulation.

Probably the most common cause of allergic cosmetic dermatitis is paraphenylenediamine, a basic ingredient in oxidation-type permanent hair dyes. Perfumes, lipsticks and sunscreening agents are among the cosmetic products more frequently causing skin sensitization.

In most instances, cutaneous allergic reactions take the form of eczematous dermatitis. In the past, however, antiperspirants that contained certain zirconium compounds produced allergic granulomatous reactions.

Aside from hair dyes and, formerly, certain nail preparations, the ingredients of the most commonly used cosmetics are weak sensitizers that produce a mild, dry, scaly eruption rather than an obvious eczematous reaction with erythema, edema and vesiculation. In most instances, dermatitis due to cosmetics involves the face, particularly the eyelids, the rims of the ears and the neck. Axillary involvement due to antiperspirants, however, is not unusual.

The principal site of a dermatitis may not be in the area of application of the cosmetic. For example, dermatitis of the eyelids may be produced by hair preparations, and the eyelids, face and neck are often involved in nail enamel dermatitis, with the paronychial area and the nail remaining unaffected. Mild cases of paraphenylenediamine dye dermatitis may initially affect the eyelids alone. Subsequently, the entire scalp, as well as widespread areas of the face, trunk and extremities, may become involved.

Primary Irritant Reactions to Cosmetics. The cosmetics that as a result of misuse are most commonly associated with primary irritant reactions are antiperspirants, depilatories and permanent wave preparations.

Cosmetic Photosensitivity Reactions. Such reactions, most commonly associated with perfumes and sunscreening agents, may occur at any site of application followed by exposure to light. Pigmentation in the affected areas (berloque dermatitis) is one type of photosensitivity reaction. Other reactions consist of an erythematous or eczematous reaction, which may be phototoxic or photoallergic.

Topical preparations contaminated with nail enamel may produce nail enamel dermatitis

Miscellaneous Reactions. Antiperspirants in particular may produce irritant follicular eruptions.

Hair Damage From Cosmetics. Chemicals used to curl or straighten the hair may cause breakage and thereby produce temporary alopecia. Mechanical curlers and rollers may produce traction alopecia.

Onychial and Paronychial Reactions to Cosmetics. Nail dystrophy and inflammatory reactions may occur from acrylic resins employed as artificial nails or nail builders. Thermoplastic resins used in ordinary nail enamel may produce dermatitis of the face and neck, but as a rule the nails and paronychial area remain unaffected.

DIAGNOSIS OF COSMETIC DERMATITIS

The proof that a cosmetic is producing a particular dermatitis is usually established by an elimination routine or patch testing or by a combination of both methods.

Cosmetic Elimination Routine

When a cosmetic dermatitis is suspected, but a specific cosmetic cannot be implicated, the following instructions may be given to the patient in order to arrest the dermatitis and to pinpoint the offending agent:

1. Stop the use of all cosmetics except lipstick, if the lips are not involved.
2. Shampoo the hair with a bland soap to remove all hair preparations, such as wave set, hair oil and other hair dressings.
3. Wash the face with an unscented soap.
4. Remove all nail products, including clear enamel.
5. Bring in all cosmetics used, both old and new, for examination and testing. This includes cosmetic sponges and powder puffs used to apply cosmetics.
6. If there has been a recent visit to the beauty parlor, obtain the names or the samples of the cosmetics that were used.
7. The cosmetic responsible for the dermatitis may be a new one or one that has been used for many years. The fact that all cosmetics that have been used have been the same for many years does not rule out a cosmetic dermatitis due to the development of allergic hypersensitivity. In addition, some ingredients may have recently been changed by the manufacturer.

The elimination routine just outlined is one of considerable help in confirming a diagnosis of cosmetic dermatitis. If the dermatitis subsides promptly, it may be assumed that one of the cosmetics eliminated contained the offending substance. After the dermatitis has subsided, one can then reintroduce individual cosmetics one at a time. The last cosmetic to be tried before symptoms reappear most probably contains the offending agent. The procedure may then be repeated with the suspected cosmetic as a final check to determine if the dermatitis is reproduced.

Once a cosmetic has been implicated as a cause of dermatitis, not only must that particular cosmetic be discarded, but also any other cosmetic that may have become mixed with, or contaminated by, the offending agent. Powder puffs and cosmetic sponges used to apply the dermatitis-producing cosmetic should be discarded. All instruments, such as tweezers and eyelash curlers, should be thoroughly cleansed before being reemployed.

Old, as well as new, preparations must be suspected in cosmetic dermatitis

When employing this elimination routine, special attention should be paid to recently acquired cosmetics. Cosmetics that have been used for a long time without difficulty, however, may suddenly, without apparent reason, cause dermatitis. For example, the manufacturer may have changed the formulation in ways that are not obvious to the user. Occasionally, deterioration due to age or improper storage may change a previously safe cosmetic into an irritant or a sensitizer.

Patients with suspected cosmetic dermatitis should be investigated for allergic reactions to rubber, because dermatitis from rubber cosmetic sponges may mimic cosmetic dermatitis. Substitution of cotton, plastic or cellulose cosmetic applicators may be instrumental in clearing so-called cosmetic dermatitis.

Patch Testing with Cosmetics

The advantage of patch testing over the elimination routine is that sometimes it is possible to identify the offending agent within 48 hours. A positive patch test reaction with a cosmetic, *providing the test has been properly performed and interpreted*, usually means that the cosmetic can produce allergic dermatitis. It is possible, however, for a cosmetic to produce a negative patch test reaction when the test is performed on the usual sites, such as the arm or back, but to produce a positive reaction when applied closer to the eruption, particularly if the thin skin of the eyelids or neck is involved and the cosmetic is a weak sensitizer. Strong sensitizers, such as hair dyes, usually give a positive reaction at the usual sites of patch testing. When a suspected cosmetic gives a negative patch test reaction, the trial-and-error method of reapplication will usually determine whether it is the offending agent.

Whenever a number of patches are applied, the cosmetic that is under strongest suspicion and that may produce a reaction should be placed away from the other patches so that its early removal, if necessary, will not disturb the remaining patches and so that a strongly positive reaction will not spread and produce false reactions at adjacent sites.

In many instances, a dermatitis-producing cosmetic may give a false negative reaction unless tests are performed with individual ingredients

Uncovered vs. Covered Patch Test Technique. Cosmetics suspected of being photosensitizers should be tested both by the covered technique and by exposure to sunlight or artificial light.

Cosmetics that contain volatile chemicals and that under normal usage are well tolerated may be primary irritants under a closed patch test. These cosmetics include hair lacquers, nail enamels, mascaras and perfumes. Such cosmetics should be allowed to remain uncovered on the skin until the volatile substances have evaporated (usually for 10 to 15 minutes). Then the patch test site may be covered. Nail enamel can be painted on a square of blotting paper and allowed to dry thoroughly before being placed against the skin under a closed patch.

Cosmetics that in use do not cause dermatitis may give false positive reactions under a covered patch because they are primary irritants when occluded. The following cosmetics should be tested uncovered: depilatories, permanent wave preparations, shampoos (soap products in general), hair tonics, alkaline hair dye mixtures, caustic agents (cuticle removers) and oxidizing agents (freckle creams).

Cronin[11] stated that the patch tests should be read at 48 hours and again at 96 hours; this latter assessment is important, because the test may become positive during the second and fourth days. Because of enhanced penetration by the closed patch test, a toxic reaction may be produced by an ingredient that is not an irritant under normal use. Such a toxic reaction may be a typical toxic soap reaction, but it can also completely simulate an allergic response.

The open test is used to evaluate a doubtful reaction; the preparation is rubbed on an area of normal skin, usually the forearm, three times a day for two days and the site is then examined. The preparation is also applied to normal controls. When a positive open test is considered to be significant, the patient should be tested with the individual ingredients of the cosmetic. Tracing the allergenic or toxic component of a cosmetic can be difficult.

THE SENSITIZER IN A COSMETIC

The elimination routine or patch testing may prove that a certain cosmetic contains a substance that has produced an allergic dermatitis in a patient. Cosmetics contain a number of ingredients, however, any one of which may be the sensitizer. Moreover, many cosmetics have in common emulsifying agents, perfumes and preservatives, which can be sensitizers. In patients with recurrent or persistent dermatitis, it may be necessary to test for sensitization to such ubiquitous agents and, if possible, to provide the patients with cosmetics free of the sensitizer. Schorr[12] emphasized that knowledge of the ingredients of cosmetic creams and lotions is essential to diagnose and treat allergic patients.

Falsely negative allergy tests to parabens, sorbic acid and other preservatives are possible when the dermatologist relies upon patch tests using the cosmetic cream or lotion as manufactured. Parabens are used in a concentration of less than 0.5 per cent, yet a patch test requires a concentration of at least 3 per cent to diagnose paraben allergy.

Sorbic acid, 0.2 per cent, is effective as a preservative in cosmetics, but a patch test with these cosmetics will also produce falsely negative responses. A concentration of at least 2 per cent is needed for diagnostic accuracy.

This seeming paradox merely reflects the limitations of our standard 48-hour patch test system. Here the patient's cutaneous exposure differs from the daily application of cosmetic and dermatologic creams or lotions. The usual concentrations may produce and extend allergic disease but may not elicit a true positive response to our present 48-hour patch test.

Preservatives, emulsifying agents and perfumes contained in cosmetics may produce allergic dermatitis and may require individual testing

HAIR DYE DERMATITIS

Hair dyeing may be accomplished with permanent oxidation type dyes, semipermanent azo and aniline dyes not requiring oxidation, metallic salts or vegetable rinses. Of this group, the oxidation type dyes are the most common sensitizers, the azo and aniline dyes are much less so, and the metallic and vegetable dyes rarely sensitize.

Oxidation Type Dyes

Most professional, and much consumer-applied, hair coloring or tinting is now done with permanent oxidation dyes, particularly paraphenylenediamine (PPDA). These dyes produce color that lasts until the hair grows out. In some countries, paraphenylenediamine and a few related intermediates are banned for use as hair dyes. In the United States, it is permitted on scalp hair but not on eyelashes or eyebrows, because an allergic reaction could cause corneal damage and blindness.

Usually hair dye preparations containing paraphenylenediamine are packaged in two bottles; one contains the dye preparation and the other contains the developer (oxidizer). The dye preparation may include the dye with modifiers (diamino anisole sulfate, hydroquinone, catechol, resorcin, pyrogallol) to stabilize shades of color, and alkali (less than 1 per cent) as ammonia, with soap and wetting agents, such as alkyl aryl sulfonates, to aid penetration. The developer is usually 20 volumes (6 per cent) hydrogen peroxide or urea peroxide.

Paraphenylenediamine is a colorless crystalline solid requiring oxygen to "develop" or become colored. In the presence of alkali, such as ammonia, oxidation is accelerated. It is a permanent dye, penetrating and coloring the hair cortex but not the cuticle, thus allowing the cuticle to retain its luster and give highlights. Such dyed hair looks natural and may be shampooed without becoming decolored. Hair dyed with it can also receive permanent waves without difficulty.

More than 95 per cent of modern oxidation hair dyes in the United States contain 1 to 8 per cent paraphenylenediamine. Other oxidation dyes may be mixed and include paratoluene diamine and methyl para-aminophenol. In addition, potassium chlorate or potassium dichromate may on occasion be used instead of the peroxides as oxidizing agents.

Paraphenylenediamine is no longer a sensitizer when oxidized. This enables individuals sensitive to it to wear wigs and fur coats dyed with it without difficulty

Patch Testing with Paraphenylenediamine

The Federal Food, Drug and Cosmetic Act, Section 601(a), provides that certain hair color preparations, such as those containing paraphenylenediamine, bear a warning to the effect that a patch test should be performed prior to each application of the dye. It is the custom in many beauty parlors to do a patch test on the initial hair dyeing procedure but to omit the test on subsequent applications.

Patch testing for allergic sensitivity to paraphenylenediamine may be performed by either the uncovered or the covered method.

Uncovered (Consumer Screening) Patch Test Method. This is the routine technique used by consumers for testing hair dye sensitivity. Instructions for such testing are included with every package of hair dye preparation. The test may be performed as follows: 5 drops of the solution from each bottle (the dye and the developer) are mixed in a small glass. The mixture is allowed to stand for 5 minutes and is then painted on the skin at the bend of the elbow where it can be easily read. The application should cover an area not less than the size of a 25-cent piece, and it should be allowed to dry and remain on the skin uncovered for 24 hours. If there is no itching or sign of irritation at the site at this time, the dye can usually be safely used on the hair. If there is any sign of irritation, such as redness, swelling, papules or vesicles, the dye should not be used.

The 2-bottle mixture should always be tested by the open method, because the alkali and the oxidizer of the mixture are primary irritants under occlusion.

Covered (Diagnostic) Patch Test Method. A 2 per cent concentration of paraphenylenediamine in petrolatum is standard for such testing. It darkens by slow oxidation and should be freshly prepared at least once yearly. Staining of the skin from a patch test with this preparation should not be confused with an irritant or allergic reaction because it is due to oxidation. Paraphenylenediamine for testing should be dispensed in a dark bottle and kept tightly closed. The completely unoxidized chemical and the black or colored end product of union with the hair probably are not sensitizers. The intermediate, partially oxidized "quinone" chemicals are sensitizers.

Evaluation of Patch Test Reactions. A 1+ to 2+ reaction to the paraphenylenediamine hair dye mixture tested by the open (consumer screening) method is of clinical significance, and usually dermatitis develops if the mixture is used.

The open patch test has proved satisfactory in identifying individuals within the general population who exhibit sufficient allergy to react to such hair dyes under use conditions

On the other hand, many individuals who show a 1+ or 2+ reaction to 1 to 2 per cent paraphenylenediamine in petrolatum tested by the covered method continue to use paraphenylenediamine-containing hair dyes without difficulty. A stronger reaction (3+ to 4+) to the covered patch test technique, however, precludes the use of these hair dyes; allergic dermatitis usually occurs if the dyes are used.

In medicolegal cases the open patch test should be performed with the actual dye mixture that was employed. If a positive reaction is obtained, the open test should be supplemented with a covered test using paraphenylenediamine alone. A positive patch test reaction by both methods proves that the paraphenylenediamine caused the dermatitis. Unless such a supplementary test is performed, one cannot be certain of the cause, because the patient has been exposed to several chemicals in the hair dyeing procedure.

Rarely, a patch test reaction with paraphenylenediamine is negative after 48 hours, and after 3 to 5 days, a reaction occurs. This may indicate that the test procedure sensitized the individual. The application of the hair dye, in the interim, produces a dermatitis despite the original negative reaction. Performing a patch test before each application of a paraphenylenediamine-containing hair dye is legally a mandatory requirement.

Treatment of Paraphenylenediamine Hair Dye Dermatitis

In mild cases, only the upper eyelids or the rims of the ears may be involved. Some individuals with minimal sensitization continue to use paraphenylenediamine hair dye for years without developing severe dermatitis. On the other hand, one may rarely observe patients who have safely used these dyes for a decade or more suddenly sustain explosive reactions, which may be accompanied by marked edema of the scalp and face. The eyelids may be completely closed and the eruption may become widespread.

In acute severe cases, the scalp should be thoroughly cleansed with a mild soap or soapless shampoo to remove excess dye. Then a 2 per cent solution of hydrogen peroxide or compresses of potassium permanganate in a 1:5000 dilution should be applied to the scalp to completely oxidize the paraphenylenediamine. The completely oxidized chemical is not a sensitizer.

A wet dressing of cold olive oil and lime water is soothing. It softens the crusts and alleviates the tight feeling of the scalp. This treatment may be followed by the application of an emulsion of equal parts of water and a water-miscible corticosteroid cream, such as Synalar or Cordran.

Some individuals with low grade sensitization to paraphenylenediamine continue to dye their hair with minimal itching or dermatitis

In the absence of contraindication, systemic corticosteroid therapy is also indicated in all severe cases.

Cross-Reactions to Paraphenylenediamine

Patients with allergic hypersensitivity to paraphenylenediamine should be warned of the possibility of cross-reaction dermatitis from immunologically related compounds, including azo and aniline dyes, local anesthetics (procaine, benzocaine), sulfonamides, paraaminosalicylic acid and sunscreens based on para-aminobenzoic acid.[13]

The spectrum of cross-sensitivity may include one or all of these compounds, and it remains the same over many years.[14] Some individuals react to paraphenylenediamine and to no cross-sensitizing chemical. Others continue to cross-react with one or more related chemicals. In my series, repeated patch tests with azo dyes and procaine, benzocaine and para-aminobenzoic acid failed to widen the cross-sensitivity pattern in individuals who originally had a narrow spectrum of cross-sensitivity. Once established, paraphenylenediamine sensitivity usually persists for many years even though the individuals are no longer apparently exposed to it.

The patient with paraphenylenediamine hypersensitivity should avoid the use of all oxidation type hair dyes. There is at present no permanent oxidation type hair dye which these patients can safely use.

Coal Tar Hair Dyes Not Requiring Oxidation

Many semipermanent dyes of coal tar origin that do not require oxidation are available. About 25 per cent of paraphenylenediamine-sensitive individuals cross-react with them. The paraphenylenediamine-sensitive patient may attempt to use such dyes, providing there is a preliminary negative patch test reaction. Certified azo dyes are used in temporary hair toners, and also in foods, medications, ballpoint pen inks, gasoline and diesel oil.

Hair Dyeing with Semipermanent Colors

In recent years there has been wide use of synthetic dyes that do not require oxidation. These dyes impart color that persists through several washings. Most manufacturers include instructions for preliminary skin testing. About 75 per cent of individuals with paraphenylenediamine-sensitivity tolerate such semipermanent colors.

Certain acid azo dyes impart only a very temporary color or merely tone down gray and brighten faded hair. About 10 per cent of individuals who are allergic to paraphenylenediamine also react to such hair dyes.

Metallic Hair Dyes

Metallic or progressive dyes are sometimes also called hair restorers. At present, dyes based on lead, bismuth, copper, iron, nickel, antimony, cobalt and silver salts are in use, with lead preparations being the most popular. These products can only be used to darken graying hair in dark-haired individuals. These dyes are not sensitizers and are safe to use providing there are no abrasions or dermatitis present on the scalp.

Vegetable Hair Dyes

Vegetable rinses, rarely used at present, usually contain natural henna, camomile or synthetic organic hennas, and combinations of henna with copper and pyrogallol. Vegetable hair dyes usually impart only a reddish color and not all hair accepts the henna color. Patients with paraphenylenediamine sensitivity tolerate henna rinses, except those with pyrogallol with which paraphenylenediamine may cross-react. Otherwise, vegetable hair dyes are nonsensitizing. Vegetable rinses are usually combined with other dyes at present.

Miscellaneous Hair Colors

Methylene blue, methyl violet or nigrosine may be used to neutralize yellow discoloration of gray hair and practically never causes dermatitis.

Wigs As a Substitute for Hair Dyeing

Wigs, now widely accepted, are made of natural or synthetic fibers and are available in any desired shade. The paraphenylenediamine-sensitive individual can thereby have a hair covering of any desired color without acquiring dermatitis even though the wig is dyed with paraphenylenediamine, because the oxidized dye is no longer a sensitizer.

PERMANENT HAIR WAVING

This process may be performed either hot or cold. In the rarely used hot method, the hair is treated with an alkaline sulfide preparation and wrapped around a rod. Heat is then applied. In the cold method, an alkaline reducing agent, usually a thioglycolate, is applied without heat. When the satisfactory amount of waving is obtained, the wave is fixed with an oxidizing agent or neutralizer (peroxide, perborate, bromates or citric acid).

Reactions to the chemicals in the process include: (1) pruritic, discrete, papulopustular and vesicular eruption scattered over the back of the scalp, about the ears and about the shoulders, (2) a solitary, deep burn (more common in old-fashioned hot waving and, if deep enough, may cause permanent alopecia) and rarely (3) an eczematous contact dermatitis of the hairline and occasionally the scalp.

Before dermatitis is ascribed to the thioglycolate or alkaline sulfide, in addition to application of these active wave-producing agents, the following steps may have been taken: (1) a preliminary shampoo, (2) use of a cleansing lotion, (3) use of the cold wave material, (4) use of the oxidizing agent or neutralizer, (5) a post-treatment shampoo and (6) application of wave-setting material (gums or resins).

The wave-setting gums or resins and perfumes may cause allergic contact dermatitis, and it is safe to perform patch tests with such agents. The thioglycolate, cleansing lotion, shampoos and oxidizing agents, however, may be primary irritants under covered patches. Allergic reactions to thioglycolate are rare. Patch tests with the sulfides or the thioglycolates are therefore rarely indicated.

Dermatitis from the thioglycolate is usually one of primary irritation and may be prevented with proper precautions. The hairline must be protected with towels. When a burning sensation occurs, the solution should be removed as completely as possible by mopping up any excess. If inflammation of the skin is present, the use of permanent wave solutions must be avoided.

In addition to dermatitis, prolonged application of permanent wave solution may cause fragmentation and splitting of the hair and even temporary baldness due to hair breakage at the scalp. Sometimes, the hair may be weakened in spite of proper use of the solution, particularly if the hair has been previously weakened by chemical bleaching, excessive exposure to sun or frequent shampooing. The patient may be reassured that alopecia is temporary and complete recovery can be expected within several weeks. When a hot waving procedure produces a localized third degree burn of the scalp with scarring, however, the patch of alopecia will persist.[15,16]

Patch Testing with Permanent Waving Solution

Ordinarily, patch tests with the salts of thioglycolic acid are not indicated, because these chemicals are not allergic sensitizers. Positive reactions with thioglycolates under covered patch tests usually are of the primary irritant variety.

Treatment of Dermatitis Due to Permanent Wave Solutions

In the acute phase, primary irritant dermatitis from excess alkali may be treated with wet boric acid compresses. If there are crusting and matting of the hair, soaking with a mixture of olive oil and lime water may be helpful. Shampooing with a mild liquid soap is permitted.

In rare instances the dermatitis following a permanent wave treatment is of the allergic variety. It is usually not caused by the thioglycolate or alkaline sulfide but by gums and resins used to set the wave or by perfumes added to mask unpleasant odors. Occasionally, dyes with sensitizing potential are added to waving preparations for esthetic effects.

Primary irritant dermatitis from thioglycolates causes burning and redness almost immediately on application. On the other hand, signs or symptoms of an allergic dermatitis due to gums, resins, perfumes and coloring agents usually do not appear until at least several hours following treatment.

Hair Breakage

Breakage of hair may occur following the application of a too strong solution of ammonium thioglycolate. For hair waving, the thioglycolates are usually used in a 6 per cent solution at a pH of 8.5 to 9. Beyond a pH of 9, breakage may occur. Alopecia may occur when a solution of the proper strength remains on the hair much longer than necessary or when the hair is too fine or has recently been bleached or dyed. It is due to breaking off of the hair shaft as with a depilatory. Since the hair papillae are not injured, the alopecia is not permanent.

DEPILATORY DERMATITIS

The popular depilatories include the thioglycolates, the sulfides and mechanical depilatories.

Thioglycolates. Calcium thioglycolate in an alkaline medium is one of the most widely used depilatories. The thioglycolate is used in a 2 to 4 per cent concentration in a pH medium of 10 to 12.5. Dermatitis from this agent appears to be less frequent than from sulfide depilatories. Calcium thioglycolate does not have the typical disagreeable hydrogen sulfide odor of the sulfides, but it does not act as rapidly. When it is not properly used, a primary irritant dermatitis may occur. Allergic sensitivity to the thioglycolates is rare.

Sulfides or Sulfhydrates. The sulfides or sulfhydrates of the alkalies or alkaline earths (sodium sulfide, barium sulfide, calcium sulfide and strontium sulfide) are also in fairly wide use as depilatories. In addition, alkaline stannite solutions, dimethylamine and alkaline solutions of salts of mercaptan carboxylic acid, or its homologues, are being used in depilatories. These preparations may be perfumed to hide the unpleasant odor. They soften keratin, are very alkaline in reaction (pH 11) and may act as primary irritants. Allergic sensitivity is rare.

Depilatory Dermatitis Due to the Thioglycolate and Sulfide Dermatitis from the chemical depilatories often presents a localized, inflamed area of skin devoid of hair. The patient usually reveals that the depilatory "stung" on application. A marked follicular reaction with a pustular folliculitis may occur in the affected area.

Mechanical Depilatories. In these depilatories, wax rosins or adhesives mechanically remove hair. The wax rosin depilatory may also contain tarry substances and perfumes. The adhesive type usually contains a plasticized rosin in a fabric, and some also contain benzocaine. Allergic dermatitis from the rosin content, the perfume or the benzocaine may occur.

DERMATITIS FROM MISCELLANEOUS HAIR PREPARATIONS

Hair Tonics. Most hair tonics are a combination of ingredients, which include rubefacients, antiseptics and so-called sebaceous gland "stimulants." The rubefacients commonly used include chloral hydrate, formic acid spirits, quinine and its salts, tincture of capsicum and tincture of cinchona. The rubefacients are primary irritants under a covered patch test.

Phenolic compounds, including halogen and alkyl derivatives, are frequently used as antiseptics in hair tonics. The related phenolic compounds, such as chlorothymol, resorcinol and beta-naphthol, are also popular ingredients. Usually less than 1 per cent of these antiseptics is added to hair tonics, with the exception of resorcinol which may be used in a 5 per cent concentration. Hair tonics containing these phenol compounds must be dispensed in dark bottles because they discolor when exposed to sunlight. The oxidized products are more irritating to the skin and scalp than are the nonoxidized phenols. These compounds are by no means rare sensitizers and may be tested by the covered method in a 2 per cent solution.

Resorcin may occasionally show cross-reactions to *hexylresorcinol.*

Other antiseptics used in hair tonics include *quinine*, *salicylic acid*, *formaldehyde* and *bichloride of mercury*. Of these antiseptics, only salicylic acid is not a sensitizer.

The following, virtually nonsensitizing hair tonic may be tried by individuals who have had difficulty with hair tonics containing irritating or sensitizing ingredients:

Salicylic acid	4.0 grams
Glycerin	4.0 ml
Alcohol 70 per cent q.s. ad.	120.0 ml

Among the materials claimed to stimulate the sebaceous glands are quinine and its salts, tincture of jaborandi leaves, pilocarpine, resorcinol and resorcinol monoacetate, cholesterol, salicylic acid, ethyl alcohol, methyl inoleate, sulfur and lecithin. The sensitizers in this group have been discussed with the antiseptics in hair tonics. The other compounds rarely act as sensitizers.

Bay rum may be used as a vehicle for the active ingredients in hair tonics. The original formula specifies Jamaica rum and oil of bay. Eugenol, one of the main constituents of oil of bay, may be a sensitizer and may show cross-reactions with balsam of Peru.

Perfumes, coloring materials and wetting agents may also act as sensitizers in hair tonics.

Hairsprays. These products are used to set or keep hair in place and are sometimes referred to as liquid hairnets. These sprays are dispensed as aerosols, which are colloidal systems consisting of very finely subdivided liquid or solid particles dispersed in a gas and are self-propellant. The most popular propellant, Freon, is a fluorinated hydrocarbon.

Most modern hairsprays are water soluble and contain polyvinyl pyrrolidine (PVP), which is not a sensitizer. Sprays containing shellac are rarely used at present.

Dermatitis from hairsprays may initially appear on the rims of the ears. Later, the eyelids, forehead, face and neck may become involved.

Hairsprays can produce minute, oval concretions on the hair shaft, which may resemble the nits of pediculosis. Sprays can also produce keratin hair casts, which may be confused with trichonodosis and monilethrix.

Shampoos. Most modern shampoos contain synthetic detergents. It has been suggested that these detergents cause diffuse alopecia in women. Anionic detergents of the alkyl benzine sulfonate type may produce itching of the scalp. Medications, solvents and essential oils, which are sensitizers, may be added to shampoos.

Shampoos may contain preservatives such as the parabens, formalin, phenylmercuric acetate, hexachlorophene, sorbic acid, sodium benzoate, alcohol and a combination of sodium o-phenyl phenate and 3, 5-dimethyl-1, 4-dichlorophenol.

Table 13–1 is a list of shampoos free of formalin.

Miranols. These amphoteric surface active agents are used widely in the cosmetic toiletry and pharmaceutical industries in Britain and the United States.

They are used primarily in hair shampoos (including baby shampoo), hair conditioning lotions, body shampoos (including bubble baths), skin creams and lotions, eye make-up and eyeliner removers, and other cosmetics with surface active agents.

Table 13-1. Shampoos Free of Formalin

Neutrogena (Neutragen A)
Therel (Spence McCord)
Polytar (Stiefel)
Ionil (Owen)

Contact dermatitis due to Miranols is rare, but awareness of these chemicals and their widespread use in the cosmetic industry is important. A patient with an allergic contact dermatitis due to Miranol has been described.[17]

Brilliantines. The liquid brilliantines are based on mineral oil, castor oil and vegetable oils, such as peanut and almond oil. The solid brilliantines and pomades are made of creams containing rosin, waxes and petrolatum. Brilliantines are usually perfumed and colored with azo dyes, which may occasionally cause dermatitis.

Setting Lotions. These preparations may contain lanolin or its derivatives and gums, mucilages or acacia, which occasionally produce allergic contact dermatitis.

Hair Conditioners. These are oily emulsions, which may include beer, eggs, lanolin and its derivatives, cholesterols, waxes, perfumes, preservatives and protein substances.

Hair Bleaches. Hydrogen peroxide is a favorite bleaching agent. Other oxidizing agents used for this purpose include sodium perborate with tartaric acid and ammonium persulfate. Oxidation is speeded up in an alkaline medium, such as ammonia. If care is not exercised, alkaline bleaching agents can cause breakage of the hair and irritant dermatitis. Ammonium persulfate has been reported as producing localized whealing and even generalized histamine reactions with syncope.[18]

Hair Straighteners. All straighteners have only a temporary effect. The simplest preparations consist of petrolatum and paraffin mixtures, which are usually heavily perfumed. Gums and waxes are also used. The use of alkalies, such as sodium hydroxide and thioglycolates, can cause hair breakage. Formaldehyde resins have also been tried without success.

Table 13–2 summarizes the cutaneous reactions to hair preparations.

Nature of Reactions to Hair Preparations

Allergic reactions usually make their appearance initially on the eyelids. The forehead, retroauricular and neck regions also become frequently involved. The fingers used to apply the preparation may be af-

Plate 9. Sensitizers in Cosmetics

1. Face Cream

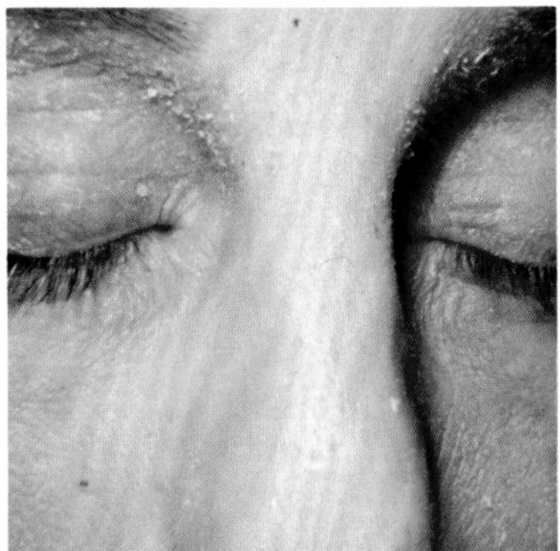

Lanolin

2. Nail Polish

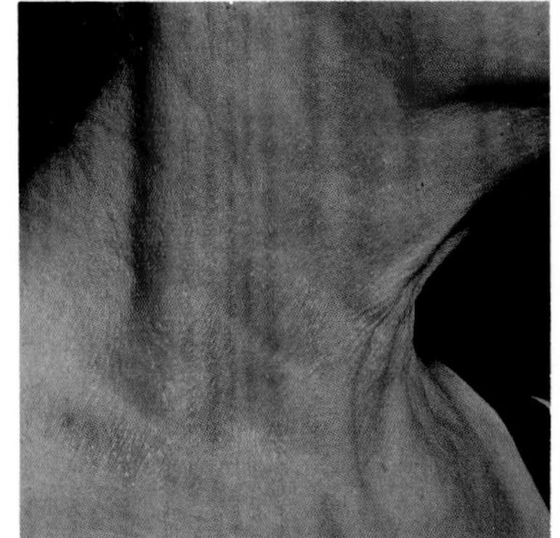

Toluene-sulfonamide Resin

3. Male Deodorant

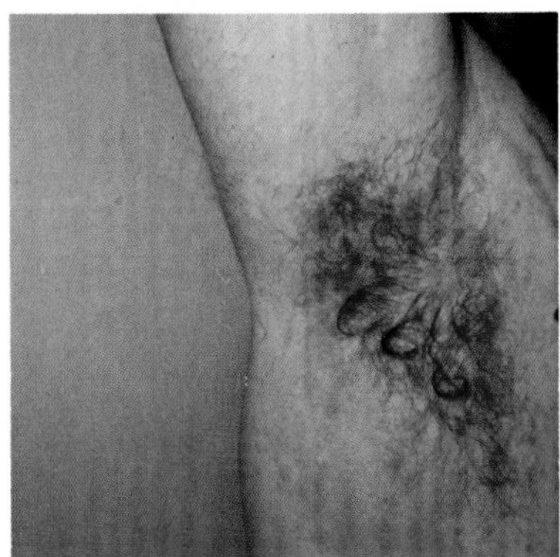

Vitamin E

4. Feminine Hygiene Spray

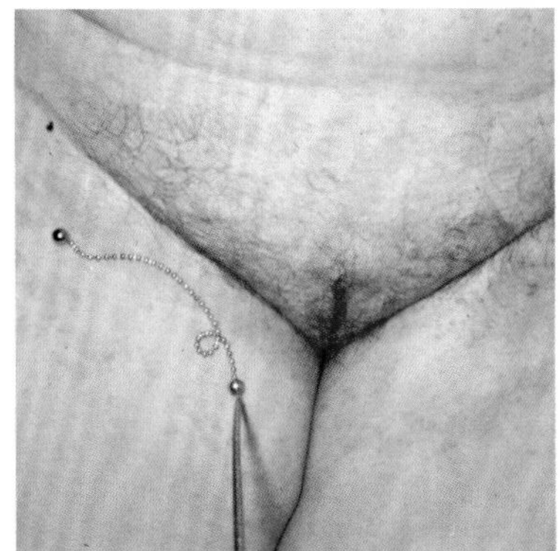

Chloroxylenol

5. Perfume

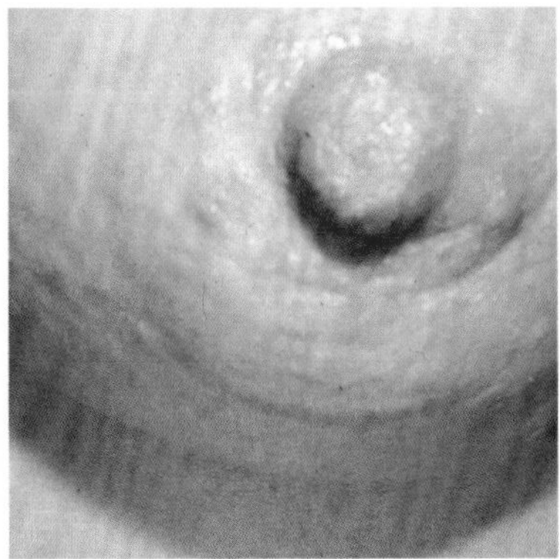

Sandalwood Oil

6. Shampoo

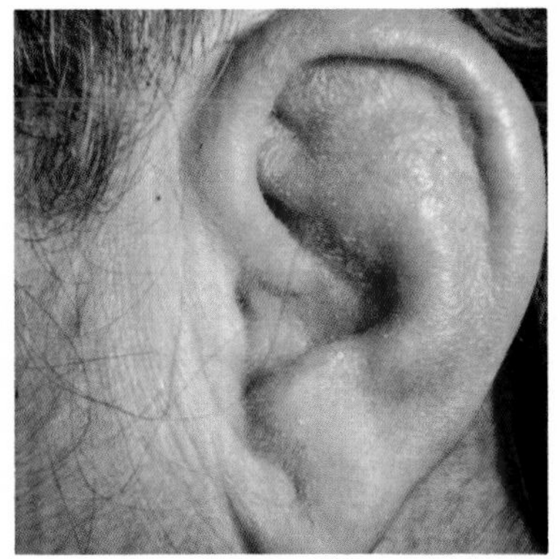

Formaldehyde

Table 13-2. Reactions to Hair Preparations

Hair Preparation	*Ingredient Responsible*	*Irritant*	*Sensitizer*	*Remarks*
Dyes				
Permanent oxidation type	Paraphenylenediamine (PPDA)		X	
Temporary rinses and tints	Azo dyes and other coal tar dyes		X	
Bleaches	Peroxides and ammonia	X		Hair breakage
	Ammonium persulfate			Urticaria and histamine reaction
Permanent wave				
Cold	Thioglycolates	X		Hair breakage
Hot	Alkaline sulfides	X		Hair breakage
Straighteners	Greases and gums			
	Thioglycolate	X		Hair breakage
Sprays	Shellac		X	
	Synthetic resins		X	
Depilatories				
Chemical	Calcium thioglycolate	X		Follicular and pustular reactions
Mechanical	Sulfides	X		
	Sulfhydrates	X		
	Mercaptans	X		
	Waxes and resins	X	X	Follicular and pustular reactions
Tonics and lotions	Cinchona tincture		X	
	Cantharides tincture	X		
	Resorcin		X	
	Perfumes (Bay rum, etc.)		X	
Shampoos	Formalin		X	
	Parabens		X	
	Hexachlorophene		X	
	Miranols		X	
	Mercurials		X	

fected with scaling, fissuring and dermatitis, particularly at the tips. Dermatitis of the scalp occurs with significant skin sensitization, such as that from oxidation hair dyes.

Nonallergic reactions, such as folliculitis and pigmentation along the hairline, may occur from impure mineral oils. Irritation from alkalines, solvents and rubefacients is not rare.

Traumatic alopecia may occur from nylon hairbrushes. Tight curlers and brush rollers may also produce a temporary alopecia.

DERMATITIS DUE TO ANTIPERSPIRANTS

Aluminum Salt Antiperspirants. In the United States, the aluminum salts are the most commonly used axillary antiperspirants. These salts, which include aluminum chloride, aluminum sulfate, aluminum chlorhydroxide and aluminum sulfocarbolate, act as mild chemical irritants, but not allergic sensitizers. Perfumes, preservatives and cream bases, however, may be sensitizers.

Aluminum chlorhydroxide in a 20 per cent solution is present in many antiperspirant preparations and is the least irritating of the aluminum salts and the least damaging to fabrics.

Where axillary dermatitis from an antiperspirant occurs, the patient often solves his own problem by switching to another brand. Some individuals do not tolerate *any* antiperspirant in a cream base, but can tolerate the same product in solutions and sprays. Certain patients who develop dermatitis from aluminum salts in a cream base find the following prescription efficient and well-tolerated:

Aluminum chloride	120. ml.
Isopropyl alcohol up to	60.0 ml.

Aluminum chlorhydroxide, which produces the least acid condition of the skin upon hydrolysis, is not readily available on prescription because most pharmacists do not have it in stock.

Some individuals do not tolerate any effective antiperspirant that is used daily. In such instances, the use of an alcoholic solution of aluminum chloride for a day, alternating with the use of the following medication, may control perspiration without producing dermatitis:

Isopropyl alcohol	12.0 ml.
Calamine and zinc lotion up to	60.0 ml.

Formaldehyde Antiperspirants. Formaldehyde, a potent sensitizer, is used much more widely in Europe as an antiperspirant than it is in the United States. Hexamethylenetetramine, which liberates formaldehyde, is the chemical most frequently used in this type of antiperspirant. It may appear under the following names: methenamine, Formamine, Hexamine, Urotropin, Cystamine, ammonioformaldehyde, Formin, Cystogen and Aminoform.

Hexamethylenetetramine is sometimes used as an accelerator in rubber compounds. I have studied patients who acquired an allergic contact dermatitis due to formaldehyde in an antiperspirant. In several such instances, the axillary dermatitis persisted because of the use of rubber dress shields that also contained a formaldehyde compound.

In general, it is advisable for women with axillary dermatitis to avoid dress shields that contain rubber. Kleinert's Stay-Rite dress shields are free of rubber and may be used in individuals with rubber sensitivity.

Zirconium Salts as Antiperspirants. Zirconium lactate and oxychloride can produce allergic granulomas in susceptible individuals.[19] The use of these zirconium salts in antiperspirants has been discontinued. Antiperspirants containing zirconyl hydroxychloride, however, are currently being used and have not caused granulomas.

Treatment of Axillary Dermatitis Due to Antiperspirants

Axillary dermatitis due to this type of contactant is often prolonged by sweating, friction and maceration. Wet dressings of Burow's solution, 1 part Burow's solution to 8 parts water, may be used in the acute phase. A corticosteroid cream or topical steroid aerosol preparation may be used between applications of wet dressings. The concurrent use of an ointment containing a nonstaining broad spectrum antibiotic, such as erythromycin (Ilotycin), may help to prevent secondary infection and to act as a deodorant while the dermatitis is being treated.

Table 13–3 is a list of cutaneous reactions to antiperspirants.

DERMATITIS DUE TO DEODORANTS

Deodorant sprays for application to the genital area have become popular. The propellant may impart an unpleasant cold sensation. These deodorants may contain antibacterial agents, such as hexachlorophene or benzalkonium chloride, which may act as irritants and rarely as sensitizers. Some cases of vulvitis have occurred.

It is claimed that deodorants mask, reduce, absorb or inhibit the odor of perspiration.[20] The most popular deodorants are said to act by an antibacterial action to prevent decomposition of sweat.[21] The aluminum salts may affect odor both by curtailing sweating and by an antibacterial effect. Many popular deodorant soaps (pHisoHex, Dial) contain the

Table 13-3. Cutaneous Reactions to Antiperspirants

Ingredient Responsible	*Irritant*	*Sensitizer*	*Remarks*
Aluminum salts	X		Folliculitis
Glutaraldehyde		X	
Formaldehyde		X	
Anticholinergics		X	
Zirconium		X	Granulomatous reaction

Table 13-4. Reactions to Axillary and Genital Deodorants

Ingredient Responsible	*Irritant*	*Sensitizer*	*Remarks*
Aluminum salts	X		
Chlorinated phenols (hexachlorophene, G-11)		X	
Benzalkonium chloride	X	X	
Neomycin		X	
Soaps containing tetrabromosalicylanilide Tetrachlorsalicylanilide		X X	Photosensitizer Photosensitizer

chlorinated phenol derivative hexachlorophene (G-11), which has an extremely low index of allergic sensitivity. The quaternary compounds are also used as deodorants and also have a low index of allergic sensitivity but may be irritating.

The oxyquinolenes are sometimes incorporated as deodorants and occasionally produce allergic contact dermatitis and may cross-react with topical medications such as iodochlorhydroxyquin (Vioform) and chlorquinaldol (Sterosan).

Neomycin sulfate has been incorporated into many preparations as an antibacterial deodorant. While intact skin usually tolerates neomycin without difficulty, damaged or eczematous skin may become sensitized to it.

Deodorant soaps containing tribromosalicylanilide or tetrachlorsalicylanilide may cause photoallergic contact dermatitis.

Table 13–4 is a list of deodorants and the irritating or sensitizing ingredients.

Irritant dermatitis of the penis and scrotum may occur in the male sexual partner if the feminine hygiene spray is applied just before intercourse

FEMININE HYGIENE SPRAYS*

Feminine hygiene sprays are composed of an antimicrobial agent, a bland emollient that acts as a carrier for the bacteriostat, perfume and propellant.

* The material on Feminine Hygiene Sprays was obtained from Gus S. Kass, Corporate Director of Research and Development, Alberto-Culver Company, Melrose Park, Illinois.

In the United States, hexachlorophene has been the preferred bacteriostat in most products, although chloroxylenol and methylbenzethonium chloride are used in at least two brands. Chlorhexidine is the antimicrobial agent in several European products. Ljunggren and Moëller reported a case of contact allergy to this agent.[22] The safety of hexachlorophene has recently been questioned by a regulatory agency of the United States Government, and its continued use in feminine hygiene deodorant sprays and cosmetic products in general is in doubt.

There is a wide choice of emollients—the carrier for the bacteriostat and the perfume, which remains on the skin. Among the preferred emollients are fatty esters, such as isopropyl myristate and palmitate, fatty alcohols, including lauryl and myristyle, glycerides and polyoxethylene derivatives of both fatty esters and fatty alcohols. The perfume components must be selected with great care, because some are irritants when applied to mucous tissues. Some deodorant sprays have both a conventional perfume compound and an encapsulated perfume that releases the fragrance slowly over a longer period of time.

The propellants in general use are the fluorinated hydrocarbons and include Propellant II (trichlorofluoromethane), Propellant 12 (dichlorodifluoromethane) and Propellant 114 (dichlorotetrafluoromethane). There is increasing use of mixtures of dichlorodifluoromethane and the hydrocarbon gas—isobutane. More important than for axillary deodorants, the propellant must not impart a chilling effect to the sensitive perineal tissues. A propellant such as trichlorofluoromethane with too low a vapor pressure could be carried in the emollient to the skin where slow evaporation could result in a chilling effect, causing discomfort and transient irritation. If the spray is held too close to the body, even the lower boiling propellants could reach the skin surface, causing erythema and possibly edema. For this reason, the instructions on most sprays caution the user to hold the can at least 6 inches from the area when spraying.

Table 13-5. Ingredients of Feminine Hygiene Sprays

Bacteriostats
Hexachlorophene
Chloroxylenol
Methylbenzethonium chloride
Chlorhexidine
Emollients
Myristates
Glycerides
Polyoxethylene derivatives
Perfumes
Propellants
Fluorinated hydrocarbons

Feminine hygiene sprays held too close to the body may readily cause erythema due to irritation by the propellant. Allergic reactions to the bacteriostat or the perfume may rarely occur

Table 13–5 is a list of ingredients in feminine hygiene sprays.

EYE MAKE-UP AND EYELID DERMATITIS

There are four kinds of eye make-up: (1) eyebrow—make-up applied to the hair of the brow; (2) eyeshadow—make-up applied below the orbital ridge, as well as to the upper and lower eyelids; (3) eyeliner—make-up applied to the lid margins; and (4) mascara—make-up applied to the cilia.

Eyebrow Make-up. Eyebrow products are a mixture of petrolatum and lanolin, paraffin, ceresin or other waxes and mineral oil along with pigments approved by the Food and Drug Administration. Eyebrow pencil is a mixture of waxes, oils and colorings in a casing, and it is used to color the eyebrows. Brush-on eyebrow cosmetics are pressed power mixtures with inert excipients, also used to color brows.

Eyeshadow. The cosmetic used to color the lids may be a cream, liquid, pressed powder or ointment. The ointments are nonaqueous mixtures of waxes and oils that are easily applied, do not easily wash off and form an oily coating. Creams, based upon stearic acid and triethanolamine, or glyceryl monostearate, with water, function as carriers for the pigment mixture. They are easily and smoothly applied and usually do not leave an oily residue. Pressed powder eyeshadow, applied with a soft brush or sponge applicator, consists primarily of talc, often with kaolin and a small amount of oil or aqueous gum as a binder.

Eyeliner. This cosmetic is used to draw a line at the base of the lid and is a suspension of pigments in an aqueous vehicle, which may contain oils. The emulsion may be based upon a hydrophilic glyceryl ester with mild soap or nonionic emulsifiers. Eyeliners can be in liquid, cake or pencil form. Pencil eyeliners are similar to eyebrow pencils but of small diameter.

Mascara. This lash coloring product is sold in cake and liquid forms. Cake mascara is usually based upon triethanolamine stearate soaps with a substantial proportion of carnauba or beeswax to make the film water-resistant. Liquid mascara is an aqueous emulsion with pigment. Water-resistant forms of mascara, in an applicator, consist of synthetic resins dissolved in a hydrocarbon solvent that has a low or intermediate boiling point.

Artificial Eyelashes. These consist of synthetic or natural fibers, including human hair, mounted on a thin fabric strip. The adhesive is a mixture of rubber latex, cellulose gums, casein solubilized with a very mild alkali or other resins and water. The adhesive is formulated to be nonirritating and to permit easy removal of the lashes by simply peeling them off. This rubber latex rarely irritates the eyelids. I have encountered no instances of allergic reactions to it.

Lash Extenders. These are liquid mascaras mixed with nylon or rayon floc (tiny fibers), which adheres to the lashes as the liquid evaporates.

According to the Federal Food, Drug and Cosmetic Act, all cosmetics to be used about the eyes are in a special category. No coal tar colors, even the certified variety, may be used near the eyes. The use of oxidation hair dyes, such as paraphenylenediamine, about the eyes has long been forbidden. Colors employed in eye make-up must be insoluble in water.

The following inorganic pigments and natural colors are most frequently incorporated into eye make-up:

Black:	Carbon black, vegetable or charcoal black
Blue:	Ultramarine or Prussian blue
Green:	Chromic oxide
Brown:	Iron oxide sienna
Yellow:	Iron oxide ochre
Red:	Carmine N.F. (an aluminum lake of cochineal pigment derived from the dried bodies of female insects called cochineals)

There are no reports of allergic sensitivity to these colors, but the vehicles and added perfumes and preservatives may be sensitizers.

Pigmentation of the mucosa of the conjunctival sacs may be related to the use of eye make-up.[23] For example, it may be due to application of eyeliners onto the mucosal edge of the lids so that the product may enter the sac.[24] The pigmentation may persist but is apparently of no significance.

Eyelid Dermatitis and Cosmetics

Cosmetic dermatitis of the eyelids may be caused not only by eye make-up but also by cosmetics used elsewhere and conveyed by the fingers to the eyelids. The extremely thin skin of the eyelids is particularly susceptible to contact dermatitis, particularly from cosmetics. Many hair preparations may produce dermatitis only on the eyelids. Nail enamel sensitivity may be manifested mainly by eyelid dermatitis.

Patch Testing for Eyelid Dermatitis

Patch tests with cosmetics are usually reliable if the dermatitis is allergic in nature, but occasionally the eyelids will react while the thicker skin of the patch test site on the back or extremity will not. Often the patient solves the problem by changing to another brand of cosmetics.

Treatment of Eyelid Dermatitis

In the treatment of cosmetic dermatitis about the eyelids, it is important to avoid irritating or potentially sensitizing substances, such as local anesthetics, antihistamines and preparations containing mercury.

Bathing with ice cold boric acid solution and removing crusts with bland oil, such as mineral or olive oil, are useful.

On the eyelids, it is preferable to use topical medications specified for ophthalmic use, because such preparations are sterile and not irritating to the mucosa.

Eyelid dermatitis often is produced by cosmetics that are not directly applied to the eyelids (e.g., nail enamel)

REACTIONS TO COSMETICS APPLIED TO THE NAILS

Most nail enamels consist of the following ingredients:

1. *A film former*, which is usually nitrocellulose. This chemical is rarely, if ever, a sensitizer. Nitrocellulose may react with resorcin in hair tonics to produce a yellowish discoloration of the nails.

2. *A thermoplastic (toluene-sulfonamide) resin* to improve the gloss and adhesion of the film. Such resin can cause allergic contact dermatitis.

3. *A plasticizer*, which is often dibutyl phthalate. Plasticizers impart flexibility, minimize shrinkage and soften and plasticize the nitrocellulose. Plasticizers are rarely sensitizers.

4. *Solvents*, such as acetates and ketones, to keep the nitrocellulose, resin and plasticizer in the liquid state. These solvents are not sensitizers, but if not permitted to evaporate before the nail enamel is applied under a covered patch test, they may cause false positive irritant reactions.

5. *Coloring substances*, which may be fluorescent or add a frosty appearance. Fluorescent dyes, including eosin, erythrosin, fluorescein and rhodamine B, may cause photosensitizing reactions. Nonfluorescent dyes, such as lithiol red, metanil yellow, bordeaux red and alizarin, are relatively insoluble organic pigments and rarely cause allergic sensitivity. Pearly iridescence is produced by the addition of a suspension of crystalline guanine (2-amino-6-hydroxy purine) obtained from fish scales (such as herring). Dermatitis from this chemical has been reported.[25]

In most cases of dermatitis due to nail enamel, the toluene-sulfonamide resin is the etiologic agent. The plasticizers and the solvents have not been implicated. The pigments and lakes used to color nail enamel are not usually sensitizers, but occasionally a photosensitizing dye may be used. Individuals sensitized to colored nail enamel usually react to the colorless type as well. It may also be the cause of dermatitis about the face and neck in a male.

Nail enamels are synthetic resins that are applied in the partially polymerized liquid state. As the resin dries, it tends to become less of a sensitizer. When completely dry, it is only a very weak allergen. Theoretically, an individual can use a nail enamel to which he is allergic without acquiring dermatitis providing the fingers do not touch the body until the enamel has dried.

In certain hypoallergenic nail enamels, the toluene-sulfonamide resin is replaced by an alkyd resin. Most individuals sensitized to ordinary nail enamel can use it without acquiring dermatitis. Nail enamel that does not contain toluene-sulfonamide resin, however, tends to peel and chip readily. The alkyd resin is a rare sensitizer.

Nail Enamel Dermatitis

Nail enamel dermatitis rarely involves the periungual areas but usually affects the face and neck and eyelids. Any portion of the skin, however, including the vulva, contacted by nail enamel may develop dermatitis in the sensitized individual. Although nail enamel dermatitis usually occurs in small localized patches, occasionally widespread areas may be involved due to "nervous" wandering of fingers with freshly enameled nails. Such extensive dermatitis is sometimes misdiagnosed as neurodermatitis.

Nail biters may develop cheilitis and angular stomatitis from nail enamel sensitivity. The use of nail enamel on stockings to stop runs and on nickel-plated costume jewelry to prevent nickel dermatitis may induce nail enamel dermatitis on the legs or the earlobes of sensitized individuals.

Once the nail enamel is removed, the dermatitis usually clears rapidly unless secondary infection or lichenification has occurred. Corticosteroid creams with or without an antibiotic expedite recovery. The patient should discard all preparations, cosmetics and others, that may have been contaminated with the nail enamel.

Toluene-sulfonamide resin is the most common cause of nail enamel dermatitis. Alkyd resins are substituted in hypoallergenic nail enamels

Patch Testing with Nail Enamel

Patch tests with nail enamel may be performed by the covered or the open method. If the closed method is used, it is wise to paint the enamel directly on the skin and to wait for about 15 minutes to allow evaporation of any volatile solvents. The test site may then be covered. In the rare instances in which photosensitivity to the dye in the nail enamel is suspected because of a history of flaring of dermatitis following exposure to sunlight, it is mandatory to perform an open patch test on an exposed portion of the skin, such as the neck.

Miscellaneous Nail Cosmetics

Nail Enamel Undercoats or Basecoats. To improve the adherence of nail enamel, small amounts of synthetic rubber compounds are incorporated into nail enamel type vehicles. These are applied prior to the application of the nail enamel.

Press-On Nails. These artificial nails, which are fashioned of synthetic resins of secret composition, can produce contact dermatitis and nail damage. Press-On nails are prepared in various shapes and colors and are merely pressed onto the natural nail. Such nails differ from acrylic nails, which have to be molded and "built-up" by the user.

Nail Hardeners. Several preparations of this type formerly contained formaldehyde, which produced dermatitis and onychia[26] and, in nail biters, produced hemorrhages of the lips.[27]

Acrylic Nail Preparations. So-called artificial fingernails have been advocated for people with short or dystrophic nails and for those who bite them. This plastic formulation, essentially the same as for acrylic dentures, is marketed under names such as Gro-nail and Glamour nail. The preparation consists of a liquid monomer (methyl methacrylate) and powder polymer (polymethyl methacrylate) to be molded onto the natural nail.

The acrylic liquid and powder used in artificial nails polymerize and harden at room temperature. These self-curing acrylic resins are created by inducing polymerization of the mixture of monomer and powder with an organic peroxide and an accelerator or promoter. The self-cured resins are not as hard as those polymerized at high temperature, and they normally contain a higher residual monomer content. Nevertheless, these resins can be fashioned into excellent artificial nails, which remain intact for several weeks.

Methyl methacrylate liquid monomer is a

Table 13-6. Reactions to Nail Preparations

Nail Preparation	*Ingredient Responsible*	*Irritant*	*Sensitizer*	*Remarks*
Nail enamel	Toluene sulfonamide resin		X	
Nail enamel removers	Solvents	X		Nail dystrophy
Artificial nails	Acrylic monomer		X	Onychia and paronychia
Nail hardeners	Formaldehyde		X	

potent sensitizer and can cause allergic contact type of eczematous reactions on the skin and the oral mucosa.[28] As predicted, the acrylic nail preparation produces many instances of allergic contact dermatitis of the skin. In addition, extremely painful onychia and paronychial reactions occur.[29] Treatment of onychia is complicated by the fact that once the acrylic nail has hardened it is practically impossible to remove it. The throbbing, swollen, painful nail is encased in a rigid plastic armor. Ice cold compresses may afford some relief, and strong sedation may be necessary for several days. Systemic corticosteroid therapy is indicated if there are no contraindications.

The dystrophic changes of the nails caused by a reaction to the acrylic monomer may persist for several months. In one instance, one year elapsed before the nails returned to normal.

Because of numerous instances of reactions to these acrylic nail preparations, few products of this type are marketed.

Swinger-Tips ("instant nail polish") are made of acrylic resins but are essentially monomer-free. No reactions have so far been reported.

Table 13–6 summarizes reactions to nail preparations.

LIPSTICK CHEILITIS

Lipstick may be regarded as more than a beauty aid, because it protects the lips from the effects of sun, wind and cold, preventing drying and chapping and possibly cancer of the lip.

The various types of lipstick are listed in the following glossary.

Lipstick Glossary

Lipstick . . . . Colored wax and oil compound in stick form, in a swivel base, used to color, lubricate and protect lips.

Sheer lipstick. . . . . A modification of lipstick that excludes indelible dyes and produces a transparent color.

Frosted lipstick . . . . Essentially the same formulation as lipstick with the addition of a pearlizing agent to impart a lustrous, frosted look to the lips.

Medicated lipstick . . . . . . Compounded with or without coloring agents, these sticks have a petrolatum, mineral wax and oil base with emollient oils. They may contain menthol, hexachlorophene and a sunscreen.

Lip gloss . . . . Usually in jars, but sometimes in tubes, these contain the same ingredients as lipstick, but usually less wax and more oil.

Lip cream . . . . A mixture of oils that melt on contact with skin similar to night creams or moisturizers.

Lip brush . . . . A brush to trace a sharp outline for the application of lipstick.

Lip pencil . . . . A colored wax mixture in wood casing for the same purpose as the brush.

Lip primer. . . . . A stick, similar to lipstick, but containing less wax, to soften the lips and serve as a base for lipstick.

Sensitizers in lipstick include perfumes, lanolin derivatives, cocoa butter and indelible dyes, such as the bromofluorescein and eosin groups. Lipsticks can produce not only cheilitis but also eyelid dermatitis

Cinnamon-flavored lipstick may produce cheilitis; in such instances cross-reactions may occur with balsam of Peru.

Lipstick Colors. The colors are mixtures that may contain natural pigments, synthetic coal tar colors and halogenated fluorescein derivatives that stain the lips and give the lipstick permanence or indelibility.

The indelible dyes used in lipstick may be photosensitizers, producing cheilitis in susceptible individuals upon exposure to sunlight. In addition, indelible lipstick may initially impart a feeling of dryness to the lips due to the use of thinner oils than in non-indelible varieties.

Cheilitis from lipstick usually appears a week or more after a new type of lipstick is used. It may, however, suddenly develop from a lipstick the patient has used for a long time without difficulty. The cheilitis usually takes the form of dryness and fissuring of the lips, particularly the vermillion border. Rarely does vesiculation or edema occur. A history of cheilitis following exposure to sunlight would tend to implicate an indelible dye if the permanent type of lipstick was being used.

Patch Testing with Lipstick

Lipstick should be tested by both open and closed methods. The site of open testing should be exposed to bright sunlight if possible. If this site is positive and the covered one negative, one concludes that a photosensitizing dye is the cause of the dermatitis.

Testing with the patient's lipstick is unreliable for the detection of eosin sensitivity. Eosin binds with keratin and the amount present in an ordinary lipstick is too small to saturate the keratin and allow eosin to penetrate through the horny layer. This is overcome by increasing the concentration of eosin to 50 per cent in a standard lipstick base or in petrolatum, and by rubbing the lipstick or eosin stick directly on the skin, thus ensuring that an adequate amount is applied. Patch testing with the patient's lipstick is always done to detect sensitivity to other components of the lipstick.

Recent refinements of eosin and lipstick dyes have reduced cheilitis from these sources

DERMATITIS FROM CREAMS, POWDERS AND ROUGE

Face Creams. Perfumes, lanolin, emollients, emulsifying agents or preservatives may be sensitizers in these cosmetics. Hormone creams containing diethylstilbestrol may produce dermatitis with cross-reactions to monobenzylether of hydroquinone.[30] Some vanishing creams are sufficiently alkaline to produce an irritant dermatitis.

Bleach Creams and Other Skin Lighteners. Ammoniated mercury from 1 to 5 per cent in ointment form is probably one of the most universally used skin lighteners. Red mercuric oxide, calomel and bichloride of mercury are also occasionally used. Allergic sensitivity to these compounds is by no means rare.

Irritation reactions, exfoliation and follicular discolorations may result from mercury creams. These preparations may also produce a grayish pigmentation of the nails. These inorganic mercurial compounds may cross-react with organic mercurials such as mercurochrome, merthiolate and mercurial diuretics.

Monobenzylether of hydroquinone, as in Benoquin Ointment and Lotion (Elder), has been applied to lighten hyperpigmented skin. In my experience, about 5 per cent of the individuals who use this compound acquire allergic contact dermatitis.

Hydroquinone, available in Eldoquin (Elder) and Artra Cream (Artra Cosmetics), is also used as a skin lightener. It appears to be less of a sensitizer than monobenzylether of hydroquinone with which it sometimes cross-reacts. Some individuals, however, are allergic to only one of these agents.

Lemon juice, citric acid, salicylic and trichloroacetic acids, which are sometimes used to bleach freckles, may be primary irritants but not sensitizers.

Bleach and freckle creams, besides containing the active depigmenting agent, may also contain perfume, lanolin, cocoa butter or almond oil, any of which may produce contact sensitivity.

Powders. Allergic reactions to modern face powders are usually traced to perfumes. Dusting powders containing antiseptics may be sensitizers.

Rouges. Modern rouges contain pigments and lakes in liquid suspensions, emulsions and creams. These colors do not bleed, are lightfast and practically never cause allergic dermatitis, although the preservatives or perfumes might.

Irritants and sensitizers in face creams include lanolin, lanolin alcohols, sulfated alcohols with sodium lauryl sulfate, preservatives (parabens, phenylmercuric acetate) and perfumes. Cosmetic dermatitis may be confused with dermatitis produced by medicated facial tissues

Facial tissues impregnated with urea-formaldehyde resins or benzalkonium chloride may produce facial dermatitis that mimics cosmetic dermatitis.

ROLE OF COLOR IN COSMETIC DERMATITIS

Practically all cosmetics contain some coloring material, which consists of dyes, pigments or lakes.

Cosmetic Dyes. Hair dyes, such as paraphenylenediamine, which require oxidation are more potent sensitizers. Azo dyes or synthetics used in rouges, powders, lipsticks and nail enamels may also occasionally cause allergic sensitization. Indelible dyes, such as acid eosin, bromo acid or fluorescein, used in certain lipsticks and nail enamels may be photosensitizers.

A certified cosmetic dye may be a sensitizer. Certification of a dye by the Food and Drug Administration simply means that the substance is not a primary irritant or a toxic substance and is free from carcinogenic properties.

Pigments. These colors used in cosmetics consist of colored or white chemical compounds that are insoluble in a particular solvent. The inorganic color pigments widely used in cosmetics include iron oxides, carbon blacks, ultramarine blues and pinks, chrome oxide green and a number of white pigments, such as purified titanium dioxide, zinc oxide, aluminum hydrate and gloss white. These inorganic pigments are not sensitizers and may be used freely even about the eyes.

Only occasionally are natural pigments of animal or vegetable origin, such as saffron, chlorophyll and carotene, used in cosmetics. These vegetable colors are practically free of sensitization potential. Carmine, a red pigment from the ground bodies of the cochineal insect, is rarely used in cosmetics, and it is very infrequently a sensitizer. A dye may be referred to as a pigment when it is used in an insoluble preparation.

Aside from hair dyes, the largest volume of colors used in cosmetics are the insoluble pigments, both certified organic and non-certifiable inorganic types. The organic and inorganic pigments may be mixed in the cosmetic, and these insoluble products practically never cause allergic sensitization.

Lakes. The term *lake*, when used in the context of cosmetics, usually refers to an organic pigment prepared by precipitating a soluble dye. Although the soluble dye may be a sensitizer, the precipitated lake is usually not one.

Occasionally, the color chemist uses the term *toner* to refer to an organic pigment that is used full strength in contrast to a lake, in which the diluent and the substratum are essential. Toners, like lakes, rarely cause allergic dermatitis.

The lakes, D and C, Red X, 31, D and C Red No. 19 and Barium Lake D and C Orange No. 117 produce allergic reactions when used in cosmetics, particularly lipstick.

PERFUMES AS A CAUSE OF DERMATITIS

There are approximately 5000 odoriferous substances in use today. The approximate concentration of perfume oils used in cosmetics generally is 0.5 per cent, in colognes and toilet water 4 per cent and in perfumes as much as 20 per cent. A complete perfume compound may consist of 10 to more than 60 basic components in three basic classifications: *natural products* from flowers, plants, roots, herbs, woods and gums; *animal products* and their extractives; and the *aromatic chemicals*, which usually account for as much as 90 per cent of the perfume compositions. A recent Russian study[31] implicated 14 perfumery substances as causes of allergic reactions.

Pinpointing a specific perfume oil as the sensitizer is a formidable task. Certain perfumes are both sensitizers and photosensitizers; others are solely photosensitizers. Patch tests with perfumes must be done not only by the usual closed patch test method, but also by the open method with exposure to light. Photosensitization is associated with a number of essential perfume oils, especially bergamot, lavender, cedarwood, neroli and petitgrain.

Gum benzoin and balsams may be added to perfumes to retard evaporation. Such fixatives may on rare occasions be sensitizers.

Clinical Appearance of Perfume Dermatitis. The extent of the dermatitis depends on the individual's pattern of application of the perfume. Some women apply the perfume only behind the ears; others apply the scent to widespread areas of the skin. Dermatitis from perfume in cosmetics, such as face creams and powders, tends to be diffuse; that due to perfumes or toilet water tends to be "streaky." Perfume dermatitis of the antecubital area may resemble atopic dermatitis.

Berloque Dermatitis. Photosensitizers of the psoralen group present in perfumes may produce photosensitization dermatitis characterized by pigmentation at the sites of application of the perfume and exposure to sunlight. Such pigmentation is usually sharply localized. If the perfume is applied with the fingers, the pigmentation will have the outline of a fingertip. The resulting pigmentation usually gradually disappears within 3 months.

Berloque dermatitis may have to be differentiated from chloasma, Riehl's melanosis and the melanosis due to exposure to oils and petrolatum.

Urticaria. In rare instances, contact with perfumes or even the inhalation of perfume may produce urticaria.

Table 13–7 is a list of 20 perfumes of 180 compounds tested that the Food and Drug Administration found most frequently involved in adverse reactions, but not necessarily of the allergic variety. This list shows the frequency of occurrence for major perfumery compound identified in investigational and complaint samples of cosmetic and perfume products.

Table 13-7. Perfumes Causing Adverse Reactions: Analysis of 138 Samples (1968-1972)

Beta-phenyl ethyl alcohol
Diethyl phthalate
Linalool
Alpha-terpineol
Geraniol
Benzyl alcohol
Citronellal
Coumarin
Benzyl acetate
Isoamyl salicylate
Hydroxy citronellal
Piperonal
Methyl ionone
Eugenol
Limonene
Caryophyllene
Cis-beta-terpineol
Alpha-methyl ionone
Menthol

Continued Use of Sensitizing Perfumes. Occasionally a patient may be permitted to use a favorite sensitizing perfume with precautions. For example, a photosensitizing perfume may be tolerated provided it is applied behind the ears or on skin not exposed to sunlight. Similarly, perfumes producing allergic contact dermatitis may often be used safely providing it is applied to the clothing or hair in such a way that there is no contact with the skin.

Chemoderms (Firmenich) in Cosmetics. Certain cosmetics may bear labels stating that they are perfumed with Chemoderm. The manufacturer describes a Chemoderm as "an especially prepared perfume for use in cosmetic, pharmaceutical, or proprietary products where the highest regard for human dermatological safety is of prime concern. These Chemoderms are carefully prepared, standardized, reproducible perfume compositions of individual aromatic chemicals and/or carefully controlled isolates of natural materials."

The Chemoderms have been reported as being relatively safe perfumes for widespread use by the public.[32] Chemoderms are available to manufacturers of cosmetics, pharmaceuticals and proprietary preparations, but not to individuals.[33]

Benzyl salicylate[34] and phenylacetaldehyde,[35] which are used in the manufacture of perfumes, recently have been shown to be sensitizers.

A positive patch test reaction to balsam of Peru, benzyl salicylate or phenylacetaldehyde may be diagnostic of perfume dermatitis

COSMETIC DERMATITIS IN MALES

The principal causes of cosmetic dermatitis in men are the following:

Self-heating shaving cream
Oxidation type hair dyes (Metallic dyes rarely sensitize)
Adhesives for hairpieces
Photodermatitis due to antibacterial soaps
Perfumed lotions and quinine in hair tonics
Sunscreens
Clear nail enamel

Other causes from toiletries include antiperspirants and deodorants.[36]

Self-Heating Shaving Cream.[37] The self-heating shaving cream has a patented valve for precise mixing of two components as they leave the container. When the nozzle is pressed, the hydrogen peroxide mixes with the pyrimidine reductant in an exothermic reaction (150 °F).

A clue that there may not always be a proper mixture of the oxidizing agent and the reductant is the warning on the aerosol can: "Do not use if the lather appears watery or soupy." Also, the label states, "The foam from the last couple of shaves will not heat up. This signals time for a new can." It is our contention that when "mismetering" occurs or when the shaving cream applied is watery or will not heat up properly, the unoxidized pyrimidine compound, or possibly the hydrogen peroxide, may produce primary irritant reactions.

The four chemicals in self-heating shaving cream capable of producing dermatitis include the pyrimidine reductant, triethanolamine (a stabilizing chemical in the soap), sodium alkyl sarcosinate (a surfactant) and hydrogen peroxide. These four compounds are very rare sensitizers but can irritate the skin in certain concentrations. In addition, some pyrimidine compounds and some medications possibly related to triethanolamine are photosensitizers.

Shaving Creams and Lotions. Brushless shaving cream is essentially a vanishing cream to which a lubricant has been added. It forms an oil-in-water emulsion. Chromic acid or chromates are added to prevent rusting of razor blades. Aerosol shave cream, which is basically a solution of soap, is the most popular type.

Allergy to after shave lotions is usually due to the perfumes used. In one instance, however, quinine was the allergen. Irritation from the alcohol used must be differentiated.

Hair Dyes. Men who gradually darken their hair with metallic hair dyes practically never acquire dermatitis. Those who use paraphenylenediamine for immediate and permanent coloring may more readily acquire allergic dermatitis.

Antibacterial (Deodorant) Soaps. For some reason, men acquire photodermatitis from such soaps much more readily than do women.

COSMETIC PIGMENTATION

Pigmentation may result from use of photosensitizers such as tar, dyes (e.g., eosin) or the essential furocoumarin plant oils (e.g., psoralens) found in bergamot oil. These substances increase melanin production and sensitize the skin to higher levels of the tanning range of ultraviolet light.

Facial pigmentation can be caused by any perfumed cosmetic. Most cosmetics contain some scent: perfumes up to 2 per cent, eau de cologne 5 per cent, cologne sticks 2.5 per cent, sachet cream 1 to 10 per cent, general cosmetics 0.5 per cent, soaps 0.2 to 2 per cent, deodorants 0.25 per cent, shampoos 0.25 per cent, sunscreens 0.25 per cent and baby lotions and powders 0.1 to 0.25 per cent.

Three types of facial pigmentation are ascribed to perfumed cosmetics: (1) berloque dermatitis; (2) diffuse melanosis of areas of the face and neck to which face cream is applied and which is increased by massage; and (3) mottled pigmentation of the face. Differential diagnosis of the pigmentation includes chloasma of pregnancy, ovarian-uterine disorders, flat pigmented nevi, Riehl's melanosis and nomelanotic pigmentations such as argyria from eyedrops with silver salts. Orange coal tar dyes used in face powders, as well as depigmenting agents containing mercury, have also caused pigmentation.

THE TERM HYPOALLERGENIC AS APPLIED TO COSMETICS

Aside from paraphenylenediamine hair dyes, preparations containing formaldehyde or its resins, and cosmetics containing photosensitizers, the bulk of cosmetics in general use are hypoallergenic, since such products have been carefully screened before being marketed. Ingredients causing reactions are soon withdrawn from the market. The term *hypoallergenic* has, therefore, very little meaning, since practically all manufacturers follow the generally accepted definition of the term.

A fair appraisal of hypoallergenic products is made by Spoor[38] who stated:

> A number of companies cater to the specific problems of the allergic woman and aid her in solving her particular cosmetic problem through her allergist or her dermatologist. Where this is so, the term "hypo-allergenic" is meaningful, and a function of value is performed. However, where such products are sold generally to the public, no significant difference exists between such products and those marketed by reputable cosmetic manufacturers. In actuality, the allergenicity in cosmetics thus distributed has been reduced to the minimum.

There are no hypoallergenic oxidation type hair dyes. There are hypoallergenic nail polishes. Manufacturers of hypoallergenic cosmetics are most helpful in solving a cosmetic problem

COSMETIC FORMULA INFORMATION

Cyril H. March, Chairman of the A.M.A. Committee on Cutaneous Health and Cosmetics, in an editorial[39] on cosmetic formula information made the following statement:

> Information concerning the ingredients of cosmetics is essential to the proper medical care of patients who are allergic to or irritated by one or more of the constituents of these products. The incidence of irritant or allergic reactions is small. Nevertheless, for those affected and for the physicians treating them, the problems of avoiding reexposure to the causative agent(s) are large.
>
> Identifying the offending product is helpful but does not suffice. What is accomplished if the patient switches to a new brand only to encounter unknowingly the same provoking ingredient?
>
> With a knowledge of the qualitative formula, a physician is in better position to carry out the specific diagnostic procedures that will identify the allergen. Since the patient's cosmetic needs and desires have not changed, the physician is then able to prescribe specially formulated cosmetic products or suggest products that are free of the specific allergen involved.
>
> Since few cosmetic labels provide any clues as to the ingredients present, and since formula information has not been readily available, this lack of information has sometimes been an obstacle to proper care of the patient.
>
> Labeling cosmetics with qualitative formulas presents many difficulties; however, a list of ingredients for a large number of cosmetics is available now through several sources of information.
>
> Poison control centers throughout the country provide information on ingredients used and concentration data. The Public Health Service will send, on request, a directory of poison control centers throughout the United States. Write Public Health Service, 1875 Connecticut Avenue NW, Washington, D.C. 20006.
>
> If no information is on file with the nearest poison control center for the particular product of interest, the center can usually provide the names of responsible scientific personnel, in the companies involved, who can supply the needed information (often around the clock).
>
> A second source of cosmetic formula information, both general and specific, is Gleason

et al.'s reference work entitled *Clinical Toxicology of Commercial Products* (Williams and Wilkins Co., Baltimore, $24.50). This publication also includes for some firms a listing through which formula information for products not listed in the book can be obtained.

While some firms may not desire to disclose formula information, they will often supply coded samples of the ingredients of a given product so that the physician can conduct patch tests on his patient. The firms will then identify the sensitizing ingredient.

It does not appear likely at this time that a central product and formula registry is practical since there is a high rate of new product marketing accompanied by an almost equally high rate of attrition. Also the formulas of a few products remain unchanged over great periods of time. Many changes in formulas are trivial (e.g., colors in lipsticks and nail polishes) and follow the dictates of fashion.

Therefore it seemed best to use the already-established data supply system of PHS poison control centers and to attempt to improve and enlarge the data.

The A.M.A. Committee on Cutaneous Health and Cosmetics has brought the need for the availability of formula information to the attention of the Scientific Advisory Committee of the Cosmetic, Toiletry and Fragrance Association. The cooperation of the cosmetics industry has been promised, particularly toward expanding the information presently available; the C.T.F.A. and the A.M.A. have agreed to publicize the availability of the sources of this information and to improve its scope and coverage.

This program is clearly of individual benefit to the patient concerned. Since it also enables one to identify the more common allergens, there is a benefit to both industry and the consumers from the avoidance of such allergens in the formulation of new cosmetic products.

In the event that a physician is unable to obtain the cosmetic formula information he needs for the proper care of his patient, the Committee on Cutaneous Health and Cosmetics stands ready to assist him.

REFERENCES

1. Kanof, N. M.: Cosmetic—A Definition in Law. Cutis, *6*, 527, 1970.
2. Sagarin, B. (ed.): *Cosmetics, Science and Technology.* New York, Interscience Publisher, Inc., 1957.
3. Wells, F. V., and Lubowe, I. I.: *Cosmetics and the Skin.* New York, Rheingold Publishing Co., 1964.
4. Middleton, A. W.: *Cosmetic Science.* London, Butterworths Scientific Publications, 1959.
5. Harry, R. G.: *Cosmetics: Their Principles and Practices.* New York, Chemical Publishing Co., 1956.
6. Schwartz, L., and Peck, S. M.: Cosmetics and Dermatitis. New York J. Med., *60*, 1940, 1960.
7. Spoor, H. J.: Establishing Efficacy of Dermatologicals to Support New Drug Applications. J. New Drugs, *5*, 127, 1965.
8. Laymon, C. W.: Cutaneous Reactions to Cosmetics and Related Substances. Minn. Med., *43*, 4, 1960.
9. Masters, B. J.: Allergies to Cosmetic Products. New York J. Med., *60*, 1934, 1960.
10. March, C. H., and Fisher, A. A.: Cutaneous Cosmetic Reactions. GP., *31*, 89, 1965.
11. Cronin, E.: Contact Dermatitis From Cosmetics. J. Soc. Cosmet. Chem., *18*, 681, 1967.
12. Schorr, W. F.: Allergic Skin Reactions from Cosmetic Preservatives. Amer. Perfum. Cosmet., *23*, 64, 1970.
13. Baer, R. L.: Cross Sensitization Phenomena. In MacKenna: *Modern Trends in Dermatology.* Second Series, 232–257. New York, Paul B. Hoeber, Inc., 1954.
14. Fisher, A. A., Pelzig, A., and Kanof, B.: The Persistence of Allergic Eczematous Sensitivity and the Cross-Sensitivity Pattern to Paraphenylenediamine. J. Invest. Derm., *30*, 9, 1958.
15. Lehman, A. J.: Health Aspects of Common Chemicals Used in Hair Waving Preparations. J.A.M.A., *141*, 842, 1949.
16. Reiches, A. J., and Lane, C. W.: Temporary Baldness Due to Cold Wave Thioglycolate Preparations. J.A.M.A., *144*, 305, 1948.
17. Verbov, J. L.: Contact Dermatitis from Miranols. Trans. St. John Hosp. Derm. Soc., *55*, 192, 1969.
18. Calnan, C. D., and Shuster, S.: Reactions to Ammonium Persulfate. Arch. Derm., *88*, 18, 1963.
19. Shelley, W. B., and Hurley, H. J.: Allergic Origin of Zirconium Deodorant Granulomas. Brit. J. Derm., *70*, 75, 1958.
20. Blank, I. H., Moreland, M., and Dawes, R. K.: The Antibacterial Activity of Aluminum Salts. Proc. Sci. Sec. Toilet Goods Assoc., *27*, 24, 1957.
21. Shehadeh, N. H., and Kligman, A. M.: The Effect of Topical Antibacterial Agents on the Bacterial Flora of the Axilla. J. Invest. Derm., *40*, 61, 1963.

22. Ljunggren, B., and Moëller, H.: Eczematous Contact Allergy to Chlorhexidine. Acta Dermatovener., *52*, 308, 1972.
23. Jervey, J. W.: Mascara Pigmentation of the Conjunctiva. Arch. Ophthal., *81*, 124, 1969.
24. Brauer, E. W.: Personal communication.
25. Stritzler, C.: Dermatitis of the Face Caused by Guanine in Pearly Nail Lacquer. Arch. Derm., *78*, 252, 1958.
26. March, C. H.: Allergic Contact Dermatitis to a New Formula to Strengthen Nails. Arch. Derm., *93*, 720, 1966.
27. Huldin, D. H.: Hemorrhages of the Lips Secondary to Nail Hardeners. Cutis, *4*, 709, 1968.
28. Fisher, A. A.: Allergic Sensitization of the Skin and Oral Mucosa to Acrylic Denture Materials. J.A.M.A., *156*, 238, 1954.
29. Fisher, A. A., Franks, A., and Glick, H.: Allergic Sensitization of the Skin and Nails to Acrylic Plastic. J. Allergy, *28*, 84, 1957.
30. Fregert, S., and Rorsman, H.: Hypersensitivity to Diethylstilbestrol: Cross-Sensitization. Acta Dermatovener., *40*, 206, 1960.
31. Gutman, S. G., and Somov, B. A.: Allergic Reactions Caused by Components of Perfumery Preparations. Vestn. Derm. Vener., *42*, 62, 1968.
32. Klarmann, E. G.: Perfume Dermatitis. Ann. Allergy, *16*, 425, 1958.
33. Osbourne, R. A., et al.: Dermatological Evaluation of Perfumes of Low Sensitizing Index. Proc. Sci. Sec. Toilet Goods Assoc., *17*, 80, 1956.
34. Rothenborg, H. W., and Hjorth, N.: Allergy to Perfumes from Toilet Soaps and Detergents in Patients with Dermatitis. Arch. Derm., *97*, 417, 1968.
35. Fregert, S.: Sensitization to Phenylacetaldehyde. Arch. Derm., *141*, 11, 1970.
36. Lazar, P.: The American Male and Dermatologic Reactions to Cosmetics. Cutis, *6*, 511, 1970.
37. Fisher, A. A., and Fine, H.: The Nature of Self-Heating Shaving Cream Dermatitis. Cutis, *6*, 516, 1970.
38. Spoor, H. H.: Skin Reactions to Cosmetics. New York J. Med., *60*, 1940, 1960.
39. March, C. H.: Cosmetic Formula Information. Editorial. J.A.M.A., *216*, 1337, 1971.

14

Dermatitis Due to Plants and Spices

Most of the dermatitis-producing plants belong to a limited number of families, and many of the plant sensitizers that have been isolated also appear to belong to closely related chemicals, such as catechols and lactones.

Many cases of plant dermatitis are occupational. The poison rhus group (ivy, oak and sumac) produces many instances of both occupational and nonoccupational dermatitis. In Europe, Primula obconica (primrose) is the principal cause of nonoccupational plant dermatitis.

In the United States, the poison ivy group produces most cases of both occupational and nonoccupational plant dermatitis, whereas in Europe, Primula obconica is the principal cause of plant dermatitis

Sex Distribution of Plant Dermatitis. Even among city dwellers, ragweed dermatitis occurs almost exclusively in men. Primula dermatitis occurs principally in women. Poison rhus reaction occurs equally in both sexes and at all ages.

Plant Sensitizers. The most recent development in the study of plant dermatitis has been the isolation of specific chemicals that are the sensitizers. It is hoped that these chemicals will become useful in hyposensitizing procedures.

Sesquiterpene Lactones. Mitchell and his coworkers[1,2] have shown that such lactones are the allergens responsible for allergic contact dermatitis caused by ragweed (Ambrosia), sneezeweed (Helenium), sagebrush, wormwood and mugwort (Artemisia), boneset (Eupatorium), poverty weed (Franseria), marsh elder (Iva), cocklebur (Xanthium), burdock (Arctium), chamomile (Anthemis), artichoke (Cynara), Gaillardia, and Chrysanthemum species (tansy, feverfew and pyrethrum).

The presence of an alpha-methylene group exocyclic to the gamma-lactone appears to be the immunochemical requisite for such dermatitis. For patch test purposes, Mitchell now uses Alantolactone 0.25 per cent in petrolatum.

Sesquiterpene lactones appear to be the specific sensitizers in chrysanthemum, pyrethrum, ragweed and other weeds

Similar lactones have been implicated as the sensitizers in Frullania, a genus of liverworts. Like ragweed dermatitis, many cases of Frullania dermatitis occur in males. Mitchell[3] has also reported that Frullania dermatitis may be due to usnic acid, which is derived from lichenized fungi. Such dermatitis occurred only during work in forest areas and was worse in wet weather. These cases may represent multiple sensitization to usnic acid, lichen chemicals and lactones.

Calnan[4] reported on two patients who developed allergic contact dermatitis from incense cedar wood (Libocedrus decurrens) used in pencils. The allergen was thymoquinone. Calnan stated there are at least 8 different cedar woods, belonging to several species, and that the terms *cedar wood dermatitis* and *cedar poisoning* are inaccurate.

Various other plants, including trees, grasses, flowers, vegetables, fruits and weeds as well as air-borne pollens can produce contact dermatitis. The term *dermatitis venenata* is usually applied in such cases.

Plant dermatitis may be classified as allergic sensitization, mechanical irritation, chemical irritation, phytophotodermatitis and pseudophytodermatitis.

The plant substances reponsible for dermatitis do not enter directly into the metabolism of the plant and are classified as secondary products. The relative proportion of these secondary products depends on vigor of growth, cultural conditions and the stage of development of the plant. Thus the amount of ragweed oleoresin increases tenfold when the plant pollinates and is at the height of growth.

Contact with certain uninjured plants may produce allergic dermatitis; other plants must be crushed to release dermatitis-producing chemicals

Another factor that may be of clinical significance is the distribution of the dermatitis-producing substances in the plant. For example, primin, the antigenic substance of the primrose, is stored in fragile cells in superficial glandular hairs and is released by casual contact. In contrast, the sensitizing substance in some daisies is stored in resin canals and released only when the plant is bruised or crushed.[5] In some plants, the sensitizers may be in the leaves and stem; in others they are found, in addition, in the flowers, pollen and roots.

ALLERGIC SENSITIZATION TO PLANTS

Most cases of plant dermatitis are the result of allergic hypersensitivity, which is dependent on immunological changes induced by previous contact with the same plant or with a closely related species.[6] Certain plants are such potent sensitizers that brief contact is sufficient to produce sensitization in a considerable proportion of those exposed. This is true for poison ivy. Sensitivity may develop within 7 to 10 days of first contact or only after many years of exposure. No plant can be dismissed as a cause of dermatitis solely because the patient has long handled it with impunity.[7]

Other plants that are fairly common sensitizers include the following:

Ambrosia. These include both giant and dwarf ragweed.

Dictamnus albus. The gas plant (fraxinella, burning bush and dittany) is a photosensitizer.

Family Compositae. The members of this family that are sensitizers include chrysanthemums and daisies.

Family Liliacae. This group consists of the tulip, hyacinth, asparagus, garlic and onion.[8]

Family Amaryllidacae. Here are included the daffodil and narcissus.

Family Umbelliferae. Carrots, celery and wild parsnips are members of this group.

Family Cannabinaceae. This family of nettles includes hops.

Family Rutaceae. The sensitizers in this family include the orange, lemon and grapefruit.

PLANT SENSITIZERS

The sensitizing substances of many plants are present mainly in the oleoresin fraction. In a few plants, the allergens are water-soluble glucosides or other aqueous fractions.[9]

Oleoresin Fraction. This fraction consists of a mixture of substances, including essential oils, terpenes, resins, phenols and camphors. The potency and amount of oleoresin increase as the growth of the plant becomes more vigorous. The oleoresin may be present throughout the plant and in the pollen. When the pollen is freely air-borne, contact dermatitis occurs without one touching the plant. In ragweed dermatitis, the contact is usually from such pollen.

Essential Oil Fraction. This fraction of oleoresin contains most of the sensitizing substances so far identified. Essential oils ordinarily occur in localized regions of the plant, e.g., predominantly in the flowers (lavender), leaves (eucalyptus), bark (cinnamon), wood (sandalwood) and peel (citrus fruits).

An essential oil is a volatile, nongreasy, nonsaponifying oil with a characteristic odor, which is obtained from plants or plant constituents by distillation. Accidental contact with the oleoresin essential oils may occur when the plant is crushed or bruised.

More than 500 compounds have been identified in essential oils. These compounds may be classified into 5 main groups:

1. Phenols and aromatic alcohols and aldehydes
2. Terpenes
3. Aliphatic and aromatic esters
4. Substituted benzene hydrocarbons (including the mustard oils)
5. Quinones

The term essential in essential oils refers to the presence of perfume essences

Of special interest to the dermatologist are phenols, aromatic alcohols and aldehydes, and terpenes. The phenols include dihydric phenols, plus catechols, resorcinols and hydroquinones. The catechols and related compounds are the sensitizing substances in the rhus (poison ivy) plants and other members of the Anacardiaceae family, which include the marking nut tree of India, the Japanese lacquer tree, the mango and the cashew nut.[10] Since the rhus plants cause most cases of allergic plant dermatitis in the United States, this group is considered separately at the end of this chapter.

Substituted Catechols. These substances, including eugenol and vanillin, are occasionally sensitizers. Eugenol is used in dentistry and is present in cinnamon oil, oil of cloves, some perfumes and soaps, and bay rum.

More complex substituted catechols are now appearing in industry. The p-tertiary butyl catechol, for example, is used in duplicating papers, in paint, in rubber manufacture, in the oil industry, and as an oxidation catalyst in the manufacture of polyester and polystyrene resins.

The chemical 2-methoxy-6-n-pentyl-p-benzoquinone is the major allergen of primrose.[11] Other plants and woods contain allergenic quinones that show cross-sensitivity to primin. This assumption is supported by the finding of a coincidence between positive reaction to Primula obconica leaf and rosewood extract.

Oranges. This fruit may be treated with ethylene gas and biphenyl, a mold retarder. In addition, the azo dye (Citrus Red 2) may be used for the peel of Florida oranges, but not those from California (J. C. Mitchell, personal communication, 1972). This azo dye is a rare sensitizer, which may be tested as 2 per cent in acetone.

The outer layer of orange peel consists of numerous oil-containing cells from which can be expressed an oil of limonene, other terpenes, linalool and a resinous residue. The natural coloring is mainly hesperidin and carotene. The terpene limonene is probably the principal sensitizer of orange peels.

Patch tests with the orange peel may lead to primary irritant reactions.

Florida oranges are dyed with Citrus Red 2, an azo dye

Lemons. This fruit may produce dermatitis in sensitized individuals because of lemon oil, which contains terpenes (limonene).[12] Allergic dermatitis may also occur in carpenters from contact with lemon wood and sawdust. In addition, an irritant dermatitis may occur in waiters and bakers from contact with citric acid, which also has been implicated in the production of aphthous ulcers.

Turpentine (Diptene). Turpentine is the concrete oleoresin (balsam) from species of pines. The irritant and sensitizing potentials vary from country to country. An individual who is sensitized may show cross-reaction with balsam of Peru, benzoin, ragweed oil, chrysanthemum and pyrethrum. The most commonly used products containing turpentine include varnishes, sealing wax, paint thinners and dry cleaning materials. Freshly distilled turpentine is less antigenic than turpentine that has been stored and become oxidized. The principal sensitizer in turpentine is a carene; pinene and limonene may be less potent sensitizers.[13]

Table 14–1 is a list of common sources of exposure to turpentine (Dr. O. Jillson, personal communication).

Terpenes. These substances are sensitizing agents in dermatitis caused by citrus fruits, celery and turpentine. Terpenes or their derivatives are present in other plants, such as chrysanthemums, and plant products, such as resins and balsams.

Table 14-1. Sources of Exposure to Turpentine

Polishes: automobile, metal, porcelain and metal, shoe, stove, silver (dip type), wood and furniture
Preservatives: paintbrush, wood
Repellants: bird
Waxes: general purpose, paste
Fertilizers
Cosmetics: liquid soaps, soap powders, bath oils, emollient creams, hair tonics, hand lotions, lilac and lily of the valley perfumes, talcum powders, suntan preparations
Cleaners: metal, general purpose
Insecticides: products with pine oil, tree sprays, dairy stock sprays, and preparations for dog and cat fleas and lice, floral garden pests, grubs, mites, moths, thrips, ticks, flies and aphids
Mange treatment
Deodorizers: cleanser type
Degreasers
Liquid starch
Paints: including anticorrosion paints
Solvents and thinners: for paints, dry cleaners and so forth
Varnishes, shellacs and lacquers
Stains and finishes
Terpineol: solvent for resins
Dutch Drops (Haarlem Oil): proprietary remedy for colds and fever
Any cleaning, cosmetic or painting product having a pine odor
Over-the-counter topical medications: Minard Liniment, Sloan's Liniment, Johnson's Anodyne, Mentholatum, Penetro Analgesic Rub, Cloverine Salve and Vicks Vapo Rub
Substances that may cross-react with turpentine: ragweed, burwood marsh elder, chrysanthemum and pyrethrin (found in disinfectants, insecticides, fungicides, soil conditioners, wood preservatives, repellents, dog and cat soaps)

In discussing the terpenes, D. S. Wilkinson (personal communication, 1970) stated that, in addition to carbohydrates, proteins and glycerides, plants contain oily substances, which are insoluble in water. Many of these essential oils are terpenes, but oils of wintergreen, aniseed and mustard are not.

The true terpenes (e.g., limonene, pinene and camphene) are hydrocarbons with the molecular formula $C_{10}H_{16}$; their alcohols, aldehydes, ketones and other related compounds are equally important and widespread (e.g., menthol and camphor).

The function of terpenes in the life of the plant is not known; they may attract or repel insects or may be waste products of metabolism. Their precursors in nature are also unknown, though two possibilities are leucine and certain carbohydrates.

Camphene is solid, but the other true terpenes are liquids, boiling between 155 and 185°C. They have strong, not unpleasant smells, and are volatile in steam.

Geraniol, $C_{10}H_{17}OH$, is a straight chain terpene alcohol. It occurs in many Indian grasses and as a glucoside in Pelargonium odorantissimum.

Citral, $C_9H_{15}CHO$, is the aldehyde of lemon grass oil.

Citronellol, $C_{10}H_{19}OH$, is an alcohol in rose oil and geranium oil. It is also a glandular secretion of the alligator.

Linalool, $C_{10}H_{17}OH$, has many botanical sources, e.g., oil of linaloe.

MONOCYCLIC TERPENES. These compounds always have 1 ring in the molecular structure.

Myrcene, $C_{10}H_{16}$, is an open chain hydrocarbon with 3 double bonds and is found in oil of bay and oil of hops.

(+) *Limonene* is found in lemon oil, oil of neroli, dill and bergamot, oil in orange peel, caraway oil and celery seed oil.

(−) *Limonene* is found in spearmint and pine needles.

Cineole occurs in wormseed oil, cajeput oil, eucalyptus oil and rosemary.

Phellandrene occurs in elemi oil, ginger grass oil, oil of cinnamon and bitter fennel oil.

(−) *Phellandrene* occurs in eucalyptus oils, pimento oils, Canada balsam oil and Japanese peppermint oil.

(+) *Phellandrene* occurs in water fennel oil and lemon oil.

Carvone, $C_{10}H_{14}O$, is a constituent of dill and caraway oils.

(−) *Menthone*, $C_{10}H_{18}$, which occurs in oil of peppermint, is a liquid.

(−) *Menthol*, $C_{10}H_{19}OH$, occurs in peppermint oils and Japanese mint oil.

DICYCLIC TERPENES. These compounds, $C_{10}H_{16}$, always have one 6-membered ring, a second closed chain, and one olefinic link.

Alpha-pinene is the principal constituent of oil of turpentine, which is obtained from members of the order Coniferae.

(+) *Camphor*, $C_{10}H_{16}O$, occurs in the camphor laurel and in feverfew oil.

Camphene occurs widely in nature, particuularly the (−) form, which is found in the oil of Abies sibirica.

Borneol, $C_{10}H_{17}OH$, occurs in many oils, such as pine oil.

Resins and Balsams. These plant products may be sensitizers. Balsams are similar to resins but are secreted following injury to the plant. Resins are acidic substances occurring either as amorphous vitreous solids or in solution in essential oils. Some are phenolic derivatives, but others are polymerization and oxidation products of terpenes. The residue remaining after distillation of crude oil of turpentine is rosin or colophony, which consists mainly of abietic acid and 1-pinearic acid. Some resins are plant exudations containing mixtures of true gums, oils and resin. *Asafoetida* is an example of such an exudation from Oriental plants of the carrot family.

Balsam of Peru. This viscid fluid has an odor resembling cinnamon or vanilla and is extracted from a tree native to El Salvador. Balsam of Peru contains 30 to 40 per cent of resins of unknown composition; the remaining 60 to 70 per cent, which is "cinnamein," consists of well-known simple chemicals, mainly benzyl benzoate, benzyl cinnamate, cinnamic acid, benzoic acid and vanillin. It also contains essential oils similar to those in citrus fruit peel. Sensitivity to balsam of Peru may extend to vanilla and cinnamon.

Balsam of Peru contains benzoate and may cross-react with vanilla and cinnamon. A reaction to balsam of Peru may indicate perfume sensitivity

Balsam of Tolu, Styrax (Storax) and Benzoin (Gum Benzoin). These resins are chemically related to balsam of Peru by their content of coniferyl alcohol esters of benzoic acid or cinnamic acid. Cross-reaction may occur between the various balsams.

Spott and Shelly[14] reported the case of a student who developed acute eczematous dermatitis in response to the application of tincture of benzoin to the skin under a cast. This was followed within 48 hours by the appearance of generalized noneczematous exanthem. The conclusion was that absorption of benzoin through the skin was responsible for both reactions. Patch tests demonstrated an eczematous reaction to benzoin, with cross-sensitivity extending to the gums of myrrh, locust, galbanum, gamboge and olibanum (frankincense).

Styrax is a balsam derived from the trunk of the trees Liquidambar orientalis and L. styraciflua. Mitchell (personal communication, 1972) observed a patient with allergic contact dermatitis from styrax in a Canadian topical preparation (Masitol).

PLANT DERMATITIS DUE TO MECHANICAL IRRITATION

Mechanical irritation may be produced by spines, thorns and specialized bristles and hairs. The large or small wounds produced by such mechanical irritation may be complicated by bacterial or fungous infection, particularly sporotrichosis. Many grasses and cereals, including barley, millet, rice and bamboo, have sharp trichomes, which may produce urticarial papules in workers handling crops or litter straw. Dogwood has t-shaped hairs, which may produce urticaria when the leaf is rubbed on the skin in the direction of the hairs.

Many European herbs of the borage family are covered with coarse, stiff hairs, which can produce an irritant dermatitis. Certain tropical plants, including palms and cacti, have spicules, which may also produce dermatitis.

The prickly pear cactus has barbs (glochidia), which can enter the skin producing a dermatitis resembling scabies. Covered parts of the body may be secondarily affected through the transfer of the broken-off barbs from primarily affected sites. In Israel, harvesting the pears of this plant produces an occupational hazard called sabra dermatitis.[15] Mechanical removal of the barbs is difficult. Peeling ointments or salicylic acid plasters may be used to bring about exfoliation of the skin with the embedded barbs.

PRIMARY IRRITANT DERMATITIS DUE TO PLANT CHEMICALS

Chemical irritation may occur from contact with fluids or crystals in either specialized hairs or other portions of the plant.[16]

Plants may injure the skin by direct chemical action. No allergic mechanism is involved, and if the degree of exposure is sufficiently great, a reaction is provoked in everyone so exposed. Variation in susceptibility is attributed to anatomical factors, notably, the thickness of the horny layer, and to climatic factors, which favor or impede the penetration of the irritant substances. Primary irritant dermatitis is particularly common in children.

Some plants have irritant hairs; others have caustic juices that are powerful primary irritants

Aside from irritant hairs, many plants contain chemicals that are strong primary irritants.

The *buttercup* is an important irritant plant.[17] It contains an unsaturated lactone, *protoanemonin*, formed by the breakdown of a glucoside in injured plants. Children chewing the leaves or stems of the injured plants may acquire blisters on the face and around the lips.

Certain members of the *daisy* family may also produce an irritant bullous eruption when crushed on the skin.

Cactus-like plants (spurges) of South Africa contain a copious milky latex in their stems, which has strong caustic properties. The *manchineel tree* of the West Indies and certain vegetables, such as tropical *gourds* and *cucumbers*, contain a juice that can irritate the skin.

Plants of the *mustard* and *radish* family contain the glucoside *sinigrin*, which is harmless in the dry state, but is converted into the irritant volatile oil of mustard in the presence of water.[18]

Pineapple juice contains *bromelin*, a proteolytic enzyme that can cause a primary irritant dermatitis.[19] The enzyme causes separation of the superficial layers of the skin and increases skin and capillary permeability. These effects resemble the mechanical damage produced by needle-shaped calcium oxalate crystals of tulip bulbs. Both the enzyme and the crystals produce itching and increased permeability of capillaries with the formation of wheals, which are suggestive of histamine liberation in the skin.

The tropical plant *Mucuna pruriens* (itch plant) is a member of the bean family. It does not occur in the United States, but it grows wild in all tropical areas. Short, barbed spicules cover its seed pods. The active itch-producing principle of the plant is a proteolytic enzyme named *mucunain*,[20] which is the principal ingredient of the "itch powder" employed by practical jokers.

PHYTOPHOTODERMATITIS

Photosensitization contact dermatitis due to plants is caused largely, if not entirely, by photosensitizing compounds related to furocoumarin.[21] Two requisites for the initiation of phytophotodermatitis are contact with a sensitizing furocoumarin in the juice of the plant, and subsequent exposure to ultraviolet radiation of wavelengths greater than 3200 Å (usually sunlight). All individuals sufficiently exposed to the plant are susceptible, because a phototoxic and not an allergic mechanism is involved.[22]

The families of plants containing the furocoumarins that can produce phytophotodermatitis include the following:

Umbelliferae: parsnip, fennel, dill, parsley, carrot, masterwort, celery, atrillal, angelica
Rutaceae: common rue, gas plant, lime bergamot, lime
Moraceae: fig
Ranunculaceae: buttercup
Cruciferae: mustard
Convolvulaceae: blin weed
Rosaceae: agrimony

Compositae: yarrow
Chenopodiaceae: goose foot
Leguminosae: bavachi
Hypericaceae: St. John's wort
Frullania: liverworts

Somner and Jillson[22] reported that the wild parsnip and gas plant readily cause photodermatitis in the northeastern United States. These authors could not produce photodermatitis with the buttercup or wild carrot.

Meadow grass dermatitis (dermatitis bullosa striata pratensis) is a phototoxic eruption produced by contact with wild parsnip and other vegetation and exposure to sunshine. A network of crisscross, striate bullae, resembling poison ivy dermatitis, is produced. The lesions develop 12 to 24 hours after the plants have been crushed on the skin and there has been subsequent exposure to sunlight. If the skin is moist, the photodynamic effect is enhanced. The bullae soon heal, leaving marked pigmentation, which may persist for many months. (See also chapter on photodermatitis.)

PSEUDOPHYTODERMATITIS

Pseudophytodermatitis is an eruption that appears to be due to plants, but in reality is produced by arthropods infesting the plants. Dyes and waxes applied to the skin of citrus fruits and plant insecticides may also produce a pseudophytodermatitis.

Pseudophytodermatitis Due to Mites

Grain Itch Mites. Pediculoides ventricosus is the North American itch mite. It feeds on various insect larvae that infest wheat, barley, rye and other grain straw and beans. The mites attack man, especially persons sleeping on straw mattresses, and may produce a generalized eruption consisting of petechiae, wheals, vesicles and pustules.[23]

Farmers, harvesters, chaff cutters, handlers of old hay, strawboard factory workers, millers, bakers, packers, unloaders and persons working in grain elevators or places where grain and straw are handled may become infested with grain itch mites.

Frequent bathing and change of clothing may prevent infestation when there is massive exposure to the mites. The wearing of clothing impregnated with benzyl benzoate may be effective. Prophylactic use of Kwell or Eurax is beneficial.

Food Mites. Tyroglyphus farinae, the flour mite, may infest not only grain stores, mills and bakeries, but also food in homes. Contact with the food produces a papular dermatitis.[24]

Tyroglyphus siro, the cheese mite, infests not only cheese but also dried fruit, sugar, roots, bulbs and copra. Grocer's itch, a pruritic papular eruption, is produced in persons handling these infested plant products. Cheese mites do not suck blood, but their migration under superficial scales of the epidermis produces pruritus and an eruption that is difficult to distinguish from that of allergic contact dermatitis.

Cheese mites have been controlled by painting the cheese with paraffin and by wiping or dipping cheese blocks with mineral oil, cotton seed oil or glycerin. Good packaging to prevent the mites from obtaining entrance to the food is important for prevention of infestation.

Mites and caterpillars on plants may be the causes of "plant dermatitis" known as pseudophytodermatitis

Miscellaneous Mites. Barley itch usually occurs in dock workers unloading barley infested with food mites. Baker's itch occurs among workers in granaries, flour mills and bakeries, particularly in small establishments that do not use mechanical processes and have few sanitary arrangements to destroy mites.

Individuals handling cotton seed in bulk may acquire a mite rash known as cotton seed itch. When the seeds are handled in bags, dermatitis does not occur. The mite in cotton seed is related to Pediculoides ventricosus. Bulb mite itch is contracted by individuals who store infested bulbs above their beds on shelves or in attics; these persons, while asleep, are attacked by the mites.[25,26]

Bakers, workers in sugar refineries or

chocolate candy factories, and those who can and pack fruits and syrups may acquire a "contact" dermatitis from the sugar mite.

Dried fruits may be infested by the mite Carpoglyphus passularum. Sorters, peelers and packers of infested prunes may acquire a follicular, papular eruption. Women sorting partly damaged dates may also be affected. Dock laborers and workmen engaged in shoveling figs for a jam factory have developed dermatitis produced by a fruit mite. A mite found on dried beans can produce dermatitis in workers handling these legumes.

Pseudophytodermatitis Due to Contact with Poison Hairs of Caterpillars[27,28]

Outdoors, exposure to caterpillars is not uncommon. In the home, caterpillars may crawl into clothes and bedding. Fomites infested with caterpillars may produce dermatitis for long periods, even in cold storage. Caterpillar dermatitis is an occupational disease in plantation workers.

Dead larvae and cocoons of caterpillars as well as debris from infested pine forests can cause dermatitis. Caterpillar dermatitis, therefore, may occur throughout the entire year. The eruption is caused by microscopic hairs containing a toxin that produces lesions in all individuals exposed. An entire community may suffer from urticaria epidemica due to caterpillars.

This type of dermatitis usually appears as an urticarial, papular eruption, but vesiculation and even necrosis may also occur. Nodular conjunctivitis and severe damage to the eyeball are serious complications.

Pseudophytodermatitis Due to Dyes

Certified azo dyes applied to the skin of oranges and grapefruits rarely cause dermatitis.

Pseudophytodermatitis Due to Waxes

Carnauba wax, from the South American palm, is used to wax oranges and is an ingredient of shoe, furniture and automobile polishes, cosmetic creams, lipsticks and solid perfumes. This wax may produce allergic contact dermatitis.[29]

Plant Insecticides

Various plant insecticides, including arsenical sprays and malathion, can produce contact dermatitis, which may initially be diagnosed as plant dermatitis.

DERMATITIS DUE TO POLLENS

Dermatitis from plant pollens, particularly that of ragweed, is a fairly common cause of plant dermatitis.[30] The shell of the pollen grain contains the allergen, a resin-like material. Reactions occur mostly in farmers, gardeners, carpenters, salesmen, field workers and others who work out of doors and have prolonged contact with pollen-bearing plants.[31]

The typical seasonal appearance is often masked because of the secondary lichenification and infection, which prolong the duration beyond the pollen seasons. In persons who have the dermatitis throughout the year, however, a careful history reveals that exacerbations occur during the pollen seasons. Often such cases masquerade as a neurodermatitis.

Pollens may contain 2 distinct antigens: (1) a protein fraction causing asthma or rhinitis and (2) an oleoresin producing contact dermatitis

The principal sites of pollen dermatitis are the exposed surfaces, namely, the face, neck, V area of the chest, arms and legs. This pattern is always suggestive of an air-borne dermatitis. Pollen dermatitis is usually subacute, but vesiculation may be found on the areas where pollen grains have adhered. The diffuse and even distribution of the eruption is attributed to the coalescing of minute individual papules produced by the grains of pollen.

Aside from the oleoresin, an aqueous protein fraction in pollen may produce asthma, hayfever and occasionally atopic dermatitis.[32] Rarely is there both an immediate urticarial sensitivity reaction (due to the protein fraction) and a delayed eczematous sensitivity reaction (due to oleoresin) to the pollen. In some patients, exacerbations of atopic dermatitis in the summer, aside from those due to humidity and sweating, are thought to be caused by inhalation of plant pollens.

Air-borne pollen dermatitis with marked involvement of the exposed areas may resemble a photosensitivity dermatitis due to plants, drugs or topical substances. Lesions on exposed areas due to simple pollen dermatitis, without photosensitivity, usually are not as sharply demarcated from normal skin as in the case of a photosensitizing dermatitis, because the pollen grains often get inside the collar and extend the dermatitis to the upper part of the chest and shoulders. Similarly, pollen grains may get inside trousers and affect the legs and even the inguinal area and genitals. Such involvement under the clothes may help differentiate simple pollen dermatitis from photosensitivity reactions. It must be remembered, however, that certain pollens, particularly ragweed, are photosensitizers as well as causes of dermatitis venenata.[33]

Ragweed dermatitis may mimic a photodermatitis

RAGWEED OIL DERMATITIS

The oleoresin that produces ragweed dermatitis is present in the pollen and the stem and leaf of the plant. Ragweed pollen has two chief components: an inner core containing the water-soluble protein fraction, which may produce allergic rhinitis or asthma, and an outer portion, which is oil-soluble and can produce allergic contact dermatitis in the sensitized individual at the time of ragweed pollination.[34] Ragweed oil dermatitis and ragweed hayfever are unrelated entities caused by different antigens of the ragweed plant. Most individuals with ragweed oil dermatitis are *not* atopic and do *not* have ragweed rhinitis or asthma.

Sensitized individuals may acquire dermatitis also by contact with the stem or leaves of the ragweed plant in the spring or summer, even before pollination takes place. In most instances, however, ragweed oil dermatitis is due to contact with air-borne pollen when the plant is at maximal growth and its oleoresin is most concentrated.[35]

Men are much more commonly affected than women in a ratio of about 20:1. Dermatitis due to air-borne pollen is seasonal, initially lasting from August to the first frost. As the patient advances in age and as the seasonal exposures continue, the dermatitis may begin in June and extend to December.

The early, uncomplicated case usually involves the face, particularly the eyelids, the sides of the neck, the sternal area and the extensor region of the arms. The dermatitis is often sharply limited by a protective undershirt. In chronic cases, it may extend to involve the trunk, groin and lower extremities and become so widespread that it resembles a generalized erythroderma. Spontaneous remissions of ragweed oil dermatitis are rare, but even the untreated patient may show variations in severity.[36]

The patient who is sensitive to ragweed oil may have associated allergic contact hypersensitivity to pyrethrum, chrysanthemum and turpentine.[37]

DERMATITIS DUE TO FLOWERS AND DECORATIVE PLANTS

Many varieties of wild and cultivated flowers may cause dermatitis.[38]

Chrysanthemum. Chrysanthemums, asters and daisies all belong to the same family of plants. Most of these flowers can produce dermatitis under certain conditions. Chrysanthemums are the most common offenders, and the resulting dermatitis usually appears in the late fall and early winter—the blooming season. Since the blooms emit a pollen, the eyelids may be the first areas involved. Many sensitized individuals also have facial involvement. Widespread chrysanthemum dermatitis is not uncommon. The diagnosis may be confirmed by a patch test. Patients who react to one species of chrysanthemum may react to others as well. For example, cross-reactions may take place with arnica, an aster.

Philodendron. This plant is widely used for interior and patio decoration. Contact dermatitis from several species, especially Philodendron cordatum, has occurred.[39] Hands and arms are usually involved. Exposure takes place when the patient washes, oils or plucks the leaves. Since the plant grows indoors, there is no relationship of the dermatitis to a particular season. A patient may have numerous attacks of dermatitis, which are not readily diagnosed.[40] Dieffenbachia, a common house plant closely related to philodendron, may also cause dermatitis.

Decorative plants such as philodendron may produce allergic contact dermatitis

Algerian Ivy. This plant may be used as a ground cover. The history usually reveals that the patient cut the ivy a day or so before the onset of the dermatitis.[41,42]

English Ivy. A dermatitis may be caused by the leaves, stems and even the roots of this ornamental plant. The lesion sometimes resembles a rhus eruption.[43]

Oleander. Dermatitis results when crushed leaves of this plant come into contact with the skin of persons who have become sensitized by previous exposure. Often children playing near shrubs are affected. Oleander poisoning due to eating the leaves also occurs, primarily in children. Since oleander is not deciduous, it may produce dermatitis at any time of year. Patch testing confirms the diagnosis.

Castor Bean. Dermatitis may occur at any time of year when there is exposure to the juice of the leaves or stems of the plants or to the beans. Castor oil extractors, fertilizer workers and farmers may acquire occupational dermatitis from handling the plants or the beans. The beans are poisonous when ingested.

Primrose Family. There are many varieties of primrose plants, any of which may cause dermatitis. The most frequent offender is Primula obconica, a common house plant in England.

Lilies. Lily rash is a papular, pruritic eruption with most severe involvement on the face, hands and forearms. Those affected are usually engaged in cutting, bunching or packing daffodils and narcissi.

Chinese Rice Paper Plant. This popular ornamental shrub may cause severe dermatitis. The toxic substance is present in a heavy yellow pollen produced in the fall and winter.

Phacelia crenulata. This plant is known as the desert or false heliotrope. It blooms profusely in March and April in the desert areas of southern Utah, New Mexico, Arizona, southeastern California and Baja peninsula. The plant produces an eruption similar to that of poison ivy dermatitis.[44]

Miscellaneous Flowers and Shrubs. Less commonly, dermatitis venenata is produced by dichondra, magnolia, tea roses, greasewood, Wigandia caracasana, daffodils, poinsettias, Ficus repens, century plants and Australian silk oak trees.[45,46]

Weed dermatitis may be confined to the hands as in milker's eczema due to weed oleoresin contaminating cows or winter fodder mixed with weeds

Tulips. These bulbs may cause a painful, dry, fissured and hyperkeratotic eczema under the free margin of the nail that extends to the fingertips and periungual region because of friction and trauma during peeling of the bulbs. The allergen of tulips is most highly concentrated in the bulbs; less is found in the stems, and the least is in the petals.

For patch testing, the epidermis of the bulb is used after the brown skin has been removed. The allergen is a lactone, which is split off the plant glucoside.[47]

Narcissus and Hyacinths. Dermatitis from these plants may be the allergic type, but it is usually an irritant reaction to bundles of needle-shaped crystals of calcium oxalate in the outer layers of the bulbs. These do not occur in tulip bulbs. The outer scales of hyacinth bulbs contain about 6 per cent calcium oxalate, and the dust on work tables has

Tulip bulb fingers may be due to trauma or an allergic reaction to a specific lactone. Narcissus and hyacinths produce "bulb fingers" mostly due to irritation from calcium oxalate crystals

a similar concentration. The crystals penetrate the skin and cause a dermatitis resembling fiber glass dermatitis. Itching can be abolished by washing with dilute acetic acid. Hyacinth itch is thus rarely of allergic origin.

DERMATITIS DUE TO TREES

Trees may contain irritants or sensitizers in the bark, wood or pollen.

Irritation Dermatitis. Sawdust and fragments of wood produced by machine tools can cause contact dermatitis. The severity depends on whether the cut fragments are hard or soft, dry or moist. As a rule, the dermatitis from cut wood is transitory and superficial.

Allergic Dermatitis. In the United States, the native woods that are cutaneous sensitizers include acacia, alder, ash, beech, birch, chestnut, cedar, elm, maple, mesquite, oak, pine, poplar, prune and spruce.

The major components of wood, such as cellulose and lignin, are not sensitizers, but the minor components, such as resins, terpenes, oils, phenols, formic acid and nitrogen-containing substances, may cause allergic contact dermatitis. In addition, certain species of poplar contain a glucoside that may be a primary irritant.

Freshly cut woods are more apt to cause a dermatitis than are older woods, but Rengas wood, used in furniture-making, may produce dermatitis only when it is old and begins to disintegrate.

Birch bark contains a fine powder on its inner aspect, which can produce a follicular acneiform eruption by mechanically plugging the follicles of exposed skin.

Tropical Woods. Working with tropical wood may result in inflammations of the oral mucosae and the respiratory system as well as acute contact dermatitis, especially of the face and extremities. The condition often occurs in persons who are exposed to high concentrations of fine sawdust. Exotic woods seem to be the most sensitizing. Obeche wood may cause contact urticaria. Teak and mansonia contain sensitizing quinones.

Some tropical woods contain quinones, which are strong sensitizers

Suskind[48] pointed out that other types of dermatitis that have been mistakenly called wood poisoning include bacterial and fungal infections, seborrheic and atopic dermatitis, and contact dermatitis from common weeds, such as poison oak. In addition, chemicals sprayed onto the wood and agents such as chloronaphthalenes impregnated into wood for protection may cause dermatitis.[49]

These woods are used in musical instruments, in boat construction, in furniture and as handles for kitchen utensils.

Fig and rubber trees, belonging to the Ficus genus of plants, contain a milky sap, which is commonly called latex. Fig tree latex may produce both allergic dermatitis and photodermatitis. Rubber latex rarely sensitizes.

Latex from other trees, such as gutta percha, chicle and balata gum, rarely cause dermatitis.

The fruit of the female ginkgo tree may produce an allergic dermatitis simulating poison ivy dermatitis.[50]

Tree Pollens. Contact dermatitis may be caused by ether-soluble portions of tree pollen oleoresin. Like ragweed oil dermatitis, tree pollen oil dermatitis is usually, in the beginning at least, confined to a short season during which the pollen is air-borne. The history usually reveals that the skin becomes clear after the pollination has ended and remains clear until the following season. Individuals sensitized to the oil fractions of the pollen, which produce allergic contact dermatitis, may not be sensitized to the aqueous protein fraction, which produces allergic rhinitis and asthma.[51]

Beekeepers can acquire an allergic contact dermatitis from bee glue (propolis) derived mainly from poplar and other tree resins.[52,53] This glue is also used as a local anesthetic in Russia. In Africa, it is used as a wood and leather varnish, and as a base for ointments, cosmetics and polishes.

DERMATITIS DUE TO VEGETABLES

The essential oils of the edible umbellifers, including carrots,[54] parsnips, parsley and celery (including celery salt),[55] may cause allergic eczematous dermatitis in sensitized individuals. Pinene, terpineol and cineole are probably the sensitizers. Some members of this family are also photosensitizers. Onions and garlic may cause a contact dermatitis that may cross-react with tulips and hyacinths.

Corn dermatitis (corn itch or corn poisoning) is an occupational eruption similar to the contact dermatitis seen in other vegetable processing or wet work with food plants.[56] Excoriations often complicate the dermatitis, and occasionally secondary infection occurs. Protective gloves and barrier creams help reduce exposure.

In addition, a photosensitivity dermatitis may appear in workers harvesting celery parasitized by fungi (rusts or smuts).[22]

DERMATITIS DUE TO LICHENS

Lichens, plants composed of fungi living in symbiosis with algae, have caused allergic contact dermatitis in foresters. The specific sensitizing substance is apparently usnic acid, which accumulates in lichenized fungi. It is chemically related to the furocoumarins, but it is apparently not a photosensitizer.[57]

So-called cedar poisoning or wood cutter's eczema may actually be a contact dermatitis due to lichens. The general population may be exposed by burning lichen-infested logs in fireplaces. Lichen mosses used to simulate trees and shrubs are the source of exposure in model railroad operators and architects. Lichens may also be employed in making clothing dyes and funeral wreaths. Litmus is derived from lichen pigment. Ointments containing usnic acid are used for treatment of skin infections, particularly in Scandinavia and Germany.

Patch tests may be performed with 1 per cent usnic acid in petrolatum.

Lichens cause allergic dermatitis. Usnic acid is the specific sensitizer

DERMATITIS FROM AQUATIC PLANTS

An irritant form of marine contact dermatitis due to certain algae has been reported.[58] During the warm summer months, the Myxophyceae, blue-green algae, produce the greenish discoloration of lakes, ponds and stagnant bodies of water by accumulation near the surface of the water. The skin irritant is probably a phycocyanin, a blue pigment specific for these algae, which distinguishes them from other plant life containing chlorophyll.

Lyngbya majuscula, a common seaweed widely distributed throughout the tropical Pacific and Indian Oceans, has also been reported as causing dermatitis.[59] It is a member of the Cyanophyceae or blue-green algae family. The eruption appears from June to September. It has a characteristic distribution on body areas covered by closely fitting swimming trunks, athletic supporters or brassieres. In all patients tested with the plant, patch tests revealed a primary irritant reaction (see also chapter on aquatic contact dermatitis).

DIAGNOSIS OF PLANT DERMATITIS

The antigenic and irritating chemicals of plants can produce a wide spectrum of reactions on the skin. Exposed skin is usually most seriously and often exclusively involved. Redness and swelling, particularly of the eyelids, is a feature. Dermatitis of the face, neck, hands and arms is common. Seasonal incidence of a dermatitis suggests a plant as the etiologic factor, except for house or greenhouse plants, which can produce dermatitis throughout the year. When there is marked sensitivity, the briefest and most casual contact with the plant may provoke a severe attack of the dermatitis.

Plant dermatitis is usually seasonal, except when produced by house and greenhouse plants

Dermatitis due to direct contact with a plant is characterized by a linear, streaked vesiculobullous eruption. Exposure to the oleoresin in air-borne pollen produces a more diffuse erythematous, papular eruption.

Strong irritants in plants can produce hemorrhagic bullae and necrosis.

Marked residual hyperpigmentation characterizes plant dermatitis due to photosensitization. Such pigmentation may help distinguish photocontact from ordinary allergic contact dermatitis.

The diagnosis of plant dermatitis is facilitated by the simple expedient of suspecting a plant as the cause in all cases of contact dermatitis. Exposure to the offending plant may have taken place at work, at home, while visiting or in public places. Occasionally individuals develop dermatitis from a plant that they have handled for years without difficulty.

Carefully executed patch tests may be valuable in the diagnosis of plant dermatitis.

GENERAL PRINCIPLES FOR PATCH TESTING WITH PLANTS

1. Aside from poison ivy and primula dermatitis, in which instances the cause is usually obvious, perform patch tests to identify the offending plant.
2. In general, avoid patch tests with poison ivy or primula, because the procedure may sensitize the patient.[60]
3. Patch test whenever possible with the actual plants to which the patient has been exposed.
4. Test initially with the leaf. If the reaction is positive, test with the flower and pollen of the same species or variety.
5. Routinely test with recently isolated lactones, casenes, pinenes and quinones to help determine the species of plants producing a dermatitis.
6. A positive patch test reaction to balsam of Peru may be an indication that a dermatitis is due to plants or spices.

TESTING FOR ALLERGIC HYPERSENSITIVITY TO PLANTS*

Testing with Oleoresins. Patch testing for hypersensitivity to plants is greatly facilitated by the use of commercial extracts especially prepared for testing. Use of these preparations prevents the application of primary irritant plant juices. Testing may be performed by the open or the closed patch test method. The closed method prevents the testing substance from accidentally being removed from the test site and may be more reliable when epidermal sensitivity is slight.[61]

Patch testing with a portion of the plant may be necessary when commercial testing materials are not available or when the antigenic substance of the plant is water-soluble and is not in the oil-soluble oleoresin fraction.

Patch tests with properly prepared plant oleoresins are valuable in establishing a diagnosis of plant dermatitis

Occasionally oleoresins of plant oils prepared for patch tests may undergo changes with time and produce false reactions. The extracts are usually reliable for a long time provided they are refrigerated. In some instances, it may be advisable to check the results of commercially prepared extracts with portions from the suspected plant.[62]

Testing with Leaves. Testing with leaves is convenient and usually simulates actual exposure. A 1-cm. square of crushed leaf from a growing plant is used for testing. Care must be taken to be certain that the leaves tested do not have a primary irritant effect on the skin. When the irritant properties of the plant are unknown, control tests must be applied to at least 3 normal persons.

Patch testing must be postponed until the dermatitis has healed, and the patches should always be applied to skin not involved in the attack. The interscapular region or arms are suitable sites. The patches are removed after 48 hours. An intense eczematous response can be regarded as indicating allergic sensitivity. The evaluation of weaker responses requires care and experience.

* Hollister-Stier Laboratories, 550 Industrial Park Drive, Yeadon, Pa. 19050, has prepared patch test trays containing the plant oleoresins of wild vegetation (grasses, trees and weeds), domesticated plants, flowers, garden vegetables, shrubs, vines and woods. These are available in 9 wild vegetation trays representing 9 botanical areas of the United States.

Useful information can also be obtained from the following sources:

Forest Products Laboratory, School of Forestry and Conservation, University of California, Berkeley, 1301 South 46th Street, Richmond, Calif. 94804.

Forest Products Laboratory, Canadian Forestry Service, Department of Fisheries and Forestry, 6620 Northwest Marine Drive, Vancouver 8, British Columbia, Canada.

Occasionally, crushed leaves and stems produce a negative patch test reaction that becomes positive if the plant material is moistened with water. This suggests that the antigen is a water-soluble substance rather than an oleoresin. In such instances, testing with the moistened plant may be more significant than testing with prepared oleoresins.

Patch tests with leaves and other parts of plants may produce severe nonspecific reactions

When the leaves of plants that ordinarily are not irritants or sensitizers are crushed, moistened and applied under a closed patch test, they may cause a nonspecific reaction not only in the patient but also in normal controls. A pruritic eczematous eruption that is produced in the patient and *not* in the controls usually indicates allergic sensitivity to the tested plants, provided the patient's skin is not in an irritable state and capable of reacting in a nonspecific manner to bland substances.

Testing with Bulbs. A thin slice of the bulb or single inner scale may be employed for patch tests. Precautions should be taken similar to those outlined for testing with leaves.

Testing to Confirm Clinical Impressions. It may be advisable to confirm the clinical diagnosis of plant dermatitis in patients whose professions require contact with plants, or who may be involved in workmen's compensation proceedings. Otherwise, the wrong plant may be incriminated and the "proof" of plant dermatitis is lacking.

Testing with Dyed Oleoresin. Many commercially prepared testing solutions are dyed green by the addition of azo dyes. False positive reactions may be obtained with such solutions, particularly in patients sensitized to paraphenylenediamine. Control dye solutions free of oleoresin are available upon request.

PATCH TESTS WITH SPECIFIC PLANTS

Ragweed. Patients with ragweed oil sensitivity invariably show a positive reaction to ragweed oil with patch tests. Most patients react to the standard test solution of 1:1000 in acetone. Some individuals, however, are so sensitive that a reaction may be obtained with a 1:10,000 dilution. Patch testing with fresh material from plants can be done if it is remembered that leaves may cause nonspecific reactions because they are rough and irritating. Patients should not be tested in the presence of a severe dermatitis in order to avoid dissemination of the eruption.

Most patch tests will yield a 48-hour delayed reaction that consists of an erythematous, edematous patch of dermatitis. At times, however, a vesicular and bullous reaction may be produced in markedly sensitive patients. Strong test reactions may be accompanied by a flare-up of the ragweed dermatitis. The inflammatory response from a strongly positive reaction may persist for several weeks.

In rare instances, the reaction is negative after 48 hours but becomes positive at the end of 5 to 7 days. The role of dermal sensitivity[63] in ragweed contact dermatitis is still a controversial subject.

Woods.[64,65] The results of patch testing with sawdust are often difficult to evaluate. There is a difference between reactions to patch tests with moist and dry sawdust, because formic acid is formed by the addition of water to the sawdust of certain woods. Dry sawdust may produce a nonspecific follicular eruption by plugging the skin follicles with particles. Freshly cut woods are sometimes more sensitizing than woods less recently cut. On the other hand, one tropical wood, Regna wood, which is used in furniture-making, is not a sensitizer until the furniture becomes old and the wood begins to disintegrate. It is best to test the patient with both moist and dry sawdust. Positive reactions to both usually signify allergic hypersensitivity to the wood.

Certain workers handle wood only after the bark has been stripped, but others are exposed to both the bark and a fine powdery material that may be present between the bark and the wood and that can cause a pronounced nonspecific follicular eruption.

English Ivy. In sensitized individuals, testing with the branch of this plant may cause a positive reaction, while the leaf produces a negative one.[43]

Phacelia Crenulata (*Desert Heliotrope*). Patch tests with dried leaves produce positive reactions in patients sensitized to this plant.[44]

Carrots. If the oleoresin of carrots is not available, patch tests may be performed with the external surface of an unpeeled raw carrot or with the surface of a slice of carrot. The reaction is usually stronger to the slice than to the outside portion.

The essential oil of carrot contains pinene, terpineol and cineole.

Many plants are photosensitizers and should be tested by both the open and the closed patch test procedures

Celery. This plant may cause an ordinary allergic contact reaction and photocontact dermatitis.[22] The sensitizing principle is an essential oil that contains limonene. The essential oil of orange, lemon, bergamot, caraway and dill also contains limonene. Cross-reactions may occur between celery, citrus fruits and balsams.

Wild Parsnips and Parsley. The dermatitis produced by these vegetables is usually due to photosensitization.[21] Moisture is necessary for the reaction. Some individuals acquire the photocontact dermatitis only when they are perspiring profusely or have become wet from water.

Exposure to sunlight within 48 hours after the moist contact with the plants is necessary for the phototoxic reaction.

Patch tests with parsnip and parsley should be performed with the vegetable moistened with water and exposed to sunlight or artificial ultraviolet radiation.

Fig Trees. Latex, the milky sap from fig trees, may produce allergic contact sensitivity and photosensitivity. In patch testing, therefore, the test area should be exposed to sunlight if there is no response to the closed patch test procedure.

Philodendron. Testing for sensitivity to this plant should be performed with crushed leaves moistened with water.[39] It is likely that the antigen is water-soluble and is in the leaves rather than on their surfaces. It has also been reported that wet philodendron plants are more apt to cause dermatitis than are the plants in the dry state.[40]

Peels of Citrus Fruits. The oil of orange peel may be tested 1 per cent in alcohol or 25 per cent in castor oil. Orange peel may be tested "as is," but if positive reactions are obtained, the test should be performed on 3 normal controls because occasionally the oil of orange peel may be a strong primary irritant. In order to avoid strong reactions, patients should be advised to remove the peel if burning or itching occurs.

Orange growers cover the oranges with a thin layer of wax, which usually is either paraffin or carnauba wax. In a patch test, the wax may protect the skin against the primary irritant or sensitizing action of the limonene and other oils in the peel. Before testing, therefore, all wax should be removed. Lemons have no similar wax film, and irritant reactions from lemon peel are more common than from orange peel.

The peel of lime should be tested by both closed and open methods with exposure to sunlight, because certain limes may be photosensitizers.

TREATMENT OF ALLERGIC CONTACT DERMATITIS DUE TO PLANTS

Contact dermatitis due to plants should be treated as outlined in the treatment of poison ivy dermatitis. Topical preventive measures are not successful. Washing of the skin with soap and water soon after exposure (within a few minutes) may remove the oleoresin and prevent dermatitis. Detoxifying agents, such as chelating chemicals and ion-exchange resins, however, are of no value. Corticosteroid ointments and sprays are also ineffective in the prophylaxis of plant dermatitis.

Further management of plant dermatitis depends on whether it is due to contact with the plant or due to air-borne pollen. Furthermore, the advice given to a professional horticulturist and florist is different from that given to the ordinary patient. It is usually wise to have the patient dispose of the offending plant, unless someone else in the household will take care of it. The amateur horticulturist usually can avoid contact with the plants to which he shows allergic hypersensitivity, but the professional gardener and florist cannot. It is important that clinical impressions be confirmed by properly performed patch tests before any advice is given to the professional.

Prolonged hyposensitization procedures may be indicated for the professional gardener or florist sensitized to chrysanthemums and other plants

When it is suspected that a florist is sensitized to chrysanthemums, he should be patch tested with all the varieties he grows. The patient usually reacts strongly to only a few, and he may be able to eliminate these varieties or have someone else handle them. Plants that cross-react with the offending plants will also have to be avoided.

Hyposensitivity procedures for allergic plant dermatitis are long and drawn out and not always successful. Such treatment may be worthwhile for the professional horticulturist, however, if he cannot avoid exposure to sensitizing plants or is unwilling to change his profession. Before prophylactic treatment is begun, sensitivity to suspected plants must always be confirmed by patch testing. Such treatment is usually worthwhile only when strongly positive patch test reactions are obtained. Patch testing at intervals after treatment has begun is generally useful to determine whether hyposensitization is occurring.

MANAGEMENT OF POLLEN DERMATITIS

Once the diagnosis of contact pollen dermatitis has been established, the patient must either reside in a part of the country where he will not be exposed to pollens to which he reacts or he must receive prophylactic treatment. Oral hyposensitization based on Shelmire's technique[30] is satisfactory in many instances of ragweed oil dermatitis.[31,37]

Oral Hyposensitization to Ragweed Dermatitis

The treatment of contact allergy to ragweed consists of daily ingestion of small amounts of the oil* from these plants over a period of several months or even years. Several rules, which are given to the patient, must be rigidly followed:

1. Treatment should be started when you are free of the skin eruption. If you have the skin rash all year, start the treatment either after the first frost or as early in the summer as possible, but not during the ragweed season.
2. Ingest gradually increasing amounts of the oil daily.
3. Decrease the number of ingested drops or stop treatment for a few days if a rash, hives or itching of the anal area develops.
4. Ingest the entire 3 bottles of oil, which is the minimal amount that will reduce your sensitivity.

The treatment set consists of three 1-oz. bottles of the specific oleoresin diluted in corn oil. The first bottle contains a 1: 100 dilution, the second bottle a 1: 50 dilution and the third bottle a 1: 25 dilution of the oleoresin. Gelatin capsules of No. 1 size are also shipped.

Oral hyposensitization for ragweed dermatitis has proved satisfactory

The patient is advised to ingest as an initial dose 1 drop of the 1:100 dilution of the oleoresin in a gelatin capsule. Warn him to avoid contaminating his fingers with the oil while filling the capsules from the dropper. Capsules are filled at the time of ingestion and are best tolerated immediately following the morning or the evening meal.

The initial dose of a drop of the 1:100 dilution is taken daily for 1 week. Two drops are ingested daily during the second week. If no symptoms of intolerance appear during these two weeks, the patient is instructed to increase the number of daily drops as rapidly as tolerance permits. Some patients can increase the dosage by 2, 3 or even more drops weekly. Some patients increase their tolerance to the point at which they can ingest a full capsule (12 drops) or more daily within a month after beginning treatment.

* The material can be obtained from the Hollister-Stier Laboratories, and consists of ragweed oleoresin diluted in corn oil.

Plate 10. Ragweed Dermatitis and Photoallergic Dermatitis Caused by Deodorants in Soaps Occur Mostly in Men

1. Ragweed Oleoresin

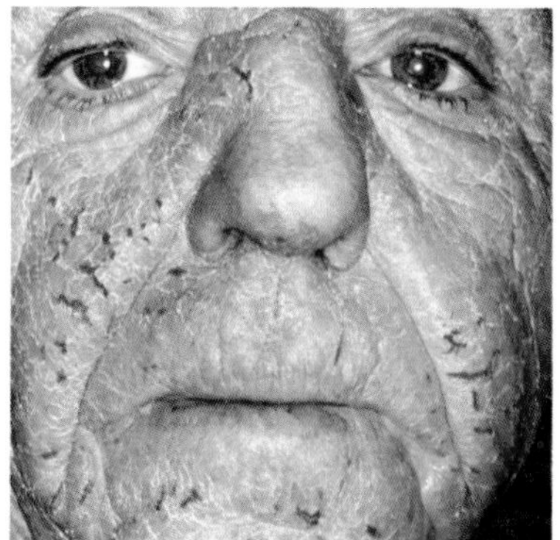

2. Photoallergic Deodorant in Soap

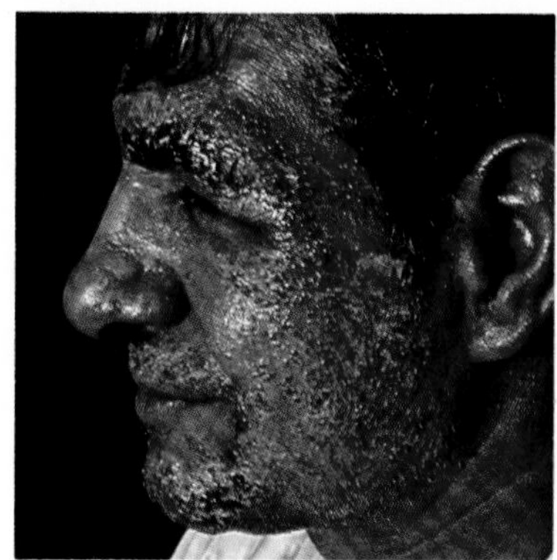

(New York Skin and Cancer Unit)

3. Ragweed

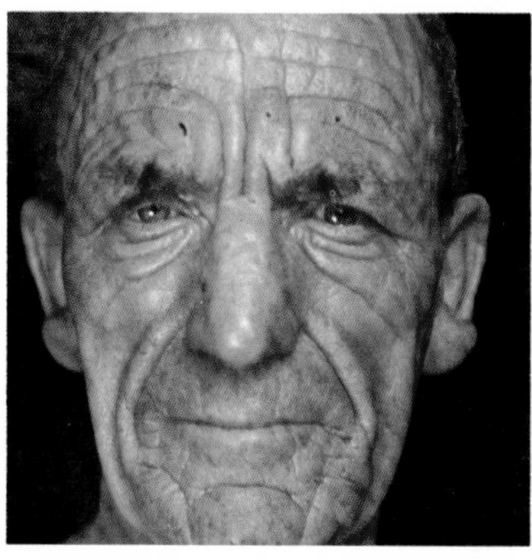

4. Photoallergic Deodorant in Soap

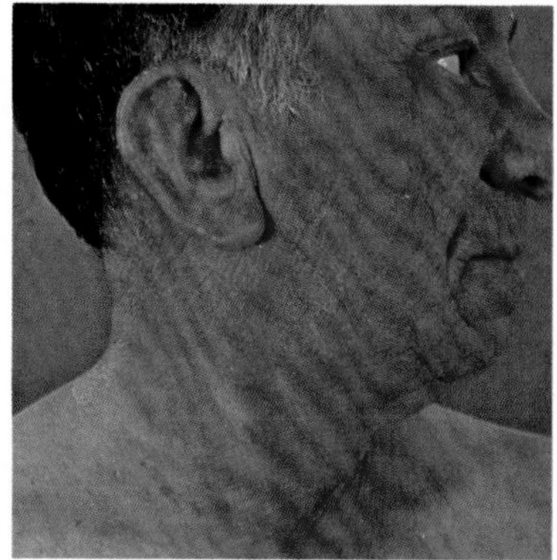

(New York Skin and Cancer Unit)

5. Ragweed

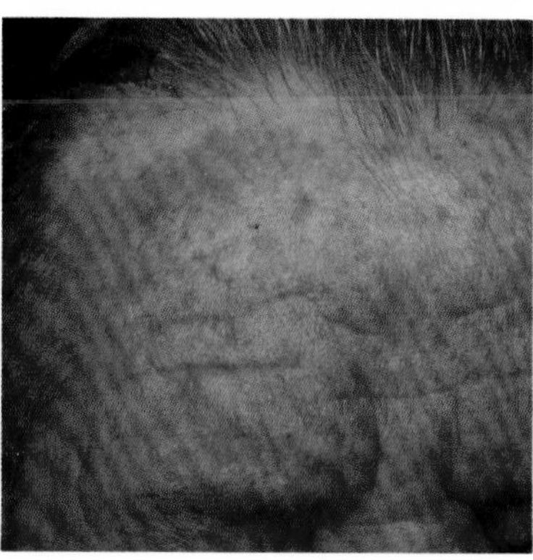

6. Photoallergic
a Persistent Light Reactor

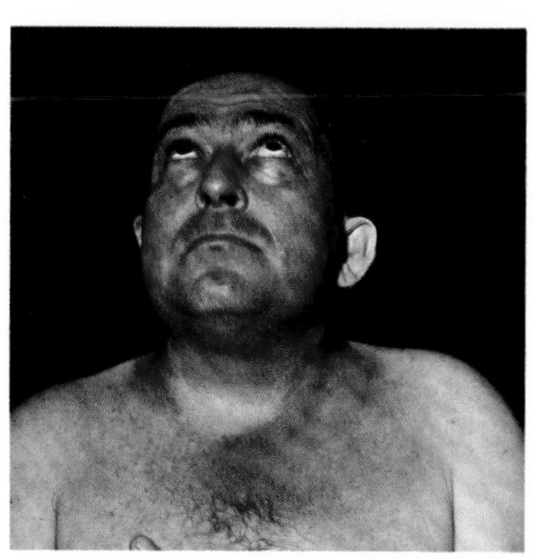

(New York Skin and Cancer Unit)

The longer the patient takes the drops, the more rapidly the dosage can be increased.

After the 1-oz. bottle of the 1:100 dilution has been ingested, the patient then begins the 1:50 dilution, starting with approximately half the maximal number of drops he was ingesting when the bottle of 1:100 dilution was finished. If he was taking 40 or 50 drops of the 1:100 dilution as a daily dose, he should start taking 20 to 25 drops of the 1:50 dilution. He should then increase the daily number of drops of this concentration as rapidly as his tolerance permits. Usually within a few weeks after beginning treatment, a patient can judge his tolerance and can determine how rapidly to increase the dosage. In the absence of pruritus ani and dermatitis, the dosage may be increased quickly.

After completion of the 1:50 dilution, the 1:25 concentration is started, again beginning with half the maximal daily dosage of the previous dilution and increasing it as tolerance permits. Patients who increase the dosage 1 drop weekly usually require 8 months or more to ingest all 3 bottles of oil. By increasing the dosage as rapidly as tolerance permits, the patient with average sensitivity can often ingest the required amount of oil in approximately 2 months. A maintenance dose of 12 drops of the 1:25 dilution of the oleoresin should be taken twice weekly indefinitely.

Pruritus ani, urticaria and dermatitis may complicate plant oral hyposensitizing treatment

Pruritus ani is the most annoying treatment complication. It occurs chiefly during the early weeks of oral therapy, and it often disappears even though the dosage is increased. This annoying symptom may be minimized by thorough cleansing of the anal region with soap and water after each bowel movement, because this itching is caused by contact of the perianal skin with the unabsorbed portion of the specific oil.

Urticaria and other skin eruptions are rarely observed if the dosage is not increased too rapidly. These eruptions are never serious, and if they occur, the patient should be advised to stop treatment until the skin has cleared (usually a few days) and then recommence it at a slightly reduced dose. Toxic manifestations of this type rarely recur, because most patients develop a tolerance for the oil. Indigestion from oral therapy may be treated with antacid remedies, such as Gelusil or Creamalin.

Individuals who start oral therapy late in the season and whose sensitivity is not sufficiently reduced by the oral treatment may develop a dermatitis from exposure to the allergenic plant. In most instances, the dermatitis will be less severe than it was prior to oral therapy. Patients should avoid exposure to the plant until after completion of oral treatment. If an eruption from direct or indirect contact with the plant does occur, oral treatment should be temporarily stopped because it may exacerbate the eruption.

Maintenance doses should be given as long as there is exposure to the plant

It is not known if reduced sensitivity to plant dermatitis is permanent. It is therefore advisable for the patient to continue taking the maintenance dose of 1 capsule (12 drops) of the 1:25 dilution of the oleoresin indefinitely.

All patients sensitive to ragweed oil should be patch tested with pyrethrum, chrysanthemum and turpentine. If strongly positive patch test reactions are obtained to any or all of these cross-reactive oleoresins, these substances should be included in the oral hyposensitizing mixture that contains the ragweed oleoresin.

Mixtures of ragweed, pyrethrum, chrysanthemums and turpentine should be given when there is evidence of clinical cross-reactivity

The advantages of hyposensitization are shorter duration of an attack of dermatitis, less spread of the eruption, and milder dermatitis. The protection is partial and relative, depending on the degree of exposure. Estimates of the duration of hyposensitivity vary from months to years.

Since spontaneous cures of pollen oil sensitivity rarely occur, hyposensitization procedures are worthwhile. Success has also been reported with an injection method.[31]

RHUS DERMATITIS

Poison Rhus Plants

In the United States, the rhus group of plants probably is responsible for more cases of allergic contact dermatitis than are all other provocatives combined.

In the eastern United States, rhus dermatitis usually occurs in the spring and summer, but in the western portion, where outdoor living is common all year, poison oak dermatitis appears at any time, regardless of the season.[66] Even in the East, however, poison ivy may be acquired from the roots of the plant throughout the year. Urban residents often acquire poison ivy dermatitis when visiting cemeteries.

Poison ivy and poison oak are the principal causes of rhus dermatitis in the United States. Poison oak (Rhus toxicodendron) is more prominent on the West Coast than elsewhere, but poison ivy (Rhus radicans) occurs throughout the United States. Poison sumac or poison dogwood (Rhus vernix) is found only in woody, swampy areas. Cross-sensitivity between the rhus plants exists, and the antigens of all of them are essentially the same.

Table 14–2 shows some distinctive characteristics of the various rhus plants.

Poison ivy, oak and sumac contain identical antigens and produce identical eruptions

Poison ivy, the most ubiquitous of the rhus group, is a versatile plant that may climb for many feet on a pole, a tree or a house. On several occasions I have discovered poison ivy being cultivated as an *ornamental* vine,

Table 14-2. Characteristics of Poison Rhus Plants*

Name	*Habitat*	*Leaves*	*Growth Features*
Common poison ivy (Rhus radicans)	U.S.A., except the extreme southwest; throughout Canada	Group of 3 leaflets; edges smooth or notched; green in summer, red in fall	Woody, ropelike vine; trailing shrub on ground or erect without support
Oakleaf poison ivy (Rhus diversiloba)	Southeastern U.S.A., from New Jersey to eastern Texas	Group of 3 leaflets; center leaf resembles oak leaf	Low shrub
Western poison oak (Rhus toxicodendron)	Pacific coast from southern California to Canada	Group of 3 leaflets; center oak leaf and side leaflets of irregular shapes	Upright shrub, can grow into large spreading clumps 6 feet tall; in forests, becomes vine up to 30 feet tall
Poison sumac (Rhus vernix)	Damp, swampy areas throughout U.S.A., particularly east of the Mississippi	Seven to 13 leaflets, arranged as pairs along a central rib with a single leaflet at the end	Coarse woodish shrub or tree, never a vine

* The *flowers* of the rhus group occur in small clusters and are usually white, greenish white or yellowish green. The *fruit* is usually white or cream colored with distinct segments like those of a peeled orange. (*Nonpoisonous sumacs have red fruit.*)

Farmer's Bulletin No. 72, issued by the U.S. Department of Agriculture, contains valuable information on the rhus plants.

growing up the side of a house as high as the second story and producing severe, recurrent poison ivy dermatitis on the unsuspecting occupants.

The leaflets of the posion ivy and oak plants always grow in groups of three, giving rise to the warning "Leaves three, leave them be!"

The poison rhus plants are related to the Japanese lacquer and cashew nut trees, the mango and the marking nut tree of India

The allergic contact dermatitis whether produced by poison ivy, poison oak or poison sumac is the same. Furthermore, since the rhus plants belong to the Anacardiaceae family, cross-reactions may occur with the following related plants and substances:

1. A furniture lacquer that may sensitize is obtained from the Japanese lacquer tree.
2. The oil from the shell of the cashew nut contains a potent sensitizer, which is destroyed by heat. Imported Haitian voodoo dolls and swizzle sticks made from cashew nuts may produce a reaction resembling poison ivy dermatitis.[67] Cashew oil may be used in the synthesis of phenolformaldehyde resins and in mucilages, varnishes and printer's ink. Components of the oil of cashew nut shells may cross-react with the fruit pulp of the ginkgo tree. The ginkgo fruit pulp may produce an eruption indistinguishable from that of poison ivy dermatitis.
3. The rind of the mango contains a catechol similar to the catechol of the poison ivy group.
4. The marking nut tree of India (Bella gutti) produces a black, tarry oleoresin used to mark laundry. Since this black ink is a potent sensitizer unaffected by boiling, it can cause repeated attacks of allergic contact dermatitis (dhobi itch) when used to mark clothing.

Dark-skinned individuals seem less susceptible than others to rhus dermatitis. It has been estimated that at least 70 per cent of the population of the United States would acquire it if exposed casually to the plants. Prolonged exposure would probably sensitize even more of the population. Although elderly individuals are not usually as susceptible to poison ivy as are younger people, I have

Table 14-3. Anacardiaceae Plants Related to the Poison Ivy Group

Common Names	*Scientific Names*	*Distribution*	*Modes of Contact*
Mango "King of the fruits" "Apple of the tropics"	Mangifera indica	Hawaii, California, Florida, India, Central America, Mediterranean	Direct—plant to skin
Lacquer tree	Rhus vernicifera	Japan, China, India	Wood boxes, bracelets, bar rails
Cashew nut shell oil		India, Africa, Central America, East Indies	Voodoo dolls, swizzle sticks, resins, mucilages, printer's ink, electric insulation
Cashew oil	Anacardium occidentale		
Indian marking nut Dhobi (washerman) itch	Bella gutti	India, Malaya	Laundry marking ink
Rengas tree Black varnish tree	Anacardium melanorrhoea	Malaya	Furniture, wood carvings
Ginkgo tree	Ginkgo biloba	Southeastern U.S.A., China, Japan, Europe	Oriental lacquer ware, stepping in seeds

seen severe poison ivy dermatitis in several individuals who were in their late 70's. Newborn infants can readily be sensitized by a single application of the oleoresin to a localized area, such as a patch test site. More than 50 per cent of infants thus sensitized showed positive patch test reactions 2 to 3 weeks after the initial sensitizing application.

Rhus dermatitis may occur in persons of all races and ages

Table 14–3 is a list of plants that contain urushiols, which are related to the poison ivy group.

Tests for the pyrocatechols in these anacardia plants (D. S. Wilkinson, personal communication) are presented in Table 14–4.

Goldstein[68] pointed out that Rengas trees, which grow primarily in Malayan jungles, furnish lumber resembling mahogany that is used for furniture. Unlike mahogany, however, Rengas sap cross-reacts with other urushiol plants and trees. If Rengas wood furniture is varnished before it is thoroughly dried, the sap may come through the varnish and cause reactions in those using it.

Indian sandal strap dermatitis may be due to the urushiol-containing sumac used to tan leather in certain Indian villages.[69]

A contact dermatitis can be caused by the oleoresin of the mango tree sap or the skin of the fruit. Ingestion of the fruit may produce anaphylactic reactions.[70]

Dermatitis-Producing Factors of the Poison Rhus Plants

The leaves, stems, seeds, flowers, berries and roots of certain plants contain a milky sap that turns into a black substance resembling varnish on exposure to air. Alcohol and other solvents can be used to extract a crude yellow-brown viscous substance from the sap. The residue remaining after evaporation of the solvents is the antigenic *oleoresin.* The term *urushiol* is often used for the oleoresins of the Anacardiaceae plants, including the poison rhus group. Urushiol is antigenic even after the plant has died.

Table 14-4. Tests for Pyrocatechols

White with lead acetate
Green to black with ferric chloride
Green to brown with alcohol and caustic soda

The dermatitis-producing principle of the oleoresin is related to the presence of *pentadecylcatechols* (PDC) which are 1,2-dihydroxy benzenes (catechols) with a 15-atom side chain in the third position.[71,72] Some investigators, however, suggest that individuals may be sensitive to another component of the oleoresin.[73] Some people with allergic hypersensitivity to pentadecylcatechols show cross-reactivity to other phenolic compounds, such as resorcinol, hexylresorcinol and the hydroquinones, but not to phenol.

A 1:10 dilution of the oleoresin in acetone usually equals a 1:1000 dilution of pentadecylcatechols in antigenicity. The oleoresin contains unstable, unsaturated compounds, however, which are probably more potent sensitizers than the stable, saturated pentadecylcatechols.

The oleoresin (urushiol) of the sap of the rhus plants contains catechols, which are the sensitizing chemicals

Aside from phenolic substances, the oleoresins contain variable mixtures of polymers of unknown chemical composition.

Nature of Rhus Dermatitis

The eruption produced by poison ivy is an allergic eczematous contact dermatitis usually characterized by redness, papules, vesicles and bullae, plus linear streaking. Occasionally, urticaria and eruptions resembling erythema multiforme, measles or scarlatina occur from systemic absorption of the poison ivy antigen.

The dermatitis is produced by exposure to some portion of the bruised plant allowing the oleoresin to contact the skin. The uninjured plant is innocuous. Pure smoke from burning the poison ivy plant is also harmless provided the particulate matter does not contain the oleoresin. Involvement of the mucous membranes, with stomatitis or proctitis, due to chewing of the leaves or overdosage in oral hyposensitization is not rare.

The fluid content of vesicles and bullae present in poison ivy dermatitis is not antigenic. Patch tests performed with it give negative reactions.

One can acquire poison ivy dermatitis from oleoresin-contaminated animals,[74] clothing, tools, golf clubs, fishing rods and baseball bats. Fomites[75] contaminated with the oleoresin in a dry atmosphere may remain antigenic for a long time, whereas a warm, moist climate favors loss of potency. Washing with soap or detergents renders oleoresin-contaminated clothing and objects harmless. The rhus oleoresin may remain under a person's fingernails unless deliberately removed by thorough cleansing. If not removed, for several days after contact with the plants, the antigen may be spread by the fingers to the covered parts of the body and even to other individuals.

Soap and water and organic solvents render rhus oleoresin harmless

After a susceptible person contacts the oleoresin, the eruption usually appears within 2 days, and delay of onset rarely exceeds 10 days. In a few cases, the skin reaction may occur within 8 hours of exposure. Such temporal differences are probably due to the degree of exposure, individual susceptibility and regional variation in cutaneous reactivity.

Rhus dermatitis usually begins with itching and redness. Streaks of erythema or papules in linear arrangement soon appear. Complications include eosinophilia, kidney damage, urticaria, dyshidrosis and marked pigmentation or leukoderma. Impetigo and pyoderma are frequent complications.

In the *differential diagnosis*, it must be remembered that arthropod bites, particularly those due to bedbugs, often cause a linear eruption. In addition, a phytophotodermatitis (dermatitis bullosa striata pratensis) due to the psoralen of plants may produce lesions consisting of bullae that are striate or irregularly linear on exposed portions of the body. The lesions develop 12 to 24 hours after plants such as celery, parsley, gas plants, lime, figs and buttercups have been crushed on the skin and there has been subsequent *exposure to sunlight*. The bullae heal, leaving pigmentation, which may persist for many months.

Rhus plants *are not photosensitizers*, and the dermatitis is distinguished by occurring on both covered and uncovered parts of the body and by not requiring sunlight for its development.

The linear configuration of poison ivy dermatitis must be differentiated from striate plant photodermatitis

Patch Testing for Poison Ivy Sensitivity

The plant oleoresin diluted 1:10 in acetone may be used for patch testing. The pure synthetic antigen, 3-pentadecylcatechol, a stable crystalline material, may also be used in various dilutions, but it is not readily available. There is also some question as to whether it contains all the antigenic materials of the poison ivy oleoresin.

Patch testing reveals that about 50 per cent of the population of the United States has been sensitized to poison ivy. There is a strong possibility that 5 to 10 per cent of non-sensitized individuals may become sensitized by being patch tested with either the synthetic antigen or the natural oleoresin.

The diagnosis of poison ivy dermatitis is usually fairly obvious, and there is not much point in proving the diagnosis by such a procedure. Patch testing with the oleoresin or pentadecylcatechol should be restricted to investigative procedures or to proving hyposensitization by prophylactic treatment.

Patch testing with rhus oleoresin should not be done routinely: this is an investigative procedure

The only objective proof of successful hyposensitization procedures, however, is a negative or weakly positive patch test reaction to poison ivy in individuals who had previously shown a strongly positive reaction to the oleoresin. The oleoresins may give intense vesicular and even bullous reactions in sensitized individuals.

General Prophylaxis of Rhus Dermatitis

The best prophylaxis for any type of allergic contact dermatitis is complete avoidance of the allergen. Patients should be taught to recognize and avoid the poison rhus group. They should carefully observe and search surrounding terrain before choosing a picnic or camping site. When a poison rhus plant is present in the garden or cannot be avoided, its chemical destruction or physical removal is indicated.[76] Farmer's Bulletin No. 2158, *Chemical Control of Brush and Trees*, issued by the U.S. Department of Agriculture, should be consulted for information on specific chemicals for destroying poison ivy or poison oak.

The best prophylaxis for rhus dermatitis is the avoidance and destruction of the rhus plants: topical prophylaxis is ineffective

Unfortunately, no topical measure is effective in the prevention of poison ivy dermatitis. Barrier creams and chelating, detoxicating and oxidizing agents are of no value.[77] All individuals exposed to these plants should thoroughly wash the entire body with soap and water. One need not use strong soaps for this purpose. Complete change of clothing is also advisable, and whenever possible, contaminated clothing should be washed with soap and water.

The poison ivy antigen enters the skin so rapidly that the oil must be totally removed within *10 minutes of exposure*. When such early washing is not feasible, however, it is worthwhile for the individual to wash at the first opportunity to remove any oleoresin remaining on the skin and thereby prevent it being transferred to other parts of the body.

Management of Mild Poison Ivy Dermatitis

Mild poison ivy dermatitis usually consists of papules and vesicles, often in linear streaks. Treatment with an antipruritic "shake" lotion, such as one consisting of phenol (1.2 ml.), menthol (0.3 gram) and calamine lotion (up to 120.0 ml.), is often sufficient. Valisone spray may be effective.

Topical preparations containing benzocaine, zirconium or antihistaminics should be avoided, because these substances are notorious sensitizers. Preparations containing iron salts should also be avoided, because they can produce a permanent tattoo. Steroid creams and ointments are not very effective in poison ivy dermatitis.

If itching is severe despite the application of the antipruritic lotion, light spraying of the affected areas with ethyl chloride often gives relief for an hour or more. Some patients find that either very cold or moderately hot water gives temporary relief from the pruritus. In this stage, Valisone spray may be effective.

Baths or showers, with a bland soap, are permitted in mild poison ivy dermatitis.

Management of Moderately Severe Poison Ivy Dermatitis

In moderately severe poison ivy dermatitis, in addition to papules, vesicles and bullae, edematous swellings of various parts of the body may be present.

Large vesicles or bullae should be opened under sterile conditions and with preservation of the roof of the lesion if possible. Cool compresses of Burow's solution (1:10) may be applied to edematous areas. Edema of the eyelids can be treated with wet dressings of cold boric acid.

On the face, lotions should usually be avoided in acute allergic dermatitis, because they tend to cake, making the skin uncomfortably stiff. Applications of wet dressings followed by zinc oxide ointment or petrolatum are better tolerated. Men with facial involvement should be allowed to shave, because the trauma of shaving causes less discomfort and irritation than does the accumulation of crusts and debris in the beard.

Baths with potassium permanganate are valuable, after vesicles or bullae are opened, for their quick drying effect and when there is the possibility of secondary infection. One teaspoonful of potassium permanganate crystals is dissolved in a tub of lukewarm water.

The patient may sit in the tub from 15 to 20 minutes. Average baths (1 cupful of plain Aveeno to a tub of water) are also cleansing and soothing.

For antipruritic and sedative effects, Temaril (5 mg.), Benadryl (50 mg.), Atarax (25 mg.) and Periactin (4 mg.) may be given to the adult before he retires to help ensure a good night's sleep.

Management of Severe Poison Ivy Dermatitis

Severe poison ivy dermatitis is characterized by widespread involvement and marked edema of the extremities and the face. Often the eyelids are so swollen that they cannot be opened. Systemic corticosteroid therapy is dramatically beneficial, provided there are no contraindications. Topical therapy is similar to that given for moderately severe cases.

Systemic corticosteroid therapy is a great boon for the treatment of poison ivy dermatitis. Such therapy should be continued for at least 3 weeks to prevent a rebound phenomenon

Schedule of Corticosteroid Therapy for Severe Poison Ivy Dermatitis

1. First and second days: Two 5-mg. prednisone tablets or the equivalent every 4 hours for 5 doses.
2. Third and fourth days: Two tablets every 4 hours for 4 doses.
3. Fifth and sixth days: Two tablets every 5 hours for 3 doses.
4. Seventh, eighth, ninth and tenth days: One tablet 4 times daily.
5. Eleventh, twelfth, thirteenth and fourteenth days: One tablet 3 times daily.
6. Fourteenth to twenty-first day: One tablet twice daily.

(In children, the doses are proportionately reduced.)

The corticosteroid therapy is spread over a *3-week period*. In many individuals who receive this therapy for a few days, the poison ivy dermatitis seems to be under control. If the therapy is stopped at this time, the patient often has a rebound reaction with return of the dermatitis to its original intensity. Such a reaction is prevented by gradually tapering off the steroid dosage over a 3-week period.

Occasionally, the patient is suffering so much when first seen that the physician may give an initial intramuscular injection of 40 mg. of Aristocort suspension or the equivalent.

For the first day or so, concurrently with the steroid therapy, one of the following may be given for sedation: 50 mg. of Benadryl, 25 mg. of Atarax or a 7½-grain capsule of chloral hydrate once or twice daily.

Specific Prophylactic Treatment of Poison Ivy

The following factors must be taken into consideration before any desensitizing procedure is attempted:[78]

1. Complete desensitization is never accomplished. The procedure is one of hyposensitization.
2. Hyposensitization should be attempted only when the need for protection is great and exposure is unavoidable, and when a previous attack of poison ivy dermatitis has been incapacitating.
3. Hyposensitization can be accomplished only over a period of several months.
4. Hyposensitization is only temporary, and the original sensitivity returns about 6 months after treatment is stopped.
5. Scientific appraisal of the efficacy of a desensitization procedure cannot be based on clinical effects alone. Only procedures that reduce positive patch test reactions are scientifically reliable.

Considering all the factors just mentioned, I have found it worthwhile to give prophylactic treatment to certain sensitive individuals in whom contact with poison ivy is inevitable because of their work or hobbies. I have found the oral hyposensitization method as introduced by Shelmire to be of moderate value.

Specific hyposensitization procedures for rhus dermatitis are worthwhile for telephone repair men, foresters and others with inevitable exposure

The prinicple of hyposensitization consists of daily ingestion of small but increasing amounts of poison ivy oleoresin, as described for ragweed oleoresin. Because four months or more usually are required for this oral hyposensitization, treatment should be started at least 4 months before the poison ivy season.

Once sufficient poison ivy oleoresin has been taken to hyposensitize the patient, a maintenance dose of a concentrated dilution of the oleoresin is given twice weekly for an indefinite period or as long as the patient will be exposed to poison ivy. Although *complete* desensitization is not obtained by any method, sensitization is reduced sufficiently to markedly benefit most of the highly sensitive individuals.

This treatment is relatively free from complications. Occasionally, pruritus ani, urticaria and mild generalized dermatitis occur, and rarely gastric distress is encountered. Such complications are usually overcome by stopping the treatment for a few days, and recommencing it at a smaller dose.

A follow-up of several patients who had taken the treatment for 1 year revealed that the original strongly positive patch test reaction to poison ivy was significantly reduced and that there was concomitant clinical improvement. Poison ivy dermatitis, when it did occur, was much milder, less extensive and lasted for a shorter period.

If poison ivy dermatitis appears during oral prophylactic treatment, the treatment should be suspended for the duration of the eruption. Other oral preparations and injectable products have their advocates and detractors.[79]

Finally, under no circumstances should an injectable poison ivy antigen preparation be given in the presence of poison ivy dermatitis. Such injections can produce severe flare-ups and widespread dissemination of the dermatitis.

It is hoped that the future will bring more effective prophylactic preparations. These substances will probably contain a synthetic antigen of the poison ivy group.

Nonspecific methods, such as the injection of measles vaccine, have been reported as temporarily reducing sensitivity to poison ivy.[80]

DERMATITIS DUE TO SPICES

At least 60 spices, with their essential oils, can produce dermatitis. Six of these are of particular interest to the dermatologist because they produce allergic contact dermatitis.

In the United States, the 5 spices that most commonly produce dermatitis are capsicum, cinnamon, cloves, nutmeg and vanilla. In Europe, laurel is apparently the most common cause.

All these spices can produce flares at the healed sites of allergic contact dermatitis when they are ingested or inhaled. In addition, spices may produce urticaria when ingested with foods or drink or when inhaled.

Spices have been used in perfumes, cosmetics and topical medications.

Highly seasoned foods were known to cause rosacea, particularly rhinophyma, more than three and a half centuries ago, a fact immortalized in the following poem:[81]

Nose, nose, nose, nose!
And who gave thee this jolly red nose!
Nutmeg, and ginger, cinnamon and cloves,
And they gave me this jolly red nose.

All the spices contain essential oils, which can irritate the skin in concentrated form. The dust that forms when spices are ground produces an irritant dermatitis mechanically as well as chemically. Many of the essential oils also are sensitizers.[82]

Many spices, particularly mustard and capsicum, can irritate the mucous membranes of the eyes and respiratory passages. The oleoresin of capsicum is such an efficient lacrimator that it is employed in the United States as tear gas.[83,84] (See also chapter on irritant reactions.)

Cayenne Pepper (Capsicum frutescens)

This pepper, from which the oleoresin of capsicum is extracted, is distributed worldwide. One patient was recently studied who had an acute eczematous dermatitis on one side of the neck after being playfully sprayed with an aerosol containing the oleoresin of capsicum at a New Year's Eve party. One year prior to this episode the patient had a stiff neck and applied Capsolin Rubefacient, which contains oleoresin of capsicum, camphor, oil of turpentine and oil of cajeput (a pungent oil from an East Indian myrtle tree). Patch tests revealed a 4+ reaction to capsicum and negative reactions to the other ingredients.

On 2 occasions the dermatitis of the neck flared following the ingestion of pickles that had been flavored with capsicum. Ginger ale and liqueurs flavored with capsicum can produce similar eczematous contact dermatitis in sensitized individuals.[85]

The oleoresin of capsicum is a powerful irritant, which may be used as a tear gas

Cinnamon and Cassia

There has been a confusion between cinnamon and cassia. When we order cinnamon toast we should, to be correct, ask for cassia toast, because cassia has almost entirely replaced cinnamon as a spice in the United States.

In Great Britain, the word *cinnamon* applies only to Cinnamomum zeylanicum and *cassia* to C. cassia. In the United States, the Food, Drug and Cosmetic Act of 1938 officially permitted the term *cinnamon* to be used for both C. zeylanicum and C. cassia, as well as other species of cassia.

The nomenclature in various countries is as follows:

	Cinnamon	*Cassia*
Spanish	Canela	Canela de la China
French	Cannelle	Cannelle de Cochinchine
German	Zimt	Zimtkassie
Swedish	Kanel	Kassia
Arabic	Qurfa	Darasini
Dutch	Kaneel	Kassia
Italian	Cannella	Cassia
Portuguese	Canela	(none known)
Russian	Koritsa	(none known)
Japanese	Seitron-Nikkei	Bokei
Chinese	Jou-Kuei (or Jou-Kwei)	Kuei (or Kwei)

Cinnamon is the bark of the cinnamon or cassia tree. The flavor is derived from oil of cinnamon, which contains cinnamic aldehyde and eugenol. Oil of cinnamon is used mainly for flavoring food, toothpaste, chewing gum, tobacco, aperitifs and bitters, and cola beverages. Because of its sensitizing properties, it is used for perfumes only to a limited extent, and always in low concentrations.

Occupational dermatitis from oil of cinnamon may occur in bakers and candy makers, but cinnamon dermatitis has also been observed among cooks and housewives.[86] Oil of cinnamon has further been reported as the cause of allergic dermatitis from ammoniated toothpaste,[87] bubble gum and lipstick. Sensitization to balsam of Peru may result in a high degree of cross-sensitivity to oil of cinnamon.[88]

Ingestion of oil of cinnamon may produce an eczematous contact type of flare-up in individuals previously sensitized by contact with the oils.[89]

Nutmeg and Mace

The nutmeg tree, Myristica fragrans, produces two closely related but separate spices, nutmeg and mace.

The terms used for nutmeg and mace in different countries are as follows:

Spanish	Nuez Moscada
French	Muscade
German	Muskatnuss
Swedish	Nuskot
Arabic	Babbasa
Dutch	Notemuskaat
Italian	Noce Moscata
Portuguese	Noz-Moscada
Russian	Oryekh Muskatny
Japanese	Nikuzuku
Chinese	Jou-Tou-K'ou

The essential oils of nutmeg and mace contain myristicin, which is highly toxic and a powerful narcotic. The fatty oils of nutmeg are used in the manufacture of soap and perfumes and may be the cause of allergic dermatitis. Blends of mace and nutmeg are used extensively for flavoring foods. Bakers may acquire allergic dermatitis from handling these spices.

When the word *mace* is mentioned in the United States, most dermatologists think of chemical Mace, referring to a tear gas. The term is an acronym derived from the chemicals involved, i.e., *M*ethylchloroform chlor*ACE*tophenone.[90] Chemical Mace is a potent sensitizer and, of course, is unrelated to mace, the spice.

Connecticut is known as the "Nutmeg State." This nickname resulted from the alleged ingenuity of Connecticut Yankee peddlers of the early nineteenth century who were facetiously charged with the sale of wooden imitation nutmegs as the genuine article to unsuspecting housewives.

For patch test purposes, capsicum and mace are tested in a 1 per cent alcoholic solution.

Cloves

The word *clove* (Syzgium aromaticum) is derived from the French, *clou*, referring to the unexpanded, nail-shaped flower bud of the tree.

Oil of clove is rich in essential oils, particularly eugenol, which are widely used in perfumes, soaps, toothpastes and mouthwashes.

Eugenol is a pale yellow liquid with a strong smell of carnation employed in the widely used zinc oxide–eugenol dental cement. It may also be combined with rosin and zinc oxide. It is the essential chemical constituent of clove oil and is also present in cinnamon oil, perfumes, soaps and bay rum. Individuals sensitized to eugenol should avoid exposure to such products. Eugenol is both a primary irritant and a sensitizer, and for patch testing a 10 per cent solution in olive oil or a 5 per cent solution in petrolatum is used.

Eugenol, one of the main constituents of oil of bay, may show cross-reactions with balsam of Peru. Sometimes oil of cloves and of cinnamon are added to bay rum. Both oils are sensitizers, and cinnamon oil may cross-react with eugenol and balsam of Peru.

Eugenol, when used in dental preparations, such as impression pastes, surgical packings and cements, may produce stomatitis venenata and allergic eczematous eruptions in dental personnel.[91]

Oil of cloves incorporated into a liniment has been reported as a cause of allergic dermatitis.[92,93] The mucilage of postage stamps may also contain clove oil, and cause glossitis in persons who lick the stamps.

Clove oil may be patch tested with a 1 per cent alcoholic solution.

Individuals sensitized to oil of cloves or eugenol may have to avoid ingestion of foods containing the spice or the essential oil in order to avoid a flare of dermatitis. Indians use cloves to flavor the betel nut. The English use oil of cloves in apple tarts. The French love onion soup with cloves. In the United States, cloves are frequently used with pork.

Vanilla and Vanillin

Vanilla is a flavoring extract made from the pod of the vanilla plant. Vanillin is a crystalline compound, which is the fragrant constituent of vanilla. The vanilla bean is the dried and fermented fruit of an orchid, Vanilla planifolia. Vanillin, a benzaldehyde, is formed from glycosides such as glucovanillyl alcohol and glucoconiferyl alcohol, the latter being converted into glucovanillin, glucose and vaniilin.

Contact dermatitis due to vanilla occurs in individuals employed in the cultivation, trade or industrial use of vanilla. One variety of vanilla dermatitis is a pseudophytodermatitis caused by mites, living on vanilla pods, of the same species as meal mites (Tyroglyphus farinae), which produce an eruption of urticarial papules, called vanilla lichen,[94] on exposed parts of the body. Vanillism, an allergic contact dermatitis acquired by workers handling the vanilla plant, produces marked edema and erythema. Rhinitis, asthma and vertigo may accompany the eruption.

Synthetic vanillin can be produced from pine tree sap, eugenol, wood pulp, sugar and coal tar. The Food and Drug Administration requires that the term *imitation vanilla* appear on the label if the product contains synthetic ingredients. If the label has the term *vanilla extract*, the product must be derived from vanilla beans. Some individuals are sensitized to synthetic vanillin and not to the natural spice, and vice versa.[82]

An unusual source of exposure to vanillin is smoking certain types of tobacco. For patch test purposes, a 10 per cent alcoholic extract of vanilla in acetone can be used.

Vanillin may be tested 10 per cent in petrolatum.

Laurel

The bay tree, Laurus nobilis, also known as sweet bay, is native to the Mediterranean region and Asia Minor. This bay tree is not related to the West Indian bay tree Pimenta acris, leaves of which are distilled to produce bay rum, or to the bayberry of coastal American dunes (Myrica pensylvanica).

Laurel oil is used in medicine and in the textile and soap industries. Laurel leaves are used in cooking because of their flavor and antioxidant properties. They are also used in meat and fish preservation, "roll mops," pickled gherkins, condensed soups and spiced sauces.

The bactericidal properties of laurel oil have been known for a long time in Germany and made use of in an ointment for abscesses. In France, laurel oil is used in only one Codex listed product (Fioravanti balsam) and in the commercial product Vegebom. Fioravanti spirit, which is also called turpentine spirit mixture, contains 0.4 per cent of L. nobilis berries, 20 per cent of larch tree turpentine and other products. Among the Vegebom preparations, only the ointment, the suppositories and an adhesive for prosthetic dentistry (Dental Vegebom) include appreciable quantities of laurel oil (1.2 per cent in the ointment).

Laurel oil is often used in the textile industry to improve the luster of felt hats. In the store, the hatband becomes contaminated when the hats are stacked and produces hatband dermatitis in the wearer.

In the United States, dermatitis from laurel is apparently extremely rare. Sensitization to laurel is not uncommon, however, in Europe. Most cases have been observed in Germany, Switzerland and France.[95]

In Germany, sensitization occurs from the use of laurel in the felt industry. In France and Switzerland, the source of exposure is ointments containing the oil of laurel (Vegebom ointment).

Cosmetics and food may also be sources of exposure. It is surprising to learn that in Strasbourg, laurel oil is a more common sensitizer than nickel or mercury.

In the United States, bay leaves are practically never used for medicinal purposes; consequently, sensitization from topical exposure is eliminated. Bay leaves are used to season some American dishes, particularly Hearty Bean Soup. Bay leaves are reported to be extremely popular in French cuisine for flavoring meats, fish, poultry, vegetables, and stews. It is conceivable that such extensive use may have sensitized some individuals.

Patch tests with laurel oil may be performed with a 2 per cent concentration in petrolatum or with a 5 per cent solution of essential oil in alcohol.

Laurel, rarely implicated in the United States, is a common sensitizer in Germany, Switzerland and France

REFERENCES

1. Mitchell, J. C., and Dupuis, G.: Allergic Contact Dermatitis From Sesquiterpenoids of the Compositae Family of Plants. Brit. J. Derm., *84*, 139, 1971.
2. Mitchell, J. C., et al.: Allergic Contact Dermatitis from Ragweeds (Ambrosia Species). The Role of Sesquiterpene Lactone. Arch. Derm., *104*, 73, 1971.
3. Mitchell, J. C.: Allergy to Frullania. Arch. Derm., *100*, 46, 1969.
4. Calnan, C. D.: Dermatitis from Cedar Wood Pencils. Trans. St. John Hosp. Derm. Soc., *58*, 43, 1972.
5. Rook, A.: Plant Dermatitis in General Practice. Practitioner, *188*, 627, 1962.
6. Rook, A.: Plant Dermatitis. The Significance of Variety-Specific Sensitization. Brit. J. Derm., *73*, 283, 1961.
7. Curtis, G. H.: Plant Dermatitis. Virginia Med. Monthly, *87*, 301, 1960.
8. Bleumink, E., et al.: Allergic Contact Dermatitis to Garlic. Brit. J. Derm., *87*, 6, 1972.
9. Cairns, R. J.: Plant Dermatoses. Trans. St. John Hosp. Derm. Soc., *59*, 137, 1964.
10. Kligman, A. M.: Poison Ivy (Rhus) Dermatitis. Arch. Derm., *77*, 149, 1958.
11. Hjorth, N., Fregert, S., and Schildknecht, H.: Cross-Sensitization Between Synthetic Primin and Related Quinones. Acta Dermatovener., *49*, 552, 1969.
12. Puglisi, V.: Dermatoses Caused by Lemons. G. Ital. Derm., *92*, 237, 1951.

13. Pirila, V., et al.: Chemical Nature of Eczematogens in Oil of Turpentine: Pattern of Sensitivity to Different Terpenes. Dermatologica, *139*, 183, 1969.
14. Spott, D. A., and Shelly, W. B.: Exanthem Due to Contact Allergen (Benzoin) Absorbed Through Skin. J.A.M.A., *214*, 1881, 1970.
15. Shanon, J., and Sagher, F.: Sabra Dermatitis. Arch. Derm., *74*, 269, 1956.
16. Woods, B.: Irritant Plants. Trans. St. John Hosp. Derm. Soc., *47*, 74, 1962.
17. Burbach, J.: The Blistering Effect of Buttercups. Nederl. T. Geneesk., *107*, 1128, 1963.
18. Muenscher, W. C.: *Poisonous Plants of the United States* (Ed. 2). New York, Macmillan Co., 1951, p. 110.
19. Polunin, I.: Pineapple Dermatoses. Brit. J. Derm., *63*, 441, 1951.
20. Shelley, W., and Arthur, R.: Studies on Cowhage (Macuna Pruriens) and its Pruritogenic Proteinase, Mucunain. Arch. Derm., *72*, 399, 1955.
21. Pathak, M. A., Daniels, F., Jr., and Fitzpatrick, T. B.: The Presently Known Distribution of Furocoumarins (Psoralens) in Plants. J. Invest. Derm., *39*, 225, 1962.
22. Somner, R. G., and Jillson, O. F.: Phytophotodermatitis (Solar Dermatitis from Plants) Gas Plant and Wild Parsnip. New Engl. J. Med., *276*, 1484, 1967.
23. Arnold, H. L., Jr., and Haramoto, F. H.: "Grain Itch" Following Fumigation for Termites. Derm. Trop., *1*, 37, 1962.
24. Baker, E. W., and Wharton, G. W.: *Acarology.* New York, Macmillan Co., 1952, p. 327.
25. Faust, E. C., Beaver, P. C., and Jung, R. C.: *Animal Agents and Vectors of Human Disease* (Ed. 2). Philadelphia, Lea & Febiger, 1962, p. 470.
26. Faust, E. C., and Russell, P. F.: *Craig and Faust's Clinical Parasitology* (Ed. 4). Philadelphia, Lea & Febiger, 1964, p. 586.
27. Micks, D. W.: Clinical Effects of the Sting of the "Puss Caterpillar" (Megalopyge Opercularis) on Man. Texas Rep. Biol. Med., *10*, 399, 1952.
28. Ziprkowski, I., Hofshi, E., and Tahori, A. S.: Caterpillar Dermatitis. Israel Med. J., *18*, 26, 1959.
29. Schwartz, L.: Cutaneous Hazards in the Citrus Fruit Industry. Arch. Derm., *37*, 631, 1938.
30. Shelmire, B.: Contact Dermatitis From Vegetation: Patch Testing and Treatment with Their Oleoresins. Southern Med. J., *33*, 337, 1940.
31. Fromer, J. L., and Jenkins, W. S.: Ragweed Oil Dermatitis. Lahey Clin. Bull., *11*, 75, 1959.
32. Tuft, L., and Heck, V. M.: Studies in Atopic Dermatitis. IV. Importance of Seasonal Inhalant Allergen, Especially Ragweed. J. Allergy, *23*, 528, 1952.
33. Curwen, W. L., and Jillson, O. F.: Light Hypersensitivity. J. Invest. Derm., *34*, 207, 1960.
34. Fromer, J. L., and Burrage, W. S.: Ragweed Oil Dermatitis. J. Allergy, *24*, 425, 1953.
35. Cohen, S. G.: Seasonal Ragweed Dermatitis. Arch. Derm., *79*, 328, 1959.
36. Canizares, O., and Trilla, E.: Dermatitis Venenata Due to Ragweed Pollen. Arch. Derm., *75*, 905, 1957.
37. Fisher, A. A.: Some Immunologic Phenomena in Treatment of and Patch Testing for Ragweed Oil Dermatitis. J. Invest. Derm., *19*, 271, 1952.
38. McCord, C. P.: The Occupational Toxicity of Cultivated Flowers. Industr. Med. Surg., *31*, 365, 1962.
39. Ayres, S., Jr., and Ayres, S.: Philodendron as a Cause of Contact Dermatitis. Arch. Derm., *78*, 330, 1958.
40. Dorsey, C.: Philodendron Dermatitis. Calif. Med., *88*, 329, 1958.
41. Dorsey, C.: Contact Dermatitis from Algerian Ivy. Arch. Derm., *75*, 671, 1957.
42. Dorsey, C.: Algerian Ivy Dermatitis (a California Disease). Calif. Med., *90*, 155, 1959.
43. Goldman, L., Preston, R., and Muegel, H.: Dermatitis Venenata from English Ivy (Hedera Helix). Arch. Derm., *74*, 311, 1956.
44. Berry, C. Z., Shapiro, S. I., and Dahlen, R. F.: Dermatitis Venenata from Phacelia Crenulata. Arch. Derm., *85*, 737, 1962.
45. Dorsey, C.: Plant Dermatitis in California. Calif. Med., *96*, 412, 1962.
46. May, S. B.: Dermatitis Due to Grevillea Robusta (Australian Silk Oak). Arch. Derm., *82*, 1006, 1960.
47. Verspyck Minjssen, G. A. W.: Pathogenesis and Causative Agent of "Tulip Finger." Brit. J. Derm., *81*, 737, 1969.
48. Suskind, R. R.: Dermatitis in the Forest Product Industries. Arch. Environ. Health, *15*, 322, 1967.
49. Weichardt, H.: Skin Lesions Caused by Wood Protecting Agents. Berufsdermatosen, *18*, 61, 1970.
50. Sowers, W. F., et al.: Ginkgo-Tree Dermatitis. Arch. Derm., *91*, 452, 1965.
51. Lovell, R. G., Matthews, K. P., and Sheldon, J. M.: Dermatitis Venenata from Tree Pollen Oils. J. Allergy, *26*, 408, 1955.
52. Bunney, M. H.: Contact Dermatitis in Beekeepers Due to Propolis (Bee Glue). Brit. J. Derm., *80*, 17, 1968.

53. Rothenberg, H. W.: Occupational Dermatitis in a Beekeeper Due to Poplar Resins in Beeswax. Arch. Derm., *95*, 381, 1967.
54. Klauder, J., and Kimmich, J.: Sensitization Dermatitis to Carrots. Arch. Derm., *74*, 149, 1956.
55. Gougerot, H., and Carteaud, A.: *Les Dermatoses Professionelles.* Paris, Norbert Maloine, 1952, p. 168.
56. Seligman, E. J., and Key, M. M.: Corn Dermatitis. Arch. Derm., *97*, 664, 1968.
57. Mitchel, S. C., and Armitage, J. S.: Dermatitis Venenata from Lichens. Arch. Environ. Health, *11*, 708, 1965.
58. Cohen, S., and Reif, C.: Cutaneous Sensitization to Blue-Green Algae. J. Allergy, *24*, 452, 1953.
59. Grauer, F., and Arnold, H. L., Jr.: Seaweed Dermatitis. Arch. Derm., *84*, 720, 1961.
60. Agrup, G., Fregert, S., and Rorsman, H.: Sensitization by Routine Patch Testing with Ether Extract of Primula Obconica. Brit. J. Derm., *81*, 897, 1969.
61. Spencer, M. C.: Open Versus Closed Patch Testing with Oleoresins. Arch. Derm., *93*, 47, 1966.
62. Williams, O., Speairs, R., and Boggs, H. W.: Hypersensitivity to March Elder: Difficulties Encountered in Patch Testing. J. Louisiana Med. Soc., *112*, 216, 1960.
63. Epstein, S.: Role of Dermal Sensitivity in Ragweed Contact Dermatitis. Arch. Derm., *82*, 48, 1960.
64. Howell, J. B., and Blair, D. S.: Eczema of the Hands from Wooden-Handled Objects. Arch. Derm., *62*, 400, 1950.
65. Schulz, K. H.: Studies on Sensitizing Effect of Components of Tropical Woods. Berufsdermatosen, *10*, 17, 1962.
66. Epstein, W. J.: Rhus Dermatitis: Fact and Fiction. Permanente Found. M. Bull., *6*, 197, 1959.
67. Orris, L.: Cashew Nut Dermatitis. New York J. Med., *58*, 279, 1958.
68. Goldstein, N.: The Ubiquitous Urushiols. Cutis, *6*, 679, 1968.
69. Pilgrim, R. E., and Fleagle, G. S.: India Sandal Strap Dermatitis. Letter to the Editor. J.A.M.A., *209*, 1906, 1969.
70. Dang, R. W., and Bell, D. B.: Anaphylactic Reaction to the Ingestion of Mango. Hawaii Med. J., *27*, 149, 1967.
71. Baer, H., et al.: The Quantitative Assay of the Active Principles of Poison Ivy by Biological and Gas Chromatographic Methods. J. Allergy, *34*, 221, 1963.
72. Auerbach, R., and Baer, H.: Comparison of the Potency of Poison Ivy Extracts With Synthetic Pentadecylcatechol in Sensitive Humans. J. Allergy, *35*, 3, 1964.
73. Mason, H. S., and Lada, A.: Immunologic Properties of Hydrourushiol-Albumin Conjugate. J. Invest. Derm., *22*, 457, 1954.
74. Muller, C. H.: Contact Dermatitis in Animals. Arch. Derm., *96*, 423, 1967.
75. Stanton, D. L., and Wilson, J. W.: Rhus Dermatitis: An Unusual Case Caused by Atomized Spray. Cutis, *8*, 553, 1971.
76. Maibach, H. I., and Epstein, W. L.: Plant Dermatitis: Fact and Fancy. Postgrad. Med., *35*, 571, 1964.
77. Mitchell, W. F.: Poison Ivy Prophylaxis: Folklore or Scientific Medicine. Ohio Med. J., *55*, 797, 1959.
78. Kligman, A. M.: Hyposensitization Against Rhus Dermatitis. A.M.A. Arch. Derm., *78*, 47, 1958.
79. Passenger, R. E.: A Clinical Evaluation of the Prophylactic Treatment of Poison Ivy Dermatitis With an Alum-Precipitated Pyridine Extract of Rhus Toxicodendron. J. Allergy, *34*, 270, 1963.
80. Blumhardt, R., et al.: Depression of Poison Ivy Skin Test by Measles Vaccine. J.A.M.A., *206*, 2739, 1968.

Spices

81. Rosengarten, F.: *The Book of Spices.* Wynnewood, Pa., Livingston Publishing Co., 1969.
82. Schwartz, I., Tulipan, L., and Birmingham, D. J.: *Occupational Diseases of the Skin* (Ed. 2). Philadelphia, Lea & Febiger, 1957, p. 466.
83. Fisher, A. A.: Dermatitis Due to Tear Gases (Lacrimators). Derm. Int., *9*, 91, 1970.
84. Gleason, M. N., et al.: *Clinical Toxicology of Commercial Products* (Ed. 3). Baltimore, Williams and Wilkins, 1969, p. 301.
85. Ormsby, O. S., and Montgomery, H.: *Diseases of the Skin* (Ed. 8). Philadelphia, Lea & Febiger, 1954, p. 239.
86. Kern, A. B.: Contact Dermatitis from Cinnamon. Arch. Derm., *81*, 599, 1960.
87. Leifer, W.: Contact Dermatitis Due to Cinnamon. Arch. Derm., *64*, 52, 1951.
88. Hjorth, N.: *Eczematous Allergy to Balsam, Allied Perfumes and Flavoring Agents.* Copenhagen, Munksgaard, 1961, p. 134.
89. Fisher, A. A.: Systemic Eczematous "Contact-Type" Dermatitis Medicamentosa. Ann. Allergy, *24*, 415, 1966.
90. Fisher A. A.: Mace—A Modern Acronym and An Ancient Nomenclature. Letter to the Editor. J.A.M.A., *212*, 320, 1970.
91. Goransson, L., et al.: Some Cases of Eugenol Hypersensitivity. Derm. Venereol. Tandlak. T., *60*, 545, 1967.

92. Gaul, L. E.: Dermatitis of the Hands from Oil of Cloves. Skin, *2*, 413, 1963.
93. Gaul, L. E.: Contact Dermatitis from Synthetic Oil of Mustard. Arch. Derm., *90*, 158, 1964.
94. Matheson, R.: *Medical Entomology* (Ed. 2). Ithaca, N. Y., Comstock Publishing Co., 1950, p. 115.
95. Foussereau, J., et al.: Contact Dermatitis from Laurel. I. Clinical Aspects. Trans. St. John Hosp. Derm. Soc., *53*, 141, 1967.

15

Contact Dermatitis in Atopic Individuals

A recent study by the International Contact Dermatitis Research Group[1] revealed that atopic persons are no more likely to develop allergic contact dermatitis than are patients with other types of endogenous eczemas, such as seborrheic or nummular eczema. The incidence of allergic dermatitis superimposed on atopic dermatitis, however, is still controverdial.[2–4]

There are patients who have atopic conditions, such as allergic asthma and rhinitis, but never suffer from atopic dermatitis. Regardless of whether atopic dermatitis is present, however, atopic individuals may acquire a contact dermatitis, which may be either the irritant or the allergic variety, or both. Atopic eczema does render the skin vulnerable to nonspecific irritants, such as heat, humidity, perspiration, dust, strong soaps, detergents and wool.

An international study revealed that individuals with atopic dermatitis are no more likely to develop allergic contact dermatitis than are patients with other types of eczema

Although atopic dermatitis does not seem to render the patient particularly susceptible to allergic contact dermatitis, a search for the presence of contactants in all instances of persistent atopic dermatitis is of importance in the management of atopic individuals.[2] This is necessary especially when the atopic dermatitis is not responding to therapy or when there are sudden flares of the eruption. In an effort to allay the itching, many individuals with atopic dermatitis are exposed to sensitizing topical medications that produce a superimposed allergic contact dermatitis.

The prompt recognition and removal of irritating and sensitizing contactants may prevent the atopic dermatitis from becoming widespread. It is surprising how often the detection and elimination of offending contactants markedly alleviate an otherwise intractable atopic dermatitis.

Allergic contact dermatitis superimposed on atopic eczema usually appears as an insidious aggravation of the eczema rather than as an acute, easily recognized epidermal eczematous contact dermatitis. The reason may be that many patients with atopic eczema receive topical or systemic corticosteroid therapy, which can modify the appearance of the dermatitis. Patients whose atopic eczema is not responding well to therapy, therefore, should be investigated for the possibility of a superimposed contact dermatitis from topical applications, particularly neomycin.

Aside from being modified by corticosteroid therapy, a superimposed contact dermatitis may not appear typical in atopic individuals because the so-called "dermal" type of contact dermatitis is especially likely to develop in such patients. Clinically, the lesion is edematous and erythematous rather than papulovesicular and may closely resemble the papular, dry form of atopic dermatitis. The allergens reported as producing "dermal" contact sensitivity include neomycin, formaldehyde, nickel and ragweed oleoresin.[5]

PATCH TESTING IN ATOPIC INDIVIDUALS

As in nonatopic individuals, the proof of allergic contact dermatitis often consists of obtaining a positive patch test reaction with a suspected contactant. There is usually a normal incidence of typical eczematous reactions to patch tests performed on patients with atopic dermatitis.[6] Atopic individuals, however, may have unique patch test reactions, such as pustular reactions and specific and nonspecific patch test responses to protein substances.

Patch testing with topical medications and their preservatives is indicated in many chronic cases of atopic dermatitis

Pustular Patch Test Reactions. There is a high incidence of papulopustular reactions to patch tests with nickel sulfate, the halogens and sodium arsenate, which probably represent some form of irritation. In contrast to true allergic patch test reactions, pustular eruptions rarely itch, do not spread beyond the patch test site and usually heal within 24 hours after the patch has been removed.[7] Although pustular patch test reactions, particularly to nickel sulfate, are more common in atopic individuals, such reactions occur frequently in the nonatopic patient and are not diagnostic evidence of the atopic state.

Nonspecific Patch Test Reactions to Protein Substances. When tested with simple chemicals, the atopic individual may show either an eczematous or a pustular reaction. In addition, atopic individuals who are patch tested with certain protein substances, such as feathers, silk and foods, may show nonspecific reactions characterized by closely aggregated, discrete, pinpoint vesicles and occasionally pustules.[8,9] There is no exudation and no crusting. Erythema and itching are minimal and are localized to the patch test site The reaction reaches its greatest intensity in 4 to 5 days. This response has been noted in atopic individuals with or without atopic dermatitis. If dermatitis is present, a positive reaction is not associated with a flare-up of the dermatitis, and the spontaneous flare phenomenon is absent.

Atopic individuals may also have a nonspecific reaction to the tuberculin patch test that is similar to that described for feathers, silk and foods. A specific, positive reaction to a tuberculin patch test consists of a group of tiny vesicles and papules on a reddened, indurated area. False positive reactions to the tuberculin test may appear as vesicles and pustules with minimal erythema and no induration.

Nonspecific pustular patch test reactions to metals and halogens and pseudo reactions to protein and tuberculin patch tests are common in atopic individuals

These nonallergic patch test reactions are probably due to an irritable skin, and indicate that the atopic individual may react nonspecifically to many protein substances. Such reactions must be carefully distinguished from true allergic changes, which are characterized by itching and a spread of the reaction beyond the borders of the test site.

Specific Allergic Patch Test Reactions to Protein Substances. Atopic individuals may rarely react in a specific manner to patch tests with molds, feathers, dander and wool. Allergic patch test reactions to the defatted pollen protein of grasses and ragweed are also occasionally obtained in atopic individuals. The specific allergic reaction to these substances differs from the nonspecific atopic patch test reaction in that the former is characterized by erythema, vesiculation, exudation and crusting. Furthermore, the reaction may spread beyond the patch test site and may be associated with a flare-up of the existing dermatitis. Such positive reactions would seem to signify that inhalation of or external contact with protein substances may cause a flare-up of atopic dermatitis.

Patch testing with protein substances is not a routine procedure, and the clinical significance of the reactions is uncertain even when they seem to be specific.

RELATIONSHIP OF CONTACT DERMATITIS TO EXPOSURE TO SPECIFIC PROTEIN ALLERGENS IN THE ATOPIC INDIVIDUAL

Contact dermatitis can be prolonged and aggravated by the intranasal, subcutaneous or surface application of specific protein allergens to which an atopic individual has been shown to be sensitive by scratch tests. For example, poison ivy dermatitis in an atopic individual may be made worse by the prophylactic injection of ragweed pollen extract or intradermal testing with protein antigens. Such injections on occasion render the atopic skin more irritable, and a concentration of a chemical that is usually innocuous may produce contact dermatitis. Furthermore, in atopic individuals with contact dermatitis, external exposure to proteins in foods, pollens and molds can produce exacerbations.[10,11] These protein substances are not primarily capable of exciting the eczematous reaction but are secondary agents. These observations seem to indicate that there is a mechanism by which specific atopens can produce a flare-up of an existing, etiologically unrelated contact dermatitis in certain susceptible individuals regardless of whether the protein atopen reaches the skin by contact, ingestion, inhalation or injection.

> **During acute phases of dermatitis, atopic individuals should not receive hay fever, asthma or other protein-desensitizing injections**

It would, therefore, be advisable for atopic individuals with contact dermatitis to avoid desensitization procedures or other injections with protein substances while the dermatitis is in the acute or subacute phase.

INHALATION OF AIR-BORNE CONTACTANTS AND ATOPIC DERMATITIS

Occasionally inhalation of pollens, dusts and animal hairs causes either a flare of atopic dermatitis or an apparent superimposed contact dermatitis. In some instances, these air-borne allergens may produce positive patch test reactions.

Champion[12] reported on 5 patients with atopic dermatitis in which exacerbations were provoked both by inhalation and by direct contact with algae. These patients also reacted to lichens, which contain algae in symbiosis with fungi. All of the patients had allergic rhinitis or asthma, often very mild in relation to the severity of the skin symptoms. Three of them also had a delayed hypersensitivity contact dermatitis from lichens, but not from algae.

It is important to investigate patients with suspected sensitivities to lichens and algae both by patch testing and by prick testing, because specific desensitization may help those with immediate wheal reactions.

Champion also stated that *contact* immediate wheal reactions may occur in atopic patients handling eggs or being licked by dogs.

SUBSTANCES THAT CAN PRODUCE BOTH ALLERGIC CONTACT DERMATITIS AND ATOPIC MANIFESTATIONS

Theoretically, there is no absolute difference between agents that cause eczematous allergy and those that engender urticarial (atopic-anaphylactoid) allergy. Under actual conditions, however, some agents generally cause eczematous allergy and rarely or never cause urticarial allergy. Many other agents generally cause urticarial allergy and rarely or never cause eczematous allergy. A small group of agents may cause both forms of hypersensitivity at the same time.[13]

> **Penicillin, quinine, sulfonamides, mercury and arsenic can produce delayed contact reactions and immediate anaphylaxis**

Some allergens alternately produce asthma and contact dermatitis. Among the drugs, penicillin, quinine, sulfonamides, mercurials and arsenicals produce both allergic contact and atopic reactions in the same individual.

These drugs can produce an eczematous contact dermatitis when applied topically and, in addition, can cause asthma, urticaria, or even anaphylactic shock when ingested or injected.[14] Fortunately, procaine (Novocain), which not infrequently produces allergic eczematous hypersensitivity, rarely produces an anaphylactic reaction in atopic individuals or even in those with the epidermal hypersensitivity to the anesthetic.[15]

Paraphenylenediamine can produce both an allergic eczematous contact dermatitis and asthma in furriers. Allergic rhinitis has been described from the inhalation of epoxy resins and the amine hardeners in a pateint who also had a contact dermatitis from processing these resins.[16]

ALLERGIC CONTACT DERMATITIS IN ATOPIC INDIVIDUALS

Allergic contact dermatitis in atopic dermatitis may appear as an eczematous eruption. If the patient is receiving topical or systemic corticosteroid therapy for an atopic dermatitis, however, the superimposed contact dermatitis may appear as an erythematous, papular, noneczematous eruption simulating the original atopic dermatitis. An allergic contact dermatitis to a topical medication therefore may not be suspected.

Superimposed contact dermatitis may make an atopic eczema appear to be intractable

Features of the "Dermal" Type of Allergic Contact Dermatitis in the Atopic Individual. Aside from being modified by corticosteroid therapy, a superimposed contact dermatitis may appear to be atypical in atopic individuals, because the so-called "dermal" type of contact dermatitis is most likely to develop in these patients.[17]

In my experience, patch tests with sensitizing contactants in atopic individuals yield positive reactions similar to those in nonatopic patients. I have not found it necessary to perform intracutaneous tests as advocated by Epstein.[17]

Allergic contact dermatitis in atopic individuals may closely mimic atopic eczema

Most cases of contact dermatitis in atopic individuals seem to be a combination of eczematous and dermal sensitivity. Usually one can demonstrate both a positive eczematous patch test reaction and a positive dermal intracutaneous test reaction in the atopic skin with superimposed allergic contact dermatitis. It is claimed, however, that occasionally the patch test reaction is negative and only an intracutaneous test reveals the dermal contact reaction.[18]

Diagnostic Features of Allergic Contact Sensitivity to Neomycin. Some investigators report that most individuals investigated for allergic contact hypersensitivity to neomycin had atopic dermatitis.[19,20]

Wereide[21] states that his study does not support the view that the atopic state (as it occurs in atopic dermatitis patients) predisposes to neomycin sensitivity. Patients with stasis dermatitis of the lower part of the leg had a significantly higher incidence of neomycin sensitivity than did any other groups with eczematous dermatitis.

In atopic dermatitis, neomycin sensitivity is often obscured by a topical neomycin-corticosteroid preparation and is usually detected only by routine patch tests

Both the classic form of allergic contact dermatitis with vesiculation and eczematization and the papular, erythematous "dermal" type of sensitivity may occur in patients with neomycin sensitivity and atopic eczema. Since neomycin is frequently prescribed in a mixture with a corticosteroid preparation, the corticosteroid may modify the appearance of the superimposed neomycin dermatitis. When an individual treated with a neomycin-containing preparation fails to improve or the eruption becomes worse, neomycin sensitivity should be suspected.

In order to prove the neomycin sensitivity,

the patient should be patch tested with the suspected topical neomycin preparation. In some instances in which allergic contact sensitivity is present, a typical positive patch test reaction is obtained with the preparation or only with a 20 per cent aqueous solution of neomycin. When the reaction to a neomycin preparation is negative, it may be worthwhile to perform an intradermal skin test with a 1:1000 solution of neomycin sulfate. A positive reaction consists of a delayed indurated papule present 48 hours after testing. In my own material, intradermal testing has rarely been necessary.

When neomycin sensitivity has been demonstrated, the patient should avoid exposure to streptomycin and kanamycin, which may cross-react with neomycin and with bacitracin, which may co-react with neomycin.

Precautions in Testing Atopic Individuals for Allergic Contact Sensitivity to Nickel. Allergic contact dermatitis due to nickel may occasionally take the "dermal" form and closely mimic atopic dermatitis. Although most cases of nickel dermatitis occur in the nonatopic population, nickel sensitivity superimposed on atopic eczema may not be readily recognized.[22]

Nickel dermatitis may often be dry and closely resemble the eruption of atopic dermatitis

Patch testing for nickel sensitivity in atopic individuals may also present the difficulty of properly interpreting pustular patch test reactions, which occur frequently in this group.

Wahlberg and Skog[23] reported that in eczema patients with nickel allergy, immunoglobulin E (IgE) and the threshold of sensitivity were determined by patch testing with dilutions of nickel sulfate ($NiSO_4$). In 4 of the 47 patients investigated, the immunoglobulin E value increased. The occurrence of atopic disease in nickel-sensitive patients was 9 per cent and among relatives 38 per cent.

Relationship of Allergic Contact Ragweed Oil Sensitivity to the Atopic State. Ragweed oil dermatitis may mimic a generalized atopic eczema, particularly the seasonal type.[24] Ragweed oil dermatitis is due to an oil-soluble oleoresin, whereas ragweed rhinitis, asthma and possibly certain cases of atopic dermatitis are due to the water-soluble protein fraction of the pollen.

In my own material, most patients with ragweed dermatitis had no atopic dermatitis or evidence of the atopic state.[25]

Ragweed rhinitis and asthma are due to atopic sensitivity to the protein fraction of the plant; ragweed dermatitis is nonatopic and is due to the oil-soluble fraction

Wool as an Irritant and Sensitizer in Patients with Atopic Dermatitis. The mechanism by which wool produces dermatitis, particularly in atopic individuals, is still controversial. Some investigators feel that the inhalation of wool is an important factor.[26] On the other hand, contact with wool, including house dust, which may be largely wool fibers, may readily irritate the atopic skin.[27] Although wool is usually a weak allergen, on rare occasion the degree of sensitivity is so great that mere contact of wool with the skin can produce urticaria.

Contact with woolen objects and dust exacerbates atopic dermatitis

Apart from allergic sensitization, wool is irritating to many individuals, particularly those with atopy.

Atopic Dermatitis Confined to the Hands or Feet. Atopic dermatitis confined to the hands may be precipitated by household or occupational irritants and sensitizers. In other instances, particularly in children, primary irritant reactions from friction, perspiration and tight shoes are factors in a recurrent dermatitis of the feet in atopic individuals.[28] Such atopic dermatitis may resemble shoe dermatitis. Occasionaly, only the dorsal aspect of the large toe is involved.

Atopic dermatitis confined to the feet may be mistaken for allergic shoe dermatitis

PREVENTION OF ALLERGIC CONTACT DERMATITIS IN ATOPIC INDIVIDUALS

Certain principles found to be useful in the prevention and control of contact dermatitis in patients with atopic dermatitis are embodied in the following precautions:

1. An attempt should be made to rule out a superimposed contact dermatitis when an atopic eczema suddenly flares up or is not responding to therapy.

2. The use of neomycin and bacitracin in patients with atopic dermatitis should be avoided. Other antibiotic ointments, such as erythromycin (Ilotycin), chlortetracycline hydrochloride (Aureomycin), tetracycline hydrochloride (Achromycin), oxytetracycline hydrochloride (Terramycin) and chloramphenicol (Chloromycetin Cream) may be used.

3. Aside from neomycin, other sensitizing therapeutic applications should be avoided, particularly in atopic individuals. The index of sensitivity for topical penicillin, ammoniated mercury, benzocaine, Furacin and antihistamine ointments is high.

4. Prior to systemic administration of quinine, sulfonamides, mercurials or arsenicals, patch testing with these drugs may be of value. A positive reaction indicating allergic eczematous sensitivity may contraindicate systemic administration, because there may be an accompanying atopic anaphylactic allergy that is not revealed by intracutaneous testing. This type of combined eczematous and anaphylactic allergy may also be present with penicillin. Patch testing with penicillin is relatively safe, but scrach and intracutaneous testing may be hazardous.

5. In the presence of acute contact dermatitis in atopic individuals, desensitizing procedures or other injections of protein substances should be avoided, because they may prolong or even spread the contact dermatitis.

INSTRUCTIONS FOR INDIVIDUALS WITH ATOPIC DERMATITIS FOR THE PREVENTION OF IRRITANT DERMATITIS

Clothing. Clothes worn close to the skin should be smooth and loose. Rough and starched cuffs and collars are irritating. Avoid contact with wool. Linen, cotton, poplin, gabardine, suede, chamois and synthetic fibers, such as orlon and nylon, are usually well-tolerated. Wash all new clothing before use, and be sure that all soaps and detergents are removed after each washing. Wear sandals or perforated shoes whenever possible. Avoid prolonged use of tennis shoes or rubbers.

Furniture and Room Furnishings. Keep rooms, especially the bedroom, as uncluttered as possible. Avoid dust-gathering draperies and carpets. Small, cotton scatter rugs are permitted. Avoid use of upholstered furniture. Plain wooden furniture is preferable.

Toys. Avoid fuzzy or woolen toys, such as teddy bears. Toys made of wood, rubber, paper or plastics are permitted.

Pets. It is best not to allow dogs, cats or birds in the house. If the presence of such pets is necessary, they must be excluded from the bedroom. Turtles and fish are permitted anywhere in the house.

Dust and Molds. Exposure to all kinds of dust must be avoided as much as possible. Dust on the skin is irritating and the inhalation of dust may also cause increased itching. Moldy objects should also be avoided for the same reasons.

Overheating and Excessive Perspiration. Indulge in activities involving minimal sweating. Swimming, particularly in salt water, seems to agree with most patients with atopic dermatitis.

Tension. Nervous excitement and tension may cause itching and scratching. If trying situations, such as school examinations or difficult business or social situations, are anticipated, taking prescribed medications beforehand may be helpful.

Scratching. Scratched skin quickly becomes inflamed and damaged with resultant retardation in healing. Patting or rubbing may be less harmful than scratching. Keep fingernails short. The application of ice or ice cold water on cotton cloths to localized areas may stop the itching.

Soaps and Cleaning Agents. Strong detergents, cleansers and solvents, such as turpentine and benzene, are particularly harmful to atopic skin. Mild soaps may be tolerated. Since one cannot predict the soap substitute that can be used, several may have to be tried, such as Soydome, Lowila, Dermolate or Aveeno Bar.

Adults with atopic dermatitis of the hands present special problems. Frequently atopic dermatitis clears with the exception of the hands, where the eruption may remain for prolonged periods. Rubber or cotton-lined gloves are used unsuccessfully, because atopic skin does not tolerate the occlusion with resulting sweat retention and maceration. The housewife with atopic dermatitis of the hands should use long-handled brushes for dishwashing, cleansing and doing most other household chores.

THE SCHOLTZ REGIMEN IN ATOPIC DERMATITIS

Ayres and Mihan[29] consider the Scholtz regimen for atopic dermatitis an approach that emphasizes a defective sweat mechanism, rather than allergic sensitivities, as the underlying cause of atopic dermatitis. Things the patient does *not* do are as important as the things he *does*.

The Scholtz regimen emphasizes the importance of defective sweat mechanism and avoidance of irritants in the management of atopic dermatitis

Table 15–1 gives the details of a modified Scholtz regimen. Psychotherapy and dietary restrictions are usually unnecessary.

Table 15-1. The Scholtz Regimen (as modified by Ayres and Mihan)

Prohibitions

- No soap on affected areas
- No water except for a 1-minute cool to lukewarm shower daily, or less often in cool weather
- No oil or grease on skin
- No strenuous exercise
- No contact with wool or use of impervious clothing
- No contact with potentially irritating household or industrial chemicals
- No oral steroids

Topical therapy

- Twice daily application of a nonlipid, soothing, softening and cleansing lotion, such as Cetaphil Lotion
- Fluocinolone acetonide 0.01% in propylene glycol (Synalar solution) applied twice daily immediately after the Cetaphil Lotion or as often as needed to relieve itching; the medication should be rubbed in gently until it disappears

Systemic therapy

- If the patient is on oral steroids, the dose should be gradually tapered over a 2-week period and discontinued
- Broad-spectrum antibiotics may be administered for short periods if there is evidence of secondary bacterial infection
- Long-acting antihistamines given twice daily are sometimes useful in treating the initial acute eruption or relapse
- Thyroid in doses of ¼ to ½ grain once or twice daily, if not contraindicated, may be given for several months
- Vitamin A, in doses of 50,000 to 100,000 units daily, may be used to potentiate the action of thyroid and reduce skin dryness

TREATMENT OF CONTACT DERMATITIS SUPERIMPOSED ON ATOPIC DERMATITIS

In general treatment for contact dermatitis complicating an atopic eczema is the same as that for contact dermatitis on nonatopic skin with the following exceptions:

1. *Wet dressings.* Potassium permanganate or silver nitrate dressings should be avoided, because they often are irritating to atopic skin. Wet dressings of a 1 per cent boric acid solution or Burow's solution, diluted 1 to 20 parts water, are better tolerated. Occasionally, even these dressings are too drying. If the inflamed skin is dry, hot and edematous, the application of a thin layer of plain petrolatum and a superimposed ice bag or ice cold water compresses may be more soothing.

2. *Tub baths.* In generalized acute cases, tub baths may be indicated. Oilated Aveeno may be more soothing than plain Aveeno or cornstarch.

3. *Topical corticosteroid therapy.* In uncomplicated atopic dermatitis, topical corticosteroid creams and ointments are often efficacious. In the presence of superimposed

contact dermatitis, however, they usually are not effective. In the acute phases of such contact dermatitis, zinc oxide ointment or plain Lassar's paste alternated with wet dressings should be used in place of topical steroid preparations. When the acute phase has subsided, topical corticosteroid medication usually again becomes useful. Occlusive dressings with Saran Wrap in general are not well-tolerated in patients with atopic dermatitis.

Occlusive therapy with Saran Wrap, helpful in many chronic dermatoses, is contraindicated in atopic dermatitis with a sweat retention syndrome

4. *Systemic Corticosteroid Therapy.* In general, one tries to avoid the use of systemic corticosteroid therapy in atopic dermatitis because of the chronicity of the disease and because the patient may become dependent on this mode of therapy. In the presence of severe or generalized contact dermatitis in the atopic individual, however, systemic corticosteroid therapy is indicated in the absence of contraindications. Such systemic therapy is particularly indicated when the contact dermatitis is of an allergic nature and the contactant has been discovered. In such instances, systemic therapy will not need to be prolonged for more than 2 or 3 weeks.

An efficient, economical method of systemic corticosteroid therapy in such cases is the administration of 60 grams of prednisone daily for 2 days, 40 mg. daily for 3 days, 30 mg. daily for 2 days, 20 mg. daily during the second week and finally 10 mg. daily during the third week. A gradual tapering off of the steroid over 2 to 3 weeks tends to avoid a severe rebound of the dermatitis, which may take place when the medication is stopped before the patient's immune reactions can take over. Children may receive 20 mg. of prednisone for 3 days and then a gradually decreasing dose for 3 weeks.

5. *Systemic antipruritic and sedative therapy.* The following medications may be tried, but the relief obtained from itching and insomnia is variable.

A. Phenobarbital, $\frac{1}{4}$ grain, and aspirin, 5 grains, given 3 or 4 times daily are often helpful. Do not use aspirin in patients with asthma or urticaria. On retiring, the patient may be given hydroxyzine hydrochloride (Atarax; Vistaril), 25 mg., or diphenhydramine hydrochloride (Benadryl), 50 mg.

B. Hydroxyzine hydrochloride, 10 mg. after each meal and on retiring, may be effective. Some patients become too drowsy in the daytime on this regimen.

C. Cyproheptadine hydrochoride (Periactin), 4 mg. twice daily, is another effective antihistamine.

D. Children may be given elixir diphenhydramine hydrochloride (Benadryl), a teaspoonful 2 or 3 times daily. Some children obtain a better antipruritic effect with syrup of trimeprazine (Temaril), 1 teaspoonful 2 or 3 times daily.

REFERENCES

1. Cronin, E., et al.: Contact Dermatitis in the Atopic. Acta Dermatovener., *50*, 183, 1970.
2. Epstein, S., and Mohajerin, A. H.: Incidence of Contact Sensitivity in Atopic Dermatitis. Arch. Derm., *90*, 284, 1964.
3. Baer, R., and Witten, V.: Editorial Comment. In *Year Book of Dermatology and Syphilography.* Chicago, Year Book Medical Publishers, 1955–1956, p. 414.
4. Fisher, A. A.: Contact Dermatitis Superimposed on Atopic Eczema. Derm. Digest, *5*, *45*, 1966.
5. Epstein, S.: Contact Dermatitis from Neomycin Due to Dermal Delayed (Tuberculin-Type) Sensitivity. Report of 10 Cases. Dermatologica, *113*, 191, 1956.
6. Sulzberger, M. B., and Witten, V. H.: Atopic Dermatitis. In L. J. A. Lowenthal (ed.): *The Enzymes.* Edinburgh, E. & S. Livingstone, 1954, p. 78.
7. Fisher, A. A., et al.: Pustular Patch-Test Reactions. A.M.A. Arch. Derm., *80*, 742, 1959.
8. Fisher, A. A.: Management of Atopic Dermatitis. New York J. Med., *66*, 236, 1966.
9. Baer, R. L.: Conference on Infantile Eczema: History, Definitions, Concepts. J. Pediat., *66*, 248, 1965.
10. Strauss, J. S., and Kligman, A. M.: The Relationship of Atopic Allergy and Dermatitis. A.M.A. Arch. Derm., *75*, 806, 1957.
11. Jadassohn, W.: Contact Dermatitis Versus Atopic Eczema. Int. Arch. Allergy, *11*, 20, 1957.

12. Champion, R. H.: Atopic Sensitivity to Algae and Lichens. Brit. J. Derm., *85*, 551, 1971.
13. Mayer, R. L.: Contact Dermatitis Versus Atopic Dermatitis. Int. Arch. Allergy, *11*, 1, 1957.
14. Fisher, A. A.: Recent Developments in the Diagnosis and Management of Drug Eruptions. Med. Clin. N. Amer., *43*, 1, 1959.
15. Fisher, A. A., and Sturm, H.: Procaine Sensitivity: The Relationship of the Allergic Eczematous Contact-Type Sensitivity to the Urticarial, Anaphylactoid Variety. Ann. Allergy, *16*, 593, 1958.
16. Morris, G. E.: Allergic Rhinitis Acquired During the Processing of Epoxy Resins. Ann. Allergy, *17*, 74, 1959.
17. Epstein, S.: Contact-Dermatitis Due to Nickel and Chromate. Observations on Dermal Delayed (Tuberculin-Type) Sensitivity. Arch. Derm., *73*, 236, 1956.
18. Baer, R. L.: Allergic Eczematous Sensitization in Man. J. Invest. Derm., *43*, 223, 1964.
19. Jillson, O. F., Curwen, W. L., and Alexander, B. R.: Problems of Contact Dermatitis in the Atopic Individual: With Reference to Neomycin and Ragweed Oil Sensitivity. Ann. Allergy, *17*, 215, 1959.
20. Patrick, J., Panzer, J. D., and Derbes, V. J.: Neomycin Sensitivity in the Normal (Nonatopic) Individual. Arch. Derm., *102*, 532, 1970.
21. Wereide, K.: Neomycin Sensitivity in Atopic Dermatitis and Other Eczematous Conditions. Acta Dermatovener, *50*, 114, 1970.
22. Fisher, A. A., and Shapiro, A.: Allergic Eczematous Contact Dermatitis Due to Metallic Nickel. J.A.M.A., *161*, 717, 1956.
23. Wahlberg, J. E., and Skog, E.: Nickel Allergy and Atopy Threshold of Nickel Sensitivity and Immunoglobulin E Determinations. Brit. J. Derm., *85*, 97, 1971.
24. Fromer, J. L., and Burrage, W. S.: Ragweed Oil Dermatitis. J. Allergy, *24*, 425, 1953.
25. Fisher, A. A.: Some Immunologic Phenomena in Treatment of and Patch Testing for Ragweed Oil Dermatitis. J. Invest. Derm., *19*, 271, 1952.
26. Osborne, E. D., and Murray, P. F.: Atopic Dermatitis: A Study of Its Natural Course and of Wool as a Dominant Factor. A.M.A. Arch. Derm. & Syph., *68*, 619, 1953.
27. Hill, L. W.: *The Treatment of Eczema in Infants and Children.* St. Louis, C. V. Mosby Co., 1956, p. 59.
28. Silvers, S. H., and Glickman, F. S.: Atopy and Eczema of Feet in Children. Amer. J. Dis. Child., *116*, 400, 1968.
29. Ayres, S., Jr., and Mihan, R.: Atopic Dermatitis—Success or Failure with the Scholtz Regimen. Aust. J. Derm., *9*, 16, 1967.

16

Noneczematous Contact Dermatitis

Irritant or allergic contact dermatitis usually presents as an eczematous process characterized by itching, redness, edema and a tendency to oozing and crusting. Occasionally, however, it may be noneczematous, with urticarial, granulomatous, acneiform, lichen planus-like, or dry, hyperkeratotic lesions.[1]

Atypical contact dermatitis may be urticarial, granulomatous, dry, hyperkeratotic, acneiform or may resemble lichen planus

CONTACT URTICARIA

Certain agents produce *allergic* urticaria upon external contact with previously sensitized skin. Other substances are *primarily urticariogenic*, producing wheals in all individuals regardless of whether there has been previous exposure.

Allergic Contact Urticaria. This is an uncommon phenomenon. In sensitized individuals, the substances listed in Table 16–1 may rarely produce localized urticaria at the site of contact.

Patients with allergic hypersensitivity to fish may react with immediate urticaria to the application of cod liver oil. Furthermore, certain patients with allergic hypersensitivity to aspirin may react with localized urticaria following the application of topical medication containing acetylsalicylic acid. Contact with ice in individuals with cold urticaria may produce an immediate urticarial reaction at the site of exposure Aquagenic urticaria, a contact sensitivity reaction to water, has been described as a variant of cholinergic urticaria.[2,3]

Allergic contact urticaria may be produced by drugs, chemicals, wool, ice, water, foods, arthropods and sea animals

Occasionally, in severe allergic contact eczematous dermatitis such as that produced by poison ivy, a concomitant urticarial eruption appears. In severe instances of allergic contact dermatitis of the scalp due to hair dyes or bleaches, a marked edematous swelling of the forehead or eyelids resembling angioedema (Quincke's edema) may appear.

Castor bean, pumice, lindane and aliphatic amine hardeners in epoxy resin users may produce contact urticaria.[4]

Air-borne materials alighting on the skin may occasionally cause contact urticaria. Such substances include chemical fumes (ammonia, formaldehyde, gaseous sulfur compounds, fresh paint), foods (particularly fried or cooked fish, which gives off odoriferous particles called osmyls), asthma-producing substances (house dust, pollens, molds, insect sprays) and cosmetics (hairsprays and perfumes).

Table 16-1. Substances Producing Allergic Contact Urticaria

Foods
Wheat
Carrots
Potato
Flour
Spices
Textiles
Wool
Silk
Animals
Dog and cat saliva
Animal danders
Arthropods
Medicaments
Horse serum
Streptomycin
Chlorpromazine
Cod liver oil
Penicillin
Alcohol
Aspirin
Industrial Exposure
Castor bean
Platinum salts
Aliphatic polyamide
Ammonia
Sulfur dioxide
Formaldehyde
Sodium sulfide
Aminothiazole
Lindane
Acrylic monomer
Exotic woods
Cosmetics
Nail polish
Hairsprays
Perfumes

Gaul[5] has described urticarial eruptions from stearyl and cetyl alcohol present in green canvas and in certain textiles.

Dr. C. D. Calnan (personal communication, 1968) described a 20-year-old girl who developed a rash when licked by dogs. Scratch tests produced negative reactions with dog hair and dander but a positive *urticarial* reaction with saliva from a beagle and a mongrel.

I have observed a similar case.

Nonallergic Contact Urticaria. This nonspecific whealing is common. Many substances that are classified as primary urticariogenic agents produce contact urticaria in all exposed individuals. Some can produce urticaria on intact skin, while others must pierce the skin for urticaria to appear.

Two therapeutic agents are capable of producing contact urticaria on intact skin:

1. *Dimethyl sulfoxide (DMSO).* This is a local analgesic, anti-inflammatory adjunct and acts as a carrier to introduce other medications into the skin. In many instances, the application of dimethyl sulfoxide produces a contact urticaria of short duration.[6]

Dimethyl sulfoxide (DMSO) and Trafuril are primary urticariogenic substances

2. *Tetrahydrofurfuryl ester of nicotinic acid (Trafuril).* This ester had been incorporated in an ointment and used as a rubefacient in inflammatory joint diseases, particularly abroad. When it is applied to the skin, the triple response of Lewis, including whealing, is produced in most individuals. In patients with atopic dermatitis, acute rheumatic fever, rheumatoid arthritis and febrile conditions, however, urticaria and erythema are not produced, but instead blanching appears.[7,8]

The ester of nicotinic acid, formerly available as Trafuril (CIBA), containing 5 per cent of the ester in a lanolin-petrolatum base, is not currently available.

Urticaria Due to Arthropods. Urticaria from casual contact with the bodies or hairs of arthropods usually is nonallergic. Bites and stings may produce allergic or nonallergic wheals or a combination of both.

Caterpillar Dermatitis. Certain caterpillars (particularly the puss caterpillar, Megalopyge opercularis) and moths (the brown-tail moth, Euproctis phaeorrhea) possess venomous, bristly hairs or spines, which can pierce intact skin and produce a nonallergic urticarial eruption in all individuals.[9] When many "stinging" hairs pierce the skin, systemic symptoms may be alarming. Prophylaxis requires destroying caterpillars on trees and shrubs with arsenic sprays and washing all clothing and bedding that may have become contaminated with hairs. Epinephrine and corticosteroids may have to be administered for systemic symptoms.

INSECT STINGS AND BITES. In all persons, the sting or bite of most insects is accompanied by a small traumatic wheal at the site of insertion of the arthropod's stinger or mouth parts. In sensitized individuals, a large wheal may develop at the site together with a systemic reaction. Generalized urticaria may be produced by antigens introduced into the skin with the insect's saliva or the venom of the stinger.

Arthropods produce urticaria by their stings and bites or by contact with their bodies or "poison" hairs

Papular Urticaria. This type of urticaria is also known as lichen urticatus, prurigo simplex and strophulus pruriginosus. Occasionally, classic urticaria and even angioedema may accompany papular urticaria. Although some cases may be due to foods or inhalants, many are an allergic response to insect bites, particularly those of the flea and the bedbug, especially in young children.

In the treatment of papular urticaria, antihistamines are helpful, and corticosteroids may give rapid relief.

Ice cold water compresses may be soothing. The following prescription is useful for its cooling, antipruritic effect. The sulfur may act as a repellent against chiggers and other mites.

Menthol	0.3 gram
Sulfur ppt.	3.6 grams
Isopropyl alcohol	40.0 ml.
Calamine lotion q.s. ad.	120.0 ml.

Infestation with Mites. Infestations with scabies mites may produce eruptions with urticarial elements. Other mites that are not parasitic in man may produce urticarial, papular lesions by their presence on or in the skin. For example, animal sarcoptes, which do not burrow in man, may nevertheless produce a papulourticarial eruption in humans.

Similarly, Tyroglyphus mites, which include cheese mites and other food mites present on dried fruits, cheese, sugar, roots, bulbs and copra, may infest individuals handling such products. Although these mites do not suck blood or feed on man, they migrate under the superficial scales of the epidermis, producing a pruritic, urticarial, papular eruption, the so-called grocer's itch or copra itch.

Many mites that are not parasitic to man may produce urticarial eruptions

Other nonparasitic mites may cause irritant dermatitis upon direct contact with human skin. Barley itch occurs in dock workers unloading infested barley. Baker's itch can occur among workers handling infested flour in granaries, flour mills and bakeries. Individuals handling cotton seed containing mites may acquire an urticarial eruption known as cotton seed itch. Bulb mite itch, characterized by papules and urticaria, occurs in workers storing infested bulbs.

Marine Animals and Plants. Several species of marine life may produce contact urticaria. Contact with the Portuguese man-of-war and other jellyfish may produce severe urticaria by releasing toxins from cells in the tentacles.[10] Ammonia neutralizes the toxin. Antihistamines, corticosteroids and epinephrine may have to be administered for systemic reactions.

*Seabather's and Swimmer's Itch.** Seabather's eruption and swimmer's itch both produce papules and occasionally urticaria.[11,12] Seabather's eruption occurs only in salt water and involves body areas covered by the bathing suit. Its etiological basis is still unknown.[13] Swimmer's itch, which occurs almost always in fresh water and on uncovered parts of the body, is produced by schistosomes. This infestation is acquired most often from the lakes of Minnesota, Wisconsin and Michigan.[14]

* The terms *seabather's* and *swimmer's itch* are confusing. For a more complete discussion of these itches and of seaweed dermatitis, see the chapter on aquatic contact dermatitis.

Needle-like Pteropods. Sea stings consisting of urticarial wheals have been experienced by persons swimming in the Gulf of Mexico. In some instances, the stings resulted from minute, needle-like pteropods, which can penetrate the swimmer's bathing suit and enter the skin.

Seaweed Dermatitis. The papules and urticarial wheals of seaweed dermatitis have a predilection for dependent body areas covered by closely fitting swimming trunks, athletic supporters or brassieres. This dermatosis is produced by a marine plant, a seaweed of Hawaii. The etiologic agent is a blue-green alga identified as Lyngbya majuscula Gomont.[15]

Portuguese man-of-war, other jellyfish, schistosomes, seaweed, pteropods and sponges may produce marine contact urticaria

Any individual who emerges from the water and complains of itching and has urticaria should be closely observed for an hour or so, in order that treatment for anaphylaxis and shock may be instituted if necessary. The topical treatment depends on what marine organism is suspected of producing symptoms and signs. (See chapter on aquatic contact dermatitis for topical treatment of marine dermatoses.)

Be prepared to treat individuals for shock who emerge from water and complain of itching and urticaria

Urticaria Due to Contact with Plants. Besides the nettle (Urens urticata), many other plants have specialized hairs and bristles containing toxic urticaria-producing substances. (See chapter on plants.)

CONTACT GRANULOMAS

Certain chemicals elicit a local sarcoid granuloma when introduced within the skin. Zirconium, talc, stearates, silica, magnesium and beryllium, having pierced the skin, may produce granulomas.[16] In addition, the pigments of tattoos, particularly chromium oxide, may cause a granulomatous reaction in sensitized individuals.

Zirconium, beryllium and chromium may produce allergic granulomas. Talc, zinc, stearate, silica and magnesium produce irritant granulomas

Allergic Contact Granulomas

Zirconium granuloma. This skin lesion, originally seen following use of zirconium compounds as deodorants,[17] continues to occur following use of these compounds for the treatment of rhus dermatitis.

The lesions usually appear 4 to 6 weeks following initial use of the zirconium preparation and are limited to the sites of contact. They appear as persistent, firm, shiny, erythematous papules the color of flesh or apple jelly, and they may be solitary, grouped or coalescent. Eczematous changes are also usually present. Pruritus is minimal or absent.[18] The histologic picture may be indistinguishable from sarcoid.[19,20]

Any defect in the protective layer of the skin enhances the development of hypersensitivity.

In the axillae, minute abrasions from shaving as well as from excess friction and sweating enhance the penetration of the zirconium salts in the deodorants. The preparations containing zirconium salts used for treatment of rhus dermatitis readily penetrate acutely inflamed skin, denuded areas, vesicles and bullae.[21]

The zirconium granulomas composed of epithelioid cells represent an acquired allergic reaction of the delayed type to zirconium in sensitized individuals.[22]

Tests for Zirconium Hypersensitivity. Either patch or intracutaneous testing may be employed to determine allergic hypersensitivity to zirconium salts.[23]

Use of zirconium salts, which are sensitizers and can cause epithelioid granulomatous reactions, should be avoided in therapeutic agents

Plate 11. Non-eczematous Contact Dermatitis

1. Lichenoid

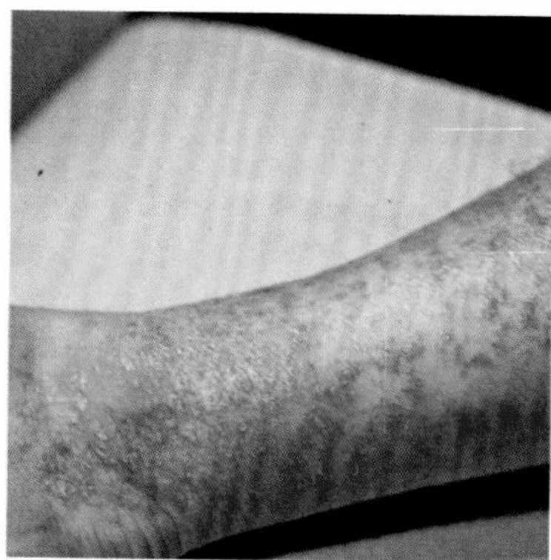

Isopropyl PPDA in Rubber Bandage

2. Follicular

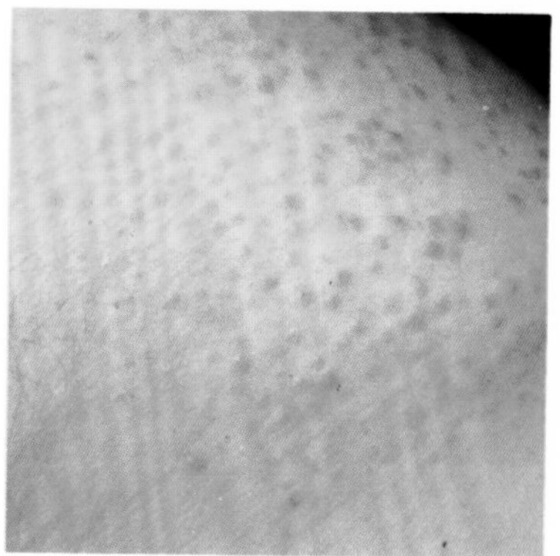

Wash and Wear Clothes
Formaldehyde Resin?

3. Zirconium Granuloma
of the Neck

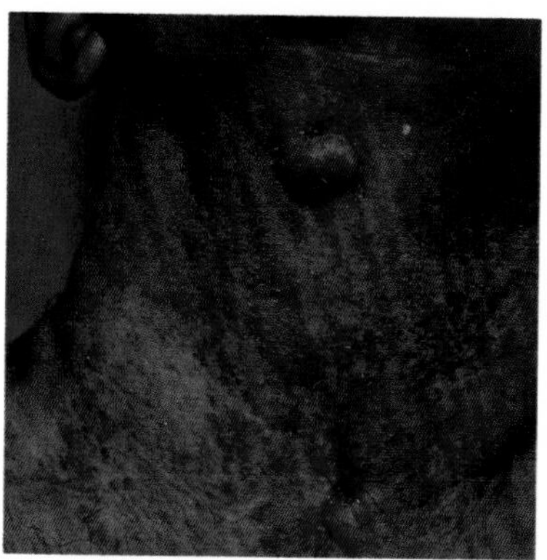

Allergic Sensitization to
Zirconium Oxide in a
Poison Ivy Remedy

4. Purpuric

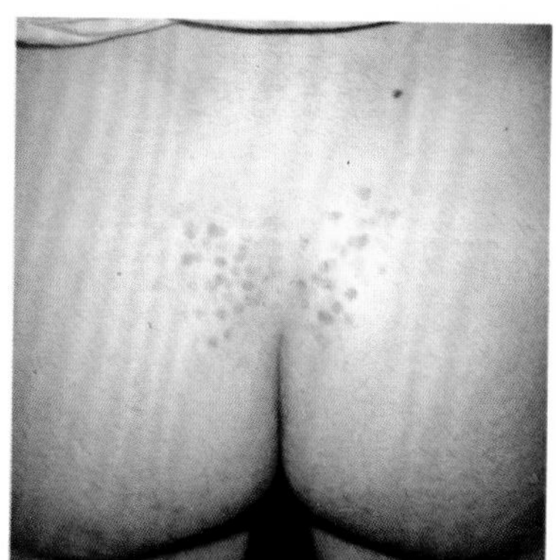

Zirconium in Poison-ivy Remedy

5. Cellulitis-like

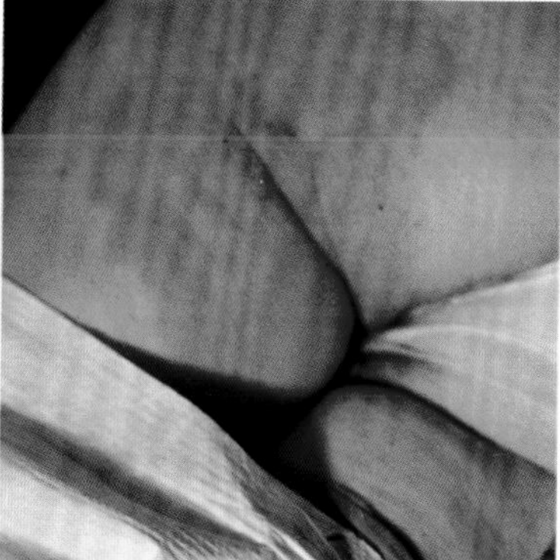

Nickel Garter Clip

6. Urticarial

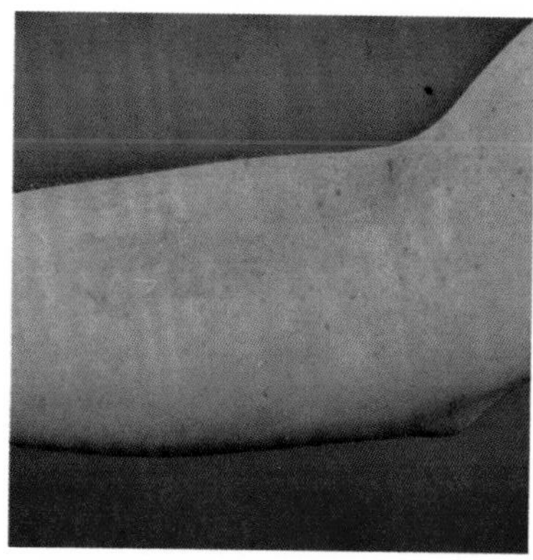

Dog Saliva
(New York Skin and Cancer Unit)

Patch Test. The zirconium preparation suspected of causing a granulomatous reaction may be rubbed into a test site that has previously been prepared by multiple scratches or denuded by a dermal curet. The test site is then covered with an occlusive dressing for 2 days. In sensitized individuals, a positive reaction consists of the development of reddish brown papules in about 4 weeks. Such papules show a sarcoid granulomatous infiltrate histologically.

Intracutaneous Test. A small wheal is made by the intracutaneous injection of a 1:10,000 dilution of sodium zirconium lactate. A positive reaction consists of a discrete papule, which appears in 8 to 14 days. In about a month, the papule clinically and histologically has the appearance of a sarcoid lesion. The papule may persist for 6 to 24 months.

Prognosis for Zirconium Granulomas. Axillary granulomas produced by the soluble zirconium lactate in deodorants usually disappear within a few months. Lesions produced by the insoluble zirconium oxide preparations used for poison ivy dermatitis usually remain unchanged for several months to years and are refractory to therapy. Temporary improvement is obtained with corticosteroids administered systemically or intralesionally.

Beryllium Granulomas. (See chapter on metals.)

Nonallergic Contact Granulomas

Sodium Stearate. The granulomatous response to sodium stearate is not based on allergic reactivity. It can be contrasted with the allergic granulomatous responses in patients with zirconium deodorant granulomas who are immunologically prepared as a result of their allergic hypersensitivity to zirconium. Most people, therefore, do not develop granuloma after skin tests with zirconium salts.

Large quantities of sodium stearate are required to elicit the granulomatous response, whereas unusually dilute preparations of the zirconium will produce it in the susceptible individual. Often even 0.0001 M solutions of zirconium salts stimulate the formation of a granuloma in the allergic individual. Less than 0.1 M concentrations of sodium stearate or sodium palmitate fail to induce such reactions.

Stearate granulomas resolve clinically within a few weeks, but allergic granulomas usually reach their peak at 3 to 6 weeks and persist for months to years. In general, allergic granulomas are still evolving when the stearate granulomas have completely resolved.

Talc Granuloma. McCallum and Hall[24] stated that treatment of the raw umbilical stump can produce pyogenic granulomas and umbilical polyps. They submit that treatment with talc or starch should be discontinued and replaced by a nonirritant and sterile substance.

Tye and co-workers[25] described hundreds of talc granulomas of the skin that developed in a 45-year-old woman. It is postulated that the talcum powder gained entrance through the skin at the sites of draining or incised furuncles.

Oil Granulomas. Bergeron and Stone[26] observed 2 cases of multiple perifollicular granulomas of the scalp produced by Egyptian Oil, a proprietary hair conditioner. Upon discontinuance of the hair condition, the lesions regressed in both patients.

Granuloma Fissuratum. Chronic irritation from glasses or dentures can produce granulomas at the site of pressure of the hard object. Such granulomas usually have a crease down the middle of the lesion.

DRY, LICHENIFIED OR HYPERKERATOTIC CONTACT DERMATITIS

Air-borne allergens and dusts tend to form dry, lichenified eruptions.

Air-borne Allergens and Irritants. Contact dermatitis from prolonged, repeated exposure to relatively small quantities of air-borne allergens, such as pollens, dusts and vapors, tends to produce diffuse, dry and lichenified eruptions without vesiculation. The exposed portions of the body as well as wrinkles and folds tend to be most markedly involved.

Ragweed Dermatitis. This type of dermatitis rarely is frankly vesicular unless the patient actually comes in contact with the plant. Exposure to the oleoresin through air-borne pollen may result in a dry, leathery dermatitis with skin so infiltrated that a lymphoblastoma is suspected.

Dermatitis Due to Dust. Dusts and their contents may produce mechanical effects, primary irritant eruptions and allergic reactions.[27]

Dust containing glass fibers can produce cuts due to its content of sharp fragments of glass. Exposed surfaces may sustain an intensely pruritic, papular eruption. The penetrating spicules of asbestos, a fibrous, silicate mineral, are mechanical irritants that can produce asbestos "corns," particularly on the palmar aspects of the fingers. Coal, rock and stone dust have an abrasive effect on the skin and can produce a lichenified, papular eruption, which may be complicated by folliculitis. Dust collecting about a collar, beltline or the ends of sleeves may be rubbed into the skin by friction, producing lichenified eruptions.

Pollens, chemical dusts and sawdust usually produce dry, lichenified dermatitis

Dermatitis due to cement dust also tends to be dry and lichenified, primarily because of its alkalinity, hygroscopic properties and abrasive effects. In addition, even when cement dermatitis is due to allergic hypersensitivity to the chromium or cobalt content, the eruption tends toward dryness rather than frank vesiculation.

Sawdust from teak, redwood, mahogany and rosewood may contain sensitizers that produce a dry dermatitis, particularly on the face, penis and scrotum, among carpenters and woodworkers. A lichenified eruption may also appear on the penis and scrotum when sawdust falls inside the clothes or is conveyed to these parts by the hands.

Other chemical dusts, fumes and vapors produce eruptions similar to sawdust dermatitis. In addition, dust and air pollutants containing pitch or tar produce follicular, keratotic and acneiform eruptions, melanosis and photosensitivity reactions.

A dermatitis resembling ichthyosis caused by a quaternary ammonium compound in an ointment has been reported from Japan.[28] The compound implicated is alkyl benzyl trimethyl ammonium chloride.

CONTACT HYPERKERATOTIC ERUPTIONS OF THE FINGERS, PALMS AND SOLES

The thick, horny layer of the fingers, palms and soles modifies the appearance of allergic contact dermatitis by minimizing the eczematous element. The dry, fissured eruptions may resemble those due to primary irritants, psoriasis, hyperkeratotic fungous infections or atopic dermatitis.

In dentists, allergic contact dermatitis due to Novocain or acrylic monomer is scaly, thickened and fissured. Affected nails may become thickened, dystrophic and separated from the nailbed.

Contact dermatitis of palms and soles may produce dystrophic nails and must be differentiated from psoriasis, atopic dermatitis and hyperkeratotic dermatophytosis

So-called tulip bulb fingers, in which the affected skin is dry, fissured and hyperkeratotic, may resemble Novocain and acrylic dermatitis. Onions, garlic and formaldehyde and its resins may produce similar eruptions on the palms and palmar surfaces of the fingers.

In nickel-sensitive individuals, the prolonged contact with nickel-plated handlebars or door handles plus pressure may produce a dry, fissured eruption of the palm. Similarly, nickel-plated arch supports may produce such changes on the soles.

ACNEIFORM ERUPTIONS DUE TO CONTACTANTS

Acneiform eruptions may be caused by prolonged contact with cutting oils, tar, chlorinated hydrocarbons and waxes. In contrast to ordinary acne, which occurs commonly on the face, chest and back, cutting oil acne appears wherever the skin becomes soaked with the oil, but particularly on the external surface of the forearms and the anterior surface of the thighs.

Chloracne due to contact with chlorinated hydrocarbons may be complicated by an acquired porphyria

Chlorinated hydrocarbons produce large comedones and form cystic lesions on the face, neck, abdomen and chest. Patients with adolescent acne tend to get severe chloracne.

In addition, hexachlorobenzene and related chemicals, such as 2,4-dichlorophenol (2,4-D) and 2,4,5-trichlorophenol (2,4,5-T), may produce an acquired porphyria in addition to chloracne.[29]

Industrially acquired acneiform eruptions are difficult to clear. Antibiotics, which are often helpful in ordinary acne, are not particularly effective in these eruptions. Proper hygiene, avoidance of the acne-producing contactant, administration of large doses of vitamin A and application of peeling sulfur lotions aid in clearing the eruption.

CONTACT EPILATING FOLLICULITIS

This type of folliculitis is produced by the penetration of sharp needles of the sugarcane bark into the hair follicles of sugarcane workers.[30] An inflammatory, follicular, pustular eruption is produced, particularly on the extremities. The borders of the scalp, the pubic area and the chest and back may also be involved. Pruritus is severe, and the involved follicle atrophies with permanent loss of hair.

An epilating folliculitis has been said to result from the wearing of wash and wear clothing.[31]

LICHENOID ERUPTIONS DUE TO CONTACT WITH COLOR FILM DEVELOPER

Certain substituted paraphenylenediamine compounds used as color film developers can produce a lichenoid eruption on skin coming in contact with these chemicals.[32] In affected individuals, acute or subacute allergic eczematous or papular dermatitis appears, then fades and is replaced by an eruption identical to that of lichen planus.[33] It subsides after several weeks, leaving marked pigmentation. Sensitization in exposed workers is fairly high and may take 1 month to 3 years to develop.

Patch test reactions to color developers such as CD2 (2-amino-5-diethylamino-toluene monohydrochloride) are positive in sensitized individuals who acquire lichenoid eruptions.[34] Patch tests with CD2 should be performed with a 1 per cent aqueous solution.

Substituted paraphenylenediamines used as color film developers may produce eruptions that are identical to those of lichen planus

The closed patch technique is most conveniently used. The patch is removed in 24 hours, and the underlying skin is washed gently with an acid-type cleanser. This removes excess chemical, which, because of its ability to become fixed to epidermal cells, might lead to sensitization. Skin reactions are read at 1 hour and again in 24 and 48 hours after removal of the patch. Evolution of the lesion over the next few days produces the typical lichenoid eruption. The brownish stain remaining on the skin after removal of the patch and subsequent washing should not be confused with a positive skin reaction.

Paraphenylenediamine does not produce this type of lichenoid eruption and does not seem to cross-react with the substituted paraphenylenediamine used as a color developer.

A lichenoid dermatitis has been produced by isopropyl aminodiphenylamine used as an antioxidant in rubber tires (Dr. C. D. Calnan, personal communication, 1971). The clinical appearance was similar to the lichenoid eruptions from color film developers. The areas of skin affected were those in contact with the rubber tires while the patient was carrying them. There was no cross-sensitization to the color film developers.

Lichenoid contact dermatitis due to substances used in developing baths for color films, namely, 2-amino-diethyl-amino toluene hydrochloride, n-n-diethyl-paraphenylenediamine and hydroxylamine hydrochloride, has been described by Dr. C. L. Meneghini (personal communication, 1971). He also described a lichenoid dermatitis on the lower extremities caused by black stocking dye in women who go into mourning for months. Positive reactions were obtained to paraphenylenediamine and para-amino compounds.

CONTACT PURPURIC ERUPTIONS

European reports describe petechial and purpuric eruptions from rough woolen socks and underwear. In some instances, residual wool oil lubricants have been implicated in this type of eruption.[35] Several reports also describe purpuric eruptions from rubber in clothing and textiles.[36–43] A purpuric eruption on the extremities following application of medication containing oxyquinoline has also been reported from France.[1]

Sedormid[44] and quinidine[45] have produced purpuric patch test reactions in individuals who had purpuric drug eruptions from the ingestion of these medicaments. Sedormid was tested as a saturated solution in propylene glycol. The patch test with quinidine consisted of a paste made by crushing a tablet of quinidine sulfate in a small volume of water. The material was left in contact with the patient's arm or back for 24 to 48 hours. The reaction is considered positive if the area of contact shows numerous small petechial hemorrhages.

Contact with Fiberglas may produce purpura, telangiectasia, folliculitis, urticaria and linear erosions in the skin creases. Clothing washed with glass fiber curtains may become contaminated with the particles and produce a purpuric contact dermatitis in the wearer.[46]

Osmundsen[47] described a dermatitis of epidemic proportions that appeared in Europe from an optical whitener in washing powders. The eruption, a reticulate pattern of faint red-brown spots with a few petechiae and dilated small vessels, may suggest a reticulosis.

Purpura produced by the suction effect of cupping is well known. A similar phenomenon due to the suction effect of plastic car seat covers was recently observed.

REFERENCES

1. Sidi, E., and Hincky, M.: *Les Manifestations Atypiques de L'Allergie de Contact.* Communication faite a la Societe Francoise d'Allergie. Seance du 20 Novembre 1956, p. 283.

Contact Urticaria

2. Shelley, W. B., and Rawnsley, H. M.: Aquagenic Urticaria. J.A.M.A., *189*, 805, 1964.
3. Chalamidas, S. L., and Charles, D. C.: Aquagenic Urticaria. Arch. Derm., *104*, 541, 1971.
4. Key, M. M.: Some Unusual Reactions in Industry. Arch. Derm., *83*, 3, 1961.
5. Gaul, L. E.: Dermatitis from Cetyl and Stearyl Alcohol. Arch. Derm., *99*, 593, 1969.
6. Stoughton, R. B., and Fritsch, W.: Dimethyl Sulfoxide and Absorption. Arch. Derm., *90*, 512, 1964.
7. McCabe, R. J.: Studies with the Local Use of the Furfuryl Ester of Nicotinic Acid. A.M.A. Arch. Derm., *74*, 522, 1956.
8. Murrell, T. W., Jr., and Taylor, W. M.: The Cutaneous Reaction to Nicotinic Acid (Niacin) —Furfuryl. A.M.A. Arch. Derm., *79*, 545, 1959.
9. Ziprowski, L., Hofshi, E., and Tahori, A. S.: Caterpillar Dermatitis. Israel Med. J., *18*, 26, 1959.
10. Ioannides, G., and Davis, J. H.: Portuguese Man-Of-War Stinging. Arch. Derm., *91*, 448, 1965.
11. Sams, W. M.: Seabather's Eruption. Arch. Derm. & Syph., *60*, 227, 1949.
12. Cort, W. W.: Schistosome Dermatitis. Amer. J. Hyg., *50*, 152, 1950.
13. Hunter, G. W., III, Molloy, J. F., and Ullman, A. F.: More Seabather's Eruption. Amer. J. Pub. Health, *53*, 1413, 1963.
14. Hutton, R. F.: Marine Dermatitis. Arch. Derm., *82*, 951, 1960.
15. Grauer, F. H., and Arnold, H. L., Jr.: Seaweed Dermatitis. Arch. Derm., *84*, 729, 1961.

Contact Granulomas

16. Shelley, W. B., et al: Intradermal Tests with Metals and Other Inorganic Elements in Sarcoidosis and Anthraco-Silicosis. J. Invest. Derm., *31*, 301, 1958.
17. Sheard, G.: Granulomatous Reactions Due to Deodorant Sticks. J.A.M.A., *164*, 1085, 1957.
18. Rubin, L.: Granulomas of Axillae Caused by Deodorants. J.A.M.A., *162*, 953, 1956.
19. Williams, R. M., and Skipworth, G. B.: Zirconium Granulomas of Glabrous Skin Following Treatment of Rhus Dermatitis. A.M.A. Arch. Derm., *80*, 273, 1959.
20. Epstein, W. L., and Allen, J. R.: Granulomatous Hypersensitivity After Use of Zirconium-Containing Poison Oak Lotions. J.A.M.A., *190*, 162, 1964.

21. Baler, G. R.: Granulomas from Topical Zirconium in Poison Ivy Dermatitis. Arch. Derm., *91*, 145, 1965.
22. Shelley, W. B., and Hurley, H. J.: Allergic Origin of Zirconium Deodorant Granuloma. Brit. J. Derm., *70*, 75, 1958.
23. LoPresti, P. J., and Hambrick, G. W.: Zirconium Granuloma Following Treatment of Rhus Dermatitis. Arch. Derm., *92*, 188, 1965.
24. McCallum, D. I., and Hall, G. F. M.: Umbilical Granulomata—with Particular Reference to Talc Granuloma. Brit. J. Derm., *83*, 151, 1970.
25. Tye, M. J., Hashimoto, K., and Fox, F.: Talc Granulomas of the Skin. J.A.M.A., *198*, 120, 1966.
26. Bergeron, J. R., and Stone, O. J.: Multiple Granulomas of the Scalp of Exogenous Origin. Cutis, *5*, 57, 1969.

Hyperkeratotic Contact Dermatitis

27. Sneddon, I. B.: Dust and the Skin. Med. Presse, *21*, 1102, 1958.
28. Skevi, M., and Mizuno, F.: Unusual Cornification in Ichthyosis-Like Dermatitis. Arch. Derm., *50*, 388, 1970.
29. Bleiberg, J., et al.: Industrially Acquired Porphyria. Arch. Derm., *99*, 793, 1964.
30. Pardo-Castello, V.: Epilating Folliculitis. Derm. Trop., *2*, 235, 1963.
31. Rudner, A.: Personal communication.

Lichenoid Contact Dermatitis

32. Buckley, W. R.: Lichenoid Eruptions Following Contact Dermatitis. A.M.A. Arch. Derm., *78*, 454, 1958.
33. Canizares, O.: Lichen Planus-Like Eruption Caused by Color Developer. A.M.A. Arch. Derm., *80*, 81, 1959.
34. Mandel, E. H.: Lichen Planus-Like Eruptions Caused by a Color-Film Developer. A.M.A. Arch. Derm., *81*, 516, 1960.

Purpuric Contact Dermatitis

35. Greenwood, R.: Dermatitis with Capillary Fragility. Arch. Derm., *81*, 947, 1960.
36. Osmundsen, P. E.: Pigmented Contact Dermatitis. Brit. J. Derm., *83*, 296, 1970.
37. Batschvarov, B., and Minkov, D. M.: Dermatitis and Purpura from Rubber in Clothing. Trans. St. John Hosp. Derm. Soc., *54*, 178, 1968.
38. Champion, R. H.: Purpura. In A. Rook, D. S. Wilkinson and F. J. G. Ebling (eds.): *Textbook of Dermatology*. Oxford, Blackwell, 1967, p. 426.
39. Doucas, C., and Kapetanakis, J.: Eczematid-Like Purpura. Dermatologica, *106*, 86, 1953.
40. Hodgson, G. A., and Hellier, F. F.: Dermatitis Caused by Shirts in B.L.A. Kir. Army Med. Cps., *87*, 110, 1946.
41. Joseph, H. L., and Maibach, H. I.: Contact Dermatitis from Spandex Brassieres. J.A.M.A., *201*, 880, 1967.
42. Mosto, S. J., and Casala, A. M.: Disseminated Puriginous Angio-Dermatitis (Itching Purpura). Arch. Derm., *91*, 351, 1965.
43. Hellier, F. F.: Dermatitis Purpura After Contact with Textiles. Hautarzt, *11*, 173, 1960.
44. Ackroyd, J. F.: The Role of Sedormid in the Immunological Reaction that Results in Platelet Lysis in Sedormid Purpura. Clin. Sci., *13*, 409, 1954.
45. Friedman, A. L., Brody, E. A., and Barr, P. S.: Immunothrombocytopenic Purpura Due to Quinidine: Report of Four New Cases with Special Observations on Patch Testing. J. Lab. Clin. Med., *48*, 205, 1956.
46. Abel, R. R.: Washing Machine and Fiberglass. Arch. Derm., *93*, 78, 1966.
47. Osmundsen, P. E.: Contact Dermatitis from an Optical Whitener in Washing Powders. Cutis, *10*, 59, 1972.

17

Systemic Eczematous Contact-Type Dermatitis

Ordinarily allergic eczematous contact dermatitis is produced by external exposure of the skin to a chemical. Occasionally, however, in sensitized individuals a systemically administered drug may reach the skin via the circulatory system and produce a hematogenous contact-type of dermatitis medicamentosa. Although the eczematous condition is produced by systemic administration, the first sensitizing exposure to the drug may have been by topical application. In such instances, an eczematous contact-type of eruption may be produced not only by the sensitizing drug, but also by drugs that are immunochemically related.

Previous ingestion of an allergen appears to have no influence on later contact sensitization in man. Ingestion of an allergen by a person previously sensitized by contact, however, may result in a variety of reactions. Most frequent reactions are focal flares at sites of previous dermatitis or occasionally dyshidrotic eruptions, but generalized eruptions may occur. Sometimes such flares may occur also from *inhalation* of the allergen.

This type of endogenic contact eczema from ingestion or systemic administration of an allergen may occasionally be accompanied by systemic effects.

Systemic or endogenic allergic contact eczema may be accompanied by systemic effects

In some sensitized patients, ingestion or parenteral administration of the contact allergen causes no reaction either in the skin or systemically. In other cases, there is a rapid response, within hours, which suggests that an immediate rather than a delayed type of hypersensitivity may be involved.

Topically applied penicillin, sulfonamides, certain broad spectrum antibiotics, antihistamines, local anesthetics, mercurials, chloral hydrate, resorcin and quinine may sensitize and subsequently produce an eczematous contact-type dermatitis upon systemic administration.[1] In addition, an eczematous dermatitis due to external sensitization by drugs such as chlorpromazine, neomycin and streptomycin may undergo exacerbation or be produced through systemic administration of immunochemically related compounds. Furthermore, the external sensitization may have been engendered by chemicals that are not drugs.[2] For example, sensitization to hydrazine hydrobromide through industrial exposure may predispose the patient to an eczematous contact-type dermatitis medicamentosa upon the administration of immunochemically related medicaments, such as isoniazid and Apresoline.[3]

Systemic contact-type dermatitis medicamentosa tends to be symmetrically distributed, as are other hematogenously produced dermatoses. In the early phases, however, the eruption often is most pronounced at sites previously involved from external exposure.

Eczematous contact dermatitis may be produced by systemic administration of a drug to an individual previously sensitized by topical application of the drug or a related chemical

ANTIBIOTICS

Topical use of penicillin and streptomycin should be avoided because of the high sensitization potential.[4] Although neomycin has been reported as producing many instances of allergic contact dermatitis, it is still used widely. The other antibiotics, such as the tetracyclines, erythromycin and chloramphenicol, rarely produce allergic contact dermatitis.

Penicillin. Topical use of penicillin is largely avoided at present because many individuals would develop contact sensitivity to the drug. Allergic contact dermatitis from penicillin occurs particularly in physicians, nurses and pharmacists who handle this antibiotic. Systemic administration of penicillin to such "externally" sensitized individuals may produce an eczematous contact-type dermatitis, which may be accompanied by urticarial anaphylactic sensitivity.

Penicillin in milk was the cause of attacks of eczema in 2 patients, both of whom were sensitive to penicillin on patch testing.[5]

Among the antibiotics, penicillin, neomycin and streptomycin have the highest potential as topical sensitizers. The other antibiotics rarely cause allergic contact dermatitis or eczematous contact-type dermatitis medicamentosa

Streptomycin. Although topical application of streptomycin is now avoided, members of the medical, nursing and pharmaceutical professions who handle the drug readily become sensitized, and subsequent systemic administration may produce a severe eczematous contact-type dermatitis medicamentosa. Since streptomycin may cross-react with neomycin, systemic administration of streptomycin may produce the eczematous contact-type dermatitis in individuals who had become sensitized to neomycin and had never been exposed to streptomycin. Streptomycin may also cross-react with kanamycin sulfate (Kantrex).

Streptomycin may be administered alone or in combination with penicillin in preparations such as Strep-Combiotic (Pfizer), Bivillimycin (Wyeth) and Wycillin (Wyeth).

Desensitization procedures by subcutaneous injection of streptomycin may be accompanied by urticaria or flares of dermatitis.

Neomycin Sulfate. This antibiotic is present not only in a host of ointments, creams and other topical medications, but has been added also to cosmetics, soaps and deodorants.[6] It has a significant capacity to produce allergic contact sensitivity.[7] Once sensitization to neomycin from topical exposure has been established, systemic administration of either streptomycin or kanamycin, both of which may cross-react with neomycin, may cause an eczematous contact-type dermatitis medicamentosa.[8]

In addition, although neomycin and bacitracin are not chemically related, in many instances there is a combined sensitivity to these two drugs. Such occurrences represent coincidental simultaneous sensitization rather than true cross-sensitivity.[9]

Pirila and Rantanen[10] gave an account of repeated eruptions in a patient sensitive to neomycin and bacitracin because of their topical use on an amputation stump. Later he developed a severe stomatitis from throat tablets containing bacitracin and from a paste containing both antibiotics used to fill an infected root canal. Oral administration of neomycin produced diarrhea and dermatitis. Ekelund and Moller[11] also produced dermatitis by the oral administration of neomycin in sensitized patients. Previous patch test sites flared.

Neomycin may be administered systemically in Bacimycin, Cremomycin, Kaomycin, Mycifradin, Paremycin, Prednicidin, Sorboquel with Neomycin, and Sulfacidin.

Neomycin shows strong cross-sensitization with paromomycin and ambutyrosin (CL-642) because of the presence of neosamine sugars in all three (Dr. W. Schorr, personal communication).

Tetracyclines. These antibiotics are safe to

apply topically, because allergic contact dermatitis rarely occurs from such usage. Eczematous eruptions of the fixed type do occasionally result from systemic administration.[12] Furthermore, cross-fixed drug eruptions from systemic use of Aureomycin, Achromycin and Terramycin have been described.[13]

In rare instances, in which allergic contact dermatitis does occur from use of Aureomycin or Achromycin ointment, the sensitizer may be the parabens added as preservatives or the certified azo dyes.

Erythromycin (*Ilotycin*, *Ilosone*, *Erythrocin*, *Pediamycin*). Topical sensitization to this antibiotic is extremely rare. Ilotycin Ointment does not contain parabens or coloring matter.

Chloramphenicol. The report by Schwank and Jirasek[14] that there was cross-sensitization between 2,4-dinitrochlorbenzene and chloramphenicol was not confirmed by Palacios et al.[15] Dr. J. E. Rasmussen (personal communication) has failed to find such cross-sensitization.

Bacitracin. Roupe and Strannegard[16] stated that a case of anaphylactic shock followed topical administration of an ointment containing bacitracin and neomycin. Antibacitracin reagins were demonstrated in sera from the patient with atopic dermatitis. There is strong evidence that the anaphylactic shock was due to hypersensitivity to bacitracin.

Atarax (*Hydroxyzine Dichloride*). Dr. J. Fregert (personal communication) reported on a patient working in the pharmaceutical industry who became sensitized to piperazine, which was being manufactured to be used mainly as a vermifuge. When this patient took Atarax, he developed a dermatitis of the upper extremities and face, which cleared when he stopped taking the drug. It is likely that piperazine is formed in the body from hydroxyzine.

Patch tests were positive to piperazine 1 per cent in water.

ANTIHISTAMINES

The antihistamines can readily sensitize the skin following topical use or occupational exposure. Although many dermatologists have discontinued topical use of antihistamines because of their high sensitizing potential, they are nevertheless still widely used.[17]

Table 17–1 is a list of currently popular topical antihistamine preparations.

The *systemic* administration of antihistamines rarely engenders sensitization, but once the patient is sensitized by *topical* application, eczematous contact-type dermatitis may occur from the antihistamine or from immunochemically related compounds.

The antihistamines Antistine, Phenergan and Pyribenzamine, which are ethylenediamine derivatives, are particularly active topical sensitizers and often produce eczematous contact-type dermatitis medicamentosa in sensitized individuals. Cross-reactions may occur with other antihistamines, such as Synopen (chlorpyramine) and Neohetramine (thonzylamine), which are also derived from ethylenediamine.

Ethylenediamine. This chemical, used as a stabilizing preservative in Mycolog Cream, is a strong sensitizer.[18] Industrial exposure

Table 17-1. Topical Antihistamines

Brand Name	*Generic Name*	*Manufacturer*
Antistine Solution	Antazoline	CIBA
Phenergan Cream	Promethazine	Wyeth
Pyribenzamine	Tripelennamine	CIBA
Caladryl Lotion and Cream	Diphenhydramine	Parke, Davis
Antopic Cream	Pyranisamine maleate	Smith-Dorsey
Neohetramine Ointment	Thonzylamine	Nepra
Thenylene Cream	Thenylpyramine	Abbott
Histadyl Ointment	Thenylpyramine (hydrochloride)	Eli Lilly
Trimeton Ointment	Prophenpyridamine	Schering
Thephorin Ointment and Lotion	Phenindamine	Hoffman-LaRoche

to it has been reported as a cause of allergic dermatitis.[19]

Sensitization to ethylenediamine may follow exposure to aminophylline (a combination of theophylline and ethylenediamine),[20] and topical use of ethylenediamine-related antihistaminics, namely, antazoline hydrochloride (Antistine Ophthalmic Solution), promethazine (Phenergan) cream and tripelennamine (Pyribenzamine) cream. Ethylenediamine tetraacetate (EDTA), a preservative in ophthalmic solutions, is another source of exposure and sensitization.[21] Systemic administration of aminophylline, tripelennamine or promethazine to ethylenediamine-sensitive individuals may result in eczematous eruptions.[22]

Systemic antihistamines rarely sensitize. Topical antihistamines are frequent sensitizers. Such topical sensitization may engender dermatitis from antihistamines and aminophylline

Antistine. This antihistamine may be used topically in the form of eye and nose drops. Following sensitization from such topical exposure to Antistine, systemic administration of the related Pyribenzamine has produced an eczematous contact-type dermatitis medicamentosa.[23] Patients with allergic hypersensitivity to Antistine may cross-react with, and show positive patch test reactions to, other antihistamines aside from Pyribenzamine, including Neo-Antergan, Diarin, Thenylene, Neohetramine, Trimeton, Benadryl and Synopen.[24]

The antihistamines Phenergan, Pyribenzamine and Antistine, derived from ethylenediamine, are potent topical sensitizers. They may cross-react with each other and the ethylene component of aminophylline

Antistine Nose Drops may be combined with Privine (naphazoline hydrochloride) and also contain phenylmercuric acetate as a preservative. When a positive patch test reaction to such nose drops is obtained, the role of the Privine or the mercury preservative may be ruled out by testing with pure Antistine crystals.

Phenergan. Phenergan Creams can produce both allergic eczematous contact dermatitis and a photocontact dermatitis.[25] Cross-reactions between Phenergan and chlorpromazine (Thorazine) have been reported many times.[26] Systemic administration of Phenergan or immunochemically related substances, such as Thephorin, Pyribenzamine and particularly chlorpromazine, may produce an eczematous contact-type dermatitis medicamentosa. Cross-reactions have also been reported between Phenergan and chemicals containing the para-amino group, including procaine.[26]

Phenergan, a potent topical sensitizer, may cross-react not only with other antihistamines, but also with Thorazine. In addition, it can produce a photocontact dermatitis

Pyribenzamine. Sensitization to this antihistaminic may occur from topical application of creams and ointments containing the compound. Pyribenzamine may cross-react with Antistine and Phenergan, both of which are derived from ethylenediamine.

There has been a single case report of a cross-reaction between Pyribenzamine and sulfapyridine based on identical pyridine rings.[27]

Antihistamines Derived from Aminalkyl Ether. These compounds include Benadryl (diphenhydramine) and Decapryn (doxylamine succinate). Dramamine (dimenhydrinate) is closely related to these antihistamines. Caladryl preparations contain Benadryl. This group of compounds are sensitizers when applied topically.

Allergic contact dermatitis due to caladryl may flare when Benadryl is administered systemically

Trimeton (Pheniramine). This drug may produce allergic contact dermatitis. Positive reactions to patch tests may cause the original eruption to flare, and ingestion of the drug in sensitized individuals may produce eczematous contact-type dermatitis.[28]

Histadyl (Methapyrilene). Histadyl Cream may produce allergic eczematous dermatitis. It apparently does not cross-react with the other antihistamines.[29]

Thephorin (Phenindamine). This antihistamine may produce allergic contact dermatitis in as high as 28 per cent of individuals exposed to it by topical application.[30–32]

PHENOTHIAZINES

All of these compounds are potential photosensitizers.

Medical and nursing personnel who inject these drugs and those handling the compounds in the pharmaceutical industry readily acquire allergic eczematous contact dermatitis from such exposure. Often a photoallergic reaction occurs in combination with the contact dermatitis.[25] Systemic administration of the phenothiazine drugs may produce an eczematous contact-type dermatitis medicamentosa in individuals sensitized by topical application. Cross-reactions readily take place between phenothiazines and related antihistamines, such as Phenergan, Theruhistin and Pyrrolazote.[33] Methylene blue, a phenothiazine dye, is also a powerful photosensitizer.

Nurses sensitized to chlorpromazine have been desensitized by taking the drug orally. Positive patch test reactions have been reported to become negative after such procedures.[34]

The phenothiazine group of drugs can produce allergic contact dermatitis, photoallergic reactions and eczematous contact-type dermatitis and may cross-react with certain antihistamines. Oral desensitization has been accomplished

PARA-AMINO COMPOUNDS

Chemicals that contain an amino group in the para position on the benzene ring are often potent sensitizers. They include paraphenylenediamine, para-aminobenzoic acid esters, para-aminosalicyclic acid, certain local anesthetics (e.g., benzocaine) and sulfanilamide.

These para-amino compounds may cross-react with one another and also with azo and aniline dyes.[35] Allergic contact dermatitis may occur readily from exposure to paraphenylenediamine in hair and fur dyes. Of the topical anesthetics in this group, benzocaine is the most notorious sensitizer. The salts of para-aminobenzoic acid used in sunscreens occasionally sensitize, but the acid is not as potent a sensitizer as are its esters. Sulfanilamide is sparingly used as a topical medication at present.

With the exception of paraphenylenediamine, the para-amino compounds may be used systemically and can produce eczematous contact-type dermatitis medicamentosa in patients who have been sensitized by topical exposure to any compound in this group. It is possible that ingestion of certified azo dyes may produce eczematous contact-type dermatitis in patients sensitized to the para-amino compounds.[36]

Paraphenylenediamine-sensitive patients may react to procaine and the sulfonamides by developing systemic contact dermatitis

Para-aminobenzoic Acid (PABA). This acid or its esters administered systemically for collagen diseases to patients who had previously been sensitized topically may react with a systemic contact dermatitis.[37]

Local Anesthetics. Some local anesthetics based on para-aminobenzoic acid are procaine (Novocain), benzocaine (Anesthesin, ethyl aminobenzoate), butethamine (Monocaine), tetracaine (Pontocaine) and butacaine (Butyn). These often cross-react with the parent substance.[38]

Procaine. This compound is used principally as a local anesthetic, but on occasion it may be administered orally for painful conditions. Parcaine (Lampar) is such an oral procaine preparation. Pronestyl, an oral and injectable product, is the amide analogue of procaine. Eczematous dermatitis medicamentosa from the systemic administration of procaine, even in individuals with allergic contact sensitivity to this anesthetic, is apparently rare.[39] Procaine-sensitive patients may show systemic dermatitis when given sulfonamides.[40]

Aminosalicylic Acid. This antituberculosis drug is present in Neopasalate, Paskalium, PAS, Di-Isopacin, Pasna Tri-Pack and PAS-C. It may cross-react not only with the para-amino group, but also with the salicylates.[41] Eczematous contact-type dermatitis medicamentosa from its administration may occur in individuals sensitized to paraphenylenediamine and other compounds of the para-amino group.

SULFONAMIDES

Cross-reactions can occur between the antibacterial sulfonamides and chemically related sulfonamides used as diuretics, oral hypoglycemics and sweetening agents. Topical application of a sulfonamide may sensitize the patient and subsequent systemic administration of a sulfonamide may produce eczematous contact-type dermatitis medicamentosa.[42]

Sulfanilamide. The systemic administration of this older sulfonamide preparation has largely been discarded. Exposure to sulfanilamide, however, may still take place from topical application of AVC Cream and Suppositories (15 per cent sulfanilamide), Vagitrol (10 per cent sulfanilamide), Otomide (5 per cent sulfanilamide) and Sulfamil Vaginal Cream (15 per cent sulfanilamide). Compounds containing sulfanilamide may be sensitizers and photoallergic agents and may cross-react with chemicals with a para-amino group.

Sulfonamide Diuretics. These thiazide and related sulfonamide compounds are photosensitizers.[43] Such thiazide sulfonamide compounds include chlorothiazide (Diuril), bendroflumethiazide (Naturetin), benzthiazide (Exna), cyclothiazide (Anhydron), hydrochlorothiazide (Esidrix, HydroDIURIL, Oretic), hydroflumethiazide (Saluron), polythiazide (Renese) and trichlormethiazide (Naqua).

Acetazolamide (Diamox), a carbonic anhydrase inhibitor, and the newer analogues, dichlorphenamide (Daranide), ethoxzolamide (Cardrase) and methazolamide (Neptazane), are now used in the management of glaucoma.

Sulfonamide Oral Hypoglycemic Agents. These sulfonylurea compounds include acetohexamide (Dymelor), chlorpropamide (Diabinese), tolbutamide (Orinase) and tolazamide (Tolinase). Eczematous or photosensitivity reactions from their ingestion are rare.

Sulfonamide Sweetening Agents. Saccharin, calcium cyclamate and sodium cyclamate are sulfonamide compounds that are artificial sweetening agents. Sucaryl and Sweeta are combinations of saccharin and cyclamate compounds.

The possibility of these sulfonamide agents causing hematogenous contact-type eruptions and photosensitivity reactions must be kept in mind.[44]

HALOGENATED HYDROXYQUINOLINES

These therapeutic agents include iodochlorhydroxyquinoline (Vioform), diiodohydroxyquinoline (Diodoquin), chlorquinaldol (Sterosan) and chlorhydroxyquinoline (Quinolor). Such preparations are commonly used topical agents. In addition, Vioform and Diodoquin may be administered systemically. Cross-sensitization between these compounds may exist. Vioform and Diodoquin administered orally may lead to an eczematous dermatitis medicamentosa in patients sensitized by topical application of any one of this group of compounds.[11,45]

Vioform, Diodoquin, Sterosan and Quinolor may cross-react. Oral Vioform and Diodoquin can produce eczematous contact-type dermatitis medicamentosa in persons topically sensitized to these halogenated quinolines

Quinolor Compound. This ointment consists of chlorhydroxyquinoline, benzoyl peroxide, menthol, methyl salicylate and eugenol in

Plate 12. Allergic Systemic (Endogenic) Contact Dermatitis "Flares" of Dermatitis Originally Produced by a Topical Agent. Dermatitis Reproduced by the Administration of a Related Drug.

1. Allergic Hand Dermatitis

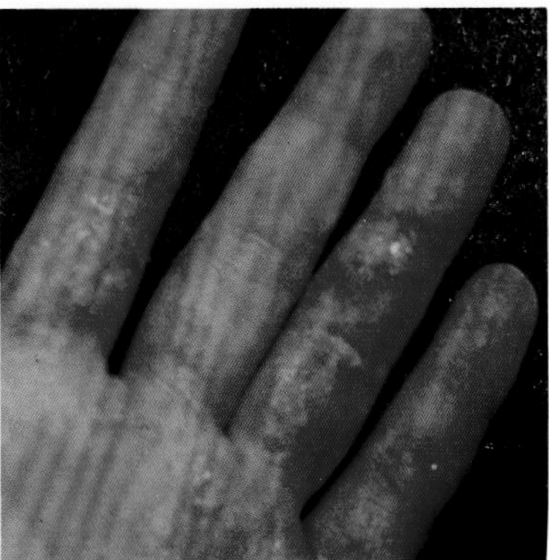

Originally Caused by Ethylenediamine in Mycolog Cream. Reproduced by the Administration of Aminophyllin.

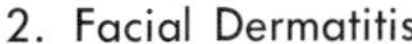

2. Facial Dermatitis

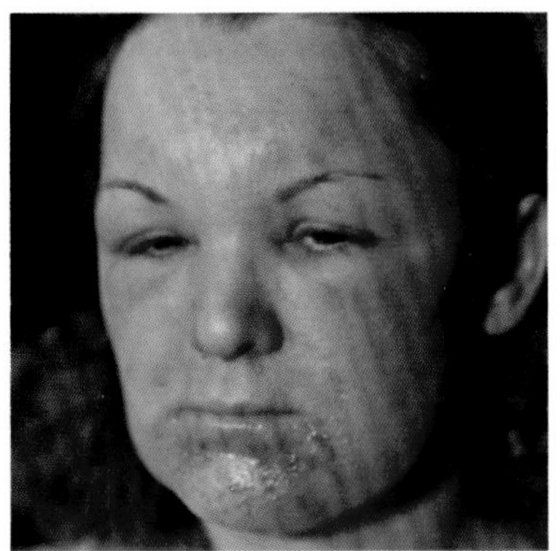

Originally Produced by Ammoniated Mercury and Reproduced by the Administration of Calomel (Mercurous Chloride). Calomel is Practically Never Used at Present, but Was Administered to this Patient by a "Country Doctor."

3. Facial Dermatitis

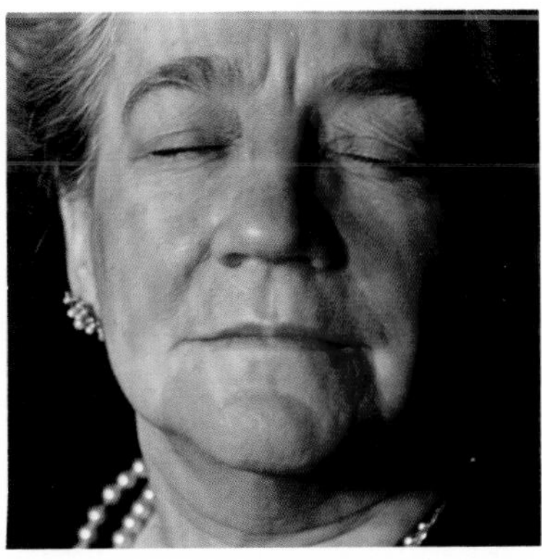

Produced by Hydrodiuril in a Patient Who, Many Years Ago, Was Sensitized to Sulfanilamide in A Cream.

Plastibase vehicle. When dermatitis occurs from its use, the chlorhydroxyquinoline is not necessarily the culprit, because the benzoyl peroxide, eugenol and Plastibase, which is a polyethylene compound related to Carbowax, can all cause allergic reactions.

MERCURIALS

Sensitization to the mercurials may be engendered by topically applied inorganic mercury, such as ammoniated or bichloride of mercury, or by organic mercurials, i.e., Mercurochrome or Merthiolate. Once the patient has been sensitized to mercury by topical exposure, the injection of a mercurial diuretic may produce an eczematous contact-type dermatitis medicamentosa. I have seen the same phenomenon in a patient who had been sensitized by ammoniated mercury and who subsequently ingested calomel (mercurous chloride).

Mercury Amalgam Dental Fillings. Individuals who have been sensitized to mercury occasionally show eczematous exacerbations where mercury amalgam fillings are used.[46] Such flare-ups may be due to absorption of minute quantities of mercury from the filling.[47] The removal of mercury amalgam fillings has been reported as clearing recalcitrant eczemas in mercury-sensitive individuals.[48]

Mercury in Tattoos. The red portions of certain tattoos consist of mercury in the form of red cinnabar. These areas may flare-up when mercurial preparations are used.[49]

CHROMIUM

Experimental administration of potassium dichromate in sensitized patients has produced flares of previous chromate dermatitis[50] with flare of positive patch test sites.[51] There is the possibility that trace amounts of chromium in food absorbed from the intestinal tract may cause dermatitis in a sensitized subject.[52]

An acute flare of a vesicular eczema of the palms occurred in a chromate-sensitive man who inhaled fumes containing chromium from an acetylene welding operation.[53]

Generalized dermatitis has been reported due to sensitivity to a chrome-cobalt removable partial denture.[54]

Ingestion of mercury or chromium in individuals sensitized to such metals may produce flares of metal dermatitis

RESORCIN

Individuals sensitized to resorcin are usually also sensitized to resorcinol monoacetate (Euresol), which is present in Ar-Ex RMS Lotion and Scalp Lotion, Resulin-F and Sulforcin Lotion.

Hexylresorcinol, which may cross-react with resorcin,[55] is present in ST 37, Sucrets, Tetrazets, Caprokol and Crystoids Anthelmintic. The ingestion of Crystoids or Caprokol could produce a contact-type dermatitis in patients sensitized to topical application of resorcin or hexylresorcinol.

Some troches, including Iso-Thirium, Listerine and Nymore, also contain hexylresorcinol.

CHLORAL HYDRATE

Sensitization from chloral hydrate in topical medications may occur from exposure to hair tonics and other scalp medications. Rectules and Calmitol Ointment contain chloral hydrate. Chlorbutanol (chlorbutol), a local anesthetic and preservative for parenteral solutions, is a chloral derivative. Chloral hydrate is also used in the manufacture of DDT, which is 1,1,1-trichloro-2-2-bis(p-chlorophenyl) ethane.

Chloral hydrate may be administered as a sedative in Aquachloral Supprettes, Beta-Chlor, En-Chlor, Fello-Sed, Felsules, Loryl, Noctagetic, Noctec and Somnos.

The ingestion of chloral hydrate by patients sensitized to it by topical exposure may result in an eczematous contact-type dermatitis medicamentosa.[56,57] Placidyl (ethchlorvynol), a condensation product of chloral hydrate, may produce a fixed drug eruption, with a flare-up upon patch testing with the drug.[58]

THIAMINE HYDROCHLORIDE (VITAMIN B_1; BETABION HYDROCHLORIDE; ANEURIN HYDROCHLORIDE)

Hypersensitivity to various vitamins has been reported, with thiamine accounting for the largest number of such cases.[59] Allergic contact dermatitis may occur in workers who fill vials in its manufacture.[60] The injection or ingestion of this vitamin in such sensitized individuals may produce an eczematous relapse in the form of a contact-type dermatitis.[61,62]

Thiamine may cross-react with coenzyme B (diphosphothiamin) and cocarboxylase.

COBIONE AND BERUBIGEN (VITAMIN B_{12})

Young et al.[63] reported on a case of sensitivity to B_{12} concentrate in which there was a delayed tuberculin-type reaction to the intradermal injection of B_{12}. Subcutaneous and intramuscular injections did not produce a flare-up of the dermatitis.

I observed a patient with cobalt sensitivity who acquired a pruritic eruption at the site of injection of Berubigen (cyanocobalamin). This area flared when vitamin B_{12} was taken orally. The patient had a strongly positive patch test reaction to cobalt chloride and a delayed positive scratch and intradermal test reaction to Berubigen. Most surprising of all, the patient had a positive patch test reaction to Berubigen alone.

HYDRAZINE HYDROBROMIDE

A large percentage of individuals who are exposed to this compound in solder flux become sensitized.[3]

It is the parent chemical of isoniazid (INH, Niconyl, Nydrazid, Rimifon, Tyvid), hydralazine (Apresoline) and phenelzine dihydrogen sulfate (Nardil), an antidepressant drug. The systemic administration of these drugs in individuals sensitized to hydrazine hydrochloride may produce eczematous contact-type dermatitis medicamentosa.

FLAVORING AGENTS

Cinnamon Oil. This oil is used for flavoring foods, cakes, toothpaste, chewing gum, tobacco, vermouth, aperitifs, bitters and beverages of the cola type. Cassia is a Chinese cinnamon. Occupational dermatitis from oil of cinnamon may occur in bakers, candy makers, cooks and housewives.

Cinnamon may cross-react with balsam of Peru.

Ingestion of oil of cinnamon may produce an eczematous contact-type flare-up in individuals previously sensitized by contact with the oil.[64]

I have observed a patient sensitized to cinnamon in a toothpaste whose dermatitis flared after drinking vermouth containing cinnamon.

Other Flavorings. Hjorth[65] reported on 2 children who were sensitive to balsam of Peru and orange peel and whose eczema flared after eating fruits and ices. Hjorth[66] also described a man with a severe hand eczema who was allergic to balsam of Peru and whose eczema flared when he ate a jar of orange marmalade. He then avoided perfumes, cola drinks, vermouth, throat tablets and cinnamon, and his hand eczema cleared. Eating vanilla sugar has also caused a flare of eczema in a patient sensitive to balsam of Peru.[67] It is possible that garlic may also have this effect.[68]

Dermatitis due to sensitization to balsam of Peru may flare with ingestion of cinnamon, oranges and other flavors

ANTABUSE (DISULFIRAM, TETRAETHYLTHIURAM DISULFIDE)

Antabuse is used as adjunctive treatment in alcoholism to help the patient remain in the state of self-imposed sobriety. When on Antabuse therapy, patients ingesting even small amounts of alcohol experience a highly unpleasant reaction, consisting of flushing, palpitations, dyspnea, hyperventilation, tachycardia, nausea and vomiting.

Disulfiram and thiram (tetramethylthiuram) are used as rubber accelerators and may show cross-reactions. Thiram is widely used as an insecticide and germicide and is present in Rezifilm (Squibb), a surgical wound dressing. Sensitization by contact with thiram may make the patient susceptible to an eczematous dermatitis medicamentosa if Antabuse is given.[69]

A patient sensitized to dipentamethylene thiuram disulfide from a rubber condom developed a violent reaction and a widespread eczema when given Antabuse (tetraethylthiuram disulfide) for the treatment of his alcoholism.[70] A similar patient was described by Pirila.[71] The reaction occurred within 4 hours, and a thiuram patch test reaction that had faded was reactivated.

FORMALDEHYDE

Sulzberger[72] showed that patients sensitized by external exposure to formaldehyde may acquire eczematous contact-type dermatitis medicamentosa from the ingestion of Urotropin (hexamethylenetetramine, methenamine), which liberates formaldehyde in an acid medium.

Methenamine-containing antiseptics, including Azolate, Mandelamine, Mandalay, Proklar, Uran, Urised, Urolita, Uro-Phosphate and Uroqid-Acid, may cause contact-type dermatitis in formaldehyde-sensitive patients.

QUININE AND QUINIDINE

It has long been known that quinine can sensitize the skin, particularly when inflammation is present.[73] Topical sensitization may take place from hair preparations containing quinine. Quinamm (National) contains quinine sulfate, as do many over-the-counter cold and headache remedies. The ingestion of such remedies and even quinine water may produce eczematous contact-type dermatitis in sensitized individuals.

Quinidine contact dermatitis has been reported in a patient whose exposure consisted of grinding the drug in the pharmaceutical industry.[74] Quinidine and quinine apparently do not cross-react.

FLUORIDES

Shea et al.[75] reported on 7 individuals with urticaria, exfoliative dermatitis, atopic dermatitis, stomatitis and gastrointestinal and respiratory allergy apparently due to fluorides in a fluoride-containing toothpaste and vitamin preparations. One individual had a positive patch test reaction to fluoride.

PATCH TESTING IN CONTACT-TYPE DERMATITIS

Patch testing with the chemicals mentioned in this chapter may be of value not only in determining the cause of an allergic contact dermatitis, but also in serving as a warning that the systemic administration of a related drug may produce an eczematous contact-type dermatitis medicamentosa. In addition, the epidermal contact-type of sensitivity may be accompanied by the urticarial, anaphylactoid variety, particularly when penicillin is the cause. A positive patch test reaction to penicillin usually precludes its systemic use. Occasionally the reactions to patch tests with penicillin and other drugs are positive when the scratch and intracutaneous test reactions are negative.

It is much safer to perform a patch test with a drug suspected of producing an eczematous dermatitis medicamentosa than to readminister even a tiny fractional dose of the drug to prove that it is the culprit. Such proof may result in a widespread, disabling eruption.

In evaluating the significance of a positive patch test reaction to a medication, one must have knowledge of immunochemically related agents. Such considerations may explain an allergic (contact-type) eczematous eruption after an exposure to one or more compounds to which an individual has never previously been exposed. The cross-reaction phenomenon may also explain the persistence of allergic reactions in some patients long after the original agent has been avoided.

Ingestion or systemic administration of an allergen that gives a positive patch test reaction can cause both dermatitis and systemic effects

When several drugs have been administered concurrently or in combination and the patient has experienced an eczematous flare-up, patch tests may be of value in discovering the culprit. For example, if the patient develops an eruption following the administration of a penicillin-streptomycin combination, the drug that causes a positive patch test reaction would be implicated.

Such patch tests are safer than scratch or intracutaneous tests.

MANAGEMENT OF ECZEMATOUS CONTACT-TYPE DERMATITIS MEDICAMENTOSA

Treatment of the presenting eczematous skin eruption is the same regardless of whether the allergen reached the skin by external exposure or by an internal systemic route.

The management of a patient with an eczematous contact-type drug eruption does not end when the eruption has finally cleared. The patient must be informed in writing of the specific drugs that caused the eruption. When taking any medication, new or old, the patient should be told to notify his physician promptly of any minor symptom, such as slight itching, rash, nausea or headache. These should serve as a clear warning that further administration may lead to disastrous results.

The patient should also be instructed not to accept any medication unless he is assured that he is not receiving the drug to which he reacted unfavorably. This is especially important if the drug is to be injected.

In addition, there should be a discussion concerning the possibility of reacting to immunochemically related medications.

Patients should have on their person information concerning their drug sensitivities. Immunochemically related drugs and chemicals should also be listed

Table 17–2 is a list of chemicals that may sensitize a patient by external contact and the corresponding immunochemically related dugs that may produce an eczematous contact-type dermatitis medicamentosa upon systemic administration.

Table 17-2. Topical Sensitizers and Immunochemically Related Drugs That Can Cause an Eruption Upon Systemic Administration

Topical Sensitizers	*Immunochemically Related Drugs*
Hydrazine hydrobromide	Isoniazid, Apresoline, Nardil
Para-amino compounds	Para-aminobenzoic acid (PABA) and related local anesthetics (benzocaine, procaine)
	Azo dyes in foods and drugs
	Dymelor, Orinase, Diabinese, sulfonamides
	Diuril, HydroDIURIL, Saluron, Renese
	Para-aminosalicylic acid (PAS)
Balsam of Peru	Cinnamon
Neomycin sulfate	Streptomycin, kanamycin
Resorcin	Hexylresorcinol (Crystoids, Caprokol)
Organic and inorganic mercurials	Mercurial diuretics
Metallic mercury	Calomel
Cobalt	Vitamin B_{12}
Thiamine	Coenzyme B (cocarboxylase)
Ethylenediamine hydrochloride	Aminophylline, Antistine, Phenergan, Pyribenzamine, Synopen, Neohetramine
Formaldehyde	Urotropin, Mandelamine, Urised
Thiram and disulfiram	Antabuse
Halogenated hydroxyquinolines	Vioform, Diodoquin
Chlorobutanol	Chloral hydrate
Iodine	Iodides, iodinated organic compounds
Benadryl	Dramamine

Whenever sensitization has taken place from topical exposure to a chemical or medicament listed in the first column, the patient should be informed of the possibility of an eczematous contact-type dermatitis medicamentosa if an immunochemically related drug listed in the second column is administered systemically. Whenever possible, such systemic exposure should be avoided and proper substitutes utilized.

REFERENCES

1. Fisher, A. A.: Recent Developments in the Diagnosis and Management of Drug Eruptions. Med. Clin. N. Amer., *3*, 3, 1959.
2. Baer, R. L.: Cutaneous Aspects of Drug Toxicity. Ann. N.Y. Acad. Sci., *123*, 364, 1965.
3. Wheeler, C. E., Penn, R. S., and Cawley, E. P.: Dermatitis from Hydrazine Hydrobromide Solder Flux. Arch. Derm., *91*, 237, 1965.
4. Rees, B. R.: Cutaneous Reactions to Antibiotics. J.A.M.A., *189*, 685, 1964.
5. Vickers, H. R., Bagratuni, L., and Alexander, S.: Dermatitis Caused by Penicillin Milk. Lancet, *61*, 351, 1958.
6. Shelley, W. B., and Cohn, M. N.: Effect of Topically Applied Antibiotic Agents on Axillary Odor. J.A.M.A., *159*, 1736, 1955.
7. Epstein, S.: Dermal Contact Dermatitis from Neomycin. Ann. Allergy, *16*, 268, 1958.
8. Epstein, S., and Wenzel, F. J.: Cross Sensitivity to Various "Mycins." Arch. Derm., *86*, 183, 1962.
9. Epstein S., and Wenzel, F. J.: Sensitivity to Neomycin and Bacitracin, Cross Sensitization or Coincidence? Acta Dermatovener., *43*, 1, 1963.
10. Pirila, V., and Rantanen, A. V.: Root Canal Treatment with Bacitracin-Neomycin as Cause of Flare-up of Allergic Eczema. Oral Surg., *13*, 589, 1960.
11. Ekelund, A., and Moller, H.: Oral Provocation in Eczematous Contact Allergy to Neomycin and Hydroxy-Quinolines. Acta Dermatovener., *49*, 422, 1969.
12. Welsh, L.: That Fixed Drug Eruption. Arch. Derm., *84*, 1012, 1961.
13. Welsh, L.: Cross-Fixed Drug Eruption from Three Antibiotics. Arch. Derm., *71*, 521, 1955.
14. Schwank, R., and Jirasek, L.: Contact Allergy to Chloramphenicol with Special Reference to Group Sensitization. Hautarzt, *14*, 24, 1963.
15. Palacios, J., et al: Lack of Cross Sensitization between 2,4-Dinitrochlorbenzene and Chloramphenicol. South. Med. J., *61*, 243, 1968.
16. Roupe, G., and Strannegard, O.: Anaphylactic Shock Elicited by Topical Administration of Bacitracin. Arch. Derm., *100*, 450, 1969.
17. Rajka, G., and Pallin, O: Sensitization to Locally Applied Antistine. Acta Dermatovener., *44*, 255, 1964.
18. Fisher, A. A., et al.: Contact Dermatitis Due to Ingredients of Vehicles. Arch. Derm., *104*, 286, 1971.
19. Wuthric, B.: Berufsekzem durch Aethylendiamine in der Kunstfaser-Industrie. Berufsdermatosen, *4*, 200, 1972.
20. Baer, R. L., Cohen, H. J., and Neidorff, A. H.: Allergic Eczematous Sensitivity to Aminophylline. Arch. Derm., *79*, 647, 1959.
21. Raymond, J. Z., and Cross, P. R.: EDTA: Preservative Dermatitis. Arch. Derm., *100*, 436, 1969.
22. Provost, T. T., and Jillson, O. F.: Ethylenediamine Contact Dermatitis. Arch. Derm., *96*, 231, 1967.
23. Sherman, W. B., and Cooke, R. A.: Dermatitis Following the Use of Pyribenzamine and Antistine. J. Allergy, *21*, 63, 1950.
24. Suurmond, D.: Patch Test Reactions to Phenergan Cream, Promethazine and Triethanolamine. Dermatologica, *133*, 503, 1966.
25. Sidi, E., Hincky, M., and Gervais, A.: Allergic Sensitization and Photosensitization to Phenergan Creams. J. Invest. Derm., *24*, 345, 1955.
26. Duperrat, B., and Lamberton, J. N.: Allergie a la Phenothiazine. Bull. Soc. Franc. Derm., *67*, 941, 1960.
27. Sidi, E., Melki, G., and Longueville, R.: Dermatitis aux Pomades Antihistaminiques. Acta Allerg., *5*, 292, 1952.
28. Epstein, E.: Dermatitis Due to Antihistamine Agents. J. Invest. Derm., *12*, 151, 1949.
29. Loverman, A. B., and Fleigelman, M. T.: Local Cutaneous Sensitivity to Methapyriline (Histadyl). Arch. Derm., *63*, 250, 1951.
30. Carryer, H. M., and Koelsche, G. G.: Use of Antihistamine Drugs. J. Invest. Derm., *13*, 25, 1949.
31. Stritlzer, C.: Studies on Topical Thephorin Therapy. J. Allergy, *21*, 432, 1950.
32. Levin, L., Kelly, J. F., and Schwartz, E.: A Clinical Evaluation of Neo-Artegan and Antistine in the Treatment of Ragweed Hay Fever. New York J. Med., *48*, 1474, 1948.
33. Epstein, S., and Rowe, R. V.: Photoallergy and Photo Cross-Sensitivity to Phenergan. J. Invest. Derm., *29*, 319, 1957.

34. Morris-Owen, R. M.: "Cover Dose" Management of Contact Sensitivity to Chlorpromazine. Brit. J. Derm., *75*, 167, 1963.
35. Fisher, A. A., Pelzig, A., and Kanof, N. B.: The Persistence of Allergic Eczematous Sensitivity Pattern to Paraphenylenediamine. J. Invest. Derm., *30*, 9, 1958.
36. Sidi, E., and Arouete, J.: Sensitization to Azo Dyes and The Para Group. Presse Med., *67*, 2069, 1959.
37. Curtis, G. H., and Crawford, P. F.: Cutaneous Sensitivity to Monoglycerol Para-Aminobenzoate: Cross-Sensitization and Bilateral Eczematization. Cleveland Clin. Quart., *18*, 35, 1951.
38. Fisher, A. A.: Paraphenylenediamine: One of the "Big Five" in Allergic Contact Dermatitis. Cutis, *1*, 171, 1965.
39. Fisher, A. A., and Sturm, H. M.: Procaine Sensitivity. The Relationship of the Allergic Eczematous Contact-Type to the Urticarial, Anaphylactoid Variety. Ann. Allergy, *16*, 593, 1958.
40. Sidi, E., and Dobkevitch-Morrill, S.: The Injection and Ingestion Test in Cross-Sensitization to the Para Group. J. Invest. Derm., *16*, 299, 1951.
41. Kierland, R. R., and Carr, D. T.: Reactions to Paraamino Salicylic Acid. Proc. Mayo Clin., *24*, 539, 1949.
42. Sulzberger, M. D., et al.: Sensitization by Topical Application of Sulfonamide. J. Allergy., *18*, 92, 1947.
43. Harber, L. C., Lashinsky, A. M., and Baer, R. L.: Photosensitivity Due to Chlorthiazide and Hydrochlorthiazide. New Engl. J. Med., *261*, 1378, 1959.
44. Seale, E.: Saccharin—A Factor in Sunlight Sensitivity. Current News in Dermatology. The Schoch Letter, Dallas, Texas, July, 1965.
45. Leifer, W., and Steiner, K.: Studies in Sensitization to Halogenated Hydroxyquinolines and Related Compounds. J. Invest. Derm., *17*, 233, 1951.
46. Fernstroem, A. I. B., Frykholm, K. O., and Huldt, S.: Mercury Allergy with Eczematous Dermatitis Due to Silver-Amalgam Fillings. Brit. Dent. J., *113*, 206, 1962.
47. Gotz, H., and Fortmann, I.: Can Amalgam Fillings Cause a Mercury Sensitization of the Skin? Z. Haut. Geschlechtskr., *26*, 34, 1959.
48. Johnson, H. H., Schonberg, I. L., and Bach, N. F.: Chronic Atopic Dermatitis, with Pronounced Mercury Sensitivity: Partial Clearing After Extraction of Teeth Containing Mercury Amalgam Fillings. Soc. Trans. A.M.A. Arch Derm. & Syph., *63*, 279, 1951.
49. Sulzberger, M. B., and Tolmach, J. A.: Allergic Flare-Up Reactions in Red Tattooing: Observations on Development and Subsidence of Mercurial Sensitivity and on Allergic Granulomatous and Sarcoid Reactions. Hautarzt, *10*, 110, 1959.
50. Fregert, S.: Sensitization to Hexa- and Trivalent Chromium. Proc. Congr. Hung. Derm. Soc., *50*, 118, 1965.
51. Schleiff, P.: Provokation des Chromatekzems zu Testzwecken durch Interne Chromsufuhr. Hautarzt, *19*, 209, 1968.
52. Shelley, W. B.: Chromium in Welding Fumes as Cause of Eczematous Hand Eruption. J.A.M.A., *189*, 772, 1964.
53. Schroeder, H. A., Balassa, J. J., and Tipton, I. H.: Abnormal Trace Metals in Man—Chromium. J. Chron. Dis., *15*, 941, 1962.
54. Brendlinger, D. L., and Tarsitano, J. J.: Generalized Dermatitis Due to a Chrome Cobalt Removable Partial Denture. J.A.D.A., *81*, 392, 1970.
55. Caron, G. A., and Calnan, C. D.: Studies in Contact Dermatitis: XIV. Resorcin. Trans. St. John Hosp. Derm. Soc., *48*, 149, 1962.
56. Baer, R. L., and Sulzberger, M. B.: Eczematous Dermatitis Due to Chloral Hydrate (following both oral administration and topical application). J. Allergy, *9*, 518, 1938.
57. Christianson, H. B., and Perry, H. O.: Reactions to Chloral Hydrate. Arch. Derm., *74*, 232, 1956.
58. Auerbach, R.: Fixed Drug Eruption: Ethchlorvynol (Placidyl). Arch. Derm., *92*, 184, 1965.
59. Combes, F. C., and Groopman, J.: Contact Dermatitis Due to Thiamine. Arch. Derm. & Syph., *61*, 858, 1950.
60. Dalton, J. E., and Pierce, J. D.: Dermatological Problems Among Pharmaceutical Workers. Arch. Derm., *64*, 667, 1951.
61. Neils, H.: Contact Dermatitis from Vitamin B_1 (Thiamine). J. Invest. Derm., *30*, 261, 1958.
62. Hjorth, N.: Contact Dermatitis from Vitamine B_1 (Thiamine). Relapse after Ingestion of Thiamine. Cross-Sensitization to Cocarboxylase. J. Invest. Derm., *30*, 261, 1958.
63. Young, W. C., Ulrich, C. W., and Fouts, P. J.: Sensitivity to B_{12} Concentrate. J.A.M.A., *143*, 893, 1950.
64. Leifer, W.: Contact Dermatitis Due to Cinnamon. Arch. Derm., *64*, 52, 1951.
65. Hjorth, N.: *Eczematous Allergy to Balsams, Allied Perfumes and Flavoring Agents.* Copenhagen, Munkgaard, 1961, p. 134.
66. Hjorth, N.: Allergy to Balsams. Spectrum, *8*, 97, 1971.

67. Pirila, V.: Endogenic Contact Eczema. Allerg. Asthma, *16*, 15, 1970.
68. Burks, J. W.: Classic Aspects of Onion and Garlic Dermatitis in Housewives. Ann. Allergy, *12*, 592, 1954.
69. Shelley, W. B.: Golf-Course Dermatitis Due to Thiram Fungicide. J.A.M.A., *188*, 415, 1964.
70. Wilson, H. T. H.: Side Effects of Disulfram. Brit. Med. J., *2*, 1610, 1962.
71. Pirila, V.: Dermatitis Due to Rubber. Proc. 11th Int. Cong. Derm., *2*, 252, 1957.
72. Sulzberger, M. B.: *Dermatologic Allergy.* Springfield, Ill., Charles C Thomas, 1940, p. 380.
73. Klaschka, F.: Discussion of High Grade Quinine Contact-Allergy. Derm. Wschr., *149*, 4, 1964.
74. Fernstroem, A. I. B.: Occupational Quinidine Contact Dermatitis. Acta Dermatovener., *45*, 129, 1965.
75. Shea, J. J., et al.: Allergy to Fluoride. Ann. Allergy, *25*, 241, 1967.

18

Contact Reactions of Mucous Membranes

Irritant and allergic reactions of mucous membranes to topical applications include stomatitis, cheilitis, conjunctivitis, vulvitis, proctitis and balanitis.

CONTACT STOMATITIS AND CHEILITIS

The oral mucosa, like the skin, is subject to two types of local reactions—primary irritation and allergic sensitization. In general, the mucosa is more resistant to primary irritants and is not as readily sensitized as is the skin, possibly because the keratin layer of the skin may contain proteins that more readily combine with simple chemical to form allergens.

The oral mucosa is constantly bathed in saliva, which washes food particles, debris, irritants and sensitizers from the mucosal surface. Saliva also plays a considerable role in digestion through the action of enzymes, such as amylase and maltase In addition, saliva may contain yeasts, which can modify the clinical picture of the stomaitis.

Mucosal reactions to contactants are modified by the presence of saliva, which cleanses, buffers and contains yeasts, and abundant vascularity

Clinical Picture of Contact Stomatitis and Cheilitis

Often the subjective symptoms of contact stomatitis are more prominent than the physical signs. Patients may complain of loss of taste, numbness, a burning sensation and soreness in the involved area. Itching is not a frequent symptom.

The appearance of the mucous membrane varies from a barely visible, mild erythema to a fiery red color with or without edema. Lingual papillae may disappear. In the presence of considerable edema, the mucosa takes on a smooth, waxy, glazed appearance. Vesiculation of the oral mucosa is rarely seen, because vesicles rupture quickly to form erosions.

In allergic reactions to denture base material, there is often a sharp line between the red, inflamed mucosa covered by the denture and the adjacent uninvolved area. The irritation of an ill-fitting plate may, however, give an appearance identical to that of allergic denture stomatitis.

Allergic stomatitis is often accompanied by cheilitis. The usual picture of allergic cheilitis, whether secondary due to stomatitis or to contactants applied directly to the lips, is one of dryness, scaliness, fissuring and angular cheilitis. Edema and vesiculation of the lips are rarely present. A riboflavin deficiency syndrome may be simulated.

In severe allergic stomatitis, the lips and circumoral skin are commonly affected. In mercury-sensitive individuals, mercurial preparations applied to the oral mucosa may produce flares of dermatitis at healed sites of previously involved skin.

ALLERGIC CONTACT STOMATITIS

There is a lower incidence of allergic contact stomatitis than of allergic contact dermatitis, probably because of the following factors:

1. With the exception of dental appliances, the period of contact of sensitizers with the buccal mucous membranes is brief.
2. Saliva dilutes and removes potential allergens and may buffer and neutralize chemicals.
3. The anatomical structure of the buccal mucosa with its extensive vascularization aids in rapid dispersion and absorption of the allergen, thereby preventing prolonged contact of the allergen with the mucosa.

When the skin is the original surface sensitized, the mucous membrane may or may not be involved on a clinical level. On the other hand, when the mucous membrane is first sensitized, the skin is usually involved also. For example, sensitization to an ingredient in a dentifrice will produce allergic stomatitis, cheilitis and circumoral dermatitis upon exposure to the allergen.

Lowney,[1] however, has shown that a series of applications of dinitrochlorobenzene (DNCB) to the buccal mucosa induces a mild contact sensitivity in some subjects and not in others. Virtually all subjects then exhibit a refractoriness to subsequent attempts to induce sensitivity or raise the level of sensitivity previously induced.

This finding, that partial tolerance to dinitrochlorobenzene can be induced in man by buccal administration of the compound, may become of importance if this technique works with other chemicals.

Although allergic contact sensitivity is usually generalized, affecting the skin and oral mucosa simultaneously, recent experiments with dinitrochlorobenzene indicate that sensitization by way of the buccal mucosa may increase skin tolerance

Allergic contact stomatitis may mimic the oral changes of a vitamin deficiency. Loss of taste, numbness and burning sensations rather than itching are prominent symptoms

In the rare instances of marked edema, difficulty in swallowing and breathing may occur.

PRIMARY IRRITATION OF THE ORAL MUCOSA BY HEAT AND CHEMICALS

Irritation Due to Heat. The oral mucosa can withstand excessively hot liquids and spicy foods with little or no evidence of irritation. Many individuals can drink tea or coffee that is close to boiling without apparent injury to the mucosa. The ingestion of hot liquids or hot foods, such as melted cheese in grilled cheese sandwiches and pizzas, however, may inflict severe, painful thermal burns with the formation of vesicles or bullae, particularly on the palate, tongue and lips. The patient may treat such burns by sucking on ice chips or by applying ice cold glycerin to the affected areas. If pain persists, Xylocaine Viscous may then be applied to painful sites.

Stomatitis Due to Chemical Injury. One of the commonest causes of chemical injury is repeated placement of aspirin tablets against a painful tooth. Prolonged contact of acetylsalicylic acid with the oral mucosa often results in superficial ulceration. Chewing gum containing aspirin may also produce oral ulceration.[2]

The prolonged use of undiluted perborate or hydrogen peroxide may also produce painful, superficial erosions of the oral mucosa. The most severe injury from chemicals occurs in individuals who swallow lye for suicidal purposes and in young children who accidentally ingest household caustics and acids. Such strong chemicals may cause severe necrosis and sloughing of the mucosa. In addition, caustic chemicals such as phenol, silver nitrate and nitric acid may be accidentally placed against the mucosa during dental procedures.

If the patient can be treated immediately after exposure to a strong chemical, the affected mucosa should first be rinsed liberally with cold water and then neutralization of the chemical should be attempted. Alkalies are neutralized by weak acetic acid or vinegar, acids by a solution of bicarbonate of soda, and phenol by alcohol.

If the chemically injured area remains painful, the patient may suck on ice chips. Subsequently, a corticosteroid ointment may be applied. Kenalog in Orabase (Squibb) adheres well to the mucosa and helps to heal the eroded area.

Aspirin tablets, chewing gum, hot foods, caustics, perborates, peroxides and antienzymes in dentifrices may produce irritation and erosions of the oral mucosa

Trauma. Prolonged, low grade irritation and trauma of the oral mucosa from jagged teeth may lead to erosions, keratinization, leukoplakia and malignant degeneration.

Uremic Stomatitis. Ten patients with uremic stomatitis have been reported.[3] Six of them died within 10 months of the onset of stomatitis. It was postulated that in these patients the stomatitis was a chemical burn caused by the action of bacterial urease on the salivary urea with subsequent liberation of ammonia.

The breakdown of salivary urea into ammonia is said to be the cause of uremic stomatitis

INGREDIENTS OF DENTIFRICES AND MOUTHWASHES

Most powder and paste dentifrices contain flavoring, coloring agents (certified dyes), abrasives and soaps or synthetic detergents, particularly "foaming" alkyl sulfates or sarcosinates. In addition, toothpastes may contain glycerine, propylene glycol, sorbital solution, alcohol and thickeners, such as tragacanth, alginate, carrageen (Irish moss) and cellulose derivatives. Some dentifrices include antiseptics, preservatives, fluorides and ammonium compounds. Saccharin and the cyclamates may be added.[4,5]

Mouthwashes are medicated liquids used for cleansing the mouth for therapeutic or cosmetic purposes and, like dentifrices, may contain alcohol, flavorings, antiseptics and preservatives.

The alkyl sulfates, sarcosinates and sulfonates are synthetic "foaming" detergents. So-called "anti-enzyme" dentifrices may contain these surfactants, which are claimed to prevent transformation of sugar to acid in the oral cavity. These surface active agents very rarely produce allergic reactions.

The abrasives in dentifrices, e.g., chalk, calcium carbonate, bentonite, pumice, hydrated aluminum, calcium phosphate, zinc oxide, sodium chloride, sodium bicarbonate

Table 18-1. Dentifrices

Product	*Manufacturer*	*Stated Ingredients*
Amm-i-dent	Block Drug	Carbamide Sodium n-lauroyl sarcosinate
Amm-i-dent with Chlorophyll	Block Drug	Carbamide Sodium n-lauroyl sarcosinate Chlorophyllins
Super Amm-i-dent with Fluoride	Block Drug	Carbamide Sodium n-lauroyl sarcosinate Sodium fluoride
Caroid	Breon	Papain
Chloresium	Rystan	Chlorophyllins
Close-up	Lever Bros.	None given
Colgate	Colgate-Palmolive	Sodium n-lauroyl sarcosinate (Gardol)
Colgate with MFP	Colgate-Palmolive	Sodium n-lauroyl sarcosinate (Gardol) Sodium monofluorophosphate (MFP)

Table 18-1. Dentifrices—(*Continued*)

Product	*Manufacturer*	*Stated Ingredients*
Crest	Procter & Gamble	Stannous fluoride (Fluoristan)
Dr. Lyon's	Glenbrook	None given
Dr. Lyon's Ammoniated	Glenbrook	Carbamide Dibasic ammonium phosphate
Dr. Lyon's Fluoride	Glenbrook	Stannous fluoride
Fact	Bristol-Myers	Stannous fluoride Sodium lauryl sulfate Hexachlorophene
Gleem II	Procter & Gamble	Sodium fluoride
Iodent No. 1 and No. 2	Iodent	None given
Kolynos Fluoride	Whitehall	Dicalcium phosphate Sodium fluoride
Kolynos Super-White	Whitehall	Dicalcium phosphate
Listerine	Warner-Lambert	Dicalcium phosphate
McLeans	Beecham	None given
McKesson Fluoride	McKesson Labs	Stannous fluoride
Mighty White	Alberto-Culver	Sodium fluoride
Neutrox	Vick	Magnesium carbonate Sodium perborate monohydrate Tricalcium phosphate Monocalcium phosphate
New Pepsodent	Lever Bros.	Alkyl sulfate (Irium)
Pepsodent	Lever Bros.	None given
Pepsodent Ammoniated	Lever Bros.	None given
Phillips	Phillips Co.	Magnesium hydroxide
Sensodyne	Block Drug	Strontium chloride
Squibb	Squibb	Magnesium hydroxide Peppermint
Super Stripe	Lever Bros.	Stannous fluoride Insoluble sodium Metaphosphate Calcium pyrophosphate
Thermodent	Leeming	Magnesium carbonate Calcium carbonate Sodium chloride Sodium sulfate Potassium sulfate Formaldehyde
Ultra Brite	Colgate-Palmolive	None given
Vince	Lactona	Sodium perborate Monohydrate (perborax) Tribasic calcium phosphate Magnesium trisilicate Calcium carbonate Sodium aluminum sulfate

and the magnesium salts, are not sensitizers. The quaternary ammonium compounds are rare sensitizers. The preservatives, essential oils, formalin, flavorings, antiseptics, antibiotic agents and alcohol are more common sensitizers.

The coloring agents (certified dyes) in modern dentifrices and mouthwashes are mostly of the aniline or azo variety. Certification of a dye relates only to its toxicity and not to its allergic potential. Allergic sensitization to these dyes is rare, and when it occurs, cross-reaction with paraphenylenediamine is present in about 25 per cent of cases. Natural colors, such as cudbear or cochineal, are rarely used at present.

The formalin in Thermodent toothpaste and the essential oils, particularly cinnamon, in dentifrices may produce allergic reactions

Table 18–1 is a list of currently popular dentifrices with their ingredients.

Table 18–2 is a list of the ingredients of mouthwashes.

Table 18-2. Widely Used Mouthwashes and Their Active Ingredients

Product	*Ingredients*
Amosan	Sodium perborate
Astringisol	Zinc chloride, fluid extract of myrrh
Cēpacol	Cetylpyridinium chloride
Chloraseptic	Borax, menthol, thymol, phenol, glycerine and chlorophyll
Colgate 100	Benzethonium chloride and alcohol
Isodine	Povidone-iodine
Kasdenol	Mono-oxychlorosene (calcium hypochlorite)
Lavoris	Zinc chloride, cinnamaldehyde, clove oil and alcohol
Listerine	Thymol, eucalyptol, methyl salicylate, menthol, boric acid, benzoic acid and alcohol
Micrin	Cetylpyridinium chloride and dequalinium (quaternary ammonium compounds), oil of peppermint, menthol and alcohol
Oral Pentacresol	Amyl-tricresols
Reef	Cetylpyridinium chloride, menthol, methyl salicylate and alcohol
Scope	Cetylpyridinium chloride and domiphen bromide (quaternary ammonium compounds), surfactants, flavorings and alcohol
Sterisol	Hexetidine
Tyrolaris	Tyrothricin and alcohol
Vince	Sodium perborate, calcium carbonate, sodium aluminum sulfate and flavorings

PRECAUTIONS FOR PATCH TESTING WITH DENTIFRICES AND MOUTHWASHES

Soaps or synthetic detergents in a dentifrice may produce primary irritant reactions under a closed patch test. Positive reactions to tests with a dentifrice or mouthwash should always be checked by testing at least 3 controls. If they also show positive reactions, the product is a primary irritant as tested.[6]

Toothpastes and powders that do not contain soap or detergents (i.e., those that do not foam or lather) usually are tested "as is" with a covered patch. Those containing soaps or detergents should be tested uncovered on the forearm. A positive reaction should be compared with the results obtained in controls.

Mouthwashes often contain alcohol and other ingredients that may partially evaporate and cause irritation under a closed patch test. In general, mouthwashes may be tested uncovered by simply rubbing the preparation into the forearm of the patient and 3 controls.

In the event that an allergic patch test reaction is obtained with a dentifrice or mouthwash, an effort should be made to ascertain *the specific sensitizing ingredient.* Such knowledge will enable the patient to avoid the sensitizer and prevent recurrent stomatitis and dermatitis.

Direct Testing of Oral Mucosa. If a dentifrice or mouthwash is suspected of causing an allergic stomatitis or cheilitis, and skin patch tests with the suspected preparation or its ingredients are negative, direct testing of the buccal mucosa may be indicated.

The suspected ingredient is incorporated into Orabase (Squibb), which is an adhering paste composed of pectin, gelatin, sodium carboxymethylcellulose and plasticized hydrocarbon gel. The mixture is applied to the inner side of the dried lip and left in place for 24 hours. Positive reactions marked by erythema of the mucosa may occur the following day, with the reaction reaching its peak at 48 hours after the allergen has been applied.

Another method of direct testing of the mucosa is that of placing the allergen inside a rubber cup that is then tied to the surface of the teeth in such a fashion that the allergen, held in the cup with collodion, is in contact with the buccal fold.

Dentures may be used to keep suspected allergens against the mucosa in those who use such appliances.

SURFACE OR TOPICAL ANESTHETICS AS MUCOSAL SENSITIZERS WITH SPECIAL REFERENCE TO BENZOCAINE

Benzocaine, a common and potent sensitizer, continues to be used in many topical anesthetic compounds.[7] The synonyms for it are Anesthesin, ethyl aminobenzoate, Anesthone and Parathesin. Benzocaine is a para-aminobenzoic acid (PABA) derivative and is chemically and immunologically related to topical anesthetics based on benzoic acid, such as cocaine.[8]

About 25 per cent of benzocaine-sensitive individuals also cross-react with paraphenylenediamine, the most popular hair dyes, the sulfonamides and the sunscreening agents based on para-aminobenzoic acid esters.

Table 18–3 shows topical preparations that contain benzocaine and should be avoided by benzocaine-sensitive individuals.

Lidocaine (Xylocaine) or dyclonine hydrochloride may be substituted when surface anesthesia is required in benzocaine-sensitive patients.

Benzocaine-sensitive patients may show cross-reactions with the following *injectable* local anesthetics, which are based on para-

Table 18-3. Benzocaine Topical Medications Used Orally

Benzocaine Ointment with Oil of Cloves (Novocol)
Benzocaine Ointment with Oil of Cloves (Oradent)
Benzodent (Vick)
Cetylite Liquid Topical Anesthetic (Cetylite)
Cetylite Spray Topical Anesthetic (Cetylite)
Novol-Benzocaine-Tetracaine Solution (Novocol)
Paracaine (Proco-Sol)
Topical Anesthetic Aerosol Spray (Graham)
Topical Anesthetic Liquid (Graham)
Topical Anesthetic Ointment (Graham)
Topical Anesthetics (Oradent)
Topicale Liquid (Premier Dental)
Topicale Ointment (Premier Dental)
Topicale Spray (Premier Dental)

aminobenzoic acid: procaine (Novocain), butethamine (Monocaine), tetracaine (Pontocaine) with 2 per cent procaine, and propoxycaine (Ravocaine) with 2 per cent procaine.

Metabutethamine (Unacaine), which is based on meta-aminobenzoic acid, and meprylcaine (Oracaine) and isobucaine (Kinacaine), which are based on benzoic acid, may also show cross-reactions with benzocaine.

Butacaine sulfate (butyn sulfate) is an aminobenzoate, which may be substituted for cocaine as a local anesthetic.

The injection of these local anesthetics into benzocaine-sensitive individuals may lead to localized swelling of the oral mucosa at the site of injection. On rare occasions, generalized urticaria or anaphylaxis will result from the injection of procaine into benzocaine-sensitive patients.[9]

Patch tests with local anesthetics do not reveal the immediate urticarial or anaphylactic type of reaction. Eyre and Nally[10] described a nasal test for screening patients with hypersensitivity to the local anesthetic lignocaine. A solution of 1 per cent lignocaine was dropped directly on the nasal mucosa, which was then examined with a nasal speculum at 2 minute intervals. A severe local reaction occurring after 2 minutes and manifested by gross mucosal swelling and erythema was considered a positive reaction. The patient on whom this test was performed had a negative patch test reaction with lignocaine and had experienced a severe allergic reaction when it was used intraorally. When the nasal test with procaine was repeated on this patient, no reaction was noted.

The authors suggest that the nasal test is a rapid, safe and easily reproducible procedure that can be used for screening purposes.

The following injectable local anesthetics do not cross-react with benzocaine and, because they are based on an amide structure, should be used in patients who are sensitive to benzocaine or to local anesthetics based on para-aminobenzoic acid, meta-aminobenzoic or benzoic acid, such as lidocaine (Xylocaine), mepivacaine (Carbocaine), prilocaine (Citanest) and pyrrocaine (Dynacaine).

Safe topical anesthetics for benzocaine-sensitive individuals include Xylocaine, Carbocaine, Citanest and Dynacaine

SENSITIZING METALS USED IN DENTISTRY WITH SPECIAL REFERENCE TO MERCURY

A wide variety of metals have been used by dentists for fillings and prostheses, including aluminum, antimony, chromium, cobalt, copper, gold, iridium, mercury, nickel, osmium, palladium, platinum, rhodium, ruthenium, silicon, silver, tin and tungsten. Mercury is probably the most common cause of allergic reactions in dentistry.

Mercury. Probably the commonest contact with mercury in the general population occurs from mercury amalgam dental fillings.

There are several contradictory reports in the literature concerning the production of allergic oral lesions in mercury-sensitized individuals from the presence of this metal in amalgams and whether or not absorption of mercury from amalgams can produce generalized dermatitis. Fernstreom et al.[11] stated that patients who had previously been sensitized to mercury and had acquired a mercury dermatitis subsequently developed a stomatitis and a flare of the dermatitis when mercury amalgam fillings were used. These patients had a prompt remission when their mercury amalgam fillings were removed. Such flares were attributed to mercury vapor, which is liberated by the silver amalgam fillings, both when the amalgam is being prepared and during insertion into the cavity. They consider the amount liberated from the filling after treatment as being negligible in comparison with the amount liberated while the filling is being inserted.

Gots and Fortmann[12] concluded that allergic reaction of the skin to mercury that is detected during routine tests is not due to the effect of amalgam fillings. Gaul[13] reported on 3 patients with mercury dermatitis in whom epidermal sensitivity to mercury was demonstrated. In all 3 patients, however, silver amalgam dental fillings, containing approximately 50 per cent metallic mercury, produced no irritation within the mouth.

Epstein[14] stated that the contact antigen formed with mercury is given specificity for the epidermis by protein conjugates characteristic of, or present only in, the epidermis and that mercury sensitivity does not extend to the oral mucosa.

Juhlin and Ohman[15] on the other hand, found that erosions of the oral mucosa occurred adjacent to amalgam fillings in mercury-sensitive individuals.

Johnson and co-workers[16] found that the removal of mercury amalgam fillings cleared recalcitrant eczemas in mercury-sensitive individuals. Sidi and Casalis[17] described mercury-sensitive patients with chronic eczema that persisted until amalgam fillings were removed.

Vickers[18] reported on a mercury-sensitive individual who developed a widespread, eczematous eruption, starting 24 to 48 hours after a mercury amalgam filling had been inserted. No oral lesions were described. Vickers speculates that the generalized dermatitis was due to mercury dropped on the mucosal surface of the mouth during the dental operation.

Spector[19] described a patient in whom there was a sudden appearance of extensive edema and urticaria involving the neck, face and upper part of the back following instillation of an amalgam filling. This reaction recurred on 2 occasions when the patient underwent dental treatment with silver amalgam. The eruption persisted for 7 to 10 days and then disappeared spontaneously without removal of the filling.

Spector performed patch tests with minute portions of the silver alloy alone, the mercury alone, and a combination of both. The patient had a negative patch test reaction to the silver alloy alone. When the mercury alone was used, the patient developed severe local erythema at the test site with vesiculation, edema and urticarial reactions on the elbows and neck. A similar reaction was noted when the combination of both was used.

The conclusion reached by Spector was that this was a rare instance of mercury sensitivity manifested by urticaria, edema and a vesiculation of the skin when mercury was used in a filling or as a patch test. In such instances of mercury sensitivity, nonmetallic or pure gold fillings are indicated.[20]

Thomson and Russell[21] described a patient who, on several occasions following mercury amalgam dental restorations, developed first an urticarial and then an eczematous eruption on her face, trunk and extremities. Her history revealed that she had previously developed an eczematous eruption on the lower part of the abdomen and thighs and a vaginitis from the use of a contraceptive jelly containing a phenylmercuric salt. Patch tests were positive to 0.1 per cent mercuric chloride and silver amalgam. The dermatitis on each occasion lasted 10 to 14 days and then subsided, although the mercury amalgam fillings were not removed.

Frykholm[22] tried to determine whether exposure to mercury in amalgam restorations can be deleterious to health. First, he tried to measure the amount of mercury that escaped from the amalgam and the amount that was absorbed. Second, he endeavored to measure the quantity of mercury excreted in the urine and feces.

Frykholm found that the average amount of mercury per millimeter of respired air in 30 minutes of treatment was 0.02 to 0.4 mg., but that the upper values occurred only if copper amalgam was used. If the fillings were coated with saliva, the amount of vapor evolved was instantly reduced. His experiments on the solubility of mercury amalgam fillings in saliva and gastric juice showed that the freshly triturated amalgam was only slightly soluble. The amount of mercury reaching the circulation appeared to be insignificant.

Frykholm concluded that amalgam restoration treatment exposes the patients to a small quantity of mercury mainly during insertion and that reports of reactions following amalgam restorations, even in mercury-sensitive persons, are uncommon, and the few cases reported usually involve a history of allergic contact to mercury.

The usual time of onset of eczema or urticaria in mercury-sensitive patients is a few hours after an amalgam filling has been inserted. The eruption usually persists for 10 to 14 days, which fits very well into Frykholm's work on mercury liberation after amalgam insertion. It is difficult to explain cases in which eczema has persisted until the amalgam was removed.

RELATIONSHIP BETWEEN ORGANIC AND INORGANIC MERCURY SENSITIVITY. The subject of cross-sensitivity between the inorganic metallic and the organic mercurials is also controversial. Fregert and Hjorth (personal communication, 1971) stated that, in Denmark, merbromin (Mercurochrome) is commonly used in surgical departments and for first aid treatment. Parallel patch tests were performed with 0.1 per cent aqueous mercuric bichloride and 5 per cent aqueous merbromin. These investigators found frequent cross-reactions between the organic and inorganic mercurial compounds.

At the University Clinic of Lund, patch tests with metallic mercury (0.5 per cent in petrolatum) were found to be reliable for detection of mercury sensitivity. Of 28 patients with positive reactions to mercuric bichloride, 25 also had positive reactions to mercury (0.5 per cent in petrolatum). These 25 were tested with 8 organic mercury compounds, and more than half showed cross-reactions between the organic and inorganic mercury compounds.

Sidi and Casalis[17] investigated a patient with a chronic eczema of the face and arms who showed positive patch test reactions to dental amalgam, inorganic mercury and Mercurochrome.

Hjorth and Trolle-Lassen stated categorically, however, that "the mercury ion does not cross-sensitize to the organic compounds."[23]

In my own experience, 3 patients with mercury sensitivity reacted to both metallic mercury and the organic and inorganic compounds. Furthermore, in patients with allergic contact sensitivity to mercury, the skin lesions may be exacerbated or reproduced by systemic administration of mercurial compounds.[24]

Nickel. Foussereau and Laugier[25] cited a case of generalized eczema that occurred after a chromium-nickel denture had been fitted. Skin tests were strongly positive to nickel and chromium, and the dermatitis subsided after the denture was removed. No mention is made of oral reactions. In my experience, metallic chromium is not a sensitizer. In most instances in which an allergic reaction is attributed to a metallic chrome object, the nickel content is the actual sensitizer. Nickel readily penetrates the micropores in chrome-plated objects.

Allergic contact stomatitis and cheilitis can occur from nickel-plated instruments used in dental procedures.[26] Many nickel-sensitive individuals have acquired allergic stomatitis and cheilitis by holding nickel-plated objects, such as needles, pins, bobby pins and metal lipstick holders between the lips.[27] Perlèche may be clearly simulated in nickel-sensitive individuals who hold nickel-plated coins, keys and other objects at the corners of their mouths. One patient developed erosions of the gums resembling aphthous ulcers from holding metal bobby pins between the teeth.[28]

Copper. Allergic sensitivity to this metal is rare. Saltzer and Wilson[29] reported on a case of allergic contact dermatitis due to copper. Frykholm et al.[30] reported that allergy to copper derived from dental alloys may produce oral lesions of lichen planus.

Gold. Elgart and Higdon[31] described a case of allergic sensitivity to gold in which the gingival mucosa sloughed from contact with a gold crown, while sites of previous gold contact dermatitis to jewelry flared. The cutaneous lesions subsided when the crown was removed.

Chrome-Cobalt Combination. Brendlinger and Tarsitano[32] described a woman with severe dermatitis and allergic reactions to several metals who recovered only after removal of a cast chrome-cobalt partial denture. Replacement with an all acrylic resin partial denture was satisfactory.

Chrome-cobalt pins used to fasten porcelain teeth to acrylic dentures may produce stomatitis in individuals sensitized to cobalt. In a recently observed case, such pins produced an extensive stomatitis and cheilitis in a cobalt-nickel sensitized individual. The reaction occurred after the acrylic portion of the denture had worn away, exposing the

Various metals used in dentures and fillings may produce stomatitis and generalized dermatitis in sensitized individuals

pins. When the pins were covered with self-curing acrylic resin, the stomatitis cleared.

Platinum. Sheard[33] stated that both metallic platinum and its salts are potent allergens and that reactions to dentist's platinum wiring may be allergic.

RESINOUS SUBSTANCES USED IN DENTISTRY

Balsam of Peru. Balsamic resin of plant origin, composed principally of cinnamic and benzoic acid esters, and resin, is a component of some cement liquids.

Copal. This substance consists of mixed resins of plant origin and is a constituent of some cavity varnishes. This resin should not be confused with Copalite (Bosworth and Co.), which is a synthetic resin.

Mastic. This substance is composed principally of masticinic acid and used in some cavity varnishes.

Rosin (colophony) and other resinous substances used in dental cement, liquids and cavity varnishes may cross-react with perfume odoriferous substances

Rosin. Also called colophony, rosin is an ingredient of many mixtures used for sealing pulp canals. Rosin in chloroform solution has been used as a varnish for pulp protection in deep cavities. It has been added to zinc oxide or to eugenol as an ingredient of pulp capping preparations, surgical packs, impression pastes and other preparations.

Dental Impression Compounds. These preparations may contain stearin, stearic acid, paraffin wax, beeswax and gutta percha with synthetic or natural resins, such as shellac, copal (kauri), coumarone-indene resins and fillers. Of these ingredients, the resin is most likely to cause sensitization stomatitis.

Some of the fluxes used contain borax, boric acid, silica and potassium fluoride. Most fluxes are strong irritants. Waxes such as paraffin, beeswax, carnauba, candelilla and petroleum are employed by dentists.

Several types of plaster containing mineral gypsum, potassium sulfate, potash alum and alizarin S are used.

ALLERGIC FACTORS IN DENTURE SORE MOUTH

Inflammatory changes of the mucous membrane beneath artificial dentures are often referred to as denture sore mouth. The oral mucosa of the palate and the maxillary edentulous alveolar ridges are the most common sites of involvement. The tissue beneath the denture may be red and edematous, and the patient may complain of soreness, rawness, dryness and burning sensations in the area in contact with the denture.

Allergic reactions of the oral mucosa may be produced to the denture base material or to its constituents, to denture cleansing materials and to denture fixing preparations.

Metals in Dentures. Patients sensitized to various metals may acquire an allergic denture sore mouth from old-fashioned metallic dentures, partial metallic dentures, metallic prostheses and metallic pins used to fasten porcelain teeth to acrylic dentures.

Acrylic Denture Materials. Most dentures today are processed from heat-cured acrylic resins. Self-curing acrylics, which harden without heat, are available for repairing and relining purposes. The heat-cured acrylic dentures rarely cause allergic reactions.[34]

Most modern dentures are processed from acrylic resins

The acrylic monomer usually contains an inhibitor, or stabilizer, such as hydroquinone, while the polymer contains an initiator, such as benzoyl peroxide, dimethyl-p-toluidine or a tertiary amine. When the monomer and polymer are mixed in the cold, the benzoyl peroxide initiates the reaction, and a hard, solid, high molecular weight polymer is produced. The mixture can also be heat cured when no initiator is required. In the heat process, the reaction is complete, but after cold cure, small amounts of monomer will probably be left unpolymerized. This residual monomer can induce stomatitis and angular cheilitis in sensitized individuals.[35]

In addition, additives in acrylic denture material may be sensitizers. For example, hydroquinone, the inhibitor in the monomer, may be the sensitzer. Benzoyl peroxide may account for some instances of methacrylate sensitivity.

Crissey[36] cited 4 instances in which hypersensitivity stomatitis venenata resulted from heat-cured acrylic dentures. The onset of symptoms followed fitting of the acrylic dentures by periods varying from 1 week to 4 years. These cases had the following features in common: (1) the clinical picture of stomatitis venenata, including angular stomatitis; (2) relief of symptoms when the dentures were removed, and subsequent flare on reinsertion; (3) positive patch test reactions (cheek) to filings from the heat-cured acrylic prostheses and the acrylic monomer; and (4) negative patch test reactions to polystyrene denture material.

Turrell[37,38] claims that inflammation of upper denture-bearing tissues is practically never due to allergy to denture base material. Turrell also made the surprising statement that "positive patch test reactions with filings from the dentures are probably not an allergic reaction to normal denture base constituents (monomer, for instance), but to such oral fluids as foods, drink, drugs, or solutions used for cleansing dentures absorbed by the latter over many years."

Furthermore, Turrell usually performed the tests by mixing the filings from the denture with the patient's own saliva. As Salo and Hirvonen[39] pointed out, patch testing with the patient's saliva often leads to false positive reactions, because such saliva often contains Candida organisms. Under an occluded patch, such saliva can produce candidiasis of the skin, which can readily be mistaken for a positive allergic patch test reaction.

In my experience, patch testing with dentures or with filings of dentures often produces false positive reactions from nonspecific pressure of hard particulate matter. Patch tests should be performed with the liquid monomer or the other basic denture materials in solution or in petrolatum.

The acrylic monomer may be a sensitizer,[40] but the heat-cured resin is not.

Acrylic dentures may also contain plasticizers (dibutyl or dimethyl phthalate), pigments (mercuric sulfate, ferric oxide, carbon black and selenium compounds), cross-linking agents (glycol dimethylacrylate and divinyl benzene) to prevent crazing and an inhibitor, such as hydroquinone.

Patients often complain of a burning sensation for several hours after first use of an acrylic denture that has been relined or repaired. Such complaints may be related to the presence of solvents such as ethyl or amyl acetate, diethyl carbonate or glycerol triacetate.

Testing for Allergic Sensitivity to Acrylic Dentures. Patch testing by strapping the denture to the forearm may lead to diagnostic errors, because redness, papulation, vesiculation and even bullae may result from nonspecific pressure effects. Patch testing with heat-cured dentures or with denture grindings may also give false reactions. Testing with the monomer and other separate ingredients avoids false positive reaction from the hardness of the denture or the sharpness of filings.

Relief of symptoms on removal of the denture and subsequent flare-up on reinsertion are not necessarily criteria of allergic acrylic denture sensitivity, because an ill-fitting denture causes the same symptoms.

Heat-cured acrylic dentures practically never produce allergic stomatitis. Cold-cured acrylic denture material may be sensitizing. Patch-testing should be performed with individual ingredients, and not with entire dentures or denture grindings

Patch Testing with Potential Sensitizers in Acrylic Dentures. The identification of specific allergens in denture materials may be difficult, because many combinations of chemicals and additives may be used. Even if a positive patch test reaction is obtained with a single chemical, the patient can often utilize dentures containing the chemical provided the denture is cured by heat. For example, dental mechanics with allergic hypersensitivity to the acrylic monomer or the hydroquinone may develop severe contact dermatitis of the hands. These individuals, nevertheless, could wear heat-cured acrylic dentures without difficulty.

In rare instances in which a patient reacts to dentures made from the usual heat-cured methyl methacrylate denture base materials, the following substitutes may be tried:

1. *Dentures made of Luxene.* These dentures are made of a copolymer of vinyl acetate and vinyl chloride plasticized with a small amount of methyl methacrylate monomer.

2. *Dentures made of polystyrene.* These dentures are made of acrylonitrile and styrene polymer.

Denture Adherent Preparations. These are made from finely powdered vegetable gums, such as karaya, acacia or tragacanth, or other agents that become mucilaginous or gelatinous upon the addition of water. Denture adherent pastes are also available and consist principally of karaya gum, petrolatum, coloring and flavoring.

Figley[42] stated that allergic sensitivity to karaya gum may result in atopic coryza, eczema, atopic dermatitis and gastrointestinal distress.

The following products contain karaya gum: Co-Re-Ga Denture Adhesive Powder, Moy Holding Powder, Perma-Grip Denture Adhesive Powder, Wernet's Powder with Neoseal, Wernet's Adhesive Cream and Fasteeth.

The following products do not contain karaya gum: Benefit Denture Adhesive, Orahesive and Fixodent. These are excellent replacements for karaya-based adhesives in karaya-sensitive individuals.

NONALLERGIC DENTURE SORE MOUTH

Trauma is the most common cause of denture sore mouth. The type in which there is an erythematous, "cluster-of-grapes" appearance is due to the suction produced by the rocking of ill-fitting dentures.[41]

Nonallergic denture sore mouth is often associated with secondary anemia, uremia and gastric disease. At menopause, women suffer from it, and many have skin that blisters readily from trauma. The first sign of pemphigus may be denture sore mouth. Only properly performed patch tests usually distinguish between the allergic and the nonallergic type.

THE ROLE OF YEASTS IN DENTURE SORE MOUTH

Salo and Hirvonen[39] concluded that denture sore mouth is often due to the combination of occlusion by the denture and yeast infection rather than to yeast infection alone. The administration of Nystatin tablets is usually curative in such cases, providing the denture sore mouth is not complicated by ill-fitting or sharp-edged dentures.

Candidiasis produced by yeasts in saliva and the occlusive effect of dentures may produce a specific type of nonallergic denture sore mouth amenable to Nystatin

ALLERGIC REACTIONS TO PRESERVATIVES IN ORAL MEDICATIONS

Certain antiseptics added to dentifrices, mouthwashes and topical oral medications and anesthetics used to retard or prevent microbial growth are sensitizers. Such chemicals include paraben (parahydroxybenzoic acid), dichlorophene (G-4), hexachlorophene (G-11), phenylmercuric sulfate, Merthiolate, ethylenediamine hydrochloride, ethylenediamine tetraacetate, the quaternary ammonium compounds, benzoic gum and benzyl benzoate.

The Parabens. The parabens (parahydroxybenzoates, parasepts) are bacteriostatic, fungistatic and antioxidant and are widely employed as preservatives. Schorr[43] and Epstein[44] emphasized that paraben-sensitivity continues to be reported increasingly in the United States.

The Food and Drug Administration[45] requires that the labels on foods and topical prescription drugs indicate the presence of parabens. This requirement does not apply to oral preparations, nonprescription drugs, cosmetics and dentifrices. Sensitive patients may therefore find it difficult to avoid contact with these agents. It is advisable for the patient with a suspected paraben sensitivity to stop using all cosmetics and dentifrices until his physician or dentist can obtain information from the manufacturer that his product does not contain parabens. Once a diagnosis of allergy to parabens is made, however, the physician can avoid prescribing formulations that contain them, and he can warn the patient not to use over-the-counter drugs in which they are likely to be incorporated.

Schamberg[46] has listed many of the products, including lidocaine (Xylocaine), that contain the parabens.

Schorr[47] published a photograph of a woman with a severe cheilitis and circumoral dermatitis who was paraben-sensitive. The eruption and cheilitis promptly disappeared when paraben-containing creams and lotions were removed from her environment.

Dichlorophene (G-4). Fisher and Lipton[48] reported that this preservative in dentifrices caused many instances of allergic cheilitis. The trade name Baxin was used for G-4 in a popular ammoniated toothpaste. Patients who became sensitized to this preservative developed stomatitis, a cherry red tongue, loss of taste and numbness. The lips became dry and scaly, and fissuring at the corners of the mouth suggested riboflavin deficiency.

Fisher and Tobin[49] found that patch tests with the Baxin-containing toothpaste were positive in individuals sensitive to G-4, causing a fine vesicular eruption within 48 hours. Control tests with 5 ammoniated dentifrices were negative. The symptoms abated 24 hours after the Baxin-containing toothpaste was discontinued, and the lesions healed in 3 days.

Preservatives in topical dental medications and dentifrices may produce allergic stomatitis and cheilitis

Hexachlorophene (G-11). This formerly widely used preservative rarely produced allergic sensitivity. Epstein[50] found cross-sensitivity between dichlorophene and hexachlorophene. Schorr[47] and Fisher and Tobin,[49] however, found no such cross-reactions.

Formaldehyde. This may be an ingredient in Thermodent dentifrice, in desensitizing agents and in Formo-Cresol, which is used in root canal therapy.

Sodium Perborate. Vilanova and Camarasa[51] found this oxidizing agent to be a common sensitizer in Spain. In the United States, it is an extremely rare sensitizer. Sodium perborate is present in Kleenite (Vick), a denture cleansing preparation.

Quaternary Ammonium Compounds. The members of this chemical family include benzalkonium chloride (Zephiran) and benzethonium chloride (Phemerol), which rarely sensitize. Huriez et al.[52] found that topical oral application may produce allergic sensitization.

Merthiolate. This widely used preservative contains not only a mercurial component, but also thiosalicylic acid. In addition, certain Merthiolate preparations contain ethylenediamine.

Phenylmercuric Nitrate. This preservative, which contains 65 per cent mercury, can produce allergic reactions.[53] It is found in several dental preparations.

Ethylenediaminetetraacetic Acid (EDTA). This agent, usually in the form of its tetrasodium or disodium-calcium salts (calcium disodium edetate, U.S.P.), is incorporated into a number of dental preparations, including chemical disinfectants and local anesthetic solutions, such as Monocaine. Raymond and Gross[54] have shown that this stabilizer is a sensitizer that may cross-react with ethylenediamine hydrochloride.

Ethylenediamine Hydrochloride. This stabilizer, present in Mycolog Cream, has produced many instances of allergic cheilitis and circumoral dermatitis.[55,56]

ANTISEPTICS USED IN DENTISTRY

These compounds include hexachlorophene (G-11), gramicidin, potassium chlorate, iodine, iodoform, chlorine compounds, thymol iodide, betadine, nitrofurazone, 8-hydroxyquinoline, sodium perborate and quaternary ammonium compounds (Zephiran).

Many organic *mercurial* antiseptics, including Mercurochrome, Merthiolate, Metaphen and Mercresin, may be used in dentistry.

Other antiseptics employed include iodine, acriflavine, benzalkonium chloride, chromic acid and chloroxylenol.

The *phenolic* compounds used for root canal work and for periapical infections include creosote and the parachlorophenols. Thymol and hexylresorcinol may show cross-reactions with resorcin.

REACTIONS TO LOZENGES AND TROCHES

These preparations may contain antibiotics, quaternary ammonium compounds, local anesthetics (particularly benzocaine), hexylresorcinol, iodine compounds or tyrothricin.

Allergic reactions to antibiotic-containing lozenges may be due to the antibiotic or to the coloring or flavoring agents.

When an oral topical medication is suspected of producing allergic contact stomatitis, testing must be performed with all the individual ingredients in the preparation, regardless of whether they are active or inert. Inert flavoring and coloring agents and preservatives are just as important causes of allergic contact stomatitis as are the active antiseptic or anesthetic chemicals present in the lozenges and troches.

Antiseptics, antibiotics, anesthetics, flavoring agents (essential oils), certified dyes in dentifrices, and topical dental medication may produce stomatitis and cheilitis

EROSIVE OR ULCERATIVE STOMATITIS DUE TO CONTACT ALLERGENS

On rare occasions, contact of the sensitized patient's oral mucosa with the specific allergen may produce erosions or ulcers rather than a diffuse stomatitis. Such lesions may be indistinguishable from aphthous ulcers.[57]

Sugarman[58] cited a case of hypersensitivity to a mint chewing gum in which the lesions were characterized by an aphthous ulcer. Kutcher et al.[59] could not confirm the finding of Tuft and Girsh[60] that aphthous ulcers were due to sensitivity to citric or acetic acid.

Cancellieri[61] listed contact sensitivity to dentifrices, teeth whiteners, mouth purifiers, chewing gum, drugs, food, acrylic resin liquid and monomers in dentures as capable of producing chronic aphthous ulcers. Fisher[24] has observed nickel-sensitive women with ulcers of the lips and oral mucosa due to the holding of nickel-plated objects, such as bobby pins or hair clips, in their mouths. Fregert et al.[62] studied a patient with allergic hypersensitivity to alcohol, as shown by positive patch test reactions, who developed a burning sensation, erythema and aphthae of the oral mucosa whenever she ingested alcoholic beverages.

Sims[63] claimed that anti-enzyme dentifrices may produce ulcerative lesions of the oral mucosa and sore tongue in patients with allergic sensitivity to the anti-enzyme. Sodium lauroyl sarcosinate, a foaming, surface-active agent in some dentifrices, has been claimed to act as an anti-enzyme. Allergic reactions to this agent have not been proved. Sensitivity to so-called anti-enzymes is probably not due to an allergic mechanism.

Aphthous-like ulcers may be produced by topical aspirin, chewing gum, essential oils, metals in dentures, alcohol and hot spicy food

ALLERGIC CONTACT CHEILITIS

The vermilion border of the lips has a modified epithelium, which is much more likely to develop allergic contact sensitivity reactions than is the oral mucosa. Allergens in contact with both the oral mucosa and the lips often produce only cheilitis.

An angular cheilitis may be the only manifestation of allergic hypersensitivity to denture materials or to mercury amalgams, and it may closely mimic a vitamin B deficiency.

Allergic cheilitis may first manifest itself merely with dryness and fissuring. Edema and crusting may supervene from contact with strong allergens over a prolonged period.

Allergic contact cheilitis may result from dental preparations, antichap agents, lipsticks, sunscreening preparations, nail polish, cigarette paper and cigarette holders, oranges, lemons, artichokes and mangoes. Patients with nickel sensitivity may develop cheilitis from holding hair pins, bobby pins or metal pencils in their mouths. Individuals who chew poison ivy leaves either inadvertently, or to produce a hyposensitization effect, often develop a severe cheilitis, sometimes accompanied by a mucositis of the tongue and mouth.

Allergic cheilitis has resulted from application of Mycolog Cream for angular cheilitis presumably due to monilia. In these instances, the actual sensitizer was the ethylenediamine stabilizer in the cream.[56]

The erythrosin in disclosing tablets (XPose and Red Cote), which are used to identify dental plaque, is a photosensitizer. If the disclosing solution made with this dye contaminates the lips and is not removed, exposure to sunlight may produce a photosensitizing cheilitis. Other disclosing solutions and tablets may contain iodine or Mercurochrome.

Cheilitis from Dentifrices

Bactericidal agents, essential oils and preservatives in toothpastes and mouthwashes may produce allergic cheilitis.[63]

Essential Oils. In dentistry, essential oils are chiefly used as pharmaceutical aids, as mild antiseptics and anodynes and as flavoring for dentifrices and mouthwashes. Several of these oils can produce allergic cheilitis.

The essential oils, particularly clove oil and cinnamon oil, may cross-react with balsam of Peru, which is used in dental cement liquids. In addition, these oils may cross-react with benzoin, rosin, vanilla and the essential oils of orange peel.[64,65]

An orange peel may be used externally for the removal of zinc oxide–eugenol cements. Orange peel may cross-react with balsam of Peru, celery, bergamot, caraway, dill and lemon turpentine.

Anise oil is used as a flavoring agent, especially to disguise substances of disagreeable taste. Loveman[66] reported a case of allergic cheilitis due to anise oil.

Cinnamon oil (cassia oil) is a very weak antiseptic. In dentistry, it is used primarily as a flavoring agent. Oil of cinnamon has further been identified as the cause of allergic cheilitis and stomatitis from toothpaste,[67,68] bubble gum and lipstick. Ingestion of oil of cinnamon in dry vermouth may provoke a flare-up of preexisting allergic contact dermatitis in sensitized individuals.[69] Cross-sensitization to balsam of Peru may result from primary sensitivity to oil of cinnamon.[69]

Many irritants and allergens in medicaments, dentifrices, cosmetics, foods and metallic objects may produce cheilitis, which may mimic vitamin B deficiency syndrome or candidiasis

Menthol, U.S.P. Menthol is used as a flavoring agent, as a component of zinc oxide–eugenol cements, and as a mint flavoring and cooling agent in toothpastes and mouthwashes, cough drops, candy, chewing gum, food, cigarettes, liqueurs and mixed drinks. Papa and Shelley[70] have described dermatitis, cheilitis and stomatitis from menthol.

Eugenol. This is the main constituent of *clove oil*, *oil of carnation*, *pimento oil* and *oil of bay*. In dentistry, eugenol is used in periodontal dressings, zinc oxide cement and impression pastes.

Goransson et al.[71] observed 3 cases of eugenol hypersensitivity. In one, a eugenol impression paste produced allergic cheilitis and stomatitis. In the other 2, an allergic eczematous reaction was produced from handling eugenol. Koch et al.[72] showed that eugenol is a potent sensitizer.

Eugenol may cross-react with balsam of Peru, diethylstilbestrol and benzoin.

Eugenol, the main ingredient in clove oil, is used in periodontal dressings, zinc oxide cement and impression pastes and may readily sensitize the mucous membrane and skin

Allergic Cheilitis Due to Cosmetics

Lipstick Cheilitis. The most common sensitizers in lipstick are the fluorescein stains or eosin indelible dyes, which may produce either a simple allergic sensitization or a photosensitizing reaction. In photosensitivity cheilitis, the eruption appears only after exposure to the sun.

Other ingredients of lipstick, such as oleyl alcohol, lanolin, antioxidants, the methyl heptane carbamate and synthetic perfume, have rarely been incriminated. Cheilitis may result in individuals previously sensitized to cinnamon flavoring in lipsticks.

In nickel-sensitive individuals, the metal lipstick container may produce allergic cheilitis.

Lipstick cheilitis occurs on the vermilion borders of the lips; the angles of the mouth are commonly spared. It may vary from a mild redness, scaling and fissuring to an edematous, crusted condition.[73]

Lip Salve Cheilitis. Lip salves have a softer base than do ordinary lipsticks and may be uncolored or colored with carmine, the aluminum lake of the pigment from cochineal obtained by precipitation with inorganic salts and aluminum. This dye, which is also present in lip rouge, has been shown by Sarkany and Everall[74] to be capable of producing allergic cheilitis.

Cheilitis Due to Nail Polish and Nail Hardeners. Patients allergic to nail polish who bite their nails may develop cheilitis and perlèche. The usual sensitizer in nail polish is a sulfanilamide-formaldehyde resin. So-called hypoallergenic nail polish contains an alkyd resin.

Huldin[75] observed 3 cases of hemorrhage of the lips in nail-biting patients who used nail hardeners, which contain formaldehyde. This phenomenon disappeared with discontinuation of the nail hardener and recurred when it was reused. Examination of the lips revealed many small (1 to 3 mm.) hemorrhages in the mid-portion of the lips, which blended out toward the angle of the mouth. Most of these changes were noted on the vermilion border of the lower lip. There were no other petechial-type lesions of the conjunctivae or the extremities.

Nail biters may develop cheilitis, perlèche and hemorrhages of the lip from nail polish and nail hardeners

Cheilitis Due to Foods

Klauder[76] described a patient with sensitivity to carrots who developed a cheilitis and perioral dermatitis when she ate this vegetable raw or cooked.

Patients who are sensitized to poison ivy may acquire an allergic cheilitis from eating mango, which contains a catechol related to poison ivy oleoresin.

Individuals who remove orange peels with their teeth may develop an allergic cheilitis from orange peel. The specific sensitizer is limonene, an essential oil. Sutton and Sutton[77] reported a case of cheilitis due to the volatile oil of oranges.

Lupton[78] described a persistent cheilitis due to coffee. In this instance, the coffee also produced a positive patch test reaction on the skin.

"SYSTEMIC" DERMATITIS ASSOCIATED WITH ALLERGIC STOMATITIS

This type of dermatitis may be produced by absorption of local anesthetics, mercury, nickel and antibiotics from the sensitized oral mucosa and has the following features:

1. The eruption is predominantly an eczematous reaction but may be urticarial.
2. The *initial* sensitizing exposure is usually from the topical application of a drug or an immunochemically related nondrug compound.[79]
3. The *eliciting* exposure is a drug injected into the oral mucosa or administered systemically.
4. The eruption tends to be symmetrical and widespread.
5. Rarely the eruption may be anaphylactoid.[80,81]

THE ANTIBIOTICS

It is generally agreed that topical use of penicillin and streptomycin should be avoided because of their high sensitization potential.[82] The tetracyclines, erythromycin and chloramphenicol rarely sensitize.

Allergens applied to the oral mucosa may produce not only local effects but also widespread dermatitis in sensitized individuals

Plate 13. Allergic Cobalt Glossitis and Chelitis Simulating Pemphigus Caused by a Denture with Exposed Chrome-cobalt Pins (New York Skin and Cancer Unit)

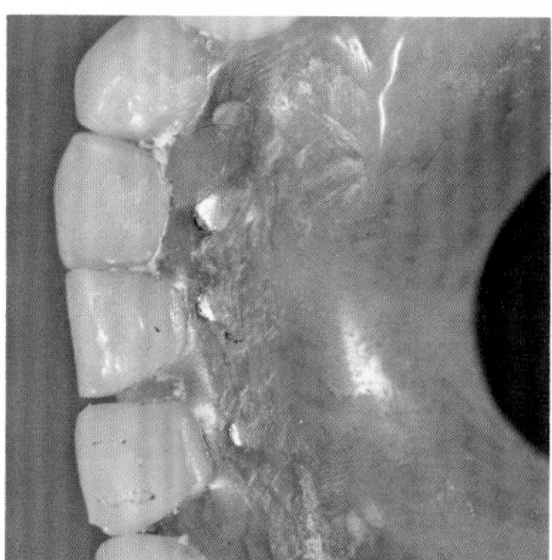

1. Note Exposed Chrome-cobalt Pins Used to Fasten Porcelain Teeth to the Acrylic Denture

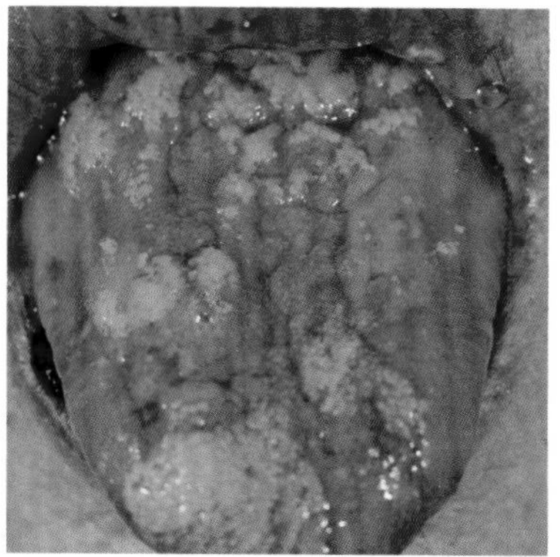

2. Allergic Glossitis in Cobalt-sensitive Patient*

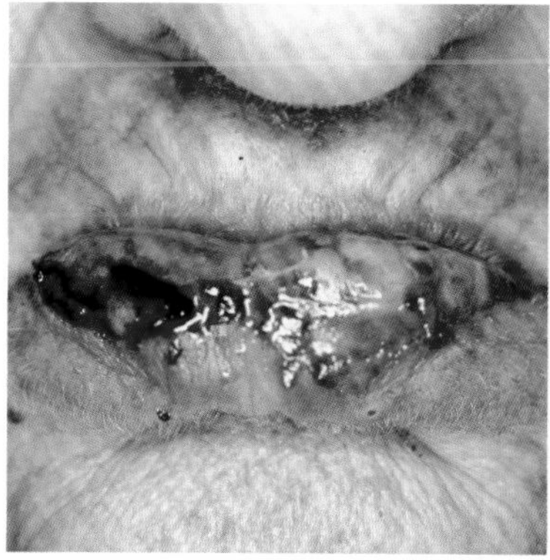

3. Allergic Cheilitis in Same Patient*

* Glossitis and cheilitis cleared when exposed pins were covered.

Neomycin Sulfate. This antibiotic is present in a host of ointments, creams and other topical medications, and it has been added to many cosmetics, soaps and deodorants. It has a significant capacity to produce allergic contact sensitivity.[83] Once sensitization to neomycin from topical exposure has been established, systemic administration of either streptomycin or kanamycin, both of which may cross-react with neomycin, may cause an eczematous contact-type dermatitis medicamentosa.

In addition, although neomycin and bacitracin are not chemically related, in many instances there is a combined sensitivity to these two drugs.[84]

Since neomycin is not readily absorbed from intact mucosa, the danger of producing a "systemic" dermatitis in individuals sensitized to topically applied neomycin is not great, except when such absorption takes place from an ulcerated oral or intestinal mucosa.

Penicillin. The topical use of penicillin is now being avoided. Contact sensitivity has been widely reported following use of topical oral penicillin preparations, such as troches.[85]

Penicillin is still occasionally used with streptomycin and other antibiotics, however, in the local treatment of infected pulp canals. Severe anaphylactoid reactions have occurred in penicillin-sensitive individuals following the endodontic use of a paste containing penicillin, bacitracin, dihydrostreptomycin and sodium caprylate.[86]

Streptomycin. Although topical application of streptomycin, like penicillin, is now being avoided, members of the medical, dental, nursing and pharmaceutical professions who handle the drug readily become sensitized. Subsequent systemic administration to such individuals may produce a severe eczematous contact-type dermatitis medicamentosa. Streptomycin may rarely cross-react with neomycin and kanamycin sulfate (Kantrex).

Streptomycin may be administered alone, or in combination with penicillin in preparations such as Strep-Combiotic (Pfizer), Bicillimycin (Wyeth) and Wycillin (Wyeth). When stomatitis or dermatitis occurs from such combinations, it is imperative to determine by skin tests whether the streptomycin or the penicillin is the sensitizer.

Tetracyclines. Undesirable oral mucosal reactions have been noted from the use of lozenges containing tetracycline, and patients being treated systemically and topically with this antibiotic may develop a transitory yellowish brown discoloration of the tongue, which is not allergic in nature.

Allergic mucosal reaction to antibiotic-containing lozenges may be due to the antibiotic or coloring or flavoring agents.[87] In 1 case of stomatitis due to Aureomycin troches, the allergic reaction was due to sensitization to a certified yellow dye in the preparation.

A few instances of hypersensitivity in connection with topical use of erythromycin have been observed.[88] Eczematous eruptions of the fixed type do occasionally result from systemic administration of tetracyclines.[89] Furthermore, cross-fixed drug reactions from systemic use of Aureomycin, Achromycin and Terramycin have been described.[90] Such reactions may produce erosions of the mouth and lips.

RELATIONSHIP BETWEEN MUCOSAL AND SKIN SENSITIZATION

Allergic contact stomatitis is usually associated with actual or potential allergic hypersensitivity of the skin. Three possible variants of cutaneous or mucosal sensitization have been described:

1. There is sensitization of the skin but not of mucous membranes.

2. There is simultaneous sensitization of the skin and the mucous membranes. Loveman[66] described a patient with dermatitis of the hand and stomatitis caused by anise oil in a denture cream. Templeton and Lunsford[91] reported cases of cheilitis and stomatitis due to hexylresorcinol toothpaste. Shelmire[92] stated that "sensitization to an external agent is always general, the skin and mucosa alike being involved." Goldman and Goldman[93] recorded 10 instances of contact stomatitis from toothpaste, denture cleaner, lavender oil, cashew nut oil, mercury, pecan and tobacco, and in 7 of these cases, cutaneous patch tests gave positive reactions.

3. There is sensitization of the mucous membranes but not the skin. This seems to be the rarest form of sensitization. Farring-

ton[94] reported a case in which contact stomatitis and glossitis followed ingestion of penicillin tablets, but cutaneous patch tests with penicillin gave negative reactions.

TESTING FOR ALLERGIC CONTACT REACTIONS OF THE ORAL MUCOSA

Many schemes have been developed to test the oral mucosa directly. Shelley[95] stated that mucosal reactions to contact allergens are rare, because the salivary flow usually prevents adequate contact, and that specific hypersensitivity of the mucosa usually can be detected by patch testing of the skin. Shelley concluded, however, that in some instances the impermeability of the epidermis prevents the demonstration of allergic hypersensitivity of the oral mucous membranes. In these rare examples, intimate contact of the mucosa with the suspected allergen for 1 hour by means of a tiny suction cup suffices to produce an allergic mucosal reaction, which consists of nonspecific inflammatory changes that may lead to erosions. If a reaction occurs, the testing should be repeated on normal controls.

Mucosal sensitization is usually accompanied by sensitization of the skin

McCarthy and Shklar[96] stated that use of the patch test in stomatitis venenata is limited because of technical difficulties in application. It has been their experience that a person who develops an oral mucosal sensitivity to any substance will demonstrate the same reaction on the skin. They stated, however, that one may exhibit a positive reaction on the skin and be nonsensitive to the same material on the oral mucous membrane.

Zegarelli and co-workers[97] stated that the results of patch tests conducted on the intact skin may be of little or no importance when the suspected allergic lesions are localized in the mouth. An oral mucosal patch test may be more informative, but it is more difficult to perform and the results have not been entirely dependable. These authors concluded that patch tests demonstrating skin hypersensitivity do not relate well to oral tissue hypersensitivity.

Forlen and Stuettgen,[98] by means of a prosthesis fixed to the teeth, found no parallels between the intensities of allergic contact reaction on the skin and mucous membranes.

Present Status of Testing the Oral Mucosa. The methods of testing the oral mucosa directly are not standardized, and interpretations of results are controversial.

THERAPY OF ALLERGIC CHEILITIS AND STOMATITIS

In mild cases, prompt removal of the specific contact allergen is all that is necessary to effect a cure.

Local Therapy. For swelling of the lips with an intact epithelium, the application of petrolatum on which is superimposed ice cold water compresses is helpful. When the swelling of the lips is accompanied by fissuring and crusting, Ilotycin (erythromycin) ointment should be applied. This is an effective, nonsensitizing antibiotic preparation.

When there is edema of the oral mucosa, sucking on ice chips is indicated. Painful erosions or ulcers may be covered with Kenalog in Orabase. If the lesions continue to be painful, Xylocaine Viscous may be applied.

According to Dr. J. Litt (personal communication), patients obtain marked relief by gargling with Benadryl Elixir and by dissolving a 250 mg. capsule of tetracycline in 2 oz. of warm water and swirling it around in the mouth for 5 minutes every 3 to 4 hours.

Systemic Therapy. When there is marked inflammatory reaction and the patient is in great distress, systemic corticosteroid therapy is indicated. An initial injection of Kenalog or Aristocort Suspension (40 mg. for the average size adult) is given. Then 3 times daily, the patient allows a Metandren Linquet (CIBA) to dissolve slowly in the mouth so that there is mucosal absorption of the corticosteroid.

THE ROLE OF CONTACTANTS IN PRURITUS ANI AND PROCTITIS

A list should be made of all the medicaments that the patient has used in the past, and particular inquiry should be made concerning the use of sensitizers such as benzocaine, neomycin and balsam of Peru. Patch tests with these topical remedies may help rule out a contact dermatitis superimposed upon the original pruritus.

The presence of hemorrhoids or fissures should lead one to inquire as to special treatment used and to determine if such treatment produced contact dermatitis. If the patient is using medicated dressing for anal hygiene, such as Tucks, medicated rectal wipes or Balneol, one must be certain that these preparations do not contain agents to which the patient is sensitized. In such instances, the patient who prefers a cooling, drying agent may use witch hazel, while the patient who prefers an oily cleanser may use cold mineral oil.

Perfumed and colored toilet paper should be avoided because of the remote possibility that the dyes or essences in it may be sensitizers.

The *ingestion* of spices, food with seeds, antibiotics, laxatives that cause a slow leakage of oil or paraffin products may cause anal itching.

Foreign bodies inserted into the rectum and rectal intercourse may produce anal irritation, which may be made worse by the use of anesthetic medications containing benzocaine.

CONTACT VULVITIS

All cleansers, douches and medications used on the vulva and in the vagina must be considered possible causes of contact vulvitis. Medications, cosmetics and other sensitizers may be conveyed by the hands to the vulva. Often sensitizing medications or douches well-tolerated by the vaginal mucosa produce vulvitis and dermatitis of the thighs. Deodorants may contain sensitizers.[99]

Irritants and Sensitizers in Douches

Table 18–4 shows examples of popular over-the-counter douches and their ingredients.[100]

Table 18-4. Over-the-Counter Vaginal Douches

Product	*Manufacturer*	*Dosage Form*	*Ingredients*
Avcen	National Drug	Powder	Dioctyl sodium sulfosuccinate Sodium citrate Citric acid Sodium chloride
B & A Hygienic Powder	Eastern Research Laboratories	Powder	Sodium bicarbonate Potassium alum Borax Oil of eucalyptus Menthol Methyl salicylate
Colagyn	Smith Laboratory	Powder	Boric acid Ammonium alum Carbolic acid Menthol Thymol Eucalyptol Aromatics
Demure	Roycemore	Liquid	Benzethonium chloride
Irrigol	Alkalol	Powder and Packettes	Sodium sulfocarbolate Sodium bicarbonate Sodium borate Salt Thymol Eucalyptol Menthol

Table 18-4. Over-the-Counter Vaginal Douches—*(Continued)*

Product	*Manufacturer*	*Dosage Form*	*Ingredients*
Koromex	Holland-Rantos	Powder and envelopes	Lactose Dendritic sodium chloride Lactic acid Urea Menthol Thymol Oil of eucalyptus Methyl salicylate Benzalkonium chloride Polyoxyethylene nonyl phenol
Kotique	Kimberly-Clark	Liquid	Benzalkonium chloride Lactic acid Sodium lactate Potassium alum Aromatics Emulsifier
Kotique	Kimberly-Clark	Powder	Benzalkonium chloride Citric acid Sodium phosphate Potassium alum Aromatics
Massengill Liquid	Masco	Liquid	Lactic acid Sodium lactate Octyl phenoxyl polyethoxyethanol Alcohol
MBA	Apco Laboratories	Powder	Magnesium sulfate Boric acid Alum Menthol Thymol Methyl salicylate Citric acid
Mu-Col	Mu-Col	Powder	Sodium borate Sodium chloride Boric acid Sodium bicarbonate Menthol Thymol Eucalyptol
Nylmerate Antiseptic Solution	Holland-Rantos	Liquid and jelly	Phenylmercuric acetate Alcohol Acetone
Trichotine	Reed & Carnrick	Powder	Sodium lauryl sulfate Sodium perborate Sodium borate Aromatics
Vagisec	Schmid	Liquid	Polyoxyethylene nonyl phenol Sodium edetate Sodium dioctyl sulfosuccinate Alcohol

Table 18-5. Sensitizers in Douches

Phenylmercuric acetate
Benzalkonium chloride
Methyl salicylate
Oxyquinolene
Oil of eucalyptus
Thymol
Aromatics (perfumes)

Most over-the-counter douches are prepared by the user. If the douches are not properly diluted, the acids or alkaline contents may cause a chemical vulvitis.

The principal acid irritants are alum, citric acid and lactic acid. Alkalies such as sodium bicarbonate or sodium borate in too high a concentration may produce vulvitis.

Table 18–5 is a list of the principal causes of allergic vulvitis from douches.

Feminine Hygiene Deodorants

Feminine hygiene deodorants, or intimate sprays, are mainly aerosols containing perfume, antibacterial agents and a hexachlorophene. (See also chapter on cosmetics.)

The deodorant spray may produce irritation and a burning sensation if not applied as directed by the manufacturer. In most instances, the sprays are well-tolerated if applied at the proper distances so that the freon propellent evaporates before it reaches the vulva or skin.

Male sexual partners may acquire dermatitis of the penis and scrotum if intercourse is attempted immediately after the spray is applied.

Table 18–6 gives examples of feminine hygiene deodorants.[100]

Feminine hygiene sprays often irritate if applied too closely. The male genitalia may be irritated by such sprays if intercourse is attempted immediately after application. Allergic reactions are rare

Table 18-6. Feminine Hygiene Deodorants

Product	*Manufacturer*	*Dosage Form*	*Ingredients*
Bidette	Young's Drug Products	Aerosol	Hexachlorophene*
Cupid's Quiver	Tawn	Aerosol	Hexachlorophene*
FDS	Alberto-Culver	Aerosol	Hexachlorophene* Isopropyl myristate Propylparaben
Feminique	Intec Lab	Aerosol	Ingredients not listed
FemMist	House of Style	Aerosol	Hexachlorophene*
Kotique	Kimberly-Clark	Aerosol	Ingredients not listed
Naturally Feminine	Johnson & Johnson	Aerosol	Methylbenzethonium chloride Low micron talc Anhydrous alcohol Isopropyl palmitate Perfume
Pristeen	Warner-Lambert	Aerosol	Hexachlorophene*
Uninhibited	Advance Design Labs	Aerosol	Hexachlorophene*
Vespré	Personal Products	Aerosol	Hexachlorophene*

* The safety of hexachlorophene has recently been questioned by the Food and Drug Administration, and its continued use in feminine hygiene deodorant sprays, and cosmetic products in general, is in doubt.

Table 18-7. Vaginal Spermicides

Product	Manufacturer	Dosage Form	Ingredients
Anvita	A. O. Schmidt	Suppositories	Boric acid, alum, thymol, monochlorthymol, phenylmercuric borate and cocoa butter
Bilco Jelly	Tablax	Jelly	Not available from manufacturer
Certane	Vogarell	Jelly	Phenylmercuric acetate, boric acid, oxyquinoline sulfate and sodium sulfodioctyl succinate
Colagyn	Smith Lab.	Jelly	Chinosol and zinc sulfocarbolate
Conceptrol	Ortho	Cream	Nonoxynol-9 as 5%
Cooper Creme	Whittaker Lab.	Cream	Trioxymethylene 0.04% and sodium oleate 0.67%
Creemoz—Improved	Larre Lab.	Cream	Boric acid, phenol, beta-naphthol, rhodinol, trioxymethylene and nonyl phenoxy polyoxyethylene ethanol
Delfen	Ortho	Cream	Nonoxynol-9 as 5%
Delfen	Ortho	Foam	Nonoxynol-9 as 12.5%
Emko Foam & Pre-Fil	Emko	Foam	Nonyl phenoxy polyoxyethylene ethanol 8%
Immolin Vaginal Cream-Jel	Schmid	Cream	Methoxypolyoxyethylene glycol 550 laurate 5% and nonyl phenoxy polyethoxyethanol 1%
Koromex	Holland-Rantos	Cream	Boric acid 2% and phenylmercuric acetate 0.02%
Koromex	Holland-Rantos	Jelly	Boric acid 2% and phenylmercuric acetate 0.02%
Koromex-A	Holland-Rantos	Jelly	Phenylmercuric acetate 0.02%, polyoxyethylene nonyl phenol 0.5% and boric acid 2%
Lactikol Creme	Durex	Cream	p-Triisopropyl phenoxy polyethoxyethanol and sodium lauryl sulfate
Lactikol Vaginal Jelly	Durex	Jelly	Glyceryl monoricinoleate, triisopropyl phenoxy polyethoxyethanol and sodium lauryl sulfate
Lanesta Gel	Esta Medical Lab.	Jelly	Chlorindanol 0.1%, sodium chloride 10%, sodium lauryl sulfate 0.2% and ricinoleic acid 1%
Lanteen Jelly	Esta Medical Lab.	Jelly	Ricinoleic acid 0.5%, hexylresorcinol 0.1% and chlorothymol 0.0077%
Lorophyn	Eaton	Jelly	Phenylmercuric acetate 0.05%, polyethylene glycol of monoiso-octyl phenyl ether 0.3% and sodium borate 3%

Table 18-7. Vaginal Spermacides—(*Continued*)

Product	*Manufacturer*	*Dosage Form*	*Ingredients*
Lorophyn	Eaton	Suppository	Phenylmercuric acetate 0.4 mg. per suppository
Marvosan Jelly	Tablax	Jelly	Not available from manufacturer
Milex Creme	Milex	Cream	Glycerol ester of ricinoleic acid, sodium lauryl sulfate, oxyquinoline sulfate and lactic acid
Ortho-Creme	Ortho	Cream	Nonoxynol-9 as 2%
Ortho-Gynol	Ortho	Jelly	p-Diisobutyl phenoxy polyethoxyethanol 1%
Preceptin	Ortho	Jelly	p-Diisobutyl phenoxy polyethoxyethanol 1%
Ramses 10-Hour Jelly	Schmid	Jelly	Dodecaethylene glycol monolaurate 5% and boric acid 1%
Zeptabs	Larre Lab.	Foaming tablets	Lactose, sodium bicarbonate, starch, acacia, tartaric acid, halazone and talc

Sensitizers in Deodorant Sprays. Hexachlorophene, the most common antiseptic in these sprays, is very rarely a sensitizer in my experience. Other quaternary ammonium salts may occasionally produce allergic reactions.[99] Perfumes may produce allergic vulvitis.

Chemical Contraceptives

Vaginal spermicides very rarely irritate the vulva but may occasionally produce allergic vulvitis. Table 18–7 lists available vaginal spermicides and their active ingredients.[101]

Table 18–8 is a list of the principal sensitizers in vaginal spermicides.

Table 18-8. Sensitizers in Vaginal Spermicides

Phenylmercuric acetate
Oxyquinoline sulfate
Quinine hydrochloride
Hexylresorcinol

Patch tests with chemical contraceptives must be interpreted with care, because some contain soapy substances that may show nonspecific irritant reactions under a closed patch. A positive patch test reaction should be followed by testing with the individual ingredients of the product.

Rubber Products

Rubber Support Pessaries and Contraceptive Diaphragms. Vaginitis and vulvitis may be produced by such rubber articles in rubber-sensitive individuals. Plastic pessaries and contraceptive devices are now available as substitutes.

Rubber Condoms. This product may produce an acute dermatitis of the vulva and inner aspect of the thighs in a rubber-sensitive woman.

A rubber condom used by the male may produce dermatitis in the rubber-sensitive female

Intrauterine Devices (IUD)

Various metals, including stainless steel and copper, are used in intrauterine devices. Stainless steel is virtually nonallergenic, and copper sensitivity is extremely rare.

Miscellaneous Causes of Vulvitis

1. *Nickel-plated* objects (pins, fasteners, zippers and clasps) on sanitary napkins may produce vulvitis in nickel-sensitive individuals.

2. *Cosmetics* may be the cause of vulvitis. For example, nail polish dermatitis will, on occasion, manifest itself on the vulvar or anal area because of contact with fingernails on which the nail polish is not yet dry.

The vulva may also be the site of perfume dermatitis from perfume or perfumed toilet tissue.

3. *Medicated soaps* containing sensitizing antiseptics can cause vulvitis.

4. *Wearing apparel.* Dyes and synthetic resins in underclothing may produce dermatitis in sensitized women. The wearing of close-fitting undergarments, such as pantyhose, panty girdles and tight sanitary napkins, may produce vulvar irritation.

CONTACT BALANITIS

The glans penis and the prepuce may acquire contact dermatitis from douches, contraceptive jellies, feminine hygiene sprays and other medicaments used by a sexual partner.

Poison ivy may cause a severe balanitis. Numerous other exposures in work and play may also be factors in producing balanitis.

Sensitizing topical applications for dermatoses, such as psoriasis or lichen planus, may produce a superimposed contact balanitis.

Rubber Condoms. These are popularly called sheaths, French Letters, prophylactics, protectives, rubbers, skins or safes.

Edema of the prepuce may be the first sign of an allergic rubber condom reaction. The eruption may spread to the shaft of the penis, the scrotum and inguinal areas and inner aspects of the thighs. Occasionally, the reaction is confined to the glans penis.

Rubber condom dermatitis[102] is usually due to sensitivity to one or more rubber antioxidants or accelerators. Occasionally, a preservative powder dusted onto the condom is the actual cause of the dermatitis. In one instance, the powder contained 10 per cent monobenzyl ether of hydroquinone (agerite alba), which not only produced balanitis and penile dermatitis but also eventually induced a leukoderma.

Some men have found by trial and error that only certain brands of rubber condoms produced reactions, while others were well-tolerated.

Table 18–9 is a list of available condoms.[101]

Patch Tests for Rubber Condom Sensitivity. Patch tests should be performed with the actual condom suspected of producing the reaction. If a powder or lubricant is present on the condom, tests should also be performed with these substances.[102]

Patch tests should also be performed with

Table 18-9. Condoms

Type	*Brand Name*	*Supplier*
Rubber—plain end packaged dry	Trojans Regular	Youngs Drug Products
	Ramses	Schmid
	Sheik	Schmid
Rubber—reservoir end packaged dry	Sheik	Schmid
	Trojan-Enz	Youngs Drug Products
	Shadow-Enz	Youngs Drug Products
Rubber—reservoir end packaged with lubricant	Trojan-Enz Lubricated	Youngs Drug Products
	Guardian	Youngs Drug Products
	Lubricated Sheik	Schmid
Lamb cecum—regular end packaged with lubricant	XXXX(Fourex) "Non-Slip"	Schmid
	Naturalamb	Youngs Drug Products

the following rubber chemicals: mercaptobenzothiazole, tetramethyl thiuram, monobenzyl ether of hydroquinone and zinc dithiocarbamate.

Patients who are allergic to tetramethyl thiuram in a rubber condom may develop a violent reaction and widespread dermatitis when given Antabuse for treatment of alcoholism.[103]

Nonrubber Condoms. Fourex and Lambskin, which are made of processed lamb cecum, are available for individuals who cannot tolerate any rubber contraceptives. Such preparations are popularly called "fishskins."

ALLERGIC CONTACT CONJUNCTIVITIS

Conjunctivitis may accompany facial and scalp dermatitis, particularly from hair dyes and cosmetics. Consultation with an ophthalmologist is required in severe conjunctival involvement. The dermatologist's skill in patch test procedures may be helpful, however, in solving cases of allergic contact conjunctivitis, particularly when due to preservatives in ophthalmic preparations. Benzalkonium chloride, ethylenediamine tetraacetate and phenylmercuric salts have been reported by dermatologists as causes of allergic conjunctivitis.

Benzalkonium Chloride (BAK). This antiseptic is present in most ophthalmic preparations and contact lens soaking solutions.[104] Theodore and Schlossman[105] stated that it may produce allergic reactions, but they did not cite specific cases confirmed by patch test reactions.

Fisher and Stillman[106] described a case of allergic contact sensitivity to benzalkonium chloride in an ophthalmic solution, which was augmented when an ophthalmologist inadvertently prescribed another solution containing this antiseptic for the treatment of conjunctivitis. Patch test reactions were strongly positive to a 1:1000 solution of benzalkonium chloride.

Table 18–10 is a list of ophthalmic products that contain benzalkonium chloride.

Ophthalmic preparations that are free of benzalkonium chloride include Soaklens (Burton, Parsons) and Vasocon (Smith, Miller & Patch).

Table 18-10. Ophthalmic Products Containing Benzalkonium Chloride

Product	*Manufacturer*
Artificial tears	
BufOpto Methulose	Professional Pharmacal
BufOpto Visculose	Professional Pharmacal
Isopto, alkaline and plain	Alcon
Lyteers	Barnes-Hind
Tearisol	Tilden-Yates
Contact lens products	
Clens	Burton, Parsons
Lensine	Murine
Liquifilm	Allergan
Soakare	Allergan
Soquette	Barnes-Hind
Wetting Solution	Alcon
Wetting Solution	Barnes-Hind
Wetting Solution	Rexall
Decongestants	
BufOpto Efricel	Professional Pharmacal
Clear Eyes	Murine
Degest	Barnes-Hind
Eye Drops	Rexall
Eye-Mo	Winthrop
Murine	Murine
Neozin	Professional Pharmacal
nTz Solution	Winthrop
OpH	Winthrop
Optihist	Tilden-Yates
Phenylzin	Tilden-Yates
Prefrin	Allergan
Prefrin Z	Allergan
Tear-Efrin	Tilden-Yates
Vasopred Ophthalmic Suspension	Smith, Miller & Patch
Visine	Leeming
Eye washes (collyria)	
BufOpto NEO-FLO	Professional Pharmacal
Dacriose	Tilden-Yates
Lavoptik	Lavoptik
Ocusol	Norwich
Op-thal-zin	Alcon
Enuclene	Alcon

Ethylenediamine Tetraacetate (EDTA). This preservative is also frequently present in ophthalmic solutions, often in conjunction with benzalkonium chloride.[54] It cross-reacts with ethylenediamine, which has sensitized many individuals through its use in Mycolog Cream. This cross-sensitivity makes the

EDTA-sensitive patient allergic to aminophylline, Phenergan, Pyribenzamine and Antistine Ophthalmic Solution.[107]

Phenylmercuric Salts. These mercury salts used in ophthalmic solutions may occasionally produce allergic reactions. Patch tests should be performed with a 0.01 per cent concentration in petrolatum. Aqueous solution may lead to false positive irritant reactions even in this dilution.

Fisher et al.[107] have emphasized that the vehicles with their preservative of topical medicaments not infrequently produce allergic reactions that can be detected only by proper patch test procedures.

REFERENCES

Stomatitis and Cheilitis

1. Lowney, E. D.: Unresponsiveness to a Contact Sensitizer in Man. J. Invest. Derm., *51*, 411, 1968.
2. Claman, H. N.: Mouth Ulcers Associated with Prolonged Chewing of Gum Containing Aspirin. J.A.M.A., *202*, 651, 1967.
3. Gruskin, S. E., Tolman, D. E., and Wagoner, R. D.: Oral Manifestations of Uremia. Minnesota Med., *53*, 495, 1970.
4. Kierland, R.: What's New. Int. J. Derm., *10*, 208, 1971.
5. *Accepted Dental Therapeutics* (Ed. 33). American Dental Assn., Chicago, 1968.
6. Fisher, A. A.: Patch Tests for Allergic Reactions to Dentifrices and Mouthwashes. Cutis, *6*, 554, 1970.
7. Thomas, J. W., and Syrop, H. M.: Allergy Problems Related to Dentistry. Ann. Allergy, *15*, 603, 1957.
8. Wilson, H.: Dermatitis from Anesthetic Ointments. Practitioner, *197*, 673, 1966.
9. Fisher, A. A., and Sturm, H. M.: Procaine Sensitivity: The Relationship of Allergic Eczematous Contact-Type Sensitivity to the Urticarial, Anaphylactoid Variety. Ann. Allergy, *16*, 595, 1958.
10. Eyre, J., and Nally, F.: Nasal Test for Hypersensitivity, Including a Positive Reaction to Lignocaine. Lancet, *1*, 264, 1971.
11. Fernstreom, A. I. B., et al.: Mercury Allergy with Eczematous Dermatitis Due to Silver-Amalgam Fillings. Brit. Dent. J., *113*, 206, 1962.
12. Gots, H., and Fortmann, I.: Can Amalgam Fillings Cause a Mercury Sensitization of the Skin? Haut. Geschlectskr., *26*, 34, 1959.
13. Gaul, L. E.: Immunity of the Oral Mucosa in Epidermal Sensitization to Mercury. Arch. Derm., *93*, 45, 1966.
14. Epstein, S.: The Antigen-Antibody Reaction in Contact Dermatitis. Ann. Allergy, *10*, 633, 1952.
15. Juhlin, L., and Ohman, S.: Allergic Reaction to Mercury in Red Tattoos and in Mercury Adjacent to Amalgam Fillings. Acta Dermatovener., *48*, 103, 1968.
16. Johnson, H. H., Schonberg, I. L., and Bach, N. F.: Chronic Atopic Dermatitis, with Pronounced Mercury Sensitivity: Partial Clearing After Extraction of Teeth Containing Mercury Amalgam Fillings. Arch. Derm. & Syph., *63*, 279, 1951.
17. Sidi, E., and Casalis, J.: Les Intolerances de la Muqueuse Buccale. Presse Med., *59*, 730, 1951.
18. Vickers, C. F.: Mercury Sensitivity. Contact Dermatitis Newsletter No. 2, 1961.
19. Spector, L. A.: Allergic Manifestations to Mercury. J.A.M.A., *42*, 320, 1951.
20. Stein, M. B., and Stein, L. J.: Personal communication regarding dental consultation in a mercury-sensitive individual.
21. Thomson, J., and Russell, J. A.: Dermatitis Due to Mercury Following Amalgam Dental Restoration. Brit. J. Derm., *82*, 292, 1970.
22. Frykholm, K. O.: On Mercury from Dental Amalgam: Its Toxic and Allergic Effects and Some Comments on Occupational Hygiene. Acta Odont. Scand., *15*, Suppl. 22, 1957.
23. Hjorth, N., and Trolle-Lassen, C.: Skin Reaction to Ointment Bases. Trans. St. John Hosp. Derm. Soc., *49*, 131, 1963.
24. Fisher, A. A.: Recent Developments in the Diagnosis and Management of Drug Eruptions. Med. Clin. N. Amer., *43*, 787, 1959.
25. Foussereau, J., and Laugier, P.: Allergic Eczema from Metallic Foreign Bodies (Tooth Fillings and Denture Alloys). Clin. Derm., *52*, 221, 1966.
26. Fisher, A. A., and Shapiro, A.: Allergic Eczematous Contact Dermatitis Due to Metallic Nickel. J.A.M.A., *161*, 717, 1956.
27. Wilson, H. T.: Nickel Dermatitis. Brit. J. Derm., *67*, 291, 1955.
28. Calnan, C. D.: Nickel Sensitivity in Women. Int. Arch. Allergy, *11*, 73, 1957.
29. Saltzer, E. J., and Wilson, J. W.: Allergic Contact Dermatitis Due to Copper. Arch. Derm., *98*, 375, 1968.
30. Frykholm, K. O., et al.: Allergy to Copper Derived from Dental Alloys as a Possible Cause of Oral Lesions of Lichen Planus. Acta Dermatovener., *49*, 268, 1969.

31. Elgart, M. L., and Higdon, R. S.: Allergic Contact Dermatitis to Gold. Arch. Derm., *103*, 649, 1971.
32. Brendlinger, D. L., and Tarsitano, J. J.: Generalized Dermatitis Due to Sensitivity to a Chrome-Cobalt Removable Partial Denture. J.A.D.A., *81*, 395, 1970.
33. Sheard, C., Jr.: Contact Dermatitis from Platinum and Related Metals. Arch. Derm., *71*, 357, 1955.
34. Fisher, A. A.: Allergic Sensitization of the Skin and Oral Mucosa to Acrylic Resin Denture Materials. J. Pros. Dent., *6*, 600, 1956.
35. Fisher, A. A.: Allergic Sensitization of the Skin and Oral Mucosa to Acrylic Denture Materials. J.A.M.A., *156*, 238, 1954.
36. Crissey, J. T.: Stomatitis, Dermatitis and Denture Materials. Arch. Derm., *92*, 45, 1965.
37. Turrell, J. J.: Allergy to Denture Materials —Fallacy or Reality. Brit. Dent. J., *120*, 415, 1966.
38. Turrell, J. J.: Angular Cheilosis and Dentures. Brit. J. Derm., *79*, 331, 1967.
39. Salo, O. P., and Hirvonen, M. L.: Yeasts as a Cause of False-Positive Reaction in Patch Tests for Allergy to Denture Materials. Brit. J. Derm., *81*, 338, 1969.
40. Nyquist, G.: Sensitivity to Methyl Methacrylate. Trans. Roy. School Dent., 1958, p. 35.
41. Mullins, J. F.: Denture Stomatitis with Inflammatory Hyperplasia. Arch. Derm., *86*, 764, 1962.
42. Figley, K. D.: Karaya Gum Hypersensitivity. J.A.M.A., *114*, 109, 1940.
43. Schorr, W. F.: Paraben Allergy. A Cause of Intractable Dermatitis. J.A.M.A., *24*, 107, 1968.
44. Epstein, S.: Paraban Sensitivity. Subtle Trouble. Ann. Allergy, *25*, 185, 1968.
45. Federal Food, Drug and Cosmetic Act, General Regulations, *1*, 106 (Subsection B), 1964.
46. Schamberg, I. L.: Allergic Contact Dermatitis to Methyl and Propyl Paraben. Arch. Derm., *95*, 626, 1967.
47. Schorr, W. F.: Allergic Reactions from Cosmetic Preservatives. Amer. Perf. Cosmet., Documentary Issue, 1970.
48. Fisher, A. A., and Lipton, M.: Allergic Stomatitis Due to "Baxin" in a Dentifrice. Arch. Derm. & Syph., *64*, 640, 1951.
49. Fisher, A. A., and Tobin, L.: Sensitivity to Compound G-4 ("Dichlorophene"). J.A.M.A., *15*, 998, 1953.
50. Epstein, E.: Hexachlorophene Sensitivity. Ann. Allergy, *24*, 437, 1966.
51. Vilanova, X., and Camarasa, G.: Present Importance of the So-Called Cutaneous Tests in the Diagnosis of Contact Eczema. Acta Dermatovener., *50*, 243, 1959.
52. Huriez, C., et al. Allergy To Quaternary Ammonium Salts. Sem. Hop. Paris, *41*, 2301, 1965.
53. Morris, G. E.: Dermatoses from Phenylmercuric Salts. Arch. Environ. Health, *1*, 53, 1960.
54. Raymond, J. Z., and Gross, P. R.: EDTA: Preservative Dermatitis. Arch. Derm., *100*, 435, 1969.
55. Provost, T. T., and Jillson, O. F.: Ethylenediamine Contact Dermatitis. Arch. Derm., *96*, 231, 1967.
56. Epstein, E., and Maibach, H. I.: Ethylenediamine Allergic Contact Dermatitis. Arch. Derm., *98*, 476, 1968.
57. Pay, D. K., and Shelley, W. B.: Necrotic Ulcerations Secondary to Oral Neomycin Troches. Arch. Derm., *91*, 136, 1965.
58. Sugarman, M. M.: Contact Allergy Due to Mint Chewing Gum. Oral Surg., *3*, 1145, 1950.
59. Kutcher, A. H., et al.: Citric Acid Sensitivity in Recurrent Ulcerative (Aphthous) Stomatitis. J. Allergy, *29*, 438, 1958.
60. Tuft, L., and Girsh, L. S.: Buccal Mucosal Tests in Patients with Canker Sores (Aphthous Stomatitis). J. Allergy, *29*, 503, 1958.
61. Cancellieri, C. P.: Chronic Aphthous Ulcers (Canker Sores) Due to Inhalant Allergen Sensitivity. J. Allergy, *29*, 503, 1958.
62. Fregert, S., et al.: Alcohol Dermatitis. Acta Dermatovener., *49*, 493, 1969.
63. Sims, W. B.: Oral Lesions Caused by Anti-Enzyme Dentifrices. U.S. Armed Forces J., *6*, 995, 1955.
64. Hjorth, N.: *Eczematous Allergy to Balsams.* Munksgaard, Copenhagen, 1961, p. 195.
65. Calap Calatayud, J.: Allergy to Balsam of Peru. Med. Esp., *61*, 119, 1969.
66. Loveman, A. B.: Stomatitis Venenata: Report of a Case of Sensitivity of the Mucous Membranes and the Skin to Oil of Anise. Arch. Derm. & Syph., *37*, 70, 1938.
67. Kern, A. N.: Contact Dermatitis from Cinnamon. Arch. Derm., *81*, 599, 1960.
68. Leifer, W.: Contact Dermatitis Due to Cinnamon. Arch. Derm., *64*, 52, 1951.
69. Leifer, W.: Contact Dermatitis Due to Cinnamon, Recurrence of Dermatitis Following Oral Administration of Cinnamon Oil. Arch. Derm. & Syph., *64*, 53, 1951.
70. Papa, C. M., and Shelley, W. B.: Menthol Hypersensitivity. J.A.M.A., *189*, 546, 1964.

71. Goransson, J., et al.: Some Cases of Eugenol Sensitivity. Svensk Tandlak. T., *60,* 545, 1967.
72. Koch, G., Magnusson, B., and Nyquist, G.: Contact Allergy to Medicaments and Materials used in Dentistry (II). Sensitivity to Eugenol and Colophony. Odont. Rev., *22,* 275, 1971.
73. Sarkany, I., and Calnan, C. D.: Lipstick Cheilitis. Trans. St. John Hosp. Derm. Soc., *39,* 27, 1957.
74. Sarkany, R. H., and Everall, J.: Cheilitis Due to Carmine in Lip Salve. Trans. St. John Hosp. Derm. Soc., *46,* 39, 1961.
75. Huldin, D. H.: Hemorrhages of the Lips Secondary to Nail Hardeners. Cutis, *4,* 709, 1968.
76. Klauder, J. V.: Sensitization to Carrots. Arch. Derm., *74,* 149, 1956.
77. Sutton, R. L., and Sutton, R. L., Jr.: *Diseases of the Skin* (Ed. 10). St. Louis, C. V. Mosby Co., 1938, p. 1484.
78. Lupton, E. S.: Cheilitis Due to Coffee. Arch. Derm., *84,* 798, 1961.
79. Fisher, A. A.: Internal Contact Dermatitis. Cutis, *5,* 407, 1969.
80. Fisher, A. A.: Systemic Eczematous "Contact-Type" Dermatitis Medicamentosa. Ann. Allergy, *24,* 415, 1966.
81. Welch, H., et al.: Severe Reactions to Antibiotics. Antibot. Med. Clin. Ther., *4,* 800, 1957.
82. Rees, B. R.: Cutaneous Reactions to Antibiotics. J.A.M.A., *189,* 685, 1964.
83. Epstein, S.: Dermal Contact Dermatitis from Neomycin. Ann. Allergy, *16,* 268, 1958.
84. Epstein, S., and Wenzel, F. J.: Sensitivity to Neomycin and Bacitracin, Cross-Sensitization or Coincidence? Acta Dermatovener., *43,* 1, 1963.
85. Farrington, J.: Stomatitis with Glossitis Following Oral Therapy with Penicillin Tablets. Arch. Derm. & Syph., *57,* 399, 1948.
86. Schmidt, G.: Penicillin Reaction in Endodontic Treatment. J.A.D.A., *52,* 196, 1956.
87. Kutcher, A. H., et al.: Reactions Following the Use of Aureomycin and Procaine Penicillin Troches: A controlled study. J. Allergy, *24,* 164, 1953.
88. Livingood, C. S., et al.: Erythromycin in Local Treatment of Cutaneous Bacterial Infections. J.A.M.A., *153,* 1266, 1953.
89. Welsh, L.: The Fixed Drug Eruption. Arch. Derm., *84,* 1012, 1961.
90. Welsh, L.: Cross-Fixed Drug Eruption from Three Antibiotics. Arch. Derm., *71,* 521, 1955.
91. Templeton, H. J., and Lunsford, C. J.: Cheilitis and Stomatitis from ST 37 Tooth Paste. Arch. Derm., *25,* 439, 1932.
92. Shelmire, B.: Contact Dermatitis from Weeds: Patch Testing with Their Oleoresins. J.A.M.A., *113,* 1085, 1939.
93. Goldman, L., and Goldman, B.: Contact Testing of the Buccal Mucous Membrane for Stomatitis Venenata. Arch. Derm., *50,* 79, 1944.
94. Farrington, J.: Modifications of the Goldman Technique for Contact Testing of the Buccal Mucosa. J. Invest. Derm., *8,* 59, 1947.
95. Shelley, W. B.: The Patch Test. J.A.M.A., *200,* 173, 1967.
96. McCarthy, P. L., and Shklar, G.: *Diseases of the Oral Mucosa: Diagnosis, Management, Therapy.* New York, Blakiston Division, McGraw-Hill Book Co., 1964, p. 157.
97. Zegarelli, E. V., Kutcher, A. H., and Hyman, G. A.: *Diagnosis of Diseases of the Mouth and Jaws.* Philadelphia, Lea & Febiger, 1969, p. 306.
98. Forlen, H. P., and Stuettgen, G.: Comparative Studies on the Allergic Reactions of the Skin and the Mucous Membranes. Hautklin, Med. Akad., Dermatologica (Basel), *112,* 417, 1961.

Vulvitis and Balanitis

99. Shmunes, E., and Levy, E. J.: Quaternary Ammonium Compound Contact Dermatitis from a Deodorant. Arch. Derm., *105,* 91, 1972.
100. Sadik, F.: O-T-C Feminine Hygiene Aid. J. Amer. Pharm. Assoc. (in press).
101. Huff, J. E., and Hernandez, L.: Contraceptive Devices. J. Amer. Pharm. Assoc. (in press).
102. Hindson, T. C.: Contact Dermatitis: Contraceptives. Trans. St. John Hosp. Derm. Soc., *52,* 1, 1966.
103. Wilson, H. T. H.: Effect of Disulfram. Brit. Med. J., *2,* 1610, 1962.

Ophthalmic Reactions

104. Dabezies, O. H., Nangle, B. S., and Reich, L.: Evaluation of a Stronger Concentration of Preservative (Benzalkonium Chloride) in Contact Lens Soaking Solution. Eye Ear Nose Throat Monthly, *45,* 78, 1966.
105. Theodore, F. H., and Schlossman, A.:

Ocular Allergy. Baltimore, Williams and Wilkins Co., 1958, p. 188.

106. Fisher, A. A., and Stillman, M.: Allergic Contact Sensitivity to Benzalkonium Chloride (BAK). Cutaneous, Ophthalmic and General Medical Implications. Arch. Derm., *106*, 169, 1972.

107. Fisher, A. A., et al.: Allergic Contact Dermatitis Due to Ingredients of Vehicles. Arch. Derm., *104*, 286, 1971.

19

Aquatic Contact Dermatitis*

It has been estimated that by the year 2000, about 80 per cent of the world population will have migrated to coastal areas. Aquatic medicine, i.e., the diagnosis and treatment of any water-related disease or injury, is becoming a specialty in its own right. We have, therefore, felt the need of adding to this text a special chapter on aquatic contact dermatitis.

DERMATITIS DUE TO NEMATOCYSTS

Nematocysts, or stinging capsules, are characteristic of all species within the phylum Coelenterata. Nematocysts are found in no other phylum.

Table 19–1 is a list of the classes within this phylum and several clinically significant species.

Table 19-1. The Phylum Coelenterata

1. Class: Hydrozoa
   - A. Order: Siphonophora
     - Species: Physalia physalis (Portuguese man-of-war); Velella velella
   - B. Order: Calycophora (glassy nectophore)
   - C. Order: Leptomedusae (feather hydroids)
   - D. Order: Milleporina
     - Millepora spp. (stinging corals [not a true coral])
2. Class: Scyphozoa (true jellyfish)
   - Order: Cubomedusae (box jellies or sea wasps)
     - Species: Chironex fleckeri; Chiropsalmus quadrigatus
3. Class: Anthozoa
   - Subclass: Zoantharia
     - Order: Actiniaria (sea anemones)
     - Order: Scleractinia (corals)

> **Nematocysts are unique to the phylum Coelenterata**

Nematocysts. These are dead organoids, sometimes called stinging cells, nettle cells or stinging capsules, which "fire" by everting a threadlike tube coiled up within the capsule. If the end of the tube, which is pointed, contacts the skin, the speed with which it has discharged carries it into the skin where it deposits its toxic substance. Both chemical and mechanical factors appear to be involved in the stimulation required to discharge a nematocyst. Not all nematocysts deposited on the skin by a tentacle fire immediately, but wait in readiness for proper stimulation at a later time. It is possible that fresh water stimulates nematocysts to explode. Friction such as rubbing with sand or cloth may cause discharge of the capsule.

Nematocyst Venom. Certain high molecular weight toxins isolated from coelenterates, including Physalia physalis, are heat labile, nondialyzable, and degraded by proteolytic

* This chapter was written in collaboration with William L. Orris, M.D., Director of Medical Services, Scripps Institution of Oceanography, University of California, San Diego.

The stinging capsules (nematocysts) deposited on the skin may inject their venom at once or lie dormant and "fire" later when stimulated by fresh water or by being rubbed by hands, sand or cloth

agents. These toxins may exhibit strong action on the heart. They appear to inhibit nerve activity by altering ionic permeability in many animal species.

Animals contacting or receiving the venom by injection may acquire urticaria, edema, pruritus, cardiac arrest, paralysis and death. Severe pain and nervous depression may occur soon after envenomization.

The pain and urticaria are probably due to the presence of serotonin, histamine or histamine-releasing agents in the venom. Paralysis and central nervous system effects are probably due to the presence of toxic proteins and peptides and secondarily to tetramine. A toxic protein-tetramine complex has been suggested to be present in coelenterate extracts.

It is possible that coelenterates release antigenic and allergenic material in their aquatic environment. The allergens in the venom thus may sensitize individuals without actual contact with the nematocysts. When a sensitized individual then comes into contact with a ruptured stinging capsule, a severe allergic reaction occurs.

Reactions Due to Contact with Nematocysts

Dermatitis resulting from contact with nematocysts varies with the toxicity of the venom. Severity varies from a mild stinging, papular eruption to a marked burning sensation accompanied by erythema and edema. Marked itching and pain may accompany severe dermatitis.[1]

Urticarial eruptions with or without anaphylactic reactions, such as edema of the throat and larynx, and marked weakness may occur. Shock and death may ensue in young victims and those with marked hypersensitivity.

Reactions to contact with nematocysts vary from mild papular eruptions to anaphylaxis and death

Table 19-2. Principles of Treatment of Contact with Nematocysts

1. Nematocysts are activated by fresh water.
2. Nematocysts are inactivated by alcohol or formalin.
3. The toxic substance is acid in reaction.
4. Involved skin should not be rubbed with anything, including the bare hand.

Treatment of Dermatitis and Allergic Reactions to Nematocysts

When an individual emerges from the sea and complains of itching or a burning sensation, he may be unaware that he had come in contact with an organism that has nematocysts. One has to presume that such contact has taken place, and the following treatment should be given, based on the principles listed in Table 19–2.

1. *Avoidance of fresh water.* Nematocysts are activated by fresh water. Putting a victim into a fresh shower after exposure could therefore result in severe intensification of symptoms and possibly shock. The patient's skin should be gently rinsed with sea water.
2. *Use of alcohol.* Any type of alcohol available, including rubbing alcohol, liquor, toilet water, cologne or perfume, should be applied to the affected areas. (Although formalin inactivates the nematocysts, it is too toxic to be used routinely.)
3. *Use of alkalies.* Five minutes after the alcohol has been applied, a mixture of sea water and baking soda should be used. Diluted ammonia water is useful in neutralizing the acid of the venom. Flour, shaving soap or shaving cream may be applied and scraped off to remove nematocysts.
4. *Use of hot salt water.* If nothing else is available, salt water heated to the limit of tolerance will help neutralize the venom.

In severe cases, especially in which children are involved, tourniquets on the exposed limbs may be life-saving. The tourniquet should always be of rubber and applied so that a finger can be slipped beneath it. Its purpose is to reduce venous return, not to stop arterial flow. It should be released for 3 or 4 minutes every hour.

Shock should be treated with epinephrine and systemic corticosteroids.

Nematocysts are activated by fresh water and mechanical stimulation, such as friction and rubbing. Alcohol inactivates the stinging capsules, and alkalies neutralize the acid venom. Hot salt water may be used if alcohol or alkalies are not available

Children, who grasp the tentacles of the Portuguese man-of-war, cry and rub their eyes, may develop acute conjunctivitis.

It is also possible to come into contact with nematocysts without encountering a coelenterate. For example, two species of nudibranch, Glaucus atlanticus and Glaucus glaucilla, eat the nematocysts and tentacles of Physalia physalis without apparent harm. The nematocysts pass through the *sea slugs* undigested and are deposited in the dorsal papillae (endosacs). Bathers coming in contact with these "armed" nudibranches may be stung by the nematocysts. This condition is called nudibranch dermatitis.

Nudibranch dermatitis is due to contact with nudibranches that have ingested nematocysts

Portuguese Man-of-War Dermatitis

The species Physalia physalis, the Portuguese man-of-war, is found throughout subtropical waters. Related species are found worldwide in tropical oceans. Large colonies (sometimes hundreds) of these hydroids drift on the surface of the water by a purple, gas-filled float, which acts as a sail.[2]

The organism drags numerous fishing tentacles, sometimes 100 feet long, which have beadlike batteries of nematocysts along their length. Upon being discharged, these stinging capsules penetrate the skin and inject a toxic substance. Swimmers may be severely stung.[2] The toxin is thought to be a multicomponent system, containing phospholipases A and B, several neutral lipids, enzymes with relatively high proteolytic activity, and biologically active peptides. Nematocysts remain capable of firing for at least several months after being detached from the coelenterate.

Contact with the tentacles of this marine organism causes a sharp sting, burning numbness, a blinding flash of pain and breathlessness. Inflammation of the skin may result, varying from lines of urticarial lesions to coagulation necrosis. Erythema, edema, itching and a burning sensation are sometimes followed by vesicular dermatitis. Systemic symptoms may occur soon after contact and consist of lacrimation, coryza, muscular pains, a feeling of constriction in the chest and dyspnea. Despite the pain involved, collapse and death are rare. Healed lesions may leave pigmented striae for weeks or months; sometimes permanent scarring results.[3]

Nematocysts detached from the tentacles of the Portuguese man-of-war are capable of discharging for several months

Velella Velella Dermatitis (By-the-Wind Sailor or Purple Sail Dermatitis)

Velella velella, a siphonophore, is a purple-edged, thin triangular sail on an oval float. It drifts on the water, much as the Portuguese man-of-war, and has trailing tentacles with nematocysts, which it uses to capture prey.

The dermatitis produced by it is a mild papulourticarial eruption.

Calycophora Dermatitis (Stinging Water Dermatitis)

A siphonophore, of the suborder Calycophora, causes a markedly pruritic eruption, which may persist for hours to several days. This small, glassy nectophore has almost the same index of refraction as sea water and can be seen only when the sunlight hits it directly. (See earlier part of chapter for treatment.)

Stinging or Fire Coral Dermatitis

The hydrozoan Millepora alcicornis looks like a coral and has nematocysts, which cause fire coral dermatitis. The organism is generally found living on the reefs, among true corals, in the tropical Pacific Ocean, Indian Ocean, Red Sea and Caribbean Sea. It is usually yellow-brown, somewhat like mustard. The wet mucus from this hydrozoan contains nematocysts.

The eruption is erythematous, papular and patchy, appears 1 to 10 hours after contact and usually subsides in 1 to 3 days. Pustules may develop in severe cases. (See earlier part of chapter for treatment.)

Feather Hydroid Dermatitis

Dermatitis may be produced by four species of the order Leptomedusae, and most commonly affected are swimmers climbing above rafts anchored off shore or swimming around pilings.

The venom of this hydrozoan affects the skin more slowly than does the jellyfish venom. Two types of skin reactions have been reported: (1) an urticarial eruption, which may develop within a few minutes or up to 2 hours after contact and (2) delayed papular, hemorrhagic or zosteriform reaction, which occurs 4 to 12 hours after contact.

Bands of dermatitis 20 cm. wide may be produced and be accompanied by erythema multiforme and morbilliform eruptions. Systemic reactions include severe abdominal muscle spasms and pain, diarrhea, rigors and fever. Marked apprehension may be noted. Recovery usually takes place within a few days.

Allergic sensitization may take place after repeated exposure. In such instances anaphylactic shock may occur.

(See earlier part of chapter for treatment.)

Jellyfish Dermatitis (Sea Nettle Dermatitis)

There are jellyfish in both salt and fresh water. The small freshwater jellyfish (Craspedacusta), one half inch or less in diameter, is similar to its saltwater relatives. The main body of the jellyfish has trailing tentacles, which may attain considerable length. These tentacles are beaded with batteries of nematocysts, which break away during storms, but remain capable of stinging for 2 or 3 months.

The symptoms and signs resulting from contact with a jellyfish vary with the toxicity of the venom of the particular species. Shock, and even death, may occur if the victim is young, particularly sensitive or stung by the deadly sea wasp, Chironex fleckeri. The severity of reaction is usually proportional to the number of nematocysts with which the victim comes into contact. The species of jellyfish can be identified by microscopic study of the nematocysts on the patient's skin and sometimes by noting the linear patterns of the lesions. One pattern is specific for a particular species of jellyfish.

Attached tentacles should be carefully removed by a person wearing gloves. Rinsing with sea water may help to remove tentacles and nematocysts.

The Commonwealth Serum Laboratories of Melbourne, Australia, have developed a Sea Wasp Antivenin, which limits the severity of the reactions to the venom of Chironex fleckeri.

The severity of reaction from contact with jellyfish nematocysts varies with the species, age of the patient, number of stinging capsules contacted and degree of allergic sensitivity

Sea Anemone Dermatitis (Sponge Fisherman's Disease or Sponge Diver's Disease)

Sea anemones belong to the phylum Coelenterata, class Anthozoa, and all species have nematocysts. The characteristics of the dermatitis produced by contact with a sea anemone depends upon the toxicity of the venom of that species.

Sargartia Dermatitis. This is the main type of sea anenome dermatitis. Sargartia may grow symbiotically at the base of sponges. It is approximately 4 cm. long and has a hollow polypoid cylinder with 2 rows of graceful tentacles radially arranged, giving it the shape of a flower.

Erythema and vesicles accompanied by itching and a burning sensation develop within a few minutes of contact. Initially, the lesion becomes red and swollen, changing later to a deep purple. Pain may be present. Headache, nausea, vomiting, fever and rigors may occur. Wounds are slow to heal, and multiple abscesses with sloughing may occur. Initial treatment is like that for jellyfish sting. Abscesses are treated with antibiotics.

Coral Dermatitis and Coral Cuts

Coral dermatitis is an eruption resulting in a pruritic erythema from being near or touching a true coral. These structures are various sizes and shapes and are formed by the cementing together of the tiny limestone exoskeletons of polyps of the order Scleractinia.

The nematocysts of true coral are usually fairly innocuous. Coral dermatitis is treated with a simple cooling lotion, such as calamine or Aveeno Lotion.

Coral cuts should be treated vigorously to prevent secondary infection and ulceration. The lesions should be carefully scrubbed with soap and water, rinsed and dried. Hydrogen peroxide should be applied and allowed to "boil" for several minutes. The wound is then dried. Isopropyl alcohol is applied, and the contents of a capsule (powder) of tetracycline are sprinkled over the wound while still wet and patted into a paste with an applicator. The paste is allowed to dry. No bandage is necessary. The crust thus formed serves as a covering on the wound, remains intact after bathing and allows the wound to heal from its outer edges.

Coral cuts should be thoroughly cleansed. Hydrogen peroxide and an antibiotic powder should be applied

DERMATITIS PRODUCED BY ECHINODERMS

The phylum Echinodermata includes sea urchins, starfish and sea cucumbers.

Sea Urchin Dermatitis

Sea urchins are spherical organisms covered with spines, the length of which varies with the species. These spines are formed by the calcification of a projection of connective tissue, are extremely brittle and break off easily in the skin. The spines of some species are venomous and may contain a neurotoxin. Some contain a dye that discolors the skin and subcutaneous tissues, giving the impression that the spine is present in the skin when actually it is not. The x-ray is diagnostic for the presence of spines.

All sea urchins have pedicellariae, or small seizing organs or fangs, intermingled among the spines. These organs are on stalks that may be shorter or longer than the spines. Venom from the pedicellariae may be injected into the skin by hooklike jaws or valves.

Fisherman, bathers and divers frequently step upon or brush against sea urchins in tropical and subtropical waters. The following reactions may result:

1. *Immediate reactions.* A severe burning pain with or without edema may occur. Some patients bleed profusely. The pain may persist for several hours.

The spines of certain sea urchins are readily phagocytosed in the tissues and dissolve without difficulty. Surgical removal of spines that do not dissolve is difficult because of their fragility. The presence of dyes also may make it difficult to see them. In the acute stage, removal of the spines should not be attempted unless they are easily seen. They should be visualized by x-ray examination before surgi cal removal is attempted.

Painful, edematous lesions should be treated with water as hot as can be tolerated, until the symptoms disappear.

Secondary infections should be treated with antibiotics. Infected, discharging wounds may be a means by which the tissues get rid of embedded spines.

2. *Delayed reactions.* Such reactions may be

delayed for 2 or 3 months after initial injury and may be nodular or diffuse.

The nodular form of granulomatous lesion consists of small, firm nodules, which may be flesh colored or the color of the dye in the spines. Such lesions may be benefited by intralesional injections of a corticosteroid. Surgery is usually indicated, however, if x-ray examination reveals the presence of spines.

Dr. C. L. Meneghini (personal communication, 1972) has prepared water–alcohol extracts from the spines of sea urchins, which gave a positive allergic delayed intradermal reaction in two fishermen with sea urchin granulomas. Controls did not develop this reaction.

Contact with sea urchin spines may produce an immediate painful edema and bleeding. After 2 or 3 months, granulomas or cyanotic swelling of fingers or toes may develop. X-ray examination should precede surgical removal of the spines

The *diffuse form* occurs mostly in the fingers and toes and takes the form of a cyanotic induration. The swelling may produce a fusiform deformity. In severe cases, the phalanges may show focal destruction with joint involvement. These patients should receive combined systemic antibiotic and corticosteroid therapy.

Starfish Dermatitis

All starfish are said to exude a toxic substance diffusible in water and alcohol. Consequently, when large numbers of starfish are present, contact with the surrounding water may produce a pruritic papulourticarial eruption. Drying lotions without alcohol (Aveeno Lotion) are soothing.

In addition, the starfish Acantaster planci (crown of thorns) can inflict a painful sting when its venomous aboral spines pierce the skin. Such injury may produce granulomatous lesions requiring surgical excision.

Sea Cucumber Dermatitis

This is a papular eruption produced by the toxic material, holothurin, in the body wall of the sea cucumber.

In personal communication to Dr. W. L. Orris, A. H. Banner, Professor of Zoology at the University of Hawaii, reported that "When my children were small they took delight in throwing apodus holothurian, Opheodesoma spectabilis, at each other. I had finally to forbid it because it caused a skin rash; whether it was from the anchor-shaped spicules or from toxic compounds, I do not know."

DERMATITIS DUE TO SPONGES

Red Sponge Dermatitis

The red sponge, Microciona prolifera, may produce erythema and edema of the hands and stiffness of the joints in oyster fishermen and others who handle it. Subsequently, bullae develop, which may become purulent. If not properly treated, the eruption may persist for several months.

A patch test with a small piece of sponge confirms the diagnosis.

The treatment is the same as for severe poison ivy dermatitis.

Fire Sponge Dermatitis

This dermatitis is produced by Tedania ignis, a brilliant vermilion or orange-red sponge that grows as a bunch of branches or "fingers" extending upward from a main base. Skin irritation is produced when the surface of the sponge is touched and especially when one of the "fingers" is broken.

The toxin of this sponge can produce a severe skin irritation similar to poison ivy dermatitis. Contact with the sponge may produce an itching or prickling sensation, which may be followed in a few hours by swelling, stiffness and pain. Affected fingers soon become stiff, and attempts at flexing them are painful. The treatment is the same as for severe poison ivy dermatitis.

The fire sponge can also produce an erythema of the extremities or an erythema multiforme type of eruption. This reaction is attributed to a pharmacologically active substance, which may also be a sensitizer.

Poison Bun Sponge Dermatitis

Contact with the sponge Fibulia nolitangere may produce a more violent reaction than that of the fire sponge. Hence, the name *nolitangere*, which means *do not touch.*

Fibulia is brown and grows in small clumps. The skin is exposed to the toxic substance when one contacts the surface of the sponge or breaks it.

Many types of sponges produce a severe poison ivy type of dermatitis with stiffness of affected fingers

Sponge Spicule Dermatitis

Certain sponges have a skeletal matrix containing silicon dioxide spicules (present in glass sponges) or calcium carbonate spicules. Both types are irritating and difficult to remove once they have penetrated the skin. Adhesive tape should be applied to the affected area, and the spicules adhere to it when it is removed. Isopropyl alcohol should then be applied.

Sponges may contain silicon dioxide or calcium carbonate spicules, which readily break off and enter the skin. The application of adhesive tape may help remove such spicules

SEAWEED DERMATITIS

The two types of seaweed dermatitis are the animal plant variety, including sea moss or sea mat dermatitis (Dogger Bank itch), and marine plant seaweed dermatitis, including Hawaiian dermatitis due to algae.

Sea Moss Dermatitis (Dogger Bank Itch)

The term *Dogger Bank itch* is usually applied to the dermatitis produced by the sea chevril, Alcyonidium hirsutum. These sea mosses or sea mats are Ectoprocta, which are found on the Dogger Bank, an immense shelf-like elevation under the North Sea between Scotland and Denmark.

Dogger Bank itch is an eczematous contact dermatitis. Positive patch test reactions with an extract from the causative marine animals and negative reactions in controls would seem to point to an allergic mechanism.

Dogger Bank itch is produced by an *animal* (sea moss) and affects exposed parts of the body; Hawaiian seaweed dermatitis is caused by a marine *plant* and affects areas of the body covered by a bathing suit.

Dogger Bank itch is due to the animal sea moss, Alcyonidium hirsutum (the sea chevril), affecting exposed parts of the body. The Hawaiian seaweed dermatitis due to plant algae affects the covered areas

Newhouse[4] described Dogger Bank itch as an allergic dermatitis due to contact with the organism Alcyonidium gelatinosum, which resembles seaweed. This itch is prevalent among Lowestoft trawlermen. Contact occurs when the alcyonidium is hauled aboard the vessel with other contents of the trawl. Patch tests with the organism were positive in the 18 men tested by Newhouse.

Although Newhouse's findings would indicate that Dogger Bank itch is an allergic dermatitis, the fact that, in some instances, all on board acquire dermatitis, except the cook, who does not appear on deck, would indicate an irritant rather than an allergic reaction.

Proper protective clothing usually prevents occurrence of the eruption.

Seaweed Dermatitis due to Algae

Seaweed dermatitis is due to contact with the marine plant Lyngbya majuscula, a blue-green alga that occurs in abundance from the intertidal zone to a depth of 100 feet, representing a hazard to sensitized swimmers.

Grauer and Arnold[5] reported 125 cases of seaweed dermatitis in Hawaii from contact with this alga. The eruption appears under the swimming garments of bathers. In males, the scrotal area is most severely involved. Cercarial dermatitis has to be differentiated from it.[6,7]

Soap and water bathing immediately after swimming and thorough washing of the bathing suit to get rid of any clinging seaweed are of prophylactic value. Cleaning the beaches of accumulated seaweed is also helpful.

Severe dermatitis may require systemic corticosteroids.

A type of seaweed dermatitis due to the marine plant Lyngbya majuscula may be prevented by soap and water bathing immediately after swimming. Bathing suits should be thoroughly washed to remove any clinging seaweed

DERMATITIS DUE TO AQUATIC WORMS

Aquatic worms that may affect the skin of man include the cercarial stage of tropical schistosomes, the adult bristle worms, and leeches.

Schistosome Cercarial Dermatitis

Because of its widespread geographical pattern, cercarial dermatitis is known as "the disease of the place." Other synonyms include clam digger's itch, swimmer's itch and sea bather's eruption. In the past, a distinction was made between swimmer's itch and sea bather's eruption.[8] Limiting the terms *swimmer's itch* to the eruption on exposed areas and *sea bather's eruption* to an eruption from ocean bathing is artificial. It would be more appropriate to speak of *schistosome cercarial dermatitis* when such organisms have been identified. The term *sea bather's eruption* will probably continue to be employed for those cases in which no specific organism has been identified.

The terms swimmer's itch and sea bather's eruption are confusing and should be dropped

Table 19–3 is a list of the hypothetical differences between the two eruptions.

The only practical method of prophylaxis, aside from not swimming in infested waters, consists of wiping the skin dry on emerging from the water. There is probably some organism that can be brushed off before it penetrates the skin, but it has not been identified. Those most familiar with sea bather's eruption believe schistosomes to be the likely culprit. Jellyfish, man-of-war, calycophora, dinoflagellates, algae, seaweed and pteropods have also been implicated.

An individual susceptibility and sensitization may be operative, because some people suffer repeatedly following exposure, while others remain unaffected.

Schistosomes, which are ordinarily harmless to man, have a cercarial stage in which they attach themselves to human skin, producing irritation. Certain birds and mammals are the definitive hosts for these schistosomes. A freshwater or saltwater snail is the intermediate host. When man interposes himself in this life cycle, he may become the accidental victim of cercarial dermatitis.[9–13]

The Nature of Schistosome Cercarial Infestation. The intricate life process, of which swimmers are the accidental victims, begins with the presence of a trematode in freshwater

Table 19-3. Contrast Between Swimmer's Itch and Sea Bather's Eruption

Factor	*Swimmer's Itch*	*Sea Bather's Eruption*
Type of water	Fresh	Salt
Part of body involved	Uncovered	Covered
Locale	Northern U.S., Canada	Florida, Cuba
Cause	Schistosome (?)	Unknown

lakes in the northern states and several Canadian provinces, including Ontario and Manitoba.

Man is an accidental host to the schistosome cercariae. Birds and mammals are definitive hosts and snails the intermediate hosts

In late June or July, the worms leave the snails and enter the free-swimming stage. The cycle is completed when cercariae penetrate the skin and enter the blood of a second host, the water fowl.

If contact is made with swimmers or bathers, the parasites pierce the skin and die soon thereafter, because humans are unsatisfactory hosts. The living or dead cercariae produce a dermatitis, which may be allergic.

Hunter[14] stated that schistosome cercarial dermatitis occurs in many parts of the world besides the United States and Canada and reported 2 cases of dermatitis from contact with water in a duck pond containing snails infested with the cercariae or C. physellae.[15] Furthermore, Hunter reproduced the dermatitis in volunteers. It was found that the cercariae attach themselves to human skin, producing an edematous, pruritic papule, which may persist for 2 weeks. Secondary infection with the formation of purulent lesions is common.

The eruption of schistosome cercarial dermatitis consists of edematous, pruritic papules, which often become purulent

Treatment. Brisk rubbing with a rough towel is usually helpful by removing the water droplets in which the cercariae are present. Children, who do not permit themselves to be dried thoroughly, and who constantly enter and leave the water, are often the most severely affected.

In mild cases, rubbing alcohol or equal parts of rubbing alcohol and calamine lotion are soothing. Severe cases may require systemic corticosteroids. The presence of infection is an indication for antibiotics.

Vigorous rubbing and thorough drying of the skin with a rough towel after emerging from infested water prevents schistosome cercarial infestations

Marine Annelid Dermatitis

A number of marine worms can produce an irritant dermatitis either by contact with their bristles or by the bite from their jaws.

Bristle Worm Dermatitis. The bristle worms of the family Amphinomidae possess tufts of silky chitinous bristles arranged in rows around their bodies. When touched, the worm contracts and the tufts of bristles rise, forming a defensive armor. When these bristles penetrate human skin, they produce a burning sensation accompanied by moderate edema, a papular eruption and even necrosis. Itching, pain and paresthesia may also be present.

The bristles must be removed by using forceps or by applying adhesive tape and removing the tape with the attached bristles. In an emergency, rubbing the affected area with sand may be effective. After removal of the bristles, diluted ammonia water or alcohol may be applied.

In various parts of the world the following worms produce a bristle worm dermatitis:

Chloeia flava (Pallas)—the Malayan coast
Chloeia viridis (Schmarda)—the West Indies, Gulf of California, Mexico south to Panama
Eurythoe companata (Pallas)—Australia and the tropical seas
Hermodice carunculata (Pallas)—tropical Eastern America and Eastern Gulf of Mexico

Worm Bites. Certain segmented worms bite with chitinous jaws, producing a stinging pain. Edema and itching may follow. The application of cold compresses or alcohol is soothing.

Marine worms may produce dermatitis from bristles entering the skin or from bites of certain species. Bristles may be removed with forceps, adhesive tape or rubbing with sand. Cold compresses or alcohol is used to treat the bites

Leeches

Leeches, parasites of the animal kingdom, may be divided in marine, freshwater and terrestrial types. Marine leeches have a saltwater habitat and feed on fishes. Freshwater leeches are present in lakes, ponds and creeks, and are still used as therapeutic agents in certain countries. Terrestrial leeches may attack sleeping soldiers and campers.

Leeches belong to the phylum Annelida (segmented worms), in which they constitute the class Hirudinea.

Leeches attach themselves to the skin, feed until engorged and then drop off. The leech bite introduces an anticoagulant, hirudin, and antigenic substances. In the unsensitized individual, the bite bleeds freely and heals slowly. If sensitization has developed, the reaction to the bite may be urticarial, bullous or necrotic. Occasionally, anaphylaxis occurs. Heldt[16] reported that the "wild" leech can cause serious allergic reactions.

Individuals walking through streams or marshes are the usual victims. In countries in which leeches are still employed medicinally, allergic reactions may complicate treatment.

Leeches produce severe skin reactions and anaphylaxis in sensitized individuals. Leeches should not be removed forcibly because their jaws may break off. Use heat or alcohol

A leech should not be removed forcibly lest its jaws remain in the wound. Heat or alcohol should be applied to force the leech to release its hold.

ERUPTIONS DUE TO VENOMOUS SPINES AND SKIN OF FISH

Fish may produce dermatitis or wounds as a result of lacerations from spines containing venom, contact with irritants on the fish skin and contact with fish that eat red feed.

Dermatitis Due to Poison Spines

Many species of fish inflict painful and dangerous lacerations by means of dorsal or caudal spines provided with complex venom glands.[17]

In warm waters, stingrays, scorpion fish, catfish, rabbit fish, Siganus species, stargazers, Uranoscopus species and toadfish are the most common causes of poison spine dermatitis.[18]

In cold waters, the weaver (Trachinus draco), the spiny dogfish (Squalus acanthicus), the Norway haddock (Sebastes norvegicus) and several species of stingray found on the Atlantic coats can inflict serious wounds.

The puncture wounds and lacerations of fish spines may produce intense pain for several hours. Edema and erythema around penetrated skin may simulate a bacterial cellulitis. The wound may, indeed, become infected and may be very slow in healing. Certain poison spines produce systemic symptoms quickly. Shock, vomiting, abdominal pain, profuse sweating and tachycardia may be followed by muscular paralysis and death.

Poison fish spines can produce severely inflamed wounds. The introduction of venom from the spines may produce shock and death

Involved extremities should be kept at rest. Infected wounds require antibiotics.

Treatment of Fish Spine Envenomization. Little is known of the chemical and pharmacological nature of fish spine venom except that it is heat-labile. Wounds from poison fish spines should therefore be treated with heat.[19]

Stingray Envenomization. The stingray has one or more sharp, barbed dorsal spines near the base of the whiplike tail, which can inflict

Plate 14. Causes of Dermatoses Acquired in an Aquatic Environment

1. Seabathers' Eruption

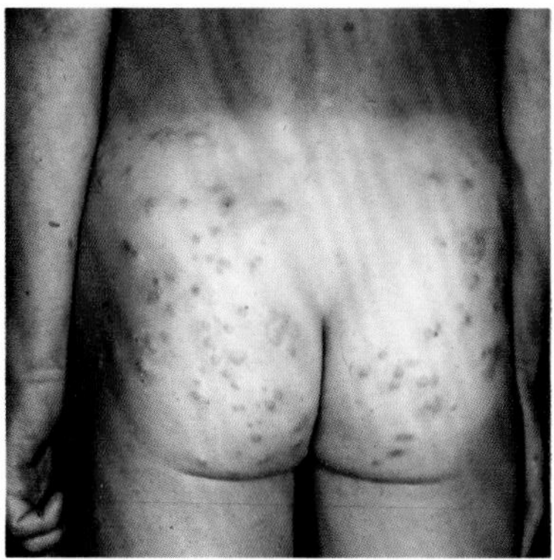

Etiology Uncertain
(Courtesy Dr. W. Sams)

2. Jellyfish Sting

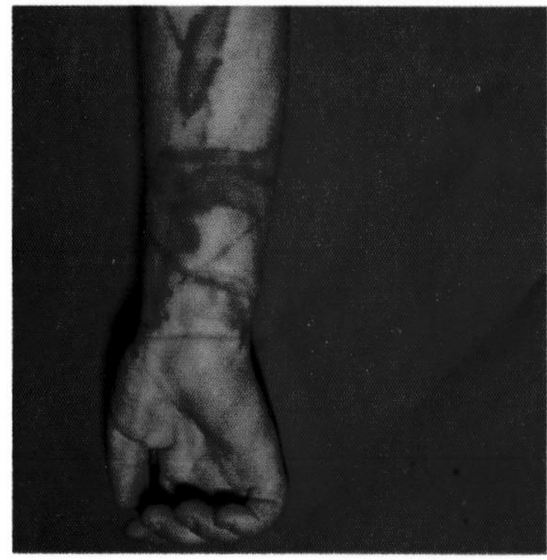

Chironex Fleckeri (Courtesy the World Life Institute, Colton, Calif.)

3. Man-of-War Stings

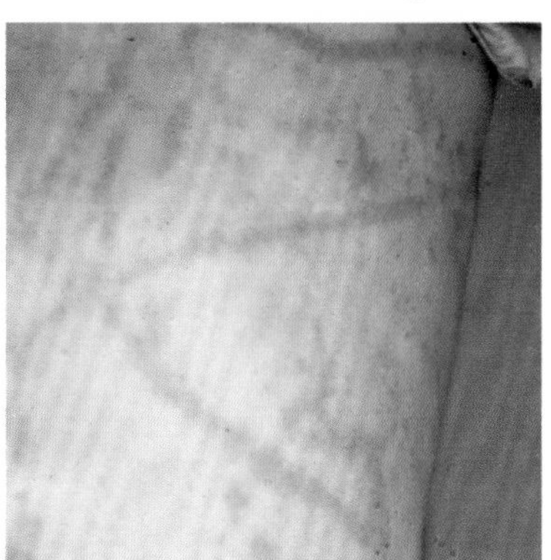

Physalia Physalia

4. Sea Anemone Dermatitis

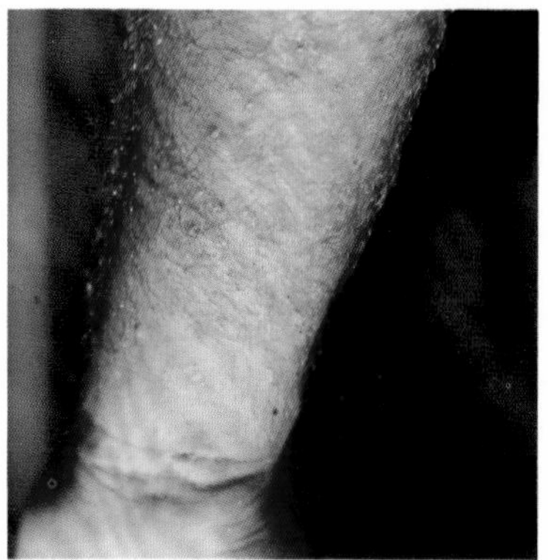

Sargaria (Courtesy the World Life Institute, Colton, Calif.)

5. Swimming Pool Granuloma

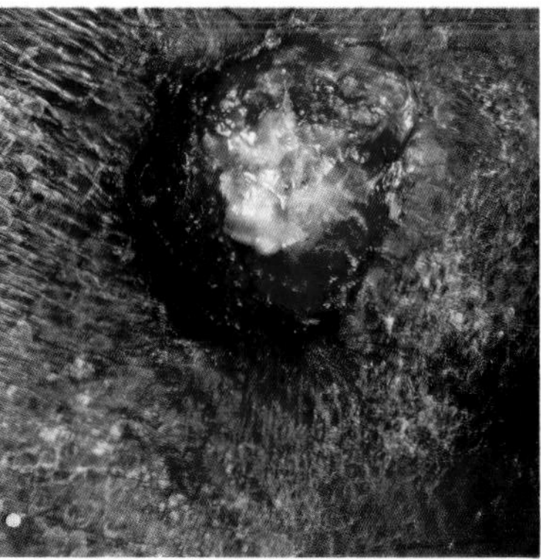

Mycobacterium Marinum
(Balanei)

6. Creeping Eruption (Larva Migrans)

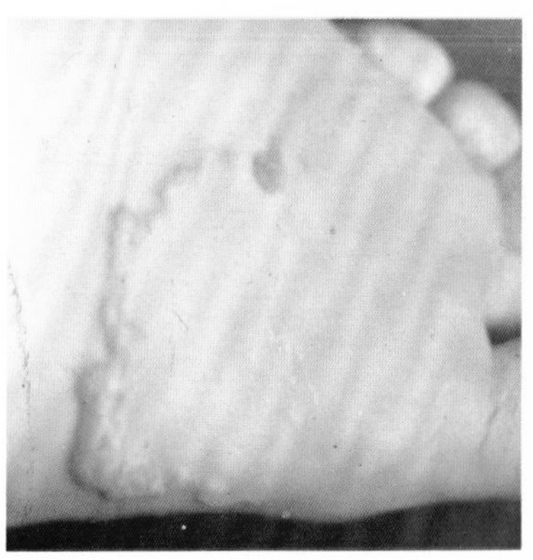

Ancyclostoma Canium
(Sand Worm)

Most aquatic venoms, including poison fish spines, are heat-labile. Emergency treatment should include immersion of affected parts in hot water or application of hot compresses

severe wounds. The venom, contained in a sheath covering the spines, enters through the wounds produced by the spines.

The wound should be debrided and heat applied immediately, preferably by immersion, or by hot wet compresses. High temperatures may be attained if the extremity is first immersed in water comfortably hot, with the addition of hotter water as acclimatization takes place. Relief from pain is usually immediate. Hot soaking should continue for at least 30 minutes and repeated if the pain returns. Occasionally, several heat treatments are necessary to neutralize all the venom present.

In severe envenomization, a tourniquet may be life-saving by slowing venous return. Elastic material should be used, applied just tight enough to allow insertion of the index finger under the tourniquet and loosened for 90 seconds every 10 minutes.

Treatment for shock may be necessary and respiratory stimulants may have to be administered.

The Commonwealth Laboratories of Melbourne, Australia, have made available an antivenin for the treatment of stonefish spine poisoning.

Dermatitis Due to Contact with Skin of Scombroid Fish

Scombroid dermatitis is due to a primary irritant found in the skin and flesh of the scombroid fish, which include tuna, skipjack and bonito. The irritant appears to be more concentrated in spoiled than in fresh fish. This dermatitis appears in workers handling scombroid fishes without wearing gloves.

Red Feed Dermatitis

Red feed is a reddish orange crustacean (Calanus species) eaten by mackerel and herring from June to September. Ingested red feed accelerates the proteolytic breakdown of the gastric wall of the fish, releasing the gastric juices. Handling of fish eating red feed results in edema, erythema and superficial ulcerations of the skin of the hands.

Cold compresses and Ilotycin Ointment are indicated.

Fish handlers can acquire an irritant occupational dermatitis from handling spoiled tuna, skipjack and bonito and from mackerel and herring that have eaten red feed, a crustacean

SEA LOUSE DERMATITIS

Sea louse dermatitis (cymothoidism) is produced by the bite of small marine crustaceans of the order Isopoda, suborder Cymothoidea, which frequent the shoal waters of temperate and tropical seas. Cymothoids usually feed upon higher marine animals but will also bite man. The bite produces punctate hemorrhages.[20]

Most cases have been reported among water skiers, skin divers and swimmers who frequent the waters of southern California.

PROTOTHECOSIS

Protothecosis is a cutaneous or disseminated infection with diverse clinical manifestations, produced by an achloric mutant of the green alga, chlorella. Several species of this mutant have been described, but only two, Prototheca segbwema and Prototheca wickerhamii, have been demonstrated as pathogens in man. The organism has been found in fresh and marine water and in sewage treatment systems.[21]

Walking barefooted in swampy areas, exposing the skin to water from contaminated water supply systems and working with aquariums predispose the individual to this disease.

The infection probably occurs from the entry of the organism through preexisting openings in the skin, producing a small, pruritic, eczematous papule. Later, a patch of atrophic, dry, depigmented skin with a well-defined border may develop. The borders of the lesions are raised and papulonodular. Verrucose lesions may appear, which resemble the "mossy foot" seen in elephantiasis.

The only treatment for this condition is complete surgical excision of the lesion prior to lymphatic dissemination of the organisms, which are highly resistant to all types of local and systemic treatment, including x-radiation.

SOAP FISH DERMATITIS

Soap fish, Rypticus saponicus, family Grammistidae, when disturbed produce a large amount of mucus that contains an irritant called grammistin.

Randal[22] reported that he temporarily stored a soap fish inside his bathing trunks to bring it to the surface. The toxic mucus of the fish produced an irritation of the urethra.

Fishermen in the Virgin Isles and Puerto Rico state that keeping soap fish in water with other fish results in the death of the other fish.

DERMATITIS AND INFECTIONS DUE TO MARINE BACTERIA

The marine bacteria that produce serious dermatitis and infection include Mycobacterium, Erysipelothrix and Pseudomonas.

Mycobacteriosis

The causative organism, Mycobacterium marinum (balnei), is an acid-fast, rod-shaped bacillus found in both fresh and sea water, and rarely on land.

Although infections occur most frequently as a result of exposure in swimming pools, aquariums[23] and fish bites[24] may also be sources.

Mycobacteriosis may be acquired from organisms in swimming pools and aquariums and from bites of fish

The organism invades the tissue through a preexisting skin lesion. The site of invasion is marked by a tender, red or bluish red nodule, which may become as large as 6 cm. in diameter and occasionally become purulent.

New lesions may continue to appear in a pattern resembling sporotrichosis.[25] Healing may take place with scarring and pigmentation.[26]

The disease usually runs a benign course with spontaneous resolution in a few months. Lesions may appear in the lungs, larynx and lymph nodes, however, and produce longstanding debility.[27]

Most granulomas resulting from mycobacteriosis heal spontaneously. Occasionally, prolonged involvement occurs, which may require surgical excision or specific chemotherapy

Mycobacteriosis Producing Swimming Pool Granulomas. In the United States, Myco. marinum (balnei) produces many instances of swimming pool granulomas.[28] Frequently the bacillus has been isolated from crevices and grooves in the cement walls of pools in which patients had been swimming. Swimming pools may harbor the bacillus even when properly chlorinated.

Swimming pool granulomas develop on the traumatized skin of the elbows, knees and dorsal aspects of the hands and feet.

After an incubation period of 3 to 4 weeks, a small red papule appears and slowly increases in size to become a hard purple nodule. It sometimes ulcerates and becomes covered with a crust or gray exudate. The lesion may eventually become verrucose. Very little pain is present. There is usually no lymphangitis or regional lymphadenopathy. Healing with scarring occurs after several months in most cases, although there are reports of lesions persisting for 4 to 45 years.[29,30]

Skin tests with a purified protein derivative (P.P.D.) of the organism are usually positive. Cross-reactivity with the purified protein derivative or other acid-fast bacteria, particularly the tubercle bacillus, is common. Culture characteristics distinguish between Myco. marinum and the tubercle bacillus.

Properly chlorinated swimming pools will, nevertheless, harbor mycobacterium marinum (balnei) and can be sources of infections producing swimming pool granulomas

Therapy of Swimming Pool Granulomas. Most lesions heal without therapy.[28] Antituberculosis therapy has been used, but the organism may be resistant to the usual antituberculosis drugs, with the exception of cycloserine and ethambutol. Surgical excision of single small lesions is sometimes indicated. Chemotherapy is recommended when multiple lesions are present. Following culture and sensitivity studies, ethioniamide (Trecator), ethambutol (Myambutol) and cycloserine (Osamycin) may be indicated.

Erysipelothrix Dermatitis

This dermatitis has various synonyms, such as erysipeloid of Rosenbach, speck finger, blubber finger and fish poisoning. The disease is common in fish handlers, but it can occur in anyone working with marine food products or aquariums.[31]

The causative organism, a gram-positive coccoid, later becomes a gram-positive bacillus. Erysipelothrix rhusiopathiae, Ery. muriseptica and Ery. erysipeloids are either variants of the same species or the same organism. It enters the skin through an opening, usually a small puncture wound on the finger. A spreading erythema develops, accompanied by pain and itching.[32]

Three forms of the disease are recognized: a relatively mild and localized form, a severe, disseminated, cutaneous form and septicemia. The localized form involves the fingers and hands. It begins as a sharply defined violet-red area around the site of infection. Prickling, itching and pain usually accompany the infection, which lasts 1 to 3 weeks. Occasionally the lesion becomes purulent.

Conservative treatment is recommended. Appropriate antibiotics should be used following culture, identification and sensitivity tests. Penicillin therapy is usually indicated. Surgery is usually contraindicated.

Pseudomonas cepacia Dermatitis

Foot lesions associated with Pseudomonas cepacia are variously known as jungle rot, foot rot and swamp rot.

The organism has been isolated from lesions of the feet, hands and groin. Invasion takes place through intact, sodden skin. Soldiers exposed to swampy, wet terrain are most frequently affected.

The lesions are characterized by maceration, hyperkeratosis and fissuring.[33] The toe webs are often involved.

Prophylaxis consists of cleanliness and dryness. Resistance to antibiotics is characteristic of Ps. cepacia. Novobiocin is active in vitro against most strains. Chloramphenicol may be given in severe cases. All strains tested have been sensitive to readily maintained levels of trimethoprim and sulfamethoxazole combined in the ratio of 20 parts sulfamethoxazole to 1 part trimethoprim.

MARINE ANIMALS THAT SHOCK ELECTRICALLY

Individuals who emerge from a marine environment *with no visible eruption* and are in a condition resembling shock may be suffering from electric shock produced by certain marine animals, including catfish, stargazers, electric eels and electric rays.

These marine animals possess electricity-generating organs that can discharge 8 to 200 volts of current. The amperage is very low, and if the victim is in good health, injury is insignificant. Contact with a large shocking marine animal may result in an electric shock strong enough to knock over or temporarily disable the victim. Contact with the animal at two points when in the water is not necessary to elicit a shock.

Recovery is usually uneventful. In severe cases, the treatment is the same as for any form of electric shock.

CREEPING ERUPTION

This form of larva migrans is briefly included in this chapter since many cases are acquired along sandy coastal areas, particularly in Florida.

The larvae of roundworms (Ancyclostoma brasiliense or canium) which infest dogs or cats produce a serpiginous tunnel as they wander about in human skin.

Cryotherapy with ethyl chloride is usually effective. Topical application of thiabendazole may be used in stubborn cases.[35]

REFERENCES

1. Stillway, L. W., and Lane, C. E.: Phospholipase in the Nematocyst Toxin of Physalia physalis. Toxicon, *9*, 193, 1971.
2. Russel, F. E.: Physalia Stings. A Report of Two Cases. Toxicon, *4*, 65, 1966.
3. Ioannides, G., and Davis, J. H.: Portuguese Man-of-War Stinging. Arch. Derm., *91*, 448, 1965.
4. Newhouse, M. L.: Dogger Bank Itch: Survey of Trawlerman. Rehabilitation, *60*, 941, 1967.
5. Grauer, F. H., and Arnold, H. L., Jr.: Seaweed Dermatitis. Arch. Derm., *84*, 720, 1961.
6. Banner, A. H.: A Dermatitis-Producing Alga in Hawaii. Hawaii Med. J., *19*, 450, 1959.
7. Schilling, R. S.: Dogger Bank Itch (Seaweed Dermatitis). Proc. Soc. Med., *59*, 1119, 1966.
8. Osmen, L. S.: Seabather's Eruption and Swimmer's Itch. Cutis, *1*, 117, 1965.
9. Hunter, G. W.: More Seabather's Eruption. Amer. J. Pub. Health, *53*, 1413, 1963.
10. Mortenson, E. W., and Mulhern, T. D.: The Occurrence of "Swimmer's Itch" in a Sierra Nevada Mountain Lake. Calif. Health, *9*, 36, 1951.
11. Simonds, W. L., Martin, W. E., and Wagner, E. D.: Fresh-Water Cercariae Dermatitis from Southern California. Amer. J. Trop. Med., *31*, 611, 1951.
12. Keh, B., and Grodhaus, G.: Swimmer's Itch at Duck Club in Yuba County, Calif. Vector News, *4*, 10, 1957.
13. Macy, R. W.: Studies in Schistosome Dermatitis in the Pacific Northwest. Northwest Med., *51*, 947, 1952.
14. Hunter, G. W.: Schistosome Dermatitis in Sacramento, Cal. Calif. Med., *100*, 427, 1964.
15. Hunter, G. W., III: Studies on Schistosomiasis. XIII. Schistosome Dermatitis in Colorado. J. Parasit., *46*, 231, 1960.
16. Heldt, J. T.: Allergy to Leeches. Henry Ford Hosp. Med. Bull., *9*, 498, 1961.
17. Halstead, B. W.: *Venoms*. Publication No. 44. Washington, D.C., American Association for the Advancement of Science, 1956.
18. Russel, F. E.: Stingray Injuries. Public Health Rep., *74*, 855, 1959.
19. Mullanney, P. V.: Treatment of Stingray Wounds. Clin. Toxicol., *3*, 613, 1970.
20. Best, W. C., and Sablan, R. G.: Cymothoidism (Sea Louse Dermatitis). Arch. Derm., *90*, 177, 1964.
21. Tindall, J. P., and Fetter, B. F.: Infection Caused by Achloric Algae (Protothecosis). Arch. Derm., *104*, 490, 1971.
22. Randal, J. E., et al.: Public Seto. Mar. Biol. Lab., *19*, 155, 1971.
23. Adams, R. A., et al.: Tropical Fish Aquariums, A Source of Mycobacterium marinum Infections Resembling Sporotrichosis. J.A.M.A., *211*, 380, 1970.
24. Flowers, D. J.: Human Infection Due to *Mycobacterium marinum* after a Dolphin Bite. J. Clin. Path., *23*, 475, 1970.
25. Dickey, R. F.: Sporotrichoid Mycobacteriosis Caused by M. marinum (balnei). Arch. Derm., *98*, 385, 1968.
26. Zeligman, I.: Mycobacterium marinum Granuloma. Arch. Derm., *106*, 26, 1972.
27. Gould, W. M., McKeenin, D. R., and Bright, R.: Mycobacterium marinum (balnei) Infection. Arch. Derm., *97*, 189, 1968.
28. Samitz, M. H.: *Cutaneous Lesions of the Lower Extremities*. Philadelphia, J. B. Lippincott, 1971, p. 62.
29. Sommer, A. F., Williams, R. M., and Mandel, A. D.: Mycobacterium balnei Infection. Arch. Derm., *86*, 316, 1962.
30. Walker, H. H., et al.: Some Characteristics of "Swimming Pool" Disease in Hawaii. Hawaii Med. J., *21*, 403, 1962.
31. Edwards, L. B., and Krohn, E. F.: Skin Sensitivity to Antigens Made From Various Acid-Fast Bacteria. Amer. J. Hyg., *66*, 253, 1957.
32. Burnett, J. W.: Uncommon Bacterial Infections of the Skin. Arch. Derm., *86*, 597, 1962.
33. Lamphier, T. A.: Erysipeloid Infection of Digits. J. Florida Med. Assoc., *58*, 39, 1971.
34. Taplin, D., and Bassett, D. C. J.: Foot Lesions Associated with Pseudomonas cepacia. Lancet, *2*, 568, 1971.
35. Davis, C. M., and Israel, R. M.: Treatment of Creeping Eruption with Topical Thiabendazole. Arch. Derm., *97*, 325, 1968.

Textbook References

Cleland, J. B., and Southcott, R. V.: *Injuries to Man from Marine Invertebrates in the Australian Region*. Canberra, Commonwealth of Australia, 1965.

Craig, C. F., and Faust, E. C.: *Clinical Parasitology*. Philadelphia, Lea & Febiger, 1948.

Faust, E. C.: *Animal Agents and Vectors of Human Disease*. Philadelphia, Lea & Febiger, 1955.

Russell, F.: *Poisonous Marine Animals*. Neptune City, N. J., T. F. H. Publications, Inc., 1971.

Sawitz, W. G.: *Medical Parasitology.* New York, Blakiston Division, McGraw-Hill Book Co., 1956.

Stitt, E. R., Clough, P. W., and Branham, S. E.: *Bacteriology, Hematology and Parasitology.* Philadelphia, Blakiston Co., 1948.

NOTES

addition to standard test tray

PCMX – para chloro meta xylenol

(found in carbolated vaseline)

Imidazolidinyl Urea } formaldehyde releasers (preservatives)

Quaternium 15 } in 1976 patch test tray.

SUNSCREENS

glyceril PABA – cross rx to caines, sulfanamides, PPDA, aniline dyes, saccharin.

amyl dimethyl PABA (ESCALOL 506) } no cross rx to caines etc.

octyl dimethyl PABA (ESCALOL 507) }

glyceryl PABA in Sea & Ski, Eclipse (latter contains benzocaine as well)

PABA of Presun ~15% cross rx to glyceryl PABA.

NOTES

NOTES

Herbicides

parachlor - (Ramrod)
alachlor - (Lasso)
patch test of 1% (commercial source) - many irritant rx.
0.5% - 0.1% conc suggested (Arch Derm July 77 - letter)

Shoe Dermatitis

mercaptobenzothiazole commonest allergen (mercaptobenzimidazole is good rubber accelerator - no cross rx c̄ thiazole)
phenolic resins & leather tanning agents (chrome & formaldehyde) - also allergens.

Appendix

Appendix

This appendix lists over 800 contact allergens plus their sources of exposure and concentrations and vehicles for proper patch testing. In addition, substances that may cross-react with the tested allergens are given. The column labeled *comment* notes allergens that may also be irritants or photosensitizers, give pustular reactions or produce noneczematous eruptions, such as the purpuric or granulomatous variety.

Since the first edition of this text was published, combinations or mixes of contactants have become available and are employed as a time-saving device both at home and abroad. It is not certain, at present, whether such mixes can be recommended for routine use because the results are difficult to interpret. A positive reaction requires the patient to be retested with the individual contactants in the mix.

The following mixes are available from Trolab, Karen Trolle-Lassen, M. Pharm., 1 Höyrups Allé-2900 Hellerup, Denmark:

RUBBER MIXES

Mercapto mix 1%

Mercaptobenzothiazole (MBT) 0.25%
n-Cyclohexylbenzothiazyl sulfenamide (CBS) 0.25%
Dibenzothiazyl disulfide (MBTS) 0.25%
Morpholinyl mercaptobenzothiazole (MDR) 0.25%

Thiuram mix 1%

Tetramethyl thiuram disulfide (TMTD) 0.25%
Tetramethyl thiuram monosulfide (TMTM) 0.25%
Tetraethyl thiuram disulfide (TETD) 0.25%
Dipentamethylene thiuram disulfide (PTD) 0.25%

PPD mix 0.6%

Phenylcyclohexyl-p-phenylenediamine 0.25%
Isopropylaminodiphenylamine identical to phenylisopropyl-p-phenylenediamine (IPPD) 0.1%
Diphenyl-p-phenylenediamine (DPPD) 0.25%

Naphthyl mix 1%

Phenyl-beta-naphthylamine (PBN) 0.5%
Di-beta-naphthyl-p-phenylenediamine (DBNPD) 0.5%

Carba mix 3%

1,3-Diphenylguanidine (DPG) 1%
Bis(diethyldithiocarbamato) zinc (ZDC) 1%
Bis(dibutyldithiocarbamato) zinc (ZBC) 1%

LOCAL ANESTHETIC (CAINE MIX) 8%

Cinchocaine chloride (dibucaine, Percain) 1%
Amethocaine chloride (tetracaine, Pontocain) 1%
Cyclomethycaine chloride (Surfacaine) 1%
Benzocaine 5%

PARABEN MIX 15%

Methyl, ethyl, propyl, butyl and benzyl parahydroxybenzoic acid, 3% each

The Hollister Stier Laboratories, 2030 Wilshire Boulevard, Los Angeles, California 90057, can supply the following mixes:

1. *Antiseptic mix:* bithionol, dichlorophene, hexachlorophene and tetrachlorosalicylanilide
2. *Caine mix:* benzocaine, Nupercaine and Surfacaine
3. *Hista mix:* Furacin, Histadyl, Pyribenzamine and Vioform
4. *Paraben mix:* ethyl, methyl and propyl parabens

5. *Rubber mix:* diphenylguanidine, mercaptobenzothiazole and tetramethyl thiuram disulfide

The paraben mix has been universally adopted.

Contact allergens are dispersed in yellow petrolatum if no other medium is mentioned.

Test allergens that are used infrequently should be stored in a dark, cool place.

The Al-test (aluminum patch test) material, which is used by the International and North American Contact Dermatitis Research Groups, may be obtained from IMECO Astra Agency Co. AB, S-151 85 Södertälje, Stockholm, Sweden.

EXPLANATION OF TERMS USED IN THE APPENDIX

1. *Primary sensitizer.* Testing with this substance may sensitize the patient. The patch test reaction usually is delayed for at least 5 days.
2. *Photosensitizer.* This substance should be tested both covered and with exposure to sunlight or ultraviolet radiation.
3. *Controls.* The substance may be a primary irritant. The patch test reaction should be checked with at least 3 normal controls.
4. *Para-amino.* This refers to chemicals that have an amino group in the para position, including paraphenylenediamine, para-aminobenzoic acid and aminosalicyclic acid. Cross-reactions occur with certain local anesthetics, sulfonamides, sunscreens and azo and aniline dyes.
5. *Sensitizes to alcohol.* Exposure to this chemical combined with the ingestion of alcohol produces an aldehyde syndrome consisting of flushing of the skin, nausea and vomiting.

KEY TO ABBREVIATIONS USED IN THE APPENDIX

acet.	—	acetone
alc.	—	alcohol 70%
aq.	—	aqueous
as is	—	undiluted
chlor.	—	chloroform
c.o.	—	castor oil
con.	—	concentration
mek.	—	methylethylketone
o.o.	—	olive oil
pdr.	—	powder
pet.	—	petrolatum
sat.	—	saturated
sol.	—	solution
veh.	—	vehicle

Contactant	Concentration and Vehicle	Exposure	Cross Reactions	Comment
Abietic acid	2% pet.	Rosins, colophony, adhesives, balsams, typewriting paper, denture adhesive powder		Forms about 80% of American rosin
Acacia (gum arabic)	As is	Ink, matches, lithography, mucilage, pharmaceutical vehicle, offset sprays in printing, adhesives, stiffener for rayon, pastry, denture adhesive powder		
Acetanilide	Pdr. as is	Analgesics, antipyretics, dye manufacture, cellulose ester varnishes		
Acetic acid	3% aq. sol.	Vinegar, flavoring agent, wart remedy, astringent mouthwash		Causes aphthous ulcer?
Acetone	10% o.o.	Industrial solvent, nail polish remover, diabetic urine, solvent for celluloid material in dentifrices		
Achromycin Ointment (Lederle)	As is	Topical medication	Tetracyclines	
Acid fuchsin	10% aq. sol.	Azo dyes	Para-amino compounds	
Acridine	Pdr. as is	Yellow dyes, acriflavine, tar		Photosensitizer
Acriflavine	1% pet.			An acridine dye
Acrylic monomer (methyl methacrylate)	10% o.o.	Synthetic resins, dentures, artificial nails, adhesives, paints, plastic, glass, sealer of screws in automobile industry, orthopedic prostheses		Can penetrate rubber gloves. May contain hydroquinone benzoyl peroxide, tertiary amines
Adhesive tape (acrylate)	As is	Dermicel (J and J), Steri-strip Brand Skin Closures, Micropore Brand Surgical Tape (3M)		Hypoallergenic
Adhesive tape (rubber)	As is			May contain rubber additives rosin and turpentine
Aerosol OT (dioctylester of sodium sulfosuccinic acid)	5% aq. sol.	Surfactant, anionic synthetic detergents, bubble baths		Controls

Akrinol Cream (acrisorcin; Schering)	As is		Hexylresorcinol	
Alantolactone	0.1% pet.	Sensitizer in Compositae plants		Known as Helenin in Denmark
Alcohol (industrial denatured)	As is			Contains methyl alcohol and acetone
Alcohol (ethyl)	70–95%		Amyl, butyl, methyl, isopropyl alcohol	Test reaction may occur very rapidly
Alcohol (isopropyl, "rubbing")	As is	Cosmetics, medicinal preparations		Denaturing agents include tartar emetic, quinine, salicylic acid, colchicine, alkaloids and azo dyes
Alcohol (methyl, methanol, wood)	As is	Chemical synthesis, antifreeze, solvent in shellac, varnish, paint remover, denaturant in denatured alcohol		*Synonyms:* methyl hydrate, methyl hydroxide, acetone, alcohol, wood spirits, wood naphtha, Columbian spirits, carrinol
Alizarin dyes: Alizarin red Alizarin 778 Alizarin sulfate	 As is 1% alc. 10% aq. sol.	 Synthetic dyes, red paints, hair dyes, chemical indicators		
Allantoin	0.5% aq. sol.	Topical medications, "healing agent," cosmetics, vaginal creams, shampoos		Uric acid derivative
Allyl glycidyl ether	1% o.o.	Reactive epoxy diluent		
Almond oil	As is	Brilliantines, hair dressings, spices, flavoring agents		
Alrosol C (fatty acid amide condensate)	5% aq. sol.	Surfactant, nonionic synthetic detergents		Controls
Alum (aluminum and potassium sulfate)	10% aq. sol.	Styptic agents, purification of water, baking powders, mouthwashes, astringents		

Contactant	Concentration and Vehicle	Exposure	Cross-Reactions	Comment
Aluminum acetate	10% aq. sol.	Mordants, siccatives, astringents, deodorants, fur dyeing, fabric finishing, waterproofing, dye compounds, disinfectants		Rare sensitizer. May produce nonspecific follicular reaction
Aluminum chlorhydroxide	10% aq. sol.	Deodorants, antiperspirants, astringents		
Aluminum chloride	2% aq. sol.	Astringents, antiseptics, antiperspirants		Rare sensitizer. Irritation from pore closure
Aluminum powder	As is	Astringents, instruments		Rare sensitizer
Aluminum sulfate	2% aq. sol.	Astringents, antiseptics, antiperspirants		Rare sensitizer. Irritation from pore closure
Aluminum sulfocarbolate	2% aq. sol.	Astringents, antiseptics, antiperspirants		Rare sensitizer. Irritation from pore closure
Amaranth pink	As is	Color elixir phenobarbital, foods, alcohol		
Amino-azobenzol	10% o.o.	Leather dyes	Para-amino compounds	
Amino-azotoluene hydrochloride	1% aq. sol.	Leather dyes	Para-amino compounds	
Amino-azotoluene	Pdr. as is	Scarlet red topical medications	Paraphenylenediamine	
Aminoethylethanolamine	1% aq. sol.	Aluminum cables		Used to solder aluminum electric wires
Aminophylline	1% aq. sol.	Pharmaceutical industry, rectal suppositories (Rectalad, Aminet, Heogen)	Phenergan, Pyribenzamine	Composed of ethylenediamine and theophylline
Ammoniated mercury	2% pet.	Topical medications	Organic and inorganic mercurials, mercury amalgam	Incompatible with sulfur and iodine
Ammonium fluoride	2% aq. sol.	Glass industry, insecticides, rust removers, dentistry, Aluminum Brite (Copper Brite Co.)		Patch tests may produce large nonspecific pustules. Keep in dark wax-coated bottle
Ammonium persulfate	2% aq. sol.	Flour and hair bleaches, disinfectants, deodorants, ammoniated dentifrices		May produce urticaria, shock by contact
Ammonium phosphate	2% aq. sol.	Ammoniated dentifrices		

Ampicillin	5% aq. sol.			Occupational hazard in nursing personnel
Amyl acetate (banana oil)	10% o.o.	Solvents, nail polish removers, waterproofing, sheet metal, enamelware, woodworking		
Amyltricresol	1% aq. sol.	A phenol mercury compound in Pentacresol Mouthwash		
Aniline	10% o.o.	Dyes, drugs, cloth marking inks, paints, paint removers	Para-amino compounds	A colorless aminobenzene
Aniline black	10% o.o.	Fur dyes	Para-amino compounds	
Aniline blue	2% pet.	Cosmetics, carbons, fur dyeing, hair dyes, nail polish, rubber, photographics, inks, colored pencils, crayons	Para-amino compounds	
Aniline dyes	2% pet.	Crayons, diaper markings, shoe polishes	Para-amino compounds	Toxic to infants when used for diaper markings
Anise oil	25% c.o.	Flavoring agents in dentistry, liqueurs (anisette), confectioneries, perfumes, soaps		Derived from seeds of carrot family
Anthracene	Pure	Tar		Photosensitizer
Anthralin ointment (Cignolin)	5% pet.	Anthra-Derm Ointment (Dermik), Anthryl (Reed & Carnrick)		Irritant when covered. Controls
Anthraquinone	Pdr. pure	Yellow vat dyes, makes seeds distasteful to birds, laxatives		From anthracine, a coal tar derivative
Antimony chloride Antimony oxide	2% aq. sol. Pure	Alloys, type metals, batteries, foils, ceramics, safety matches, ant pastes, textiles, tartar emetic, Fuadin, base for paints, vitreous enamels, fireproofing plastics		Irritant and toxic
Antimony sulfide	2% aq. sol.	Matches, putty		
Antipyrine	As is	Auralgan Ear Drops (Ayerst), Tympagesic Ear Drops (Warren-Teed)		Auralgan also contains benzocaine and hydroquinoline

Contactant	Concentration and Vehicle	Exposure	Cross-Reactions	Comment
Antistine (antazoline)	0.5% aq. sol.	Eye and nose drops	Pyribenzamine, Neo-antergan, Diatrin, Neohetramine, Trimeton, Benadryl, aminophylline	Derivative of ethylene-diamine
Antivy (CIBA)	As is (patch-scratch)			Contains zirconium oxide. Allergic granuloma
Aquaphor (Duke Lab.)	As is		Lanolin	Cholesterolated Vaseline and lanolin alcohol. Cholesterolated absorbent ointment base
Aracel C (Sorbitan sesquioleate)	5% aq. sol.			In Polysorb Hydrate
Araldite 502	0.1% acet.	Low molecular weight epoxy resins		
Araldite 6060	10% acet.	High molecular weight epoxy resins		
Arctic Syntex M (sodium monoglyceride sulfide)	5% aq. sol.	Surfactant, synthetic detergents		Controls
Argyrol	10% aq. sol. (open)	Antiseptics		
Arlacel A (mannide monooleate)	5% aq. sol.	Surfactant, nonionic synthetic detergents		Controls
Arnica, Tincture of	20% alc.	Rubefacients	Chrysanthemum	Arnica and chrysanthemum, belonging to the aster family
Arning's Tincture	As is (open)		Balsam of Peru	Contains anthrarobin, tumenol ammonium, ether, tincture of benzoin
Arsenate (potassium)	1% aq. sol.	Fowler's solution		
Arsenate (sodium)	5% aq. sol.	Insecticides, ant poisons, weed killers, wallpaper paints, glass, ceramics	Other arsenicals	Frequent pustular patch test reaction
Arsenic trioxide (white arsenic)	5% in starch pdr.	Insecticides, soaps, hair tonics, depilatories, caustics, weed killers, poison baits, fungicides, glasses, enamels, alloys	Sodium arsenate	Frequent pustular patch test reaction

Asterol (diamthazole)	As is	Antifungal agents		
Aureomycin Ointment, Powder (Lederle)	As is		Tetracyclines	
Azo dyes	2% pet.	Foods, drugs, cosmetics, clothes, ballpoint pens, ink	Para-amino compounds	
Bacitracin	As is	Wybiotic Troches, Tyrotrace, Baciguent, Baci-Wax, Mycitracin, Epimycin A, Bacimycin, Cortisporin, Polysporin, Neo-polycin, Neosporin, Tetrazets		May co-react with neomycin
Balsam of Peru	10% pet.	Topical medications, cements, liquids in dentistry, Anusol Suppositories (Warner-Chilcott), Rectocaine Suppositories (Moore Kirk), Endacaine Compound Suppositories, Granulex, Rectal Medicone Suppositories and Ointment, Wyanoids HC, Calmol 4, Melynor Ointment (Davies Rose Hoyt), cosmetics, hair tonics, perfumes, flavoring industry, china painting, oil painting	Benzoin, rosin, benzoic acid, benzyl alcohol, cinnamic acid, essential oils, orange peel, eugenol, cinnamon, clove	An important sensitizer in Scandinavia
Balsam of tolu	1% alc.	Cough mixtures, throat lozenges, benzoin tincture, tolu varnish, coating for pills, perfumes	Benzoin tincture, balsam of Peru	
Barium sulfide	2% aq. sol.	Depilatories		
Bay rum	As is	Hair tonics	Eugenol, clove oil, cinnamon oil	Combination of Jamaica rum and oil of bay
Bee glue (propolis)	As is			May contain raw beeswax
Beeswax (cera alba [bleached], cera flava [unbleached])	As is	Adhesives, plasters, textile waterproofing agent, ointments, cosmetics, polishes, cosmetic stiffeners		May be contaminated with bee glue

Contactant	Concentration and Vehicle	Exposure	Cross-Reaction	Comment
Beeswax-turpentine mixture	5% pet.	Eyeglass frames		To produce smooth gloss on plastics
Benadryl (diphenhydramine hydrochloride; Parke, Davis)	As is	Caladryl Ointment (Parke, Davis)	Antistine, Dramamine	
Benomyl (benlate)	1% pet.	Insecticide		
Benoquin (monobenzone; Elder)	As is	Depigmenting agent	Hydroquinone	Contains monobenzylether of hydroquinone
Benzaldehyde	5% pet.	Oil of bitter almond, preservatives, biologicals	Vanilla, balsam of Peru	
Benzalkonium chloride	1:1000 aq. sol.	Antiseptic detergents, mouthwashes, preservative in ophthalmic solutions, Zephiran solution, medicated paper tissues (Zephiran towelettes)		
Benzene (benzol)	5% o.o.	Coal tar distillates, motor fuels, commercial solvents		Synonyms: phenyl hydride, coal tar naphtha
Benzene hexachloride	5% pet.	Insecticide Kwell (Reed & Carnrick)		May cause chloracne, porphyria
Benzethonium chloride (Phemerol)	1:1000 aq. sol.	Antiseptic detergents		Present in Colgate mouthwash, feminine hygiene sprays
Benzidine (para-diamino-diphenyl)	As is	Tests for blood, derivatives are optical bleaches		
Benzine	50% o.o.	Petroleum solvents		Synonyms: petroleum benzene, petroleum ether
Benzocaine	5% pet.	Numerous topical anesthetic compounds (see text)	Procaine, butethamine, tetracaine, butacaine, meapaine, orthoform, neo-orthoform, paraphenylenediamine, sulfonamides, para-aminosalicylic acid, para-aminobenzoic acid	Synonyms: anethesin, ethyl aminobenzoate, Anesthone, parathesin

Benzoic acid	5% pet.	Balsam of Peru, Whitfield's ointment, essential oils, mouthwashes, preservatives for fruit, pharmaceuticals		Extremely rare sensitizer
Benzoin	10% alc.	Tincture of benzoin, compound tincture of benzoin, Arning's tincture, benzoinated lard (adeps benzoatus), antioxidant in creams, perfumes, expectorants, throat lozenges, raw beeswax, bee glue, preservative in adhesives, gums of myrrh, locust, golbam	Balsam of Peru, benzyl cinnamate, benzyl alcohol, eugenol, vanilla, alpha-pinene	
Benzophenone (Sulsobenzone)	5% pet.	Sunscreens (Solbar, Sunguard, Uval), textiles, plastics, rubber products, paints, varnishes, cosmetics		May produce urticarial and contact sensitivity. Synonyms: Spectra Sorb UV 284
Benzoyl peroxide	1% pet.	Polyester and acrylic resins, Quinolor Ointment (Squibb), burn dusting powder, flour improver, benzoyl peroxide ointment. *Acne medications:* Persadox, Benoxyl, Loroxide, Vanoxide, Oxy 5, Oxy 5 HC	Benzoic acid derivatives, cinnamon, cocaine, Surfacaine, Metacaine	
Benzyl alcohol	5% pet.	Essential oils, balsam of Peru, food flavorings, perfumes, antiseptic and local anesthetics		
Benzyl benzoate	5% pet.	Balsam of Peru, balsam of tolu, perfumes, nail polish plasticizer, Topocide (Lilly)		
Benzyl salicylate	2% pet.	Perfumes, detergents, sunscreens (methoxsalen), psoralens		May enhance photosensitization
Bergamot, oil of	10% pet.	Eau de Cologne Shalimar, hair tonics, toilet water, china painting, ceramics		A photosensitizer. Test open and closed
Beryllium nitrate	1% aq. sol.	Cathode tube and fluorescent lights, alloys, electrical equipment, ceramics, fluorophors		

Contactant	Concentration and Vehicle	Exposure	Cross-Reactions	Comment
Betadine (providone-iodine; Purdue Frederick)	As is			Iodine in polyvinyl pyrrolidine
Betanaphthol	10% o.o.	Glues, adhesive solvent, book binding, mouthwashes, hair tonics		
Bis(diethyl and dibutyl-dithiocarbamato) zinc	1% pet.	Rubber		
Bismark brown	Pure	Dyeing silks, wools, leathers	Para-amino compounds	
Bisphenol A	1% acet.	Epoxy resin converter, antioxidant, component of oil-soluble phenolic resins	Diethylstilbestrol, organic silicone compounds, monobenzylether of hydroquinone	
Bithionol (bisphenol), (Actamer)	1% pet.	Antiseptic no longer used	Chlorinated salicylanilides	Photosensitizer
Bitter almond, oil of	10% o.o.		Benzoin, balsam of Peru	A benzaldehyde poison
Blue Ointment	As is (open)			25% mercury in pet.
Borax (sodium borate)	Sat. aq. sol.	Refrigerant, antiseptics, soaps, detergents, abrasives, bath salts, cosmetics, flux		
Boric acid	Pdr. as is	Antiseptics, detergents, cosmetics		
Brilliant green	2% aq. sol.	Dyes		
British antilewisite (BAL; 2-3, dithiopropanol; dimercaprol)	As is	Chelating agents		
Bromo acid	As is	Lipstick dyes		A photosensitizer
9-Bromofluorene	Do not test	Chemistry laboratory		Erythema multiform reaction
Brucine	1% pet.	Denatured alcohol		A strychnine compound
BTC (lauryl dimethyl benzyl-ammonium chloride)	5% aq. sol.	Surfactant, cationic synthetic detergents, bubble baths		Controls
Burow's solution (liquor aluminum acetatis)	10% aq. sol.	Astringents, antiseptics		Very rarely sensitizes
Butesin picrate	As is	Local anesthetic, antiseptic	Procaine, benzocaine	
Butethamine (Monocaine)	1% aq. sol.	Local anesthetic	Procaine, benzocaine	Based on para-aminobenzoic acid

Butyl acetate	25% o.o.	Solvents, nail polish removers		
Butyl glycidyl ether	1% o.o.	Reactive epoxy resin diluent		
Butyn sulfate (butacaine; Abbott)	1% aq. sol.	Topical anesthetic	Procaine, benzocaine	Based on para-aminobenzoic acid
Butyrolactone (Antara)	As is	Organic solvent		Useful solvent for patch testing of resins
Cadmium sulfide (Capsebon)	1% aq. sol.	Tattoos, photo-conducting material, forms pink pigment in acrylic dentures with cadmium selenide		Photoallergic
Calcium chloride	2% aq. sol.	EEG Electrode Paste, dehydrating agents, antimildew		A primary irritant
Calcium oxide (quicklime)	Do not patch test	Unslaked lime, caustic lime, burnt lime		Not a sensitizer. Burns skin when moistened. See also lime, slaked
Calcium thioglycollate	5% aq. sol.	Depilatories		
Camomile, oil of	25% o.o.	Cosmetics, mirror manufacturing, vegetable hair dyes		
Camphor oil Camphor powder	10% pet. As is	Used in dentistry as camphorated chlorophenol, preservatives, plasticizer, nail polish, lacquers, varnishes, moth repellents, embalming fluids, explosives, pharmaceuticals		Some camphors contain oil of laurel
Canada balsam	As is	Cement for lenses, fine lacquers, mounting slides	Turpentine, balsam of Peru	
Cantharidin	1% alc.	Skin vesicant, rubefacient in hair tonics, Cantharone (Ingram), wart remedy Verrusol (C & M)		
Capsicum, tincture of	1% alc.	Hair tonics, rubefacient, tear gas (On Guard)		
Captan	1% pet.	Pesticide	Phaltan	A dicarboximide
Caraway seed oil	25% c.o.	Spices in baking, liqueurs, soaps, flavor in dentifrices		

Contactant	*Concentration and Vehicle*	*Exposure*	*Cross-Reactions*	*Comment*
Carbamide (urea)	10% aq. sol.	Therapeutic agent, Ammident, Colgate and Dr. Lyons toothpaste		
Carbitol (diethylene glycol)	10% aq. sol.	Solvents, stabilizer of emulsions		
Carbocaine Hydrochloride (mepivacaine; Winthrop)	2% aq. sol.	Local anesthetics		Not based on para-aminobenzoic acid
Carbolfuchsin paint (Castellani's paint)	As is (open)			Contains resorcin. Keep in dark bottle
Carbon disulfide	10% o.o.	Industrial solvents, laboratories, rayon industry		
Carbon paper	As is	Typing, lithography, blue printing, photocopying		*Reported sensitizers:* Triphenyl phosphate, oleyl alcohol, nigrosine
Carbon tetrachloride	10% o.o.	Solvents, floor waxes, cleansers, fire extinguisher fluids, insecticide sprays		Synonyms: carbon tet, tetrachloromethane and perchloromethane
Carbowax	As is	Cosmetics, pharmaceutical vehicles		Solid polyethylene glycols
Carboxylase (co-carboxylase, coenzyme B)	10% aq. sol.	Manufacture of thiamine	Thiamine chloride	
Carbromal (bromodiethylacetylurea)	Pdr. as is, or 1% in propylene glycol	Carbrital (Parke, Davis), Taborea (Table Rock)	Barbiturates	Purpuric patch test
Carmine dye	As is	Rouge, lip pomade, ink, stains, food		Contains cochineal, a dried insect
Carnation oil	10% aq. sol.	Eugenol, "Flubber" putty, flavoring agent		
Carnauba wax	As is	Orange skin protective, old phonograph records, furniture, shoe and floor waxes, candles, electrical insulation, cosmetics, lipsticks, cologne sticks		Obtained from South American palm trees. A solid that becomes fluid when rubbed with a circular motion
Casalic green	As is	Chromium oxide powder, green tattoos		

Cashew nut oil	3% alc.	Voodoo dolls, swizzle sticks, mucilage, printer's ink, varnishes	Rhus and other Anacardiaceae	
Cassia flavor	5% o.o.	Chinese cinnamon		
Catechol	3% o.o.	Plastic industry, rubber	Resorcin, hydroquinone	
CD_2 (amino diethylamino monohydrochloride; diethyl paraphenylenediamine)	1% aq. sol.	Color film developers		Lichen planus type of eruption
Cedarwood oil	10% o.o.	Essential perfume oil		A photosensitizer
Cement (clay and limestone)	As is (open)	Construction industry		May contain cobalt, nickel and chromates
Ceramol	30% pet.			Blend of cetyl and stearyl alcohol with sodium lauryl sulfate
Ceresin (ozokerite)	Pure	Cosmetic stiffeners		
Cetyl alcohol	30% pet.	Fatty alcohol present in lanolin, Chloromycetin Cream, Vioform HC Lotion, Neo-Cord-Dome Lotion, Pragmatar		Synonyms: hexadecyl or palmityl alcohol
Cetyl pyridinium bromide	1:1000 aq. sol.			Used in Hungarian contraceptives
Cetyl pyridinium chloride (Ceepryn)	1:1000 aq. sol.	Cēpacol, Micrin, Reef, Scope		A quaternary ammonium compound
Chloracetamide	1% aq. sol.	Preservative in cosmetics and pharmaceuticals		
Chloral hydrate	10% aq. sol.	Hair tonics, suppositories, Calmitol Ointment, veterinary anesthetics	Chlorobutanol	
Chloramine	2% aq. sol.	Water disinfectants		
Chloramphenicol (Chloromycetin [Parke, Davis])	Pdr. as is	Antibiotic cream, Genetris Pessaries		
Chloracetopenone (CN)	1% acet. (open)	Tear gas		Test open. A severe irritant and primary sensitizer
Chlorobenzylidene malonitrile (CS)	1% alc. (open)	Tear gas		Test open. A severe irritant and primary sensitizer
Chlordane	5% acet.	Insecticides		

Contactant	*Concentration and Vehicle*	*Exposure*	*Cross-Reactions*	*Comment*
Chlorinated alkalies	0.5% aq. sol.	Javelle water, Labarraque's solution, Carrel-Dakin's solution, Clorox, chlorinated lime		
Chlorinated naphthalene	As is	Electric wires, motors, electrical equipment, transformers		Produces acneiform eruptions
Chlorobenzene	5% o.o.	Insecticides		Produces acneiform eruptions
Chlorobutanol	As is	Dentalone (Parke, Davis), sedative dressing (Krutchen), local anesthetics, preservative for parenteral solutions and pharmaceuticals, biological fluids	Chloral hydrate	
Chlorocresol	5% pet.	Valisone Cream, topical medications, pesticides	Chloroxylenol	
Chloroform	40% o.o.	Solvent for gutta percha, gum copal, acrylic dentures, Ultra Brite and McLean's Toothpaste, anesthetics, liniments		
p-Chloro-o-cresol	0.1% alc.	Pesticides		
Chloro-2-phenylphenol (Dowicide 32)	1% pet. (open and closed)	Liquid soap, disinfectants, fungicides		Photosensitizer
Chlorophyll	5% o.o.	Deodorizers		
Chlorophyllins	5% aq. sol.	Deodorizers, cosmetics, suntan preparations, Green Mint Mouthwash		
Chloroquin	Pdr. as is	Pharmaceuticals	Atabrine	
Chlorosalicylamide	1% white pet.	Antimycotic agent (Jadit)		Photosensitizer
Chlorothion	1% alc. (open)	Insecticides		

Chlorothymol	2% aq. sol.	N.F. Antiseptic Solution. *Antiseptic solutions:* Gray Cross, C.S.I. *Foot powders:* Upjohn Medicated, Dr. Solvey, Ward's Foot Balm, K4. *Douches:* Lanteen, Verazeptol. *Liniments:* Neurabalm, Balsam of Myrrh, Rex Rub. Key Nose Drops. Formula DC Vaginal Jelly. *With benzocaine:* Idol, Lanocaine		
Chloroxylenol	2% pet.	Chloroxylenol Solution B.P., Absorbine, Jr., Redux EGG Paste, Nullo Foot Cream, Rezamid Cream Lotion, Acne Aid, Cenathesin, First aid petroleum jelly. *Sprays:* Feminine hygiene "My Own" (Emko), Unburn, Unguentine, Top Brass, Stopette Deodorant. *Powders:* ZeaSORB, Desitin, Aveeno	Chlorocresol	Synonyms: p-chloro-meta-xylenol; 4-chloro-3,5-xylenol; Ottasept; PCMX; Bezytol
Chlorpromazine chloride (Thorazine)	1% pet.	Medical, nursing and chemistry personnel	Phenothiazines	Photoallergic and phototoxic
Chromium sulfate	2% aq. sol.	Textile inks, paints, varnishes, leather processing, lithographing, fur dyeing, electroplating, blueprinting		
Chromium trichloride	0.5% aq. sol.	See Chromium sulfate		Use 1/100 for intradermal testing
Chrysarobin	0.03% pet.	Topical medications		Obtained from goa powder (Indian tree)
Chrysoidine brown	As is	Leather dyes	Para-amino compounds	
Cidex	1% aq. sol.	Cold sterilizing solution		Is 2% buffered glutaraldehyde
Cinchona, tincture of	1% alc.	Hair tonics, rubefacients		
Cinnabar (red mercuric sulfide)	3% pet.	Red tattoos, topical medications		Only mercurial compatible with sulfur

Contactant	*Concentration and Vehicle*	*Exposure*	*Cross-Reactions*	*Comment*
Cinnamates (2-ethoxyethyl-p-methoxy)	1% pet.	Sunscreens		
Cinnamic acid	5% pet.	Styrax, balsam of Peru, menthyl and benzyl cinnamates in sunscreens: RVPaque (Elder), SunDare Lotion (Texas Pharmacal), Sun Bath (Revlon), Sun Tan Gelee (Rexall)		
Cinnamic aldehyde	2% pet.	Cinnamon oil, cassia oil, cinnamon powder, patchouli oil, flavoring agents, toilet soaps, perfumes	Balsam of Peru, benzoin	
Cinnamon oil	0.5% pet.	Cassia bark, flavoring agents, vermouths, gum, toothpastes, confections, cola beverages, tobacco, bubble gum, lipsticks	Balsam of Peru	
Citric Acid	1% aq. sol.	Transfusions, nicotine stain remover, astringent mouthwash		Cause of aphthous ulcers?
Citronella oil (lemon grass oil)	As is	Perfumes, insect repellents		
Citrus Red 2	2% acet.	Dye for Florida orange peel		An azo dye
Clorox	5% aq. sol.	Detergents, chlorinated alkalies		
Clove oil	1% pet.	Eugenol, antiseptics, local anesthetics, mucilage, perfumes, condiments, chewing gum	Balsam of Peru, diethylstilbestrol, benzoin	
Coal tar	5% pet.	Adhesives, creosotes, insecticides, phenols, wood working, preservation of wood		Photosensitizing
Cobalt chloride	2% aq. sol.	Tattoos, pottery, clays, cements, hematinics, alloys, anodes, glass enamels, adhesives, fly paper, hair dyes, carbides, pigments	Vitamin B_{12}	Vitamin B_{12} (Cobione) is a cobalt compound
Cobalt naphthenate	5% aq. sol.	Polyester resins		

Cobalt sulfate	2% aq. sol.	Alloys, dyeing, lacquers, glass, paints, oilcloth colors, enamels, permanent ink for porcelain		
Cobaltous aluminate (azure or cobalt blue)	2% aq. sol.	Blue tattoo pigment		
Cocaine	1% aq. sol.			Based on benzoic acid
Cocaine liquid	1% aq. sol.	Topical anesthetics, mydriatic	Surfacaine, Metycaine	Based on benzoic acid
Cocoanut oil	Pure	Soaps, oleomargarine, cooking fat, baking ingredients, confections		
Cocoanut soap (sodium salt)	5% aq. sol.	Surfactant, synthetic detergents, bubble baths		Control
Cocobolo wood	As is	Musical instruments, kitchen utensil handles, wood-working industry		
Coins, U.S.A.	As is	Penny Nickel Dime Quarter Half dollar	95% copper, 5% zinc 75% copper, 25% nickel 90% copper, 8% nickel 90% copper, 8% nickel 60% copper, 40% nickel (All U.S. coins except the penny give a positive dimethylglyoxime test reaction)	
Collodion	As is			Contains ether, absolute ethyl alcohol and pyroxylin
Collodion, flexible	As is			Contains colophony (rosin) and castor oil
Colocynth extract	1% alc.	Denaturing agent in alcohol		
Colophony	See Rosin			
Coniferyl benzoate	1% pet.	Benzoin	Benzyl cinnamate, benzyl alcohol, eugenol, benzoin, vanilla	
Copper sulfate	5% aq. sol.	Insecticides, fungicides, food processing, fertilizers, mordant in fur dyeing, coins, alloys, D'Alibour solution		A rare sensitizer

Contactant	*Concentration and Vehicle*	*Exposure*	*Cross-Reactions*	*Comment*
Coriander, oil of	10% c.o.	Flavoring agents		
Cottonseed oil	As is	Cosmetics, margarine, vegetable shortening		
Coumarin	5% pet.	Flavorings (including vanilla), perfumes, cosmetics, optical bleaches		A cinnamic acid derivative
Creosote (creosote oil)	10% o.o.	Expectorants, preserving wood, waterproofing, lumber industry		A photosensitizer
Cresol	1% aq. sol.	Antiseptics		
Crystal violet	1% aq. sol.	Gentian violet		
Cutting oil	As is or 50% o.o.			Controls. May contain additives
Cyclaine (hexylcaine hydrochloride; Merck Sharp & Dohme)	1% aq. sol.	Local anesthetics	Procaine	
Cyclohexamde (actidione)	1% pet.	Culture media, garden spray	Neomycin	
Cyclohexanol peroxide	0.5% pet.	Polyester resin hardener		
n-Cyclohexyl benzothiazyl sulfenamide	1% pet.	Rubber		
Dangard	0.25% pet.	Q.E D. Shampoo sold by barbers		
DDT (dichlorodiphenyl-trichloroethane)	1% pet.	Insecticides, chlorobenzene derivatives		May produce chloracne and possibly porphyria
Decyl alcohol	5% pet.	Lanolin		An aliphatic alcohol
Depilatories	As is (open)			Controls
Dequalinium	0.1% aq. sol.	Micrin Mouthwash, antiseptics		A quaternary ammonium compound
Desenex (WTS-Pharmacraft)	As is	Antifungal agents		Rare sensitizer
Detergent 1011 (secondary amide of lauric acid)	5% aq. eol.	Surfactant, nonionic synthetic detergents		Controls
Detergent, enzyme	0.25%			Test the pure subtilisms 0.1% aq.
Diallyl phthalate	0.1% acet.	Polyester resin industry		A strong irritant

Diaminodiphenylmethane	0.1% pet.	Rubber antioxidant, epoxy resin curing agent, intermediate in germicides, surface active agents, pharmaceuticals, corrosion inhibitors, phosphate insecticides	Paraphenylenediamine	
Diazonium	1% alc. (open)	Phosphate insecticides		
Diazonium compounds	10% aq. sol.	Ozalid photocopy paper		Contains 4-nn′-diethyl amino benzene diazonium chloride
Dibenzothiazyl disulfide	1% pet.	Rubber		
Di-beta-naphtyl paraphenylenediamine	1% pet.	Rubber		
Dibromsalan (dibromosalicylanilide)	1% pet.	Deodorant soaps, White Lifebuoy		Photoallergic
Dibutyl phthalate	5% pet.	Plasticizer for synthetic resins, nail lacquer		
Dibutyl tin maleate	1% pet.	Plasticizer in plastic (Elastiglass)		
Dichlorobenzene	5% chloroform	Mothballs		A primary sensitizer
Dichlorodiphenyl (methyl carbinol)	5% acet. (open)	Organic insecticides		
1,2,4-Dichloronitrobenzene (dinitrochlorobenzine)	0.1% acet.	Algicide in air conditioner NALCO-205		A primary sensitizer
Dichlorophene (G4)	2% aq. sol.	Fungicides, antimildew agents, preservative in creams, dentifrices		
Diethylenetriamine	0.1% aq. sol.	Epoxy resin amine		
Diethylethanolamine	0.1% aq. sol.	Amine polyurethane catalyst		
Diethyl-meta-toluamide (DEET)	5% alc. (open)	Black Flag, Off, 7–11, RVPellent (Elder)		May produce bullous eruption
Diethylparaphenylenediamine (CD_2)	1% aq. sol.	Color film developers		Lichen planus reaction
Diethylstibestrol	0.1% in ethyl alc.	Aquarant "E" (Webster), Furestrol Suppositories (Eaton), diethylstilbestrol suppositories (Lilly)	Dienestrol, hexestrol, bisphenol A, monobenzylether of hydroquinone, eugenol, stilbene benzophenone	
Difluorodiphenyltrichloroethane	5% acet.	Insecticides		

Contactant	*Concentration and Vehicle*	*Exposure*	*Cross-Reactions*	*Comment*
Difolantan	1:1000 aq.	Fungicide for farm crops		Derivative of dicarboximide
Digalloyltrioleate	3% pet.	A-Fil, Neo-A-Fil (Texas Pharmacal), Sunprotectol (Lamond)		Sunscreens may be photosensitive
Dihydrostreptomycin	5% aq. sol.	Pharmaceutical and nursing personnel	Neomycin, kanamycin	
Dihydroxyacetone	10% aq. sol.	Man Tan, Magictan, Positan, Tan-O-Rama, Tansation, Tanfastic		Rare sensitizer
Dihydroxyphenyl	1% pet.	Rubber		
Diisopropyl fluorophosphate	1% alc. (open)	Insecticides		
Dilan	5% acet. (open)	Insecticides		
Dimethylaniline	10% alc.	Polyester resin accelerator		
Dimethylglyoxime	10% in Carbowax	Chemical test for nickel		
Dimethyl paratoluidine	2% pet.	Accelerators, acrylic resins		
Dimethyl phthalate	As is	Plasticizer for synthetic resins, insect repellents		
Dimethyl sulfate	*Do not* test			Forms sulfuric acid
Dimethyl sulfoxide (DMSO)	90% aq. sol.	Industrial solvents, topical medicaments		Primary urticariogenic agent
Dimethyloldihydroxy ethylene urea	10% pet.	Crease resistant, drip dry clothing		
Dimethylol urea formaldehyde	10% pet.	Crease resistant, drip dry clothing		
Dimite dichlorodiphenylethanol	5% acet. (open)	Insecticides		
Dinitrochlorobenzene (DNCB)	0.1% acet.	Investigative sensitizer, Algacide in water cooling systems	Chloromycetin (chloramphenicol)	A primary sensitizer
Dioctyl phthalate	1% pet.	Plastics and rubber		
Dioctyl sodium sulfosuccinate	5% aq. sol.	Wetting compounds, anionic surfactant		
Diodoquin (diiodohydroxyquin; Searle)	As is	Amebicides	Vioform, Quinolor, Sterosan	
Dipentamethylene thiuram disulfide	1% pet.	Rubber		
Diphenyl	Pure	Dielectrics		

Diphenylcyclopropenone	0.1% acet.	Chemistry experiments	
Diphenylguanidine	1% pet.	Rubber accelerator	
Diphenylparaphenylenediamine	1% pet.	Rubber accelerator	
Dithionone	1% pet.	Pesticide	Merck product
Divinyl benzene (styrene)	1% o.o.	See Styrene	
Domiphen bromide	0.1% aq. sol.	Quaternary compound in Scope Mouthwash	
Dowicide(s)	1% pet.	Germicides, fungicides, antiseptics, disinfectants	A series of phenolic substances
Dowicide A (sodium-o-phenyl phenate)	1% pet.	Dowicide A, B and G used in paper money	Not absorbed through skin. An oil solution (5%) is well-tolerated on human skin, but aqueous solutions of the sodium salt are irritating in concentrations exceeding 0.5%
Dowicide B (sodium 2,3,5-trichlorophenate)	1% pet.	Water-soluble fungicide	
Dowicide C (sodium chloro-o-phenyl phenate	1% pet.	Water-soluble antiseptic	
Dowicide D (2-chloro-4-phenyl-phenol sodium)	1% pet.	Germicide	
Dowicide E (2-bromo-4-phenyl-phenol sodium)	1% pet.	Fungicide	
Dowicide F (sodium tetrachlorophenate)	1% pet.	Used as germicide, antiseptic, fungicide	
Dowicide G (sodium pentachlorophenate)	1% pet.	Industrial antiseptic	
Dowicide H (sodium tetrachlorophenoxide)	1% pet.	Industrial antiseptic	
Dowicide 1 (o-phenyl phenol)	1% pet.	Germicide, antiseptic, fungicide	

Contactant	*Concentration and Vehicle*	*Exposure*	*Cross-Reactions*	*Comment*
Dowicide 3 (chloro-o-phenyl phenol)	1% pet.	Germicide, antiseptic, fungicide		
Dowicide 4 (2-chloro-4-phenyl phenol)	1% pet.	High-efficiency germicide		
Dowicide 6 (tetrachlorophenol)	1% pet.	Germicide, antiseptic, fungicide		
Dowicide 7 (pentachlorophenol)	1% pet.	Oil-soluble antiseptic, germicide, fungicide		
Duponol WA (sodium lauryl sulfate)	5% aq. sol.	Surfactant, anionic synthetic detergents		Controls
Duraspan (International Latex)	As is	Polyurethane elastomer (spandex)		
Dyclone (dyclonine hydrochloride; Dow Chemical)	1% aq. sol.	Local anesthetics		Not based on para-aminobenzoic acid
Dyes				
Certified	2% pet.	Foods, drugs, cosmetics	Para-amino compounds	
Disperse Orange 3	1% pet.	Nylon dyes		
Disperse Yellow 3				
Ecogaine	2% aq. sol.	Local anesthetics	Procaine, benzocaine	Based on para-aminobenzoic acid
Edathamil (calcium EDTA versenate)	25% aq. sol.	Chelating agent		
Eldoquin (Elder)	See Hydroquinone			
Emulsifying wax	20% pet.			
Eosin	As is (open)	Fluorescent dyes		A photosensitizer
Ephedrine	1% o.o.	Nose drops		
Epichlorhydrin	0.1% alc.	Epoxy resin	Propene oxide	
Epon 828	1% acet.	Epoxy resins		
Epon 1001	10% acet.	Epoxy resins		
Epoxy glue hardener	0.5% pet.	One part of 2 tube preparation, household glue, collages, sculptures		May contain triethylenetetramine or diaminodiphenylmethane

Epoxy glue resin	1% acet.			
Erythrosin	As is (open)	Fluorescent dyes		A photosensitizer
Esoterica (Mitchum)	As is	Skin-lightening cream		Contains ammoniated mercury
Essential oils	1% alc. or 2% pet.	Flavor in dentifrices, mouthwashes, medicinal elixirs, perfumes		
Ether	60% o.o.	Anesthetics, solvents		
Ethoxyethyl-p-methoxycinnamate	5% pet.	Sunscreen		Photosensitivity
Ethoxyquin	0.5% aq.	Apple packing		A quinoline
Ethyl acetate	5% mek.	Solvent for varnishes, lacquers and nitrocellulose plastics, component of nail polish removers		Trace amounts in foods and alcoholic beverages
Ethyl cetab (cetylethyldimethyl-ammonium bromide)	5% aq. sol.	Surfactant, cationic synthetic detergents		Controls
Ethylenediamine hydrochloride	1% pet.	Mycolog Cream, parent substance of certain antihistamines and aminophylline; dyes, rubber, fungicides, waxes, resins, insecticides, asphalt; present in Tincture Merthiolate (Lilly)	Aminophylline, Phenergan, Pyribenzamine, Antistine, Ethylenediamine tetraacetate	
Ethylenediamine tetraacetate (Versene)	1% aq. sol.	Stabilizing agent in many ophthalmic solutions, chelating agent	Ethylenediamine hydrochloride	
Ethylene dichloride	50% o.o.	Solvents, plastics, rubber, insecticides, hobby crafts		
Ethylene glycol monomethyl ether acetate (Egmea)	1% mek.	Used to cement nose pads to eyeglass frames		May contain traces of ethyl acetate
Ethylene oxide	Do not test	Sterilizing gas for surgical instruments, towels, sheets, gloves, anesthesia masks, chemical reactor		Powerful vesicant
1,3-Ethylhexanediol	As is	Insect repellent		
Ethyl parahydroxybenzoate	5% pet.	Preservative in pharmaceuticals, cosmetics, foods, cleansers		
Eucalyptus oil	1% alc.	Gutta percha for root canal fillings	Balsam of Peru, benzoin, vanilla, oil of orange peel	

Contactant	*Concentration and Vehicle*	*Exposure*	*Cross-Reactions*	*Comment*
Eugenol	5% pet.	Oil of carnation (hyacinth), oil of bay, pimento oil (allspice), clove oil, flower oils, cinnamon oil, food spices, perfumes, zinc oxide dental cement, flavoring agent, dental impression agent		Derived from clove oil
Eurax Cream and Lotion (10% n-ethyl-o-crotonotoluide; Geigy)	As is	Scabicide		
Eyeglass frames, plastic	Shavings (controls)			*Possible allergens:* cellulose acetate, cellulose propionate, resorcinol monobenzoate, p-tertiarybutyl phenol, azo dyes, beeswax-turpentine mixture, ethylene glycol, ethylene oxide and ethyl acetate
Eyeglass nose pad				Ethylene glycol monomethyl ether acetate (welds nose pad to eyeglass frames)
Fentichlor	1% pet. (open and closed)	Antiseptic and fungicide, cosmetics, pharmaceuticals		A photosensitizer
Ferric chloride	2% aq. sol.	Monsel's solution, styptic		Very rare sensitizer
Flit	25% o.o.	Insecticide		
Fluorescein	1% alc.	Dyes, eyeglass cleaner		Photosensitizer
Formaldehyde resins				
Urea formaldehyde	10% pet.	Plastics, textile finishes		
Melamine formaldehyde	10% pet.			
Others	1% pet. or 1% isopropyl alcohol	Glues, plastics, textile finishes		

Formalin (40% sol. of formaldehyde gas)	2% aq. sol.	*Cosmetics:* shampoos, antiperspirants, Sub-Rosa Cream Deodorant, nail hardener, nail polish, resins, Thermodent Toothpaste, soaps, permanent wave lotions. *Medical:* root canal preparation (Forno-Cresol) disinfectant, wart remedies, fungicides, insecticides, tissue fixative, embalming fluid, denatured alcohol, orthopedic casts, renal dialysis unit, vaccines. *Industrial:* tanning white leather, textile finish (antiwrinkle), synthetic gums and adhesives, synthetic resins and rubber, paper, photography, antimildew in leather, glues, wet strength paper	Glutaraldehyde ?	Hexamethylenetetramine (methenamine) liberates formaldehyde in the presence of acids
Formic acid spirits	1% aq. sol.	Hair tonics		
Fowler's solution (potassium arsenite solution)	As is			Equivalent to 1% arsenic trioxide
Fumaronitrile	Do not test	Plasticizer for vinyl resin herbicide, soil fumigant		A potent irritant and vesicant. May also be allergen.
Furacin (nitrofurazone; Eaton)	As is	Topical bacterial agent	Carbowax	Water-soluble Furacin preparations have a base of polyethylene glycols
Garamycin (Gentamycin)	20% pet.	Antiseptic topical medication	Neomycin, kanamycin	
Garlic	Aq. extract		Balsam of Peru, tars, onion	Controls
Gasoline	50% o.o.			
Gentian violet (methylrosaniline chloride)	1% aq. sol.	Stain, indicator, antiseptics, vaginal creams, tablets, aerosols	Rivanol	Intradermal test with 0.05 ml. of a 1:5000 dilution
Geraniol	10% pet.	Flavoring agent		
Ginger oil	25% c.o.	Condiments, candy gastric medications, rubefacient		

Contactant	*Concentration and Vehicle*	*Exposure*	*Cross-Reactions*	*Comment*
Ginkgo fruit pulp	1:10 acet.		Rhus, cashew	Ginkgo tree is a member of Anacardium genus
Glospan (Globe Manufacturing Co.)	As is	Polyurethane elastomer (spandex)		Lycra spandex is free of mercaptobenzothiazole
Glue	As is open or 10% acet.	Furniture, shoes, books, toys, waterproofing		Rubber, epoxies, chromates, formaldehyde, polyvinyl acetate resins
Glutaraldehyde	1% aq. sol.	Tissue fixative, antiperspirants, antiseptics, tanning agent for soft leather, embalming fluids, shampoo preservative, dentifrices	Formaldehyde?	Tans and dries skin
Glycerin	As is	Emollient, pharmaceutical vehicle, mounting medium in microscopy		Very rare sensitizer
Glyceryl monooleate	30% pet.	Emulsifier, soaps, cosmetics		
Glyceryl monostearate	30% pet.	Emulsifier, cosmetics, food products, medicinals		
Glycol	10% aq. sol.	Solvents for water-insoluble chemicals, pharmaceuticals		
Glycol dimethacrylate	5% o.o.	Synthetic resins		Prevents crazing, cracking of resins
Gly-Oxide	As is	Mouthwash providing hydrogen peroxide		Contains urea peroxide
Gold chloride	1% aq. sol.	Photographers		Pustular patch test reaction
Gold cohesive	As is	Dentistry		
Gold leaf	As is	Gilding, topical ulcer medication		
Gold sodium thiosulfate	2% aq. sol.	Medicinal for lupus erythematosus, arthritis		
Gold trichloride	1% aq. sol.	Jewelry		
Gramicidin	As is	Antibacterial topical agent, mouthwashes		
Graphite (black lead)	As is	Lead pencils, crucibles, rubber surfaces, lubricants		

Guaiacol	10% o.o.			
Guanine (2-amino-6-hydroxy purine)	As is	Pearly nail lacquer		Obtained from fish scales
Guignet's green (chromium oxide)	2% aq. sol.	Green tattoo pigment		
Gum(s)	As is	Resinous plant exudates		Contains carbohydrates forming mucilaginous substances with water
Gum arabic (acacia)	As is	See Acacia		
Gutta percha	As is	Resins, rosins, root canal mixtures		Latex of Malaysian trees contains more resin than does rubber
Hair lotions and tonics	As is (open)			May contain: *rubefacients*—chloral hydrate, formic acid spirits, quinine salts, tincture capsicum or cinchona, cantharidin; *phenolic compounds*—chlorthymol, resorcinol, betanaphthol; *other antiseptics*—salicylic acid, formaldehyde, mercury bichloride; *tars*—coal tar derivatives, oil of cade; *vehicles*—alcohol and volatile solvents, perfumes
Henna	As is	Vegetable dye, synthetic henna (Lawsonia, hydroxynaphthoquinone—the coloring matter of henna leaves)		Rarely sensitizes
Hexachlorophene (G-11)	1% pet.	Soaps, detergents, creams, oils, pharmaceuticals	Bithionol, chlorinated salicylanilides	Now restricted by FDA primarily to prescription items
Hexamethylenetetramine (methenamine)	1% pet.	Many proprietary urinary antiseptics often combined with mandelic acid. Also a rubber accelerator	Formaldehyde	Liberates formaldehyde in the presence of acids

Contactant	*Concentration and Vehicle*	*Exposure*	*Cross-Reaction*	*Comment*
Hexetidine	1% aq. sol.	Antibacterial agent in Sterisol mouthwash, douches		Synonyms: ethylhexyl, hexahydro, methyl-imidaso, imidasolel
Hexylresorcinol	1% pet.	Contraceptives, Sucrettes, Tetrazets, ST 37, Crystoids, Caprikol (Merck), Akrinol Cream, Listerine, Lanteen Jelly (Esta), Nymore	Resorcin	
Holocaine (phenacaine)	1% aq. sol.	Local anesthetics	Benzocaine, procaine	
Homatropine	1% aq. sol.	Eye drops		
Hyamine 1622 (p-diisobutyl phenoxyethoxy ethyldimethyl benzylammonium chloride)	5% aq. sol.	Surfactant, cationic synthetic detergents, bubble baths, Clesk Lotion (Dara), Quinette Inserts (Arnar-Stone)		
Hydralizine hydrochloride or sulfate	1% aq. sol. or 1% pet.	Wide industrial exposure, metal, plastics, rubber products, rocket fuel, photography, insecticides, fungicides, preservatives. Parent substance for drugs listed in adjacent column	Apresoline, isonicotinic acid, hydrazide, phenylhydrazine, Nardil (derived from hydrazine hydrobromide)	
Hydrochloric acid	1% aq. sol.	Chemical industry, Acidulin (Lilly), Convertin (Ascher), Muripsin (Norgine), Normacid (Stuart)		Rarely sensitizes
Hydrocortisone	20% pet.			
Hydrocortisone acetate or free alcohol	2% pet			
Hydrofluoric acid	0.2% aq. sol.	Corrosive agents, glass etching, electric lamp manufacturing, dry cleaning		Pustular patch test reaction
Hydrogen peroxide solution	3% aq. sol.	Bleaches, oxidizing agents, antiseptics		
Hydrogen sulfide	10% aq. sol.	Petroleum refineries, tunnels, mines, rayon plants		

Hydrophilic ointment U.S.P.	As is			Contains sodium lauryl sulfate, propylene glycol, stearyl alcohol, methyl paraben, propyl paraben, white petrolatum, distilled water
Modified				Modified hydrophilic ointment contains glycerin instead of propylene glycol
Hydrophilic petrolatum (U.S.P.)	As is			Contains stearyl alcohol, cholesterol, white wax, white petrolatum
Hydroquinone	1% pet.	Rubber inhibitor polyester, acrylic, photography, Eldoquin and Eldopaque (Elder), Artra (White), Derma-blanch (Brayten)	Resorcin, pyrocatechol, monobenzylether of hydroquinone	Depigmenting agent
Hydroquinone, monobenzylether of	See Monobenzylether of hydroquinone			
Hypochloride	10% aq. sol.	Kasenol Mouthwash, Oxychlorosene		
Ichthyol (ichthammol; sulfonated bitumen)	10% pet.	Topical medications, Derma Medicone (Medicone), Ichthymall (Mallinckrodt)		Rarely sensitizes
Igepal (nonylphenoxy polyethylene oxyethanol)	5% aq. sol.	Surfactant, synthetic detergents, bubble baths		Controls
Igepon T.H.C. (sodium oleyl laurate)	5% aq. sol.	Surfactant, synthetic detergents, bubble baths		Controls
Indalone	As is (open)	Insect repellents		
Indane	5% acet. (open)	Insecticides: chlordane, heptachlor, aldrin, dieldrin, endrin, diendrin		
Indigo	10% aq. sol.	Tattoos, stains, blue dye		

Contactant	*Concentration and Vehicle*	*Exposure*	*Cross-Reactions*	*Comment*
Ink(s)	As is			Acid and basic dyes, iron salts, tannic acid, gallates, phenol, silver nitrate, alkalies, castor oil
Ink eradicator	As is (open)			Active agents are tin chloride, sodium bisulfite, sodium hypochlorite, sodium chloride
Iodine crystals	0.5% aq. sol.		Iodoform, radiopaque iodine, iodized medications, thymol iodide	Old iodine solutions exposed to light are irritants. Incompatible with sulfur and mercury.
Iodine, tincture of	As is (open)		Same as Iodine crystals	Is an irritant when covered
Iodochlorhydroxyquin	3% pet.	Vioform, Sterosan		
Iodoform (formyl triiodide)	25% pet.	Local anesthetics, antiseptics	Iodine, formaldehyde	
Ioprep	As is (open)			Irritant when occluded
Irgasan CF3 (Cloflucarban [Geigy])	0.5% pet.	Safeguard soap; used abroad as bacteriostat in vinyl gloves; shampoos		A carbanilide
Irgasan DP 300 (Triclosan [Geigy]; 2,4,4-trichloro-2-hydroxy-diphenyl ether)	0.5% pet.	Surgical scrub soaps; Dial, Colgate P300, Palmolive and Calgan antiseptic soaps; Right Guard, Calm and Dial underarm deodorants and antiperspirants; commercial laundry products, disposable paper products, paper lining for rodent cages, industrial fabric softener, fabric bacteriostat		Widely used bacteriostat
Irish moss (carrageen)	As is	Cosmetics, wave sets, dentifrices, mucilage		Trade names: Sea Kem, Viscarin, Chondrus extract
Isobutyl-p-aminobenzoate	5% pet.	Sunscreen		
Isocyanate monomer	1% acet.	Polyurethane resins		

Isodine	As is	Mouthwash		Like Betadine, is iodine in PVP
Isopropyl myristate	10% alc. or 2% pet.	Cosmetics, pharmaceuticals, Decaspray, aerosol sprays		Alcohol ester of fatty acid
Isopropyl-n-phenyl paraphenylenediamine	0.1% pet.	Rubber Antioxidant	Hair dye, paraphenylenediamine	May cause lichenoid or purpuric eruptions. *Trade names:* Cysone, Eastone, Fleezwax, Flexaone, Santoflex, Nonox-2A
Isothane (laurylisoquinolinium bromide)	5% aq. sol.	Surfactant, cationic synthetic detergents, bubble baths		Controls
Jaborandi leaves, tincture of	As is (open)	Hair tonics		
Javelle water (potassium hypochlorite)	10% aq. sol.	Disinfecting and bleaching agents		European preparations may contain dichromates
Juniper tar (oil of cade)	25% c.o.	Alma-Tar (Schieffelin)		
Karaya gum (Sterculia gum)	As is	Hair-waving lotions, denture adhesive powders, cement for ileostomy appliances, furniture polishes		
Kerosene	60% o.o.	Solvents, curing tobacco, heating, cooking, lighting, waterless hand cleansers		
Ketone	As is	Organic solvents		
Krameria, tincture of (tinctura rhatanhiae)	5% alc.	Poultices for hemorrhoids, oral and mucosal astringents, combined with tincture myrrh		Primary sensitizer
Kwell (Reed & Carnrick)	As is	Pediculosis remedy		Contains benzene hexachloride
Lactic acid	3% aq. sol.	Astringent mouthwash		
Lanolin	As is	Wool fat, wool wax, adhesives, cosmetics, pharmaceuticals		Wool alcohols may be the specific sensitizers
Latex	As is	Rubber, gutta percha, chicle, balata, fig		Fig tree latex is a sensitizer and photosensitizer
Laurel oil	2% pet.	Flavoring agent, felt hats, camphor laurel, plastics, perfumes		

Contactant	*Concentration and Vehicle*	*Exposure*	*Cross-Reactions*	*Comment*
Lauryl alcohol	5% pet.	Lanolin		An aliphatic alcohol
Lauryl gallate	5% pet.	Antioxidant in margarine and cosmetics		
Lavender oil	1% alc. or pet.	Colognes, cosmetics, soaps, china, ceramics and paintings	Balsam of Peru, rosin, wood tar	A photosensitizer, essential oil
Lead acetate	1% aq. sol.	Dyeing and printing cottons, weighing silks, laboratory determinations		
Lead arsenate	Pure	Fungicides, insecticides		
Lead chloride	Pure	Fur processing, felt processing, mordants, printing, solder and flux		
Lead oxide (red lead)	2% aq. sol.	Matches, glazes for ceramics, paints		
Lime, slaked (calcium hydroxide)	As is	Hydrated lime		Controls. See also Calcium oxide (quicklime)
Limonene, oil of	1% alc.	Orange, lemon peel, perfumes, lemon wood	Turpentine, celery, bergamot, dill	Main sensitizer of orange and lemon peel
Linalool, oil of	10% pet.	Flavoring in dentifrices		
Lindane	1% pet.	Pesticide		Hexachlorocyclohexane, gamma-hexane
Linseed oil	As is	Paints, varnishes, sculpturing, furniture polishes, refinishing waxes, carron oil, putty		
Lipstick	As is			Indelible variety may photosensitize
Lycra (DuPont)	As is	Polyurethane elastomer (spandex)		
Lysol (compound cresol solution)	1% aq. sol.	Disinfectant		
Mace, oil of (nutmeg)	1% alc.	Flavoring agent		
Mafenide acetate	8% in pet.	Burn remedy (Sulfamylon Cream)		
Magnesium peroxide	As is	Oxidizing agent—McLean's Toothpaste		
Malachite green	2% aq. sol.	Dye		

Malathion	1% alc. (open) 0.5% pet.	Insecticides		A primary sensitizer
Maleic anhydride	1% aq. sol.	Epoxy resin		
Manganese oxide	Pure	Pigment in rubber goods, alloy in iron and steel, dry batteries, brick, pottery, dyeing industry, drying paints and varnishes, glass making, printing, dyeing textiles		
Mastic	As is	Varnishes, styptic, astringent, cements, microscopy, dentistry		Resin of European mastic tree
Matches and match boxes (striking surfaces)	As is			Principal ingredients are potassium chlorate, red phosphorus, phosphorus sesquisulfide (phosphorus trisulfide), antimony sulfide, chromates, red lead, glue, cornstarch, coloring agents, rosin, paraffin
Melamine formaldehyde	10% pet.	Clothing finishes, epoxy resins, synthetic resins		
Menthol	1% pet.	Flavoring agents, rubefacients, dusting powders, douches, foods, cigarettes, liqueurs, mixed drinks, Listerine, Reef, Chloraseptic, face cream, toothpaste, mint candies, cough drops, aerosol room spray		
Mercaptans	Pure	Depilatories, glue	Thioglycolic acid, BAL (dimercaprol)	
Mercaptobenzothiazole	1% pet.	Rubber accelerator		
Mercolized cream (Dearborn)	As is	Skin lightener cream		Contains ammoniated mercury
Mercresin Tincture (Upjohn)	As is (open)		Organic and inorganic mercurials	Irritant when covered. Contains organic mercury and cresol

Contactant	*Concentration and Vehicle*	*Exposure*	*Cross-Reactions*	*Comment*
Mercurochrome Solution (merbromin; Hynson, Westcott & Dunning)	As is	Organic mercurial antiseptic	Organic and inorganic mercurials	
Mercurous chloride (calomel)	Pdr. pure	Topical and systemic medicaments	Organic and inorganic mercurials	May produce eczematous "contact-type" dermatitis medicamentosa
Mercury (metallic)	0.5% pet.	Dentistry, thermometer		
Mercury bichloride	0.05% aq. sol.	Disinfectants, processing artificial silk, bronzing, dental laboratories, electric wiring, electroplating, electric equipment, paints, electric storage batteries, reagents, embalming fluid, fur processing, felt curing, engraving, printing, thermometers, metal work, mirror finishing, lamp bulbs, photography, photogravure, insecticides, skin lighteners	Organic and inorganic mercurials	May cause nonspecific pustular patch test reactions
Mercury-salicylic ointment	As is (open)	Topical medications		May irritate glabrous skin
Merthiolate (thimerosal)	0.1% aq. sol.	Preservative in cosmetics, topical medications, dentifrices, germicides		Contains an organic mercurial and thiosalicylic acid. Tincture of Merthiolate contains ethylenediamine
Metacide	1% alc. (open)	Insecticides		
Metaphen (nitromersol; Abbott)	0.5% alc.	Germicides	Inorganic mercurials	
Metaphenylenediamine	0.1% aq. sol.	Epoxy hardeners		
Methoxychlor	5% acet.	Insecticides		
8-Methoxypsoralen	1% alc.	Plants of Umbelliferae family, perfume oils (oil of bergamot), Trisoralen (Elder)		A photosensitizer
Methyl acetate	10% o.o.	Organic solvents		

Methyl alcohol (methanol)	Pure as is	Solvents, thinners, artificial leather manufacture, dry cleaning, antifreeze, rubber cement, celluloid, gums, resins, chemical processing		Synonyms: methyl hydrate, methyl hydroxide, acetone, alcohol, wood spirits, wood naphtha, carbinol, Columbian spirits, colonial spirits
Methylbenzethonium chloride	0.1% aq. sol.	Germicides, disinfectants, Diaparene (Breon)		Quaternary ammonium disinfectant
Methyl bromide	Do not test	Fire extinguisher, fluid, refrigerants, fumigants		Severe irritant
Methyl cellulose	As is	Binder in dentifrices		
Methyl dichlorobenzene sulfonate	5% pet.	Dental impression material		
Methylene blue	As is	Dyes, platinum bleach	Phenothiazines	A photosensitizer
Methyl ethyl ketone	As is (open)	Solvents		
Methyl ethyl ketone peroxide	0.5% acet.	Polyester resin catalyst		
Methyl heptene carbonate	0.1% alc.	Perfumes, blend fixatives in lipsticks, soaps		
Methyl morpholine	0.1% aq. sol.	Polyurethane catalyst		
Methyl orange	5% aq. sol.	Indicator		
Methyl parahydroxybenzoate	5% pet.	Preservatives, pharmaceuticals, cosmetics, food, cleansers		
Methyl salicylate	2% o.o.	Flavoring in dentifrices, Listerine, Reef, oil of wintergreen, rubefacients		A primary sensitizer
Metol	1% pet.	Photography		p-Methylaminophenol sulfate
Metycaine (piperocaine; Lilly)	1% aq. sol.	Local anesthetics, suppositories, ophthalmic ointment		Based on benzoic acid, not on para-aminobenzoic acid
Miranol HM (lauroyl imidazoline)	5% aq. sol.	Surfactant, synthetic detergents, bubble baths		Controls
Miranol SM (capryl imidazoline derivative)	5% aq. sol.	Surfactant, synthetic detergents, bubble baths		Controls

Contactant	Concentration and Vehicle	Exposure	Cross-Reactions	Comment
Mirbane oil (nitrobenzene)	25% c.o.	Substitute for oil of bitter almonds, manufacturing aniline dyes		
Monobenzylether of hydroquinone (agerite alba; monobenzone)	1% pet.	Rubber antioxidant, depigmenting agent, Benoquin (Elder)	Hydroquinone	Sensitizer and producer of leukoderma
Monoglycerol para-aminobenzoate	5% pet.	Sunscreening agents	Para-amino compounds	A photosensitizer
Monosulph (sulfated castor oil)	5% aq. sol.	Surfactant, synthetic detergents, bubble baths		Controls
Monsel's solution	As is (open)	Styptic		Contains approximately 20% iron
Morphine	1% aq. sol.			Primarily urticariogenic on scratch or intracutaneous testing
Morpholinylmercaptobenzothiazole	1% pet.	Rubber		
Mucilage	As is			Plant substances forming adhesive liquids with water
Mustard oil	0.1% pet.	Flavoring in food products, soaps, drugs		
Myristyl alcohol	5% pet.	Lanolin		
Myrrh, tincture	10% alc.	Astringosol and Odora Lorvic Disinfectants		
Nacconol NRSF (alkylaryl sulfonate)	5% aq. sol.	Surfactant, anionic synthetic detergents, bubble baths		Controls
Nail polish	As is			Sulfonamide resin most common sensitizer. Dye may be photosensitizer
Naphtha	50% o.o.	Solvents, dry cleaning agents, varnishes, fuel		
Naphthalene	Pure as is	Mothballs, moth flakes, deodorant cakes, synthetic intermediate		

Neomycin	20% pet.	Topical medications, cosmetics, soaps, deodorants	Streptomycin, kanamycin, co-reacts with bacitracin	If reaction to patch test is negative, check with 1/100 intradermal testing
Neoprene	20% in equal parts of toluene and ethyl acetate	Rubber industry		
Neroli, oil of	10% o.o.	Essential perfume oil, liqueurs		A photosensitizer
Nesacaine (chloroprocaine hydrochloride; Strasenburgh)	2% aq. sol.	Local anesthetics	Para-amino compounds	
Neutral red	0.05% alc.	Dye added to quaternary ammonium salts to control pH		Neutral red is red at pH 6.8 and yellow at 8.0
Neutronyx 600 (aromatic polyglycol ether condensate)	5% aq. sol.	Surfactant, nonionic synthetic detergents, bubble baths		Controls
Nickel sulfate	5% aq. sol.	Hairpins, curlers, bobby pins, eyelash curlers, earrings, eyeglass frames, nickel coins, dental instruments, metal lipstick holders, clasps of necklaces, zippers, medallions, metal identification tags, wire support of brassiere cups, garter clasps, metal chairs, handles of doors, handbags, carriages, umbrellas, thimbles, needles, scissors, pens, watchbands, metallic eyelets of shoes, metal arch supports, safety pins on sanitary napkins, hair dyes and bleaches, electric wiring, telephone wiring, silver work, mordant in dyes, insecticides, fungicides, nickel plating, nickel-containing alloys		Pustular patch test reactions
Nicotine sulfate	5% aq. sol.	Agricultural sprays, insecticides, "black leaf"		Do not test with nicotine base
Nigrosine	As is	Dye, varnish leather, platinum blond hair bleach		

Contactant	Concentration and Vehicle	Exposure	Cross-Reactions	Comment
Nigrosine base (Solvent black 7)	1% pet. or 1% mek.	Carbon paper, shoe polish, crayons, typewriter ribbon, inks, leather finish		
Ninol 2012 (fatty acid alkanolamine condensate)	5% aq. sol.	Surfactant, nonionic synthetic detergents, bubble baths		Controls
Nitric acid	Do not test	Explosives, dyes, celluloid manufacture, artificial pearls, precious stones		Powerful irritant
Nitrobenzene (oil of mirbane; artificial oil of bitter almonds)	10% o.o.	Shoe dyes, flavoring in foods, soaps, perfumes		Odor like that of oil of bitter almonds
Nitrofurazone	1% pet.	Antibacterial agent, mouthwashes, Furacin (Eaton)		
Nitrogen mustard	As is	Topical agent for mycosis fungoides		May produce urticaria and anaphylaxis
Nitrose dimethyl aniline	1% alc.	Dye		Primary sensitizer
Nonic 218	5% aq. sol.	Surfactant, nonionic synthetic detergents, bubble baths		Control
Norhidroquaiaretic acid	2% pet.	Fat antioxidant		
Novocain (procaine; Winthrop)	2% aq. sol.		Para-aminobenzoic acid esters	Does not cross-react with Xylocaine. Based on para-aminobenzoic acid
Nutmeg oil (mace)	1% alc.	Condiments, flavoring agent		
Nylon dyes	1% pet.			Disperse Orange 3 and Yellow 3
Nystatin	3% alc.	Mycolog Cream, Nystaform-HC, Mycostatin, Nilstat, Nysta-Dome, Achrostatin, Declostatin, Florotic, Myconef, O-V Statin, Tetrex-F		Rare sensitizer
Octyl alcohol	5% pet.	Lanolin		
2-Octyl dodecanol	30% pet.	Lanolin		
Oleyl alcohol	30% pet.	Lanolin, hair lotions, brilliantines, cosmetics, superfatting agent, solvent for essential oils	Stearyl alcohol	

Optical bleaches	1% aq. sol.	"Whiter-than-white" detergent, blancophores, stilbene derivative, Solium methyl umbelliferones		
Orange peel	As is	May be covered with carnauba wax, colored with azo dye (Citrus Red 2), sprayed with arsenic		Controls. Orange peel may be irritant under patch
Orange peel, oil of	1% alc.	Colognes, perfumes, baking, candies, beverages	Turpentine, celery, bergamot, caraway, dill, balsam of Peru	Contains terpenes, oil of limonene, carotene
Orcinol (dihydroxytoluene)	2% alc.	Antiseptic	Resorcinol	5-Methyl resorcinol
Orris root	Pdr. pure	Dentifrices, perfumes, teething rings, adhesives, back plasters		
Orthoform	25% pet.	Topical anesthetics	Para-amino compounds	Based on para-aminobenzoic acid, primary sensitizer
Orvus WA (sodium lauryl sulfate)	5% aq. sol.	Surfactant, anionic synthetic detergents, bubble baths		Controls
Ovotran	5% acet.	Insecticides		
Oxaine (oxethazine; Wyeth)	2% aq. sol.	Gastrointestinal topical anesthetics	Para-amino compounds	
Oxalic acid	5% aq. sol.	Bleaches, stain removers, rust removers, metal cleansers		
Oxychlorosene	1% aq. sol.	Hypochlorite in Kasdenol Mouthwash		
Oxyquinoline sulfate	1% pet.	Contraceptive, antiseptic		
Ozokerite (ceresin)	As is	Cosmetics, candles, waxes		
Paints	As is (open) or 10% pet.			
Pancreatin	As is	Enzyme mixture, Pycopay Toothpaste		
Panthenol (pantothenol)	30% pet.	Vitamin B_5, Aquasol A, Panthoderm		Alcohol of pantothenic acid
Paper money	As is		U.S. paper bills may contain formaldehyde and Dowicides (chlorinated phenols) to prevent mildew	
Para-aminobenzene	0.25% pet.	Organic dye	Paraphenylenediamine	

Contactant	*Concentration and Vehicle*	*Exposure*	*Cross-Reactions*	*Comment*
Para-aminobenzoic acid (aminobenzoic acid)	10% pet.	Pabafilm sunscreening agent, Solar Cream (Doak), synthesis of local anesthetics, vitamin B complex, brewer's yeast	Paraphenylenediamine, procaine, sulfonamides, azo dyes, benzocaine	The acid is less soluble and less sensitizing than are its salts
Para-aminophenol	10% pet.	Analgesics, fur dyes	Paraphenylenediamine	
Paraben mixture	15% pet.	Preservative in topical agents, cosmetics, foods, cleansers		3% each of ethyl, methyl, propyl, butyl and propyl parahydroxybenzoic acid
Parachlorophenol	1% aq. sol.			
Paradichlorobenzene	1% alc.	Mothproofing, toilet bowls, deodorants		May produce purpura
Paraffin	Pure	Petrolatum (soft yellow paraffin)		
Parahydroxybenzoic acid (methyl and ethyl propyl parabens)	5% pet.	Parabens as preservatives in pharmaceuticals, cosmetics, foods		Sensitizer in topical creams
Para-oxon	1% alc. (open)	Insecticides		
Paraphenylenediamine (PPDA)	2% pet. in a dark bottle	Hair dyes, fur dyes, leather processing, rubber vulcanizing, printer's ink, photographic work, x-ray fluids, lithographing	Azo and aniline dyes,, procaine, benzocaine, para-aminobenzoic acid, HydroDIURIL, carbutamide, sulfonamides, para-aminosalicylic acid	Many weakly positive patch test reactions are *not* significant
Pararosaniline	Sat. sol.	Dye		
Para-tertiary butyl phenol	1% pet.	Adhesive, resins, duplicating paper, rubber industry, leather industry		May cause leukoderma
Parathion	1% alc. (open)	Insecticides		
Paratoluenediamine sulfate	1% pet.	Chemistry laboratories		
Paris green (Schweinfurt or emerald green)	2% acet.	Paint pigment, wood preservative, insecticide sprays		Copper acetoarsenite compound
Parsnip, parsley (wild)	As is (moist)			Photosensitizer
Patchouli, oil of	1% pet.	Cosmetics, perfume		

Pearl essence Natural	As is	Frosted nail polish		A suspension of guanine crystals (from fish scales) in amyl acetate or acetone
Synthetic	As is	Lacquers, plastics		Metal stearates, lead, barium hypophosphites, bismuth oxychloride, metallic silver, zinc ammonium phosphate and hydrolysis of products of titanium chloride on protein films
Pencil colors				*Lead* (graphite) is not a sensitizer. *Indelible pencils*—methyl or crystal violet—are not sensitizers. Green and yellow colored *pencils* may contain lead chromate
Penicillin (powder or ointment)	As is	Topical use, pharmaceuticals, nursing and medical professions, cheese processers, fruit handlers		Contact allergy may be accompanied by anaphylactic variety
Pentachlorophenol	1% aq. sol.	Weed killers, insecticides, wood preservatives, adhesives		
3-Pentadecylcatechol	0.1% acet.	Anacardiaceae: rhus, mango, cashew, India nut marking tree		A primary sensitizer
Pentoxol	As is	Organic solvents		
Peppermint oil	1% pet.	Flavoring agent, perfumes	Balsam of Peru, rosin, wood	An essential oil
Perchlorethylene (tetrachloroethylene)	25% o.o.	Dry cleaning		Sensitizes to alcohol
Perfumes	As is (open and closed		Balsam of Peru, Benzyl salicylate, Phenyl-acetaldehyde	May produce berloque dermatitis
Permanent wave solutions	10% aq. sol.			Rare sensitizers
Permanganate, potassium	1% aq. sol.	Oxidizing agents, neutralizer of alkaloids, disinfectants		

Contactant	Concentration and Vehicle	Exposure	Cross-Reactions	Comment
Peroxide catalysts Acetyl Benzoyl peroxide Cumene hydroperoxide Cyclohexanone Lauroyl Methylethylketone	0.5% acet. or 1% pet.	Polyester resins		
Petitgrain	10% o.o.	Perfume oil		A photosensitizer
Petrolatum	As is	Vaseline, soft yellow paraffin		Best vehicle for most patch test substances
Petroleum	20% o.o.	Insecticides, rodenticides, gasoline, solvents		
Phemerol chloride (benzethonium chloride)	0.1% aq. sol.	Antiseptic detergent		
Phenanthrene	Pdr. pure	Tar		A photosensitizer
Phenergan Cream (Wyeth)	As is		Promethazine, phenothiazine (Thorazine, Thephorin, Pyribenzamine)	A photosensitizer
Phenol (carbolic acid)	1% aq. sol.	Dermal Chemabrasive (Budkon), Carbolated Vaseline, carbolfuchsin, Chloraseptic Lozenges and Mouthwash (Eaton), P&S Liquid and Ointment, Panscol Ointment (Baker)	Resorcin, cresols, hydroquinone	
Phenolformaldehyde	5% pet. or 1% alc.	Clothing, finishes, epoxy resins		
Phenolic compounds	1% aq. sol.	Mouthwashes		Amyl, heptyl and actyl phenols in mouthwashes
Phenolphthalein	Pdr. as is	Indicator, laxative		Test at site of fixed drug eruption

Phenothiazine	1% aq. sol. (photo-sensitizer—test open and closed)	Veterinarian anthelmintic, fly control, methylene blue	Phenergan	Present in Sparine, Thorazine, Compazine, Stelazine, Temaril, Largon, Tindal, Dartal, Mellaril, Vesprin, Prolixin, Repoise, Dermitil
Phenoxy ethoxy ethanol	0.5%	Contraceptives		
Phenylacetaldehyde	2% pet. or 0.5% alc.	Perfumes, flavoring agents		
Phenylbetanaphthylamine	1% pet.	Rubber antioxidant		
Phenylcycloparaphenylenediamine	1% pet.	Rubber		
Phenylglycidyl ether	1% o.o.	Epoxy resin		
Phenylisopropyl paraphenylenediamine	0.1% pet.	Rubber		Can cause lichenoid or purpuric eruptions
Phenylmercuric acetate	0.05% pet.	Fungicides, germicides, preservatives in cosmetics, contraceptives, Nylmerate (Holland-Rantos)	Organic and inorganic mercurials	May be a primary irritant in 0.1% aq. sol.
Phenylmercuric nitrate	0.05% pet.	Preservatives, vaginal cream, contraceptives, Pher-Mer-Nite, Merpectogel		
Phenyl salicylate (salol)	As is	Plastics, lacquers, adhesives, waxes, polishes, suntan oils, plasticizers		
Phosphorus trisulfide (phosphorus sesquisulfide)	0.5% pet.	Safety matchboxes, matches, ignition paper, diesel motors, high-pressure lubricants, asphalt		
Phthalic anhydride	1% alc.	Epoxy resins		A primary sensitizer
Picric acid (trinitrophenol)	5% aq. sol.	Dye industry, explosives, artificial flowers, antiseptics		
Picryl chloride	1% acet.			A primary sensitizer
Pimiento	10% c.o.	Flavoring agent		
Pine oil	Pure	Disinfectants, deodorants, liquid scrub soaps		Controls
Pine tar	25% pet.			

Contactant	*Concentration and Vehicle*	*Exposure*	*Cross-Reactions*	*Comment*
Piperazine	1% aq. sol.	Vermifuges, Antepar, Pipizan, Multifuge, Perin, Ascarey		May flare from ingestion of Atarax (hydroxyzine hydrochloride)
Pitch	As is (open)	Various tars		A photosensitizer
Plants	As is—leaf, flower, pollen bulb			Risk of false positive reaction
Plaster of Paris (gypsum; calcium sulfate)	As is	Cast, moldings		Some reinforced with formaldehyde resin
Plastibase (Squibb)	As is	Quinolor Ointment	Carbowax	Contains 5% polyethylene plastic resin
Plastic(s)				
Monomer	0.1–1% acet. or pet.			
Polymer	As is			
Plastic cement	As is (open)	Industrial, toys, models, glue sniffers		Contains volatile hydrocarbons and solvents, formaldehyde, formaldehyde resins, nitrocellulose
Platinum bleaches for hair	As is	Methyl violet, methylene blue, nigrosine		Applied after peroxide bleach
Platinum chloride	1% aq. sol.			May cause a pustular reaction
Plexoderm (Crookes-Barnes)	As is		Balsam of Peru	Contains salicylic acid, allantoin and styrax
Poison ivy extract or oleoresin	0.1% acet.	Identical to poison sumac and poison oak	Oleoresin of Japanese lacquer tree, cashew nut, mango fruit, India ink tree, ginkgo tree	A primary sensitizer
Polyester monomer	10% acet.	Polyester resin		
Polyethylene glycol	10% aq. sol.	Polyethylene glycol ointment (U.S.P.), Furacin (Eaton), Plastibase (Squibb), Carbowax, hair dressings		Nos. 200 to 700 are liquids. Nos. 1000 to 6000 are solids (Carbowax)

Polymethyl methacrylate (acrylic polymer powder)	As is	Dentistry, synthetic resins		Acrylic *monomer* may sensitize; the *polymer* very rarely does so
Polymyxin B sulfate	As is	Numerous topical medications		Rare sensitizer
Polysorb-80 U.S.P.	As is	Emulsifier and dispersing agent in dentifrices		
Polysorb Hydrate (Fougera)	As is			Sorbitan sesquioleate in wax-petrolatum
Polysulfide liquid polymer	1% acet.	Epoxy resin plasticizer		
Polyvinyl pyrrolidone	As is	Hair lacquers, cosmetics, pharmaceuticals, Betadine, Isodine		Not a sensitizer
Pontamine black powder	As is (pure)	Fur dyes		
Pontocaine (tetracaine hydrochloride; Winthrop)	2% aq. sol.	Local anesthetics		
Potassium carbonate	1% aq. sol.	Soaps, cleaning agents, lye, Drano, Pronto		
Potassium chlorate	1% aq. sol.	Matches, oxidizer in mouthwashes		
Potassium dichromate	0.25% aq. sol.	*General:* leather, bleaches, matches, yellow paints, spackle compounds, detergents. *Industrial:* fur industry, photography, photoengraving, lithography, electroplating, tanning agents, mordants in dyeing, yellow and orange paints, ink manufacture, stainless steel, chrome plating, match making, polishing steel, diesel engine radiator fluid, welding, acetylene workers, cement, rubber, glass, linoleum, wood impregnated with chromated zinc chloride, alloys, containing chrome, antirust compounds	Trivalent chromium compounds	Sensitizer, also irritant and producer of chrome ulcers. False positive reactions common in patients with acute dermatitis or irritable skin
Potassium hydroxide	0.5% aq. sol.	Soaps, cleaning agents, cuticle remover		

Contactant	*Concentration and Vehicle*	*Exposure*	*Cross-Reactions*	*Comment*
Potassium iodide	30% pet.	Photographic emulsions, animal and poultry feed, table salt, medications		Halogens often produce pustular patch test reactions. Control test in Duhring's disease with potassium bromide
Potassium persulfate	2.5% aq. sol.	Bleaches, germicides		
Potosan	1% alc. (open)	Insecticides		
Pramoxine hydrochloride (4-n-butoxyphenyl gamma-morpholinopropyl ether hydrochloride)	1% aq. sol.	Topical anesthetics: Anugesic Ointment and Suppositories (Warner-Chilcott), Aural Acute (Saron), Drotic Ear Drops (Ascher), Phorm Ointment (Ascher), Tronothane Hydrochloride (Abbott), Vio-Hydrocortisone Cream (North American Pharmacal)		
Primrose (Primula obconica)				
Expressed	25% aq. sol.	Main English plant sensitizer	Daisy family	Primary sensitizer
Leaf	As is	Main English plant sensitizer	Daisy family	Primary sensitizer
Procaine hydrochloride (Novocain)	2% aq. sol.		Benzocaine, para-aminobenzoic acid, para-aminosalicylic acid, paraphenylenediamine	Does *not* cross react with Xylocaine
Proflavine dihydrochloride	1% pet.	Topical fluorescent dye		Advocated for herpes simplex. Caution: a sensitizer
Propantheline bromide	1% aq. sol.	Pro-Banthīne (Searle) when incorporated in topical agents as an antiperspirant		Treatment of axillary hyperhidrosis
Propylene glycol	10% aq. sol.	Vehicle for 5-fluorouracil, humectant, cosmetics, Synalar Solution, Lidosporin	Balsam of Peru	
Propyl parahydroxybenzoate (propyl paraben)	5% pet.	Preservative in topical agents, cosmetics, foods, cleansers		

Psoriasis Lotion (Rexall)	As is			Mercuric oleate
Pyrethrum powder	As is	Insecticides, mothproofing	Chrysanthemum, turpentine, ragweed	Contains pyrethrins and cinerins
Pyribenzamine hydrochloride (tripelennamine)	As is	Antihistamine	Sulfapyradine, phenothiazine, Antistine, Phenergan	An ethylenediamine derivative
Pyridine	30% o.o.	Tar		A photosensitizer
Pyrocatechol	2% in 95% alc.		Hydroquinone, resorcin	
Pyrogallol	3% aq. sol.	Hair dyes, tars	Resorcin	
Quassin (extract of Jamaica bitter wood)	2% acet.	Lacquers, paper, waterproofing, denatured alcohol		Contains sucrose octa-acetate
Quaternary ammonium compounds	0.1% aq.	Cetrimide, antiseptic detergents such as Phemerol, Zephiran, Ceepryn, Diaprene		Rare sensitizers, may cause ulceration of genitalia in concentrated solutions
Quicklime (unslaked lime; calcium oxide)	Caustic; do not test	Mortar, cement, fertilizers, soap, glass, metals, depilatories, manufacture of calcium cyanide, calcium carbide		See Lime, slaked and Calcium oxide
Quillaja	1% alc.	Emulsifying agent, solution of coal tar, cosmetics		Derived from South American rosaceous tree bark
Quince seed	As is	Hair straighteners, mucilage, gums, cosmetics		
Quinidine sulfate	Sat. aq. sol.	Pharmaceutical industry, contraceptives		Eczematous or purpuric patch test reaction
Quinine sulfate or hydrochloride	1% aq. sol.	Contraceptives, sunscreens, hair tonics, quinine tablets, vermouth, gin, vodka, denatured alcohol		
Quinolor Compound Ointment (Squibb)	Half strength with pet.		Vioform, Sterosan, Diodoquin	Contains chlorhydroxyquinoline, benzoyl peroxide, methyl salicylate, menthol and eugenol in Plastibase vehicle. Some preparations contain eucalyptol, white thyme oil

Contactant	Concentration and Vehicle	Exposure	Cross-Reaction	Comment
Quotane Ointment and Lotion (dimethisoquin hydrochloride; Smith, Kline & French)	As is	Topical anesthetic		Not related to para-aminobenzoic acid
Ragweed	1:1000 acet.		Chrysanthemum, pyrethrum, turpentine	Plant leaves and pollen may also be used for testing
Rapeseed oil (Factice)	As is	Adhesives, lubricant		
Red mercuric oxide	3% pet.	Antiseptics, bleaching agents	Organic and inorganic mercurials	
Resorcin	5% pet.	Acne remedies, hair tonics, suppositories, eye drops, tanning, explosives, resins, dyes, cosmetics, freckle cream, dyeing and printing	Euresol, phenol, hexylresorcinol, orcinol, hydroquinone, pyrocatechol, pyrogallol, hydroxyquinone	Deteriorates when exposed to light. Dispense in dark bottle.
Resorcin green	3% aq. sol.	Azo dye	Para-amino compounds	
Resorcinol monoacetate (Euresol [Knoll])	5% aq. sol.	Clantis (Dara), Resulin Resorcitate (Schieffelin), Sulforcin (Texas Pharmacal), RMS Lotion (Ar-Ex), Acne-Dome (Dome)	Resorcin	
Resorcinol monobenzoate	1% pet.	Colored eyeglass frames	Balsam of Peru	Ultraviolet inhibitor
Rezifilm (Squibb)	As is			Contains tetramethyl-thiuram disulfide
Rhodamine	As is	Red lipstick dye		A photosensitizer
Rhulicream, Rhulispray, Rhulitol (Lederle)	As is (patch scratch)	Topical agent for plant dermatitis		Allergic granuloma from zirconium
Riasol (Shield)	As is	Proprietary preparation for psoriasis		Mercury as cocoanut oil soap
Rigithane 112	1% alc.	Polyurethane resins		
Rigithane catalyst	10% aq. sol.	Polyurethane resins		
Roccal (alkyldimethyl-benzyl-ammonium chloride)	1% aq. sol.	Surfactants, cationic synthetic detergents, bubble baths		Controls
Rodannitrobenzene	1% pet.	Pesticides	Paraphenylenediamine	

Rosaniline (basic fuchsin)	2% aq. sol.	Therapeutic dye		
Rose bengal	As is	Dyes		Photosensitizing
Rose, oil of	1% alc.	Perfume, unguentum aquae rosae		
Rosin (colophony): gum rosin (from turpentine), wood rosin (from pine stump)	10% pet.	Yellow bar soap, adhesive tape, insulating tape, Scotch Tape, glossy paper, flypaper, polish, paints, inks, epilating wax, rosin bags for ball players, rosin for violin bows	Balsam of Peru, turpentine (gum rosin)	Contains abietic acid and 1-pinearic acid
Rotenone powder	5% in talcum	Insecticide		From roots of rotenone-bearing plants (Derris and Lonchocarpus)
Rubber accelerators	1% pet.	Mercaptobenzothiazole, tetramethylthiuram monosulfide, diphenylguanidine		Of the rubber accelerators, these are the most common sensitizers
Rubber antioxidants	1% pet.	Monobenzylether of hydroquinone, phenyl-beta-naphthylamine, isopropyl paraphenylenediamine		Of the rubber antioxidants, these are the most common sensitizers
Rubber, finished products	As is	Rubber box toes of shoes, rubber cements, dress shields, elastic in hairnets, panties, dental plates, edge of eyelash curler, kneeling pads, rubber support pessary and diaphragms, dental sheeting, head rests, condoms, rubberbands, finger guards, art gum erasers, stethoscopes, rubber hand grip of vibrators, aprons, mammary prostheses, goggles, adhesive tape, "Flubber" (a putty-like toy), tire treads, tubes, wire insulation, drug sundries, calendered stocks		Rubber accelerators and antioxidants are the most common cause of rubber dermatitis
Rubber peptizer	1% pet.	Thio-beta-naphthol		Keeps rubber soft

Contactant	Concentration and Vehicle	Exposure	Cross-Reactions	Comment
Rust removers	Do not test (see comment)			Contains irritants such as naphtha, ammonium sulfide, oxalic acid, hydrofluoric acid, concentrated solution of phosphoric acid, inorganic heavy metal salts. For testing, see individual chemicals or begin with 1% solutions and use controls
Salicylates	2% o.o.		Aminosalicylic acid	Amyl, benzyl, glyceryl, menthyl, ethylhexyl phenyl and propylene salicylates may be used as sunscreens
Salicylic acid	1% pet.	Many topical agents, including Whitfield's ointment		Rare sensitizer. Salicylic acid and mercury combinations may be irritants when covered
Saligenin (salicyl alcohol)	2% aq. sol.	Topical local anesthetics		Rarely sensitizes
Sassafras oil	2% o.o.	Flavoring agents		
Sawdust	As is			Test dry and moist
Scarlet red (aminoazotoluene)	As is	Dye, therapeutic agent for burns and ulcers	Para-amino compounds	
Sedormid	Sat. sol. in propylene glycol	This drug is not being made at present		Purpuric patch test reaction
Selenium sulfide	2% aq. sol.	Selsun (Abbott), glass, photoelectric cells, coloring of acrylic dentures		
Selsun (Abbott)	5% aq. sol.	Therapeutic shampoo		Contains selenium sulfide

Sesame oil	50% o.o.	Vehicle for intramuscular medications, synergist for pyrethrins, cosmetics	
Shampoos	5% aq. sol. (open) 2% aq. sol. (closed)		Controls
Shellac	As is	Paint, varnish, hair dressings, waxes	May have methyl alcohol and arsenic trisulfide. Controls
Shoe polish	5% pet.		
Silicone fluids (dimethyl polysiloxanes)	As is	Cosmetics, greases, antifog agent, eyeglasses, glass	May cause blepharitis, lacrimation
Silver bromide	2% aq. sol.	Photography, mirror finishing	
Silver nitrate	2% aq. sol. (open)	Caustic pencils and hair dyes	Pustular patch test reaction
Siroil (Siroil)	As is	Proprietary psoriasis remedy	Contains mercury
Soaps	1% aq. sol.		Controls
Sodium alginate (algin)	As is	Emulsifiers, mucilage, ice cream, wave sets	
Sodium alkyl sulfate	2% aq. sol.	Foaming surfactant in detergents, Ultrabrite, Gleem, McLeans, Pepsodent	
Sodium arsenate	10% aq. sol.	Arsenical soaps, insecticides, hair tonics	
Sodium bisulfite	10% aq. sol.	Antioxidant in food	
Sodium carbonate	10% aq. sol.	Soap additives	
Sodium diethyldithiocarbamate	10% in Carbowax	Treatment of nickel carbonyl poisoning	
Sodium fluoride	0.5 aq. sol.	Glass etchings, dentifrices	Pustular patch test reaction common
Sodium fusidate	2% aq. sol.	Fucidin Ointment	
Sodium hydroxide	Do not test	Soaps, cleaning agents, lye—Drano, Pronto	Powerful irritant
Sodium hypochlorite	2% aq. sol.	Bleaching solutions, cleansing agents	Controls

Contactant	Concentration and Vehicle	Exposure	Cross-Reactions	Comment
Sodium lauryl sulfate (duponal C)	5% aq. sol.	Emulsifying agent in cosmetics, pharmaceuticals, "foaming" dentifrices		Fatty alcohol sulfate. Primary irritant. Controls
Sodium monofluorophosphate	0.5% aq. sol.	Surfactant (Colgate Toothpaste)		Pustular patch test reactions
Sodium monoglyceride sulfonate	2% aq. sol.	Surfactant (Gleem Toothpaste)		Controls
Sodium n-lauroyl sarcosinate	2% aq. sol.	Antienzyme, dentifrices, emulsifiers, surfactant in cosmetics, pharmaceuticals		Controls
Sodium perborate	Pdr. as is	Dentures, household cleansers, cold hair-waving neutralizers, mouthwashes, Vince, Amosan		
Sodium stearate	1% aq. sol.	Cosmetics		Controls
Sodium sulfide	2% aq. sol.	Bleaching agent for cotton, paper, stain remover for tetryl and and potassium permanganate, preservative for dyes and foods, Wandex (Research Supplies)		Controls
Sodium thiosulfate	5% aq. sol.	Fungicides, stain removers, hair dye developers, Tinver, Komed Lotion, Microsyn		
Solithane 113	1% alc.	Polyurethane prepolymer		
Solithane catalysts				
C–113–300	1% alc.	Polyurethane catalyst		
C–113–328	2% aq. sol.	Polyurethane catalyst		
Sorbic acid	5% pet.	Preservative, Hytone Cream (Dermik), Aristocort Cream (Lederle)		Present in many fruits, especially strawberries
Sorbital	10% aq. sol.	Humectants, cosmetics, pharmaceuticals		
Sorsis Cream (Ar-Ex)	As is	Topical agent for psoriasis		Contains ammoniated mercury

Span 20 (sorbitan monolaurate)	5% aq. sol.	Surfactant, nonionic synthetic detergents, bubble baths		Controls
Span 80 (sorbitan monooleate)	5% aq. sol.	Surfactant, nonionic synthetic detergents, bubble baths		Controls
Spandelle (Firestone)	As is	Polyurethane elastomer (spandex)		Not a sensitizer
Sparklers				*Green sparklers* contain barium nitrate, potassium perchlorate and aluminum powder; *red sparklers* contain strontium carbonate, nitrate, potassium perchlorate and aluminum powder
Spearmint oil	1% alc.	Flavoring agents		
Spermaceti	As is	Cosmetics, pharmaceuticals, candles		
Spice, oil of	5% pet.			
Stannous fluoride	0.5% aq. sol.	Dentifrices, including Crest, Cue, Fact, Superstripe, Dr. Lyons Fluoride, McKesson Fluoride		Pustular patch test reaction
Stearic acid	1% aq. sol.	Cosmetics, soaps		Pustular patch test reaction common
Stearyl alcohol	3% liq. paraffin	Lanolin, aliphatic alcohol in lanolin, cosmetics, textile finishes, antifoam agent, lubricant	Oleyl alcohol	May cause contact urticaria
Sterosan Cream (Geigy) (chlorquinaldol)	As is	Bacteriostatic and fungistatic cream and ointment	Vioform, Diodoquin, Quinolor	Free of iodine
Stilbene triazine	0.5% aq. sol.	Optical bleaches, brightening agents, soaps, detergents, cosmetics, textiles		Photosensitizer
Stoddard Solvent (high flash point petroleum distillate)	25% o.o.	Dry cleaning, paint thinner		
Streptomycin	2.5% aq. sol.	Medical, nursing and pharmaceutical personnel	Dihydrostreptomycin, kanamycin, neomycin	
Strontium chloride	2% aq. sol.	Sensodyne dentifrice		

Contactant	*Concentration and Vehicle*	*Exposure*	*Cross-Reactions*	*Comment*
Strontium sulfide	2% aq. sol.	Depilatories		
Styrax USO (storax)	2% pet.	Plexoderm, perfumes, cosmetics, topical medication	Benzoin, styrene, balsam of Peru	A balsam with cinnamic acid
Styrene (vinyl benzene)	1% o.o.	Synthetic rubber, alkyd, acrylic and polyester resins, extractive of storax balsam, compound tincture of benzoin, soaps	Benzoin compounds	
Styrene oxide	1% o.o.	Reactive epoxy diluent		
Subtilins	0.1% aq. sol.	Detergent enzymes		
Sulfacetamide, topical	As is	Sultrin (Ortho), many ophthalmic and acne topical medications		Rarely sensitizes
Sulfanilamide, topical	As is	AVC, Otomide, Vagitrol, Sufamil	Para-amino compounds	A photosensitizer
Sulfobromophthalein	5% aq. sol.	Diagnostic dyes		Anaphylactic or immediate rather than delayed allergens
Sulfonamide	As is	Blexcon (Madland), Gantrisin (Roche), Vagitrol (Syntex)	Para-amino compounds	Sulfonamide diuretics may be photosensitizers
Sulfonamide-formaldehyde resin	10% pet.	Main sensitizer in nail lacquer		
Sulfonated imidazole	0.5% aq. sol.	Optical bleaches, brightening agents, soaps, detergents, cosmetics, textiles		Photosensitizer
Sulfur	5% pet.	Topical medications, gunpowder, matches, bleaches, insecticides, fungicides		*Precipitated* sulfur contains calcium sulfide; *sublimed* sulfur is a pure yellow sulfur powder. Incompatible with iodine and mercury
Sulfuric acid	2% aq. sol.			
Sulisobenzone (2-hydroxy-4-methoxy-benzophenone-5-sulfonic acid)	10% pet.	Sungard, Uval, Spectra Sorb UV 284, Uvinulms-40		Sunscreen
Surfacaine (cyclomethycaine; Lilly)	1% pet.	Topical anesthetic, Surfacaine Compound, Surfadil		Not based on para-aminobenzoic acid
Synthetic detergents	2% aq. sol.			Controls

Talc (talcum) U.S.P.	As is	Cosmetics, pharmaceuticals	May produce granulomas in wounds
Tannic acid	1% aq. sol.	Mordant in dyes, sizing paper and silk, polished fabrics, tortoise shell frames, rubber manufacture, tanning leather, photography, sunscreens and medicines for burns, Dalidyne (Dalin), Astringent lotion, Onycho-Phytex (Unimed), artificial nail preparation, tannic jelly	Rare sensitizer
Tar			
Coal	5% pet.	Alphosyl, Balnetar, Carbo-Cort, Daxalan, Ionil T, Polytar, Pragmatar, Sebical Tar Shampoo, Sebutone, Supertah, Tarbonis, Tar Distillate, Tarpaste, Topigel, Tropsor Lotion, Unguentum Bossi, Ze-Tar-Quin, Zetar Shampoo and Emulsion	Photosensitizer
Coal tar solution	As is	Liquor carbonis detergens, Epidol, Tridentar (Spirt), Hydro-Tar (Schieffelin), Pentarcort (Dalin), Methatar (Borden), Ulcortar (Ulmer), Cor-Tar-Quin Cream and Lotion (Dome)	Photosensitizers. Contains coal tar, Quillaja bark, alcohol
Wood	12% (3% each of pine, beech, juniper and birch)	Almay-Tar (Schieffelin), oil of cade (juniper tar)	Not photosensitizers
Tartar emetic	3% aq. sol.	Dye mordant, counterirritant, denaturing agent in rubbing alcohol	
Tashan Cream (Hoffman-La Roche)	As is		The vitamin E in this preparation reported to be a sensitizer. See Vitamin E

Contactant	*Concentration and Vehicle*	*Exposure*	*Cross-Reactions*	*Comment*
Tattoo pigments	As is			*Black:* carbon, iron oxide, logwood (may contain potassium dichromate). *Blue:* cobaltous aluminate. *Brown:* ferric sulfate. *Flesh:* iron oxide. *Green:* Chromium oxide, chromium sesquioxide (casalis green), hydrous chromium oxide (Guignet's green), copper salts mixed with azo dyes. *Red:* cadmium selenide, cinnabar, sienna. *Violet:* manganese violet. *White:* Zinc oxide. *Yellow:* cadmium sulfide
Tegon	0.1% aq. sol.	European antiseptic detergent		Dodecylic aminoethyl glycine hydrochloride
Tertiary butyl catechol	1% acet.	Polyester resin inhibitor, antioxidant, lubricating oils, paint, rubber, plastics		May produce leukoderma
Tertiary butyl phenol	1% acet.	Detergents, synthetic oils, disinfectants		May produce leukoderma
p-Tertiary butyl phenol formaldehyde	1% pet.	Resins, blues		
Tetrabromofluorescein	As is	Dye in lipsticks		Photosensitizer
Tetracaine (Pontocaine [Winthrop])	2% aq. sol.	Local anesthetics, PNS suppositories (Winthrop), Vertussin Loz-tablets (Warren-Teed), Rectodyne Ointment (Semed)	Procaine, benzocaine	Based on para-aminobenzoic acid
Tetrachlorodiphenylethane (TDE)	5% acet.	Insecticides		

Tetrachlorosalicylanilide (TCSA, Impregon)	0.5% pet.	Antiseptic used in soaps	Tribromosalicylanilide, bithionol, hexachlorophene	A photosensitizer
Tetraethylthiuram disulfide (disulfiram, Antabuse)	1% pet.	Rubber industry, medications	Thiram	Sensitizes to alcohol
Tetralin (tetrahydronaphthalene)	25% o.o.	Plumbing, steam fitting		
Tetramethylthiuram disulfide (thiram, febram, fermate)	1% pet.	Rubber industry, insecticides, fungicides, germicides, Rezifilm (Squibb)	Disulfiram, Antabuse	Sensitizes to alcohol
Tetramethylthiuram monosulfide	1% pet.	Rubber accelerator	Tetrathiuram disulfides, carbamates	Sensitizes to alcohol
Tetryl	Sat. sol. in ether	Munitions		Produces yellow stain; often causes folliculitis
Thallium sulfate	1% aq. sol.	Rodenticides, insecticides, depilatories		Toxic hair loss
Thephorin (phenindamine tartrate; Hoffman–La Roche)	As is			Potential topical sensitizer
Thermometer fluids	As is (open)			*Clinical:* mercury. *Indoor and outdoor:* triethyl phosphate, toluene, xylene, alcohol
Thiamine chloride (vitamin B_1)	50% aq. sol.	Pharmaceuticals	Cocarboxylase (coenzyme B)	
Thimerosal	See Merthiolate			
Thio-beta-naphthol	1% pet.	Rubber peptizer		
Thioglycolic acid	10% aq. sol.	Depilatories		
Thiokol polysulfide polymers	1% acet.	Epoxy resin systems		
Thiophenol	0.1% alc.	Merthiolate (Lilly)		Sensitizer in thiosalicylic acid
Thiosalicylic acid	0.1% alc.	Merthiolate (Lilly)		
Thorazine (Smith Kline & French)	1% pet.	Medical, nursing, pharmaceutical personnel handling and injecting the drug. Excreted in urine (contaminated linen)	Phenothiazine drugs, Phenergan, Theruhistin, Pyrrolazote	Photosensitizer

Contactant	Concentration and Vehicle	Exposure	Cross-Reactions	Comment
Thyme, oil of	25% c.o.	Waterproofing, flavoring agent, Quinolor Compound (Squibb)		
Thymol (isopropyl metacresol)	1% pet.	Dentifrices, mouthwashes, antiseptics, antimildew, Listerine, Chloraseptic, douches		
Thymol iodide	25% pet.	Antiseptics		
Tiger Balm	As is	Chinese proprietary ointment	Balsam of Peru	Contains balsams
Tin (stannic chloride)	10% aq. sol.	Metal, plating		
Tinactin (Schering)	As is	Fungicide		Contains tolnaftate 1%, butylated hydroxytoluene polyethylene glycol
Titanium tetrachloride	Do not test			Vesicant
Tobacco	As is			
Toilet water	As is			Photosensitizer
Tolnaftate	1% pet.	Tinactin Solution		Iso-z-naphthyl-m-n-dimethylthiocarbanilate
Toluene	50% o.o.	Solvents, rubber, adhesives, dyes, perfumes, thermometer fluids, nonclinical thermometer fluids		
p-Toluenesulfonyl chloride	0.5% alc.	Furan plastics, dye manufacture, synthetic tanning		
Toluidine	10% o.o.	Aniline		
Toluxol	50% o.o.	Organic solvents		
Toothpastes and powders				
Soapless	As is			Controls
With soap or detergent	2% aq. sol.			
Topocide (Lilly)	As is	Miticide, insecticide		Benzyl benzoate, benzocaine and DDT
Tragacanth	1% aq. sol.	Powders, cosmetics, candy manufacture, calico printing, drying agent, drug filler, sizing paper, printing, wave-setting fluids		Vegetable gum

Trenimon (2,3,5-triethylene-imino-1,4-benzoquinone)	0.05% pet.	Chemotherapeutic agent		
Triacetin (glyceryl triacetate)	As is	Cigarette filters, Enzactin (Ayerst), antifungal agent		
Triazine	0.5% aq. sol.	Film hardener		
Tribromosalicylanilide (TBS)	1% pet.	Antiseptic in soaps—Green Lifebuoy, Praise, Safeguard	Tetrachlorosalicylanilide, bithionol, hexachlorophene	A photosensitizer
Trichloroacetic acid	Do not test			Primary irritant
Trichloroethylene (ethylene trichloride, acetylene trichloride)	5% o.o.	Metal degreasing, solvent for oils, greases, paints, varnishes, dye; leather manufacturing, dry cleaning, refrigerant, anesthetics, insecticides, perfumes		Sensitizes to alcohol
Tricresylphosphate (tritolyl phosphate)	5% pet.	*Plasticizer:* vinyl films, resins, polyester, cellulose, nail lacquer. *Lead scavenger:* in gasoline, fire retardant. *Carbon paper*	Triphenylphosphate	
Triethylenediamine	0.1% aq. sol. 0.5% pet.	Polyurethane resin catalyst, epoxy hardener		
Triethylenetetramine	0.1% aq. sol. 0.5% pet.	Epoxy resin		
Trimeton Ointment (prophenpyridamine; Schering)	As is	Tripoton, Inhiston	Antistine	
Trinitrobenzene	1% acet.			Primary sensitizer
Trinitrotoluene	As is	Explosives		Causes yellow discoloration
Tri-Ortho-Cresyl-Phosphate	5% acet.	Plastic coatings, fireproofers, lubricants, gasoline		In Morocco, vegetable oil adulterated with this compound produced paralysis in thousands
Triphenylmethane	1% pet.	Dyes		
Triphenyl phosphate	5% pet.	Cellulose acetate carbon paper		
Trisodium phosphate	2% aq. sol.	A "builder" added to detergents and soaps		

Contactant	Concentration and Vehicle	Exposure	Cross-Reactions	Comment
Triton 25 (para-octyl phenol ethylene oxide)	0.1% aq. sol.	Wetting agent in cosmetic and pharmaceutical preparations, textiles, metal cleaning, dry cleaning solvent, solvent in ballpoint inks		
Triton X-100 (alkylated aryl polyether alcohol)	5% aq. sol.	Surfactant, nonionic synthetic detergents, bubble baths		Controls
Triton X-200 (sodium salt of alkylated aryl polyether sulfonate)	5% aq. sol.	Surfactant, anionic synthetic detergents, bubble baths		Controls
Triton X-400 (stearyldimethyl-benzylammonium chloride)	5% aq. sol.	Surfactant, cationic synthetic detergents, bubble baths		Controls
Turkey Red Oil	1% o.o.	Surfactant, agricultural textile industry		
Turpentine	10% o.o. or (turpentine peroxides) 0.3% pet.	Synthetic resins, pine oleoresins, furniture and stove polish, varnish, wax solvent, cleaning fluid, paint thinner, adhesives, insecticides. *Liniments:* Sloans, Minards, Johnson's Anodyne, Mentholatum, Penetromide	Chrysanthemum, ragweed, pyrethrum, colophony (rosin), balsams (pine and spruce)	Sensitizer is alpha-carene or alpha-pinene
Tween 20 (sorbitan monolaurate polyoxyethylene derivative)	5% aq. sol.	Surfactant, nonionic synthetic detergents, bubble baths		Controls
Tween 80 (sorbitan monooleate polyoxyethylene derivative)	5% aq. sol.	Surfactant, nonionic synthetic detergents, bubble baths		Controls
Tylosin (Tylan)	1% aq. sol.	Animal feed		Antibiotic
Tyrothricin	As is	Tyrolaris Mouthwash, Creams and Ointments, Isodettes, Otalgine Drops (Purdue Frederick)		
Ultrawet K (sodium aralkyl sulfonate)	5% aq. sol.	Surfactant, synthetic detergents, bubble baths		Controls
Umbelliferone (7-hydroxycoumarin)	2% pet.	Sunscreening agents, optical bleaches	Furocoumarin	A cinnamic acid derivative. Photosensitizer

Undecylenic acid	As is	Sweat, topical antifungal medications		Rare sensitizer
Unguentum Bossi (Doak)	As is	Psoriasis remedy		Contains ammoniated mercury, tar and sulfosalicylic acid
Urea (carbamide)	10% aq. sol.	Amino Cerv (Milex), Carbamine (Key Pharmaceuticals), Carmol Cream (Ingram), Debrox (International Pharmaceutical), Gly-Oxide (International Pharmaceutical), Kerid Drops (Blair), Otomide (Schering), Panafil Ointment (Rystan), Panafil-White Ointment (Rystan), Ureaphil (Abbott), Stilbamidine, deodorants, dentifrices, hand creams (Aquacare), formaldehyde resins		Rare sensitizer. Urea frost (urea particles of face in uremia). Cause of ammoniacal dermatitis and stomatitis. Tsyrkunol, L: Occupational Skin Diseases in Workers Engaged in Production of Nitrogen-Mineral Fertilizers. P. Westnder.-Vener., *6*, 31, 1963. Synthetic urea is an irritant
Urea formaldehyde	10% pet.	Plastics, finishes		
Urea peroxide (Gly-Oxide)	As is			
Uric acid	1% aq. sol.	Allantoin (a derivative of uric acid)		Rarely sensitizes
Usnic acid	1% pet.	Lichens, lichen mosses, clothing dyes, litmus paper	Furocoumarins	
Vanilla (alcoholic extract)	10% acet.	Flavoring agent in foods, tobacco, beverages, perfumes	Balsam of Peru, benzoin, oil of cloves	Vanilla lichen—a dermatitis due to mites infesting vanilla pods
Vanillin	10% pet.	Aromatic crystalline principle of vanilla	Balsam of Peru, benzoin, oil of cloves, eugenol	Vanillism—allergic dermatitis, rhinitis and asthma from vanilla
Vegetable gums	As is			Karaya, gum arabic (acacia) and tragacanth are the most sensitizing gums
Vermouth	As is (open)	Handlers and imbibers		Some vermouths contain oil of cinnamon and quinine

Contactant	*Concentration and Vehicle*	*Exposure*	*Cross-Reactions*	*Comment*
Vinegar	As is	Condiments, preservative, fermenting beer, cider, malt, wine, lead subacetate		Acetic acid content causes aphthous ulcers ?
Vinyl benzene (styrene)	1% o.o.	See Styrene		
Vinyl films	As is			Sensitizers in vinyl films may be *plasticizers*, such as tricresylphosphate, dioctyl-phthalate, ester of adipic acid, and epoxy resins, or *stabilizers*, such as dibutyl tin maleate
Vioform Ointment, Cream, Lotion (iodochlorhydroxyquin; CIBA)	As is	*Related compounds:* Entero-Vioform (CIBA), HEB-Cort V Cream and Lotion (Barnes-Hind), Hysone (Mallard), Lidaform-HC Creme and Lotion (Dome), Nystaform Ointment (Dome), Nystaform-HC Ointment and Lotion (Dome), Pentarcort (Dalin), Racetico Cream (Lemmon), Vioform Inserts (CIBA), Vioform-Hydrocortisone (CIBA), Vio-Hydrosone Cream (North American Pharmacal), Quinoform, 1- Quinn Dermaform, Domeform, Torofor (Torch), HEB-Cort, Hyquin Cream, Topigel	Diodoquin, Sterosan, Quinolor Ointment	Iodine containing hydroxyquinoline
Vitamin A	0.1% pet.	Hand and cosmetic creams, vitamin A and D ointment		
Vitamin A acid (Tretinoin)	0.1% pet.	Topical acne medications		An irritant

Vitamin B_1 (thiamine chloride, Betabion Hydrochloride, Aneurin Hydrochloride)	50% aq. sol.	Pharmaceutical industry	Cocarboxylase, coenzyme B (diphosphothiamin)	Sensitized workers flare and acquire "systemic" contact dermatitis after ingestion or injection of thiamine chloride
Vitamin B_6 (pyridoxine; 2-methyl-3-nitro-4-methoxyly-methyl-5-cyano-6-chlopyridine)	10% aq. sol.	Pharmaceutical industry	Pyridine derivatives in production of castor oil	Berufdermatosen, *13*, 28, 1965. Allergic contact dermatitis in production of B_6 and of castor oil, another pyridine derivative
Vitamin B_{12} (cyanocobalamine, Betalin 12, Berubigen, Cobione)	As is		Cobalt	0.4% of B_{12} molecule is cobalt. See text for cobalt patient whose dermatitis flared from injection of B_{12}. Positive patch test reactions obtained with injectable B_{12} preparations
Vitamin E (alpha-tocopherol)	As is	Tashan Cream, Vitamin E Deodorant Spray (Mennen), Vitamin E Soap (Altabra from Italy)		Brodkin, R. H., et al.: Sensitivity to Topically Applied Vitamin E (in Tashan Cream). Arch Derm., *90*, 76, 1965
Vitamin E Deodorant Spray (Mennen)	As is			Contains propellent, Alcohol SD-40, vitamin E, silicone fluid and perfume. (The sensitizer in many cases proved to be vitamin E in this spray)
Vitamin K (Menadiol sodium diphosphate [Kappadione, Synkayvite]; menadione sodium bisulfite [Hykinone])	0.1% aq. sol.	Production of vitamin K		Jirasek, L.: Hypersensitivity to Vitamin K. Cesk. Derm., *40*, 17, 1965
White henna (magnesium carbonate)	As is	Hair bleaches		

Contactant	*Concentration and Vehicle*	*Exposure*	*Cross-Reactions*	*Comment*
White spirits	25% o.o.	Solvent, thinner, turpentine substitute		
Wintergreen, oil of (gaultheria oil)	1% alc.	Flavoring agent, rubefacient, antiseptic, Banalg Liniment (Cole), Ger-O-Foam (Geriatric), Panalgesic (Poythress)	Salicylates	Rich in methyl salicylate
Witch hazel (Hamamelis)	As is	Topical medications, rubefacient, Tucks Pads, Cream, Ointment (Fuller); Hazel-Balm (Arnar-Stone)		Contains tannins and 70–80% alcohol
Wood (sawdust)	As is			Risk of false positive reaction. Controls
Wood tars		See Tar, wood		
Wool alcohols	30% pet.	Lanolin		Main sensitizer in lanolin
Xylene (benzene, toluene, cumene, mesitylene)	50% o.o.	Solvents, paint removers, lacquers, degreasing cleansers, insecticides, pesticides		
Xylocaine (lidocaine; diethylaminoacet-2,6-xylidide hydrochloride)	2% aq. sol.	Local anesthetic, solution, ointment, jelly, suppositories		Have not as yet encountered allergic dermatitis from this anesthetic
Xylol	50% o.o.	Organic solvents		
Zephiran chloride (benzalkonium; Winthrop)	1:1000 aq. sol.	Cationic antiseptic detergent, antirust powder and tablets		
Zinc chloride	2% aq. sol.	Astringents, plumbing, welding, wood preservative		
Zinc oxide	Pure	Adhesives, paints, galvanizing, zinc plating, drying agents, dental cements, automobile tires, white ointments and powders, cosmetics		Rare sensitizer. May cause black dermographism

Zinc peroxide	As is	Oxidizing medications, bleaches, healing agents, deodorants, astringents	
Zinc phenolsulfonate	1% alc.	Astringents, cosmetics, deodorants (Secret, Top Brass, Arrid, Hi & Dry, Manpower)	
Zinc stearate	As is		May cause irritant granulomas
Zinc sulfate	5% aq. sol.	Astringent, styptic pencil	
Zinc sulfocarbolate	5% aq. sol.	Astringents, Right Guard Deodorant	
Zineb	1% pet.	Pesticide	Ethylene-bis(dithiocarbamate) zinc
Ziradryl (Parke, Davis)	As is (patch-scratch)	Topical agent for plant dermatitis	Zirconium oxide, Benadryl. Allergic granuloma
Zircobarb Lotion (Vogel)	As is (patch-scratch)	Topical agent for plant dermatitis	Hydrous zirconium. Allergic granuloma
Zirconium lactate, sodium	4% pet. (patch-scratch or 1:10,000 intracutaneous)	Antiperspirants	Allergic granuloma
Zirconium oxide	Pdr. as is (patch-scratch)	Ziradyl, Zirium, Zirnox, Rhulihist, Rhulicream, Rhulitol, Ivarest, Allergesic, Zotox	Allergic granuloma
Zirconium silicate	As is (patch-scratch)	Pepsodent Toothpaste	
Zirconyl hydrochloride	As is	Secret Roll-on Deodorant	"Safe" zirconium?
Zirium (Ulmer)	As is (patch-scratch)	Topical agent for poison ivy dermatitis	Zirconium oxide and thenylpyramine. Allergic granuloma
Zirnox (Bristol)	As is (patch-scratch)	Topical agent for plant dermatitis	Allergic granuloma

Index

Page numbers followed by t refer to tables.